Pneumonia: Diagnosis and Treatment

Pneumonia: Diagnosis and Treatment

Edited by Russell Peterson

hayle medical
New York

Hayle Medical,
750 Third Avenue, 9th Floor,
New York, NY 10017, USA

Visit us on the World Wide Web at:
www.haylemedical.com

ISBN: 978-1-63241-862-3

Cataloging-in-Publication Data

Pneumonia : diagnosis and treatment / edited by Russell Peterson.
p. cm.
Includes bibliographical references and index.
ISBN 978-1-63241-862-3
1. Pneumonia. 2. Pneumonia--Diagnosis. 3. Pneumonia--Treatment. I. Peterson, Russell.
RC771 .P54 2020
616.241--dc23

Table of Contents

Preface IX

Chapter 1 **Aboriginal and non-Aboriginal children in Western Australia carry different serotypes of pneumococci with different antimicrobial susceptibility profiles** 1
Eileen M. Dunne, Kylie Carville, Thomas V. Riley, Jacinta Bowman, Amanda J. Leach, Allan W. Cripps, Denise Murphy, Peter Jacoby and Deborah Lehmann

Chapter 2 **Necrotizing pneumonia: an emerging problem in children?** 10
I. Brent Masters, Alan F. Isles and Keith Grimwood

Chapter 3 **Pulmonary infections in the returned traveller** 29
Ashleigh Trimble, V. Moffat and A. M. Collins

Chapter 4 **Childhood pneumonia and meningitis in the Eastern Highlands Province, Papua New Guinea in the era of conjugate vaccines: study methods and challenges** 39
Christopher C. Blyth, Rebecca Ford, Joycelyn Sapura, Tonny Kumani, Geraldine Masiria, John Kave, Lapule Yuasi, Andrew Greenhill, Ilomo Hwaihwanje, Amanda Lang, Deborah Lehmann and William Pomat

Chapter 5 **Encouraging rational antibiotic use in childhood pneumonia: a focus on Vietnam and the Western Pacific Region** 49
Nguyen T. K. Phuong, Tran T. Hoang, Pham H. Van, Lolyta Tu, Stephen M. Graham and Ben J. Marais

Chapter 6 **Global burden of childhood tuberculosis** 58
Helen E. Jenkins

Chapter 7 **Atypical bacterial pneumonia in the HIV-infected population** 65
Breanne M. Head, Adriana Trajtman, Zulma V. Rueda, Lázaro Vélez and Yoav Keynan

Chapter 8 **Pneumococcal conjugate vaccine implementation in middle-income countries** 72
Serena Tricarico, Hannah C. McNeil, David W. Cleary, Michael G. Head, Victor Lim, Ivan Kok Seng Yap, Chong Chun Wie, Cheng Siang Tan, Mohd Nor Norazmi, Ismail Aziah, Eddy Seong Guan Cheah, Saul N. Faust, Johanna M. C. Jefferies, Paul J. Roderick, Michael Moore, Ho Ming Yuen, Marie-Louise Newell, Nuala McGrath, C. Patrick Doncaster, Alex R. Kraaijeveld, Jeremy S. Webb and Stuart C. Clarke

Chapter 9 **Predictors of pneumococcal carriage and the effect of the 13-valent pneumococcal conjugate vaccination in the Western Australian Aboriginal population** 87
Deirdre A. Collins, Anke Hoskins, Thomas Snelling, Kalpani Senasinghe, Jacinta Bowman, Natalie A. Stemberger, Amanda J. Leach and Deborah Lehmann

Chapter 10 **Increased risk of pneumonia in residents living near poultry farms: does the upper respiratory tract microbiota play a role?** **98**
Lidwien A. M. Smit, Gert Jan Boender, Wouter A. A. de Steenhuijsen Piters, Thomas J. Hagenaars, Elisabeth G. W. Huijskens, John W. A. Rossen, Marion Koopmans, Gonnie Nodelijk, Elisabeth A. M. Sanders, Joris Yzermans, Debby Bogaert and Dick Heederik

Chapter 11 **How and when to use common biomarkers in community-acquired pneumonia** **107**
Erica J. Shaddock

Chapter 12 **Risk factors for community-acquired pneumonia among adults** **114**
Esther Muthumbi, Brett S. Lowe, Cyprian Muyodi, Esther Getambu, Fergus Gleeson and J. Anthony G. Scott

Chapter 13 **Impact of viral multiplex real-time PCR on management of respiratory tract infection** **123**
Lena M. Mayer, Christian Kahlert, Frank Rassouli, Pietro Vernazza and Werner C. Albrich

Chapter 14 **Tuberculosis and pneumonia in HIV-infected children** **139**
Helena Rabie and Pierre Goussard

Chapter 15 **Development of PCRSeq Typing—a novel molecular assay for typing of *Streptococcus pneumoniae*** **149**
Geetha Nagaraj, Feroze Ganaie, Vandana Govindan and Kadahalli Lingegowda Ravikumar

Chapter 16 **Non-adherence to community oral-antibiotic treatment in children with fast-breathing pneumonia in Malawi– secondary analysis of a prospective cohort study** **159**
Rebecca Nightingale, Tim Colbourn, David Mukanga, Limangeni Mankhambo, Norman Lufesi, Eric D. McCollum and Carina King

Chapter 17 **Economic burden of community-acquired pneumonia among elderly patients** **167**
Keiko Konomura, Hideaki Nagai and Manabu Akazawa

Chapter 18 **Corynebacteria as a cause of pulmonary infection** **177**
Katharine Yang, Robert L. Kruse, Weijie V. Lin and Daniel M. Musher

Chapter 19 **Cilostazol for the prevention of pneumonia** **185**
Hirotaka Nakashima, Kazuhisa Watanabe, Hiroyuki Umegaki, Yusuke Suzuki and Masafumi Kuzuya

Chapter 20 **The association between pre-hospital antibiotic therapy and subsequent in-hospital mortality in adults presenting with community-acquired pneumonia** **192**
Biswajit Chakrabarti, Dan Wootton, Steven Lane, Elizabeth Kanwar, Joseph Somers, Jacyln Proctor, Nancy Prospero and Mark Woodhead

Chapter 21 **Decreased relative risk of pneumococcal pneumonia during the last decade 201**
Carlos M. Luna, Laura Pulido, Michael S. Niederman, Alberto Casey, Diego Burgos, Sebastián D. Leiva Agüero, Alejandra Grosso, Evangelina Membriani, Andrea C. Entrocassi, Marcelo Rodríquez Fermepin, Carlos A. Vay, Susana Garcia and Angela Famiglietti

Chapter 22 **Rationale and methods of a randomized controlled trial of immunogenicity, safety and impact on carriage of pneumococcal conjugate and polysaccharide vaccines in infants 209**
Deborah Lehmann, Wendy Kirarock, Anita H. J. van den Biggelaar, Megan Passey, Peter Jacoby, Gerard Saleu, Geraldine Masiria, Birunu Nivio, Andrew Greenhill, Tilda Orami, Jacinta Francis, Rebecca Ford, Lea-Ann Kirkham, Vela Solomon, Peter C. Richmond and William S. Pomat

Permissions

List of Contributors

Index

Preface

Pneumonia is an inflammatory condition of the alveoli of the lung. It typically starts as an upper respiratory tract infection, which moves into the lower respiratory tract. Pneumonia can be diagnosed based on a chest X-ray and examination of physical signs. In individuals requiring hospitalization, chest radiography, blood tests and pulse oximetry are generally performed. Oral antibiotics, analgesics, fluids and rest are sufficient for complete resolution of the disease. In the elderly, or individuals with difficulty breathing or other medical conditions, treatment requires advanced care. A first dose of antibiotics is required as soon as possible. A combination of corticosteroids and antibiotics can significantly improve outcomes. Neuraminidase inhibitors are used for the treatment of viral pneumonia. Most of the topics introduced in this book cover new techniques in the diagnosis and treatment of pneumonia. It will also provide interesting topics for research, which interested readers can take up. This book aims to serve as a resource guide for students and experts alike.

This book has been the outcome of endless efforts put in by authors and researchers on various issues and topics within the field. The book is a comprehensive collection of significant researches that are addressed in a variety of chapters. It will surely enhance the knowledge of the field among readers across the globe.

It gives us an immense pleasure to thank our researchers and authors for their efforts to submit their piece of writing before the deadlines. Finally in the end, I would like to thank my family and colleagues who have been a great source of inspiration and support.

Editor

1

Aboriginal and non-Aboriginal children in Western Australia carry different serotypes of pneumococci with different antimicrobial susceptibility profiles

Eileen M. Dunne[1], Kylie Carville[2], Thomas V. Riley[3,4], Jacinta Bowman[4], Amanda J. Leach[5], Allan W. Cripps[6], Denise Murphy[7^], Peter Jacoby[8], Deborah Lehmann[8*] for the Kalgoorlie Otitis Media Research Project Team

Abstract

Background: Carriage of *Streptococcus pneumoniae* is considered a precursor to pneumococcal diseases including pneumonia. As part of the Kalgoorlie Otitis Media Research Project, we characterised pneumococci isolated from the nasopharynx of Western Australian Aboriginal and non-Aboriginal children.

Methods: Between 1999 and 2005, 100 Aboriginal and 180 non-Aboriginal children were followed from birth to two years, with nasopharyngeal aspirates collected at ages 1–3 and 6–8 weeks, then at 4, 6, 12, 18 and 24 months. Introduction of 7-valent pneumococcal conjugate vaccine (7vPCV) in 2001 enabled evaluation of its impact on carriage in study participants according to vaccines doses received. Pneumococcal serotyping was performed by Quellung and antimicrobial susceptibility by disk diffusion and Etest®. Molecular epidemiology of pneumococcal isolates was investigated by pulse-field gel electrophoresis and multilocus sequence typing.

Results: Overall, the prevalence of 7vPCV serotypes was similar for Aboriginal and non-Aboriginal children (19 % vs. 16 %), but the prevalence of non-vaccine serotypes was higher in Aboriginal children (22 % vs. 7 %). A multi-resistant 6B clone (ST90) was found only in non-Aboriginal children. Aboriginal children who received three doses of 7vPCV had lower odds of carrying 7vPCV serotypes (odds ratio [OR] 0.19, 95 % CI 0.08–0.44) and higher odds of carrying non-vaccine serotypes (OR 2.37, 95 % CI 1.13–4.99) than unvaccinated Aboriginal children; this finding was not observed in non-Aboriginal children.

Conclusions: This unique study shows important differences in pneumococcal serotypes, genotypes, and antimicrobial susceptibility between Aboriginal and non-Aboriginal children living in the same geographic area before widespread 7vPCV use, and highlights the need for ongoing post-vaccination surveillance in outback Australia.

Keywords: *Streptococcus pneumoniae*, Carriage, Serotypes, Pneumococcal conjugate vaccine, Aboriginal

* Correspondence: Deborah.lehmann@telethonkids.org.au
^Deceased
[8]Telethon Kids Institute, The University of Western Australia, Subiaco, WA, Australia
Full list of author information is available at the end of the article

Background

Pneumonia is a major cause of childhood morbidity and mortality worldwide and is estimated to be the second leading cause of death for children under the age of five, behind preterm birth complications [1]. Although the majority of disease burden occurs in Africa and south Asia, indigenous peoples living in high-income countries also have high rates of pneumonia [2, 3]. *Streptococcus pneumoniae* (the pneumococcus) is the predominant cause of community-acquired pneumonia [4, 5]. Pneumococci commonly reside in the nasopharynx of healthy young children [6, 7], and there are links between pneumococcal colonisation and invasive pneumococcal disease, pneumonia, and otitis media (OM) [8–10]. Studies in Australia have reported higher rates of pneumococcal carriage and disease in Aboriginal than in non-Aboriginal populations, and pneumococcal carriage occurs earlier in Aboriginal children [11–13]. However, there are no comparative data on pneumococcal serotypes and antimicrobial susceptibility in Aboriginal and non-Aboriginal children living in the same geographic region, either in Australia or elsewhere.

The pneumococcus is a highly diverse species, with variations in capsule structure giving rise to over 90 known serotypes. The use of pneumococcal conjugate vaccines (PCVs) in children can prevent invasive pneumococcal disease [14, 15] and OM [16, 17] caused by vaccine serotypes, as well as pneumonia [18, 19]. PCVs also reduce carriage of vaccine serotypes, but typically this reduction is associated with increased carriage of non-vaccine serotypes [6, 7, 20–22]. 7vPCV (which includes serotypes 4, 6B, 9V, 14, 18C, 19F and 23F) was included in the Australian immunisation schedule in 2001 for Aboriginal and high risk children, and in 2005 for all other children. This was replaced by PCV13 (7vPCV + serotypes 1, 3, 5, 6A, 7F, 19A) in 2011 [23].

As part of an investigation into causal pathways to OM, the Kalgoorlie Otitis Media Research Project examined bacterial carriage in young Aboriginal and non-Aboriginal children in the Kalgoorlie–Boulder area, Western Australia [11, 24]. Pneumococcal carriage rates were high in Aboriginal children: 18 % in the first month of life, and ranging between 51 and 67 % from age 3 months onwards. Equivalent figures for non-Aboriginal children were 3 % and 26–37 %, respectively [11]. The number of children in the household was positively associated with pneumococcal carriage for both Aboriginal and non-Aboriginal children, and day care attendance was a risk factor for carriage in non-Aboriginal children [25]. Here, our aim is to describe the serotypes, antimicrobial susceptibility, and molecular epidemiology of pneumococci isolated from the nasopharynx during the Kalgoorlie Otitis Media Research Project and the impact of 7vPCV on upper respiratory tract carriage among participants in this study. We hypothesise that there are differences in the serotypes and characteristics of pneumococci carried by Aboriginal and non-Aboriginal children.

Methods

Study design

The design of the Kalgoorlie Otitis Media Research Project has been described elsewhere [11, 24]. Briefly, between April 1999 and January 2003, 100 Aboriginal and 180 non-Aboriginal children residing in the Kalgoorlie–Boulder area were enrolled soon after birth. Written informed consent was provided by participants' guardians. Nasopharyngeal aspirates (NPAs) were collected at ages 1–3 and 6–8 weeks, and at 4, 6, 12, 18 and 24 months as previously described [11]. NPAs were added to 1 ml skim milk-tryptone-glucose-glycerol broth and placed immediately at −20 ° C until transfer to −70 ° C within 72 hours. NPAs were collected, rather than nasopharyngeal swabs, to facilitate viral as well as bacterial detection, and have been shown to have similar pneumococcal isolation rates to nasopharyngeal swabs [26]. In July 2001, 7vPCV was introduced into the routine immunisation schedule for all Australian Aboriginal children to be given at ages 2, 4 and 6 months with a catch-up program for all Aboriginal children aged <2 years. A booster of 23-valent pneumococcal polysaccharide vaccine (23vPPV) was recommended for Aboriginal children at age 18 months. In the absence of a universal 7vPCV program for non-Aboriginal children during the study period, from October 2001 we also offered the same 3-dose schedule of 7vPCV to non-Aboriginal study participants. Vaccination characteristics of the study population are shown in Additional file 1: Table S1.

Primary culture and serotyping of pneumococci

Selective media were used to isolate *S. pneumoniae* [11] and 4 colonies, preferably morphologically different colonies, were subcultured. Serotyping using the Quellung reaction was performed on all 4 subcultured colonies, with any identified serotypes reported once per sample and defined as 'distinct pneumococcal isolates'.

Antimicrobial susceptibility

Antimicrobial susceptibility testing was performed on one subcultured pneumococcal isolate from each sample, and also on any additional serotype or morphologically distinct isolate identified in the sample. We used disc diffusion [27] and the minimum inhibitory concentration (MIC) for penicillin- or ceftriaxone-resistant strains determined by Etest® (bioMerieux, USA) according to the recommended breakpoints at the time of testing [28]. Isolates were classified as penicillin susceptible (MIC ≤ 0.064 μg/ml), penicillin intermediate resistant (MIC > 0.064, ≤ 1.0 μg/ml) or penicillin resistant (MIC > 1 μg/ml). Isolates were classified as ceftriaxone susceptible (MIC ≥ 1.0 μg/ml), ceftriaxone intermediate resistant (MIC 2 μg/ml) or ceftriaxone resistant (MIC ≤ 4 μg/ml).

Pulse field gel electrophoresis

Pulse field gel electrophoresis (PFGE) typing was performed as previously described [29] on a subset of 199 pneumococcal isolates that were available for investigation in May 2003. These isolates were from samples collected between April 1999 and April 2002. Isolates were from 99 children: 53 non-Aboriginal children contributed 97 pneumococci and 46 Aboriginal children contributed 102 pneumococci. A single isolate per sample was typed and the pneumococcal isolates represented a range of serotypes.

Multilocus sequence typing

To further investigate a multiresistant 6B clone identified by PFGE, multilocus sequence typing (MLST) was performed on a subset of 6B isolates ($n = 12$) using a mass spectrometry based method [30]. Isolates were selected based upon antimicrobial susceptibility profiles with approximately half from Aboriginal and half from non-Aboriginal children. As serotype 19A is commonly associated with serotype replacement following 7vPCV introduction [31], twelve 19A isolates from this study and six 19A isolates collected in Kalgoorlie during 2008 as part of pneumococcal surveillance in Western Australian Aboriginal people [32] were also analysed by MLST.

Data analysis

Statistical analyses were performed using SPSS (version 15.0 for Windows) and the level of statistical significance was set at $p < 0.05$. The Mann–Whitney U test was used to compare the age of Aboriginal and non-Aboriginal children at vaccination and time from vaccination to sample collection. Pearson's chi square was used to test differences in total vaccine doses received between Aboriginal and non-Aboriginal children. The modified Wald method was used to calculate confidence intervals of proportions using GraphPad (GraphPad Software Inc, USA) and the Z test used to compare proportions.

When investigating the effect of vaccination on carriage, to avoid potential bias related to health-seeking behaviour (e.g. delayed attendance for immunisation), the cohort was restricted to include data from those children who never received 7vPCV during the study period and those who received their first dose of 7vPCV before age 12 months. Among 7vPCV recipients, only samples collected >14 days after 7vPCV administration were considered post-vaccine to allow for the immunologic response to develop. Logistic regression modeling was used to assess the relationship between 7vPCV vaccination and pneumococcal carriage whilst adjusting for age. The models incorporated Generalized Estimating Equations (GEEs) to account for loss of independence due to repeated sampling of individuals. The regression analysis was performed separately for Aboriginal and non-Aboriginal children. Non-typeable pneumococci were excluded from this analysis.

Results

A total of 506 nasopharyngeal samples were collected from Aboriginal children and 1,045 from non-Aboriginal children. The median number of samples collected was 6 for both Aboriginal and non-Aboriginal children. The median age at first sample collection was 15 days for Aboriginal children and 17 days for non-Aboriginal children. Information on vaccination status is presented in Additional file 1: Table S1. The overall pneumococcal carriage rates (% of samples containing any pneumococcus) were 49.2 % for Aboriginal children and 24.9 % for non-Aboriginal children, with carriage rates increasing with age as previously reported [11]. A total of 547 distinct pneumococcal isolates were identified and subject to further analysis.

Pneumococcal serotypes

The prevalence (% of samples) of pneumococcal serotypes (7vPCV serotypes, non-7v PCV13 serotypes, and non-vaccine types) in study participants is shown in Fig. 1, with full data available in Additional file 1: Table S2. Overall, 18.8 % (95 % CI 15.6–22.4) of samples from Aboriginal children contained 7vPCV serotypes compared to 15.7 % (95 % CI 13.6–18.0) of samples from non-Aboriginal children. There were no significant differences in the prevalence of 7vPCV between Aboriginal and non-Aboriginal groups when examined in different age groups (<6 months 17 % vs 10 %, 6 - <12 months 21 % vs 23 %, and ≥12 months 22 % in both). There were also no differences in prevalence of the most common serotype, namely 6B, between Aboriginal and non-Aboriginal children in the 3 age groups (<6 months 3-4 %, 6- < 12 months 11 %, ≥12 months 8-10 %). Data for other individual serotypes were too sparse to investigate in different age groups. For the additional six serotypes contained in 13vPCV, rates were 9.7 % (95 % CI 7.4–12.6) from Aboriginal children and 2.7 % (95 % CI 1.8–3.9) from non-Aboriginal children (note that serotype 5 was not detected in this study). Non-vaccine serotypes were more common in samples from Aboriginal children (21.9 % [95 % CI 18.5–25.8]) compared to non-Aboriginal children (7.1 % [95 % CI 5.7–8.8]), with similar patterns in different age groups. A broader range of serotypes was seen in Aboriginal children (33 different serotypes in 506 samples) than in non-Aboriginal children (29 serotypes in 1,045 samples, $p = 0.0004$). Serotypes 6A, 19A, 16F, 11A, 33F, 9V, and non-typeable pneumococci were more commonly found in samples from Aboriginal than non-

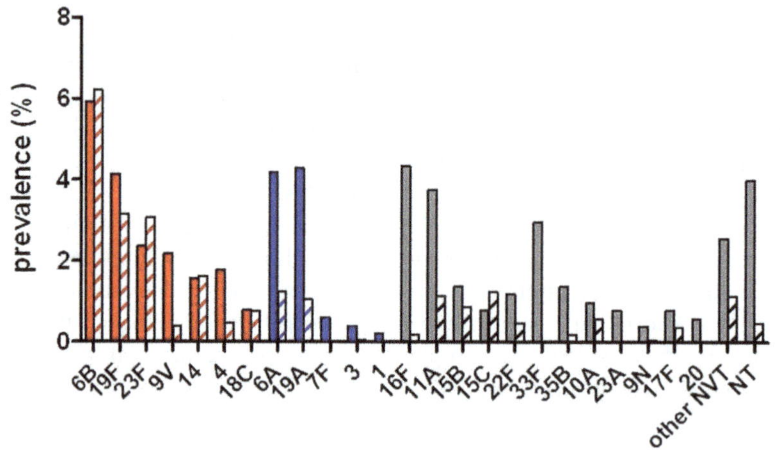

Fig. 1 Prevalence (% of samples) of pneumococcal serotypes in carriage samples collected from Aboriginal (solid bars) and non-Aboriginal (hashed bars) study participants (1999–2005). 7vPCV serotypes are shown in red, with the additional serotypes contained in 13vPCV shown in blue and non-vaccine types (NVT) shown in grey. NT = non-typeable

Aboriginal children. Twenty-five (4.9 %) samples from Aboriginal children yielded multiple pneumococcal serotypes (24 samples with two different serotypes and one sample with three different serotypes). Twelve (1.1 %) samples from non-Aboriginal children produced two different serotypes.

Antimicrobial susceptibility

A total of 526 pneumococcal isolates from 507 samples were tested for susceptibility to penicillin, erythromycin, tetracycline, cotrimoxazole, chloramphenicol, and ceftriaxone. Rifampicin and vancomycin susceptibility was tested for on 478 and 479 isolates, respectively. All isolates were susceptible to ceftriaxone, rifampicin, and vancomycin. Results for other antimicrobials are summarised in Table 1, with detailed results by serotype shown in Additional file 1: Tables S3 and S4. Overall, 127 (24.1 %) isolates showed reduced susceptibility to penicillin, 73 (13.9 %) to erythromycin, 78 (14.8 %) to tetracycline and 147 (27.9 %) to cotrimoxazole. There were differences in antimicrobial susceptibility between pneumococci isolated from Aboriginal and non-Aboriginal children. All isolates from Aboriginal children were susceptible to chloramphenicol, whereas 13.2 % of isolates from non-Aboriginal children displayed reduced susceptibility. Reduced penicillin susceptibility of serotypes 19F and 19A was more common and that of serotype 6B less common in Aboriginal than in non-Aboriginal children (19F: 70 % vs. 39 %; 19A 64 % vs. 18 %;

Table 1 Reduced antimicrobial susceptibility of *Streptococcus pneumoniae* in nasopharyngeal samples from Aboriginal and non-Aboriginal children

Isolate type	Number of isolates	% with reduced susceptibility to antimicrobial agent				
		Penicillin[a]	Erythromycin	Tetracycline	Cotrimoxazole	Chloramphenicol
7vPCV types						
Aboriginal	92	31.5	7.6	17.4	35.9	0.0
Non-Aboriginal	162	35.2	26.5	27.2	43.8	21.6
Non-vaccine types						
Aboriginal	151	15.2	4.0	3.3	4.6	0.0
Non-Aboriginal	97	3.1	6.2	3.1	13.4	0.0
Non-typeable						
Aboriginal	18	66.7	50.0	27.8	72.2	0.0
Non-Aboriginal	5	60.0	40.0	60.0	80.0	0.0
All pneumococci						
Aboriginal	261	24.5	8.4	10.7	22.6	0.0
Non-Aboriginal[b]	265	23.8	19.2	18.9	33.2	13.2

[a]Pneumococci showed intermediate resistance to penicillin (MIC 0.065-1.0 μg/mL) except for 1 serotype 23F isolate that showed MIC =1.5 μg/mL
[b]Includes 1 isolate not serotyped

6B 21 % vs. 59 %). Cotrimoxazole resistance was present in almost half of the serotype 6B isolates from Aboriginal children and 74 % of those from non-Aboriginal children. Of note, 65 % of non-typeable pneumococci isolated from Aboriginal and non-Aboriginal children had reduced susceptibility to penicillin and 74 % had reduced susceptibility to cotrimoxazole. Overall, 5 % of 503 serotypeable pneumococci were resistant to two antimicrobials and a further 9 % to three antimicrobials. Equivalent figures for 23 non-typeable pneumococci were 30 % and 43 %, respectively.

There were 33 isolates (serotypes 6B, $n = 27$; 23F, $n = 5$; 19F, $n = 1$) from 20 non-Aboriginal children, which showed reduced susceptibility to penicillin, tetracycline, erythromycin, cotrimoxazole and chloramphenicol (6.3 % of all isolates, 12.5 % of isolates from non-Aboriginal children). This multi-resistance pattern was not seen in any isolates from Aboriginal children.

Molecular epidemiology

Using PFGE, 67 different molecular types of *S. pneumoniae* were identified among the 199 isolates examined (Additional file 1: Table S5). Of these, 30 were represented once and 14 types were seen five or more times. All 7vPCV serotypes in this population were quite variable except 18C. Only one molecular type (72) was found in both a vaccine (6B) and a non-vaccine (10A) serotype; these isolates were not from the same child.

MLST was performed on 12 serotype 6B isolates and 18 serotype 19A isolates (6 of which were collected in 2008) (Table 2). The multiresistant 6B clone identified as molecular type 58 by PFGE was revealed to be ST90, a globally distributed clone also known as Spain^{6B}-2. Interestingly, ST90 was only found in non-Aboriginal children, whereas ST185, a globally distributed clone known as S. Africa^{6B}-8 was isolated from both Aboriginal and non-Aboriginal children.

The 6B isolates clustered into two broad clonal complexes, one related to ST385 and one related to ST90. These two clonal complexes were evenly distributed throughout the study period. Most of the 19A isolates were related to ST199, although one 19A isolate was ST162, which is mainly associated with serotypes 9V and 19F [33]. Three isolates with distinct PFGE molecular types were all ST199. The six more recent 19A isolates examined belonged to ST202 and ST320. No serotype 6B isolates were identified in 2008 following widespread use of 7vPCV.

Pneumococcal carriage and vaccination

A higher proportion of Aboriginal than non-Aboriginal children received 7vPCV, they were older than non-Aboriginal children at time of receiving each dose of

Table 2 Genotypes and antimicrobial resistance of select 6B and 19A isolates

Isolates (*n*)	Ethnicity	Serotype	Antimicrobial resistance[a]	PFGE type[b]	Sequence Type[c]
1	Aboriginal	6B	cotrimoxazole *(I)*, tetracycline *(R)*	59	385
1	Aboriginal	6B	tetracycline *(R)*	ND	385
4	Aboriginal (3), non-Aboriginal (1)	6B	cotrimoxazole *(R)*	60 (2), ND (2)	185 (DLV 385)
1	Aboriginal	6B	cotrimoxazole *(R)*	ND	4276 (DLV 385)
4	Non-Aboriginal	6B	multiresistant	58, ND	90
1	Non-Aboriginal	6B	multiresistant	ND	10265[d+] (SLV 90)
1	Aboriginal	19A	none	30	199
1	Aboriginal	19A	none	28	199
1	Non-Aboriginal	19A	none	11	199
1	Aboriginal	19A	cotrimoxazole *(R)*	31	876 (SLV 199)
1	Non-Aboriginal	19A	cotrimoxazole *(R)*	ND	10264[d] (DLV 199)
2	Aboriginal, non-Aboriginal	19A	none	18	172
1	Aboriginal	19A	none	34	10262[d]
2	Aboriginal	19A	none	ND	10263[d] (SLV 10262)
1	Non-Aboriginal	19A	cotrimoxazole *(R)*	ND	162
4 (3 from 2008)	Aboriginal	19A	cotrimoxazole *(R)*, tetracycline *(R)*	ND	202
3 (from 2008)	Aboriginal	19A	multiresistant	ND	320

[a] *I* Intermediate, *R* Resistant, *multiresistant* resistant to cotrimoxazole, erythromycin, and tetracycline, and chloramphenicol and/or penicillin
[b] *ND* not determined
[c] *SLV* single locus variant, *DLV* double locus variant
[d] *ST* first reported in this study

7vPCV and there was no difference in time from receiving 7vPCV to sample collection between Aboriginal and non-Aboriginal children (Additional file 1: Table S1). Table 3 shows pneumococcal carriage in unimmunised children and according to number of doses among those who received their first dose of 7vPCV before age 12 months. Serotypes were grouped as 7vPCV and non-7vPCV types for this analysis as numbers were too small to analyse individually for most serotypes. Similarly, children receiving 1 and 2 doses of 7vPCV were grouped due to small numbers. There were 415 samples from Aboriginal children and 1,010 samples from non-Aboriginal children included in this analysis (82 % and 97 % of all study samples, respectively). From this cohort of Aboriginal children, pneumococci were isolated from 105 (40.9 %) samples from unvaccinated children, 44 (57.1 %) samples from those who had received one or two doses of 7vPCV, and 53 (65.4 %) samples from those who had received 3 doses. Equivalent numbers for the non-Aboriginal children were 183 (22.3 %), 33 (37.1 %), and 33 (32.4 %), respectively. Note that the increased pneumococcal carriage with more doses is related to the increase in carriage prevalence with age during the first year of life [11].

A higher proportion of samples from Aboriginal children had non-7vPCV serotypes after receiving 3 doses of vaccine (46.9 %, 95 % CI 36.4–57.7 %) compared with samples from those who were not vaccinated (24.5 %, 95 % CI 19.6–30.1 %), while carriage of 7vPCV serotypes was lower following 3 doses of vaccine than in unvaccinated children (9.9 % [95 % CI 4.9–18.5 %] vs. 17.9 % [95 % CI 13.7–23.1 %]). In contrast, similar proportions of 7vPCV and non-7vPCV pneumococcal serotypes were found in unvaccinated and fully vaccinated non-Aboriginal children. After controlling for age and accounting for repeated sampling, the odds of isolating 7vPCV pneumococcal serotypes in samples from Aboriginal children were about five times less after three doses of vaccine than in samples from unvaccinated children, and the odds of isolating non-7vPCV types were 2.5 times greater (Table 4). Similar results were not seen with samples taken from non-Aboriginal children. However, non-Aboriginal children who received 1–2 doses of 7vPCV had an increased odds of carrying 7vPCV serotypes.

Discussion

To our knowledge, this is the only study to date comparing the characteristics of pneumococci isolated from the upper respiratory tract in indigenous children with those in non-indigenous children living in the same geographic area, and notably in an arid zone of Australia, for which there is a dearth of any carriage data. In addition to higher carriage rates, the distribution of pneumococcal serotypes was more diverse, and carriage of non-typeable strains and simultaneous carriage of multiple serotypes were more common in Aboriginal than in non-Aboriginal children.

The serotype distribution and antimicrobial susceptibility patterns differed between Aboriginal and non-Aboriginal children. Of note, non-PCV7 serotypes 16F, 19A, 6A, and 33F (known to be replacement serotypes following widespread use of PCVs [34, 35]) were more common in Aboriginal than in non-Aboriginal children. These differences may relate, in part at least, to vaccination status: more Aboriginal children received three doses of 7vPCV, and these fully vaccinated children were less likely to carry 7vPCV serotypes (Table 4), providing evidence of vaccine impact on carriage. However, unvaccinated Aboriginal children had higher carriage rates overall and higher carriage of non-7vPCV serotypes (more serotype diversity) than unvaccinated non-Aboriginal children, indicating some baseline differences in pneumococcal carriage.

Non-Aboriginal children receiving 1 or 2 doses of 7vPCV had increased odds of carrying 7vPCV serotypes when compared to those who had had no 7vPCV. This finding was unexpected and the reasons are unclear. It may relate

Table 3 Proportion of samples with 7vPCV or non-7vPCV serotypes in Aboriginal and non-Aboriginal children who received 0, 1–2, or 3 doses of 7vPCV

		Doses			Total
		0	1-2	3	
Aboriginal	Samples (n)	257 (%)[a]	77 (%)	81 (%)	415 (%)
	7vPCV serotypes	46 (17.9)	16 (20.8)	8 (9.9)	70 (16.9)
	Non-7vPCV serotypes	63 (24.5)	27 (35.1)	38 (46.9)	128 (30.8)
Non-Aboriginal	Samples (n)	819 (%)	89 (%)	102 (%)	1010 (%)
	7vPCV serotypes	110 (13.4)	24 (27.0)	18 (17.6)	152 (15.0)
	Non-7vPCV serotypes	72 (8.8)	11 (12.4)	14 (13.7)	97 (9.6)

[a]% = proportion of samples

Note: To avoid potential bias related to health service utilization, data presented here are from children who either never received 7vPCV or received their first dose of 7vPCV before age 12 months. Among 7vPCV recipients, only samples collected >14 days after 7vPCV administration were considered post-vaccine Some nasopharyngeal aspirates included more than one 7vPCV or non-7vPCV serotypes or both 7vPCV and non-7vPCV serotypes. Non-typeable pneumococci were excluded

Table 4 Odds Ratios for carriage of *S. pneumoniae* serotypes in nasopharyngeal samples by vaccine doses received

Serotype	Dose 1/2 OR[a] (95 % CI)		Dose 3 OR (95 % CI)	
	Aboriginal	Non-Aboriginal	Aboriginal	Non-Aboriginal
7vPCV serotypes	0.90 (0.43, 1.88)	1.93 (1.13, 3.32)	0.19 (0.08, 0.44)	0.83 (0.41, 1.66)
Non-7vPCV serotypes	1.83 (1.04, 3.20)	1.25 (0.57, 2.74)	2.50 (1.17, 5.35)	1.19 (0.65, 2.17)

[a]OR odds ratio from logistic regression, adjusting for age and age-squared and accounting for repeated sampling of individuals, with unvaccinated as the reference category. Non-typeable pneumococci were excluded

to temporal variation in carriage of certain serotypes or association between health-seeking behaviour and carriage (i.e. a small proportion of non-Aboriginal parents chose to have their children vaccinated and those who were vaccinated may have been more sickly and more likely to carry pneumococci), or the lack of herd effects in this community as 7vPCV was not included in the national immunization schedule for non-Aboriginal children during the study period. But the small number of non-Aboriginal children in this study who received 7vPCV precludes further analysis.

Generally, reduced susceptibility to antimicrobial agents was observed more often in *S. pneumoniae* carried by non-Aboriginal than Aboriginal children, with all multi-resistant strains isolated from non-Aboriginal children. An exception was serotype 19F which was more commonly resistant when carried by Aboriginal children. The antimicrobial prescription frequency was similar in Aboriginal and non-Aboriginal children in the study, but there are no available data on specific antimicrobial agents [36]. The reasons for the differences in susceptibility to antimicrobial agents are unclear, but may relate to differences in circulating pneumococcal clonal types between the two population groups or potential differences in the classes of antibiotics prescribed.

Carriage of serotype 6B was common in both Aboriginal and non-Aboriginal children, but the multi-resistant clone ST90 was only observed in non-Aboriginal children. A multiple-drug resistant clone of 6B was known to be circulating in Australia from 1988 to 1997 [37]; however, no MLST results are available from this time period so it is not known whether this clone was related to ST90. Reduced susceptibility to antimicrobials was commonly observed in non-typeable isolates from both populations, consistent with reports identifying non-typeable pneumococci as a major reservoir for antimicrobial resistance genes [38, 39].

As expected, the widespread use of PCV in more recent years has altered serotype prevalence in carriage. Surveillance of pneumococcal carriage in Aboriginal people in Western Australia from 2008 to 2011 found a 7 % prevalence in 7vPCV serotypes across varying age groups, with serotypes 19A, 16F and 6C the most common in children under five years old [32]. Further shifts in serotype distribution and a reduction in carriage of 19A have been reported following the switch to PCV13 in 2011 [40]. MLST analysis of serotype 19A isolates suggests that circulating strains may have changed following 7vPCV introduction. Only a small number of isolates was examined, so expanded molecular epidemiological studies would be needed to investigate whether selective pressure following PCV introduction results in clonal expansion, as has been observed in other settings [41].

Limitations of this study include the fact that antiserum to serotype 6C (required to differentiate between 6A and 6C) was not available at the time of sample analysis, so this serotype would not have been detected. It is also likely that simultaneous carriage of multiple serotypes was underestimated [42]. Non-typeable pneumococci were not subject to genetic analysis, therefore could represent both isolates not producing capsule and "true" non-typeable pneumococci that lack capsule synthesis genes. More sophisticated serotyping methodologies are now available [43]. Antibiotic susceptibility data were not examined according to vaccine status, due to small numbers within each dosing group.

An overall reduction in invasive pneumococcal disease (IPD) and a reduction in IPD caused by 7vPCV serotypes have been observed in the post-PCV years in Australia, although IPD due to non-vaccine serotypes has increased [13, 44]. The switch to PCV13 in 2011 has led to further reductions in IPD, particularly in children under five years of age [45]. Although a gap still remains, the disparity in pneumonia hospitalisations between Australian Aboriginal and non-Aboriginal children has declined over time, likely due in part to PCV introduction [46].

Conclusions

This study identified important differences in pneumococcal serotypes, genotypes, and antimicrobial susceptibility between Aboriginal and non-Aboriginal children living in the same region before widespread 7vPCV use. Ongoing surveillance of pneumococcal carriage is warranted to monitor potential increases in antimicrobial resistance and changes in serotype distribution that could impact on pneumococcal disease and health outcomes, and to help in the continual development of effective vaccines. Data reported here provide a useful baseline comparator, as well as insight into some of the differences in *S. pneumoniae* carried by Aboriginal and non-Aboriginal children in Australia.

Additional file

Additional file 1: Table S1. 7vPCV vaccination characteristics of the study participants. **Table S2.** Prevalences of pneumococcal serotypes found in the respiratory tract of study participants 1999–2005. **Table S3.** Reduced antimicrobial susceptibility of *Streptococcus pneumoniae* in nasopharyngeal samples from Aboriginal children reported by serotype. **Table S4.** Reduced antimicrobial susceptibility of *Streptococcus pneumoniae* in nasopharyngeal samples from non-Aboriginal children reported by serotype. **Table S5.** The molecular type by pulse-field gel electrophoresis (PFGE) of 199 *S. pneumoniae* isolates reported by serotype. (DOCX 26 kb)

Abbreviations

23vPPV: 23-valent pneumococcal polysaccharide vaccine; 7vPCV: 7-valent pneumococcal conjugate vaccine; CI: confidence interval; IPD: invasive pneumococcal disease; MIC: minimum inhibitory concentration; MLST: multilocus sequence typing; NPA: nasopharyngeal aspirate; OM: otitis media; OR: odds ratio; PCV: pneumococcal conjugate vaccine; PFGE: pulse field gel electrophoresis

Acknowledgements

This study resulted from the collaborative work of the Kalgoorlie Otitis Media Research Project Team (listed in reference # [11]); however, we particularly thank crucial field staff: Dimity Elsbury, the late Janine Finucane, Annette Stokes and Ruth Monck. We thank Lyn O'Reilly for assistance with bacterial typing.

Funding

This study was funded through the Australian National Health and Medical Research Council project grant #212044 and two Healthway grants (#6028 and #10564). DL was funded through National Health and Medical Research Council program grant #353514. Wyeth Australia provided Prevenar™ for non-Aboriginal study participants. MLST work was supported by the Victorian Government's Operational Infrastructure Support Program. AJL was supported by a National Health and Medical Research Council Career Development Award (#283312). KC was supported through the Masters of Applied Epidemiology program funded by the Australian Government. The funders had no role in study design, collection and analysis of data, decision to publish, or writing of the manuscript.

Authors' contributions

Conception, generation and design of the research plan: DL, TVR, AJL, AWC, PJ Data collection: KC, JB, DM, EMD Data analysis: PJ, EMD, DL Drafting of manuscript: EMD, DL. All authors performed critical review of the manuscript.

Competing interests

DL has previously been a member of the GSK Australia Pneumococcal-*Haemophilus influenzae*-Protein D conjugate vaccine ("Phid-CV") Advisory Panel, has received support from Pfizer Australia and GSK Australia to attend conferences, has received an honorarium from Merck Vaccines to give a seminar at their offices in Pennsylvania and to attend a conference, and is an investigator on an investigator-initiated research grant funded by Pfizer Australia. AJL has received research funding and support to attend conferences from GlaxoSmithKline and Pfizer Australia. AWC has previously been a member of the GSK Advisory Panel for the 10 valent pneumococcal conjugate vaccine and presented at Symposia. He received an honorarium from GSK to undertake these activities. He has also chaired a Symposium on pneumonia for Pfizer Australia. No honorarium was accepted. All other authors have no competing interests.

Margaret Hospital Ethics Committee and the Confidentiality of Health Information Committee of the Health Department of WA. Written informed consent was provided by participants' guardians.

Author details

[1]Pneumococcal Research, Murdoch Childrens Research Institute, Parkville, VIC, Australia. [2]Victorian Infectious Disease Reference Laboratory at the Peter Doherty Institute for Infection and Immunity, Melbourne, VIC, Australia. [3]Microbiology & Immunology, School of Pathology & Laboratory Medicine, The University of Western Australia, Crawley, WA, Australia. [4]Department of Microbiology, PathWest Laboratory Medicine, Queen Elizabeth II Medical Centre, Nedlands, WA, Australia. [5]Child Health Division, Menzies School of Health Research, Darwin, NT, Australia. [6]School of Medicine and Menzies Health Institute Queensland, Griffith University, Southport, QLD, Australia. [7]Public Health Bacteriology Laboratory, Centre for Public Health Sciences, Coopers Plains, QLD, Australia. [8]Telethon Kids Institute, The University of Western Australia, Subiaco, WA, Australia.

References

1. Liu L, Oza S, Hogan D, Perin J, Rudan I, Lawn JE, et al. Global, regional, and national causes of child mortality in 2000–13, with projections to inform post-2015 priorities: an updated systematic analysis. Lancet. 2015;385:430–40. PMID:25280870.
2. O'Grady KA, Taylor-Thomson DM, Chang AB, Torzillo PJ, Morris PS, Mackenzie GA, et al. Rates of radiologically confirmed pneumonia as defined by the World Health Organization in Northern Territory Indigenous children. Med J Aust. 2010;192:592–5. PMID:20477736.
3. Alaghehbandan R, Gates KD, MacDonald D. Hospitalization due to pneumonia among Innu, Inuit and non-Aboriginal communities, Newfoundland and Labrador, Canada. Int J Infect Dis. 2007;11:23–8. PMID: 16533615, http://dx.doi.org/10.1016/j.ijid.2005.09.003.
4. File TM. Community-acquired pneumonia. Lancet. 2003;362:1991–2001. PMID:14683661.
5. Michelow IC, Olsen K, Lozano J, Rollins NK, Duffy LB, Ziegler T, et al. Epidemiology and clinical characteristics of community-acquired pneumonia in hospitalized children. Pediatrics. 2004;113:701–7. PMID:15060215.
6. Ghaffar F, Barton T, Lozano J, Muniz LS, Hicks P, Gan V, et al. Effect of the 7-valent pneumococcal conjugate vaccine on nasopharyngeal colonization by *Streptococcus pneumoniae* in the first 2 years of life. Clin Infect Dis. 2004;39: 930–8. PMID:15472842, http://dx.doi.org/10.1086/423379.
7. Millar EV, O'Brien KL, Watt JP, Bronsdon MA, Dallas J, Whitney CG, et al. Effect of community-wide conjugate pneumococcal vaccine use in infancy on nasopharyngeal carriage through 3 years of age: a cross-sectional study in a high-risk population. Clin Infect Dis. 2006;43:8–15. PMID:16758412, http://dx.doi.org/10.1086/504802.
8. Leach AJ, Boswell JB, Asche V, Nienhuys TG, Mathews JD. Bacterial colonization of the nasopharynx predicts very early onset and persistence of otitis media in Australian Aboriginal infants. Pediatr Infect Dis J. 1994;13: 983–9. PMID:7845752, http://dx.doi.org/10.1097/00006454-199411000-00009.
9. Simell B, Auranen K, Käyhty H, Goldblatt D, Dagan R, O'Brien KL, Group PC. The fundamental link between pneumococcal carriage and disease. Expert Rev Vaccines. 2012;11:841–55. PMID:22913260, http://dx.doi.org/10.1586/erv.12.53.
10. Ruohola A, Pettigrew MM, Lindholm L, Jalava J, Räisänen KS, Vainionpää R, et al. Bacterial and viral interactions within the nasopharynx contribute to the risk of acute otitis media. J Infect. 2013;66:247–54. PMID:23266462, http://dx.doi.org/10.1016/j.jinf.2012.12.002.
11. Watson K, Carville K, Bowman J, Jacoby P, Riley TV, Leach AJ, Kalgoorlie Otitis Media Research Project Team, et al. Upper respiratory tract bacterial carriage in Aboriginal and non-Aboriginal children in a semi-arid area of Western Australia. Pediatr Infect Dis J. 2006;25:782–90. PMID:16940834, http://dx.doi.org/10.1097/01.inf.0000232705.49634.68.
12. Barry C, Krause VL, Cook HM, Menzies RI. Invasive pneumococcal disease in Australia 2007 and 2008. Commun Dis Intell Q Rep. 2012;36:E151–65. PMID:23186214.
13. Lehmann D, Willis J, Moore HC, Giele C, Murphy D, Keil AD, et al. The changing epidemiology of invasive pneumococcal disease in Aboriginal and non-Aboriginal Western Australians from 1997 through 2007 and emergence of nonvaccine serotypes. Clin Infect Dis. 2010;50:1477–86. PMID:20420501, http://dx.doi.org/10.1086/652440.

14. Black S, Shinefield H, Fireman B, Lewis E, Ray P, Hansen JR, Northern California Kaiser Permanente Vaccine Study Center Group, et al. Efficacy, safety and immunogenicity of heptavalent pneumococcal conjugate vaccine in children. Pediatr Infect Dis J. 2000;19:187–95. PMID:10749457, http://dx.doi.org/10.1097/00006454-200003000-00003.
15. Hennessy TW, Singleton RJ, Bulkow LR, Bruden DL, Hurlburt DA, Parks D, et al. Impact of heptavalent pneumococcal conjugate vaccine on invasive disease, antimicrobial resistance and colonization in Alaska Natives: progress towards elimination of a health disparity. Vaccine. 2005;23:5464–73. PMID:16188350, http://dx.doi.org/10.1016/j.vaccine.2005.08.100.
16. Eskola J, Kilpi T, Palmu A, Jokinen J, Haapakoski J, Herva E, Finnish Otitis Media Study Group, et al. Efficacy of a pneumococcal conjugate vaccine against acute otitis media. N Engl J Med. 2001;344:403–9. PMID:11172176, http://dx.doi.org/10.1056/NEJM200102083440602.
17. Ben-Shimol S, Givon-Lavi N, Leibovitz E, Raiz S, Greenberg D, Dagan R. Near-elimination of otitis media caused by 13-valent pneumococcal conjugate vaccine (PCV) serotypes in southern Israel shortly after sequential introduction of 7-valent/13-valent PCV. Clin Infect Dis. 2014;59:1724–32. PMID:25159581, http://dx.doi.org/10.1093/cid/ciu683.
18. Black SB, Shinefield HR, Ling S, Hansen J, Fireman B, Spring D, et al. Effectiveness of heptavalent pneumococcal conjugate vaccine in children younger than five years of age for prevention of pneumonia. Pediatr Infect Dis J. 2002;21:810–5. PMID:12352800, http://dx.doi.org/10.1097/00006454-200209000-00005.
19. Lucero MG, Nohynek H, Williams G, Tallo V, Simões EA, Lupisan S, et al. Efficacy of an 11-valent pneumococcal conjugate vaccine against radiologically confirmed pneumonia among children less than 2 years of age in the Philippines: a randomized, double-blind, placebo-controlled trial. Pediatr Infect Dis J. 2009;28:455–62. PMID:19483514, http://dx.doi.org/10.1097/INF.0b013e31819637af.
20. Pelton SI, Loughlin AM, Marchant CD. Seven valent pneumococcal conjugate vaccine immunization in two Boston communities: changes in serotypes and antimicrobial susceptibility among *Streptococcus pneumoniae* isolates. Pediatr Infect Dis J. 2004;23:1015–22. PMID:15545856, http://dx.doi.org/10.1097/01.inf.0000143645.58215.f0.
21. Leach AJ, Morris PS, McCallum GB, Wilson CA, Stubbs L, Beissbarth J, et al. Emerging pneumococcal carriage serotypes in a high-risk population receiving universal 7-valent pneumococcal conjugate vaccine and 23-valent polysaccharide vaccine since 2001. BMC Infect Dis. 2009;9:121. PMID: 19650933, http://dx.doi.org/10.1186/1471-2334-9-121.
22. van Hoek AJ, Sheppard CL, Andrews NJ, Waight PA, Slack MPE, Harrison TG, et al. Pneumococcal carriage in children and adults two years after introduction of the thirteen valent pneumococcal conjugate vaccine in England. Vaccine. 2014;32(34):4349–55.
23. Australian Technical Advisory Group on Immunisation. The Australian Immunisation Handbook. 10th ed. Canberra: Australian Government Department of Health; 2013.
24. Lehmann D, Arumugaswamy A, Elsbury D, Finucane J, Stokes A, Monck R, et al. The Kalgoorlie Otitis Media Research Project: rationale, methods, population characteristics and ethical considerations. Paediatr Perinat Epidemiol. 2008;22: 60–71. PMID:18173785, http://dx.doi.org/10.1111/j.1365-3016.2007.00891.x.
25. Jacoby P, Carville KS, Hall G, Riley TV, Bowman J, Leach AJ, Kalgoorlie Otitis Media Research Project Team, et al. Crowding and other strong predictors of upper respiratory tract carriage of otitis media-related bacteria in Australian Aboriginal and non-Aboriginal children. Pediatr Infect Dis J. 2011;30:480–5. PMID:21593705.
26. Carville KS, Bowman JM, Lehmann D, Riley TV. Comparison between nasal swabs and nasopharyngeal aspirates for, and effect of time in transit on, isolation of *Streptococcus pneumoniae, Staphylococcus aureus, Haemophilus influenzae*, and *Moraxella catarrhalis*. J Clin Microbiol. 2007;45:244–5. PMID: 17079497, http://dx.doi.org/10.1128/JCM.01131-06.
27. National Committee for Clinical Laboratory Standards. Performance standards for antimicrobial disk susceptibility tests; approved standard, 7th edition Pennsylvania, USA NCCLS; 2000.
28. National Committee for Clinical Laboratory Standards. Performance standards for antimicrobial susceptibility testing; twelfth informational supplement. Pennsylvania, USA: NCCLS; 2002.
29. Sá-Leão R, Tomasz A, Sanches IS, Nunes S, Alves CR, Avô AB, et al. Genetic diversity and clonal patterns among antibiotic-susceptible and -resistant *Streptococcus pneumoniae* colonizing children: day care centers as autonomous epidemiological units. J Clin Microbiol. 2000;38:4137–44. PMID:11060081.
30. Dunne EM, Ong EK, Moser RJ, Siba PM, Phuanukoonnon S, Greenhill AR, et al. Multilocus sequence typing of *Streptococcus pneumoniae* by use of mass spectrometry. J Clin Microbiol. 2011;49:3756–60. PMID:21880964, http://dx.doi.org/10.1128/JCM.05113-11.
31. Hanage WP. Serotype replacement in invasive pneumococcal disease: where do we go from here? J Infect Dis. 2007;196:1282–4. PMID:17922390, http://dx.doi.org/10.1086/521630.
32. Collins DA, Hoskins A, Bowman J, Jones J, Stemberger NA, Richmond PC, et al. High nasopharyngeal carriage of non-vaccine serotypes in Western Australian aboriginal people following 10 years of pneumococcal conjugate vaccination. PLoS ONE. 2013;8:e82280. PMID:24349245, http://dx.doi.org/10.1371/journal.pone.0082280.
33. Brueggemann AB, Griffiths DT, Meats E, Peto T, Crook DW, Spratt BG. Clonal relationships between invasive and carriage *Streptococcus pneumoniae* and serotype- and clone-specific differences in invasive disease potential. J Infect Dis. 2003;187(9):1424–32.
34. Hicks LA, Harrison LH, Flannery B, Hadler JL, Schaffner W, Craig AS, et al. Incidence of pneumococcal disease due to non-pneumococcal conjugate vaccine (PCV7) serotypes in the United States during the era of widespread PCV7 vaccination, 1998–2004. J Infect Dis. 2007;196:1346–54. PMID: 17922399, http://dx.doi.org/10.1086/521626.
35. Grivea IN, Priftis KN, Giotas A, Kotzia D, Tsantouli AG, Douros K, et al. Dynamics of pneumococcal carriage among day-care center attendees during the transition from the 7-valent to the higher-valent pneumococcal conjugate vaccines in Greece. Vaccine. 2014;32:6513–20. PMID:25252194, http://dx.doi.org/10.1016/j.vaccine.2014.09.016.
36. Murigu N. Utilisation of health services by Aboriginal and non-Aboriginal children in the Kalgoorlie Boulder region of Western Australia: Curtin University. 2008.
37. Carlisle JB, Gratten M, Leach AJ. Molecular epidemiology of multiple drug resistant type 6B *Streptococcus pneumoniae* in the Northern Territory and Queensland, Australia. Epidemiol Infect. 2001;126:25–9. PMID:11293678, http://dx.doi.org/10.1017/S0950268801005106.
38. Chewapreecha C, Harris SR, Croucher NJ, Turner C, Marttinen P, Cheng L, et al. Dense genomic sampling identifies highways of pneumococcal recombination. Nat Genet. 2014;46:305–9. PMID:24509479, http://dx.doi.org/10.1038/ng.2895.
39. Marsh R, Smith-Vaughan H, Hare KM, Binks M, Kong F, Warning J, et al. The nonserotypeable pneumococcus: phenotypic dynamics in the era of anticapsular vaccines. J Clin Microbiol. 2010;48:831–5. PMID:20042626, http://dx.doi.org/10.1128/JCM.01701-09.
40. Hoskins A, Collins D, Senasinghe K, Bowman J, Stemberger NA, Jones J, et al. Pneumococcal carriage rates remain high in Western Australian Aboriginal people: 12 years and two vaccines later. Pneumonia. 2014;3:290 [Abstract ISPPD - 0352].
41. Mahjoub-Messai F, Doit C, Koeck J-L, Billard T, Evrard B, Bidet P, et al. Population snapshot of *Streptococcus pneumoniae* serotype 19A isolates before and after introduction of Seven-Valent Pneumococcal Vaccination for French children. J Clin Microbiol. 2009;47(3):837–40.
42. Huebner RE, Dagan R, Porath N, Wasas AD, Klugman KP. Lack of utility of serotyping multiple colonies for detection of simultaneous nasopharyngeal carriage of different pneumococcal serotypes. Pediatr Infect Dis J. 2000; 19:1017–20. PMID:11055610, http://dx.doi.org/10.1097/00006454-200010000-00019.
43. Satzke C, Dunne EM, Porter BD, Klugman KP, Mulholland EK. PneuCarriage project group The PneuCarriage Project: a multi-centre comparative study to identify the best serotyping methods for examining pneumococcal carriage in vaccine evaluation studies. PLoS Med. 2015;12, e1001903. PMID: 26575033, http://dx.doi.org/10.1371/journal.pmed.1001903.
44. Williams SR, Mernagh PJ, Lee MH, Tan JT. Changing epidemiology of invasive pneumococcal disease in Australian children after introduction of a 7-valent pneumococcal conjugate vaccine. Med J Aust. 2011;194:116–20. PMID:21299484.
45. de Kluyver R, Enhanced Invasive Pneumococcal Disease Surveillance Working Group. Invasive pneumococcal disease surveillance Australia, 1 January to 31 March 2015. Commun Dis Intell Q Rep. 2015;39(2):E308–11.
46. Moore HC, Lehmann D, de Klerk N, Jacoby P, Richmond PC. Reduction in disparity for pneumonia hospitalisations between Australian indigenous and non-Indigenous children. J Epidemiol Community Health. 2012;66:489–94. PMID:21258115, http://dx.doi.org/10.1136/jech.2010.122762.

2

Necrotizing pneumonia: an emerging problem in children?

I. Brent Masters[1], Alan F. Isles[1] and Keith Grimwood[2,3]*

Abstract

Background: In children, necrotizing pneumonia (NP) is an uncommon, severe complication of pneumonia. It is characterized by destruction of the underlying lung parenchyma resulting in multiple small, thin-walled cavities and is often accompanied by empyema and bronchopleural fistulae.

Review: NP in children was first reported in children in 1994, and since then there has been a gradual increase in cases, which is partially explained by greater physician awareness and use of contrast computed tomography (CT) scans, and by temporal changes in circulating respiratory pathogens and antibiotic prescribing. The most common pathogens detected in children with NP are pneumococci and *Staphylococcus aureus*. The underlying disease mechanisms are poorly understood, but likely relate to multiple host susceptibility and bacterial virulence factors, with viral–bacterial interactions also possibly having a role. Most cases are in previously healthy young children who, despite adequate antibiotic therapy for bacterial pneumonia, remain febrile and unwell. Many also have evidence of pleural effusion, empyema, or pyopneumothorax, which has undergone drainage or surgical intervention without clinical improvement. The diagnosis is generally made by chest imaging, with CT scans being the most sensitive, showing loss of normal pulmonary architecture, decreased parenchymal enhancement and multiple thin-walled cavities. Blood culture and culture and molecular testing of pleural fluid provide a microbiologic diagnosis in as many as 50% of cases. Prolonged antibiotics, draining pleural fluid and gas that causes mass effects, and maintaining ventilation, circulation, nutrition, fluid, and electrolyte balance are critical components of therapy. Despite its serious nature, death is uncommon, with good clinical, radiographic and functional recovery achieved in the 5–6 months following diagnosis. Increased knowledge of NP's pathogenesis will assist more rapid diagnosis and improve treatment and, ultimately, prevention.

Conclusion: It is important to consider that our understanding of NP is limited to individual case reports or small case series, and treatment data from randomized-controlled trials are lacking. Furthermore, case series are retrospective and usually confined to single centers. Consequently, these studies may not be representative of patients in other locations, especially when allowing for temporal changes in pathogen behaviour and differences in immunization schedules and antibiotic prescribing practices.

Keywords: Necrotizing pneumonia, Child, *Streptococcus Pneumoniae*, *Staphylococcus aureus*, Panton-Valentine leukocidin, Empyema, Bronchopleural fistulae

* Correspondence: k.grimwood@griffith.edu.au
[2]School of Medicine and Menzies Health Institute Queensland, Gold Coast campus, Griffith University, Building G40, Southport Gold Coast, QLD, Australia
[3]Departments of Infectious Diseases and Paediatrics, Gold Coast Health, Southport Gold Coast, QLD, Australia
Full list of author information is available at the end of the article

Background

Necrotizing pneumonia (NP) is an uncommon, but severe complication of pneumonia. It is characterized by progressive pneumonic illness in a previously healthy child despite appropriate antibiotic therapy, and runs a protracted clinical course [1]. The diagnosis is made by chest imaging studies showing one or more small thin-walled cavities within areas of pulmonary consolidation. Pathological examinations from autopsies or resected lung specimens reveal pulmonary inflammation, alveolar consolidation and thrombosis of intrapulmonary vessels with accompanying necrosis and multiple small cavities [1, 2]. It is speculated that reduced blood flow from thrombosed vessels decreases antibiotic concentrations within the affected lung tissue, leading to persistent infection and further destruction of pulmonary tissue. NP lies on a spectrum between pulmonary abscess and pulmonary gangrene, and is accompanied frequently by empyema and bronchopleural fistulae (BPF) [2].

First reported in adults with severe pneumonia in the 1940s, NP was not described in children until 1994 when a small case series of four patients was published [3]. Since then, descriptions of NP have included individual case reports [4–12] and small retrospective series of 2–18 cases [13–27] with few publications involving larger numbers of affected children. Although still regarded as uncommon, the incidence of NP (as with other more common forms of complicated pneumonia, parapneumonic effusion [PPE] and empyema) may be increasing [18, 22, 28–32]. NP may be complicating 0.8–7% of all cases of community-acquired pneumonia (CAP) [29, 30, 33–35] and up to 20% of those with empyema admitted to tertiary pediatric hospitals [18]. Therefore, it is timely to review NP in children. To do so, the authors searched PubMed for articles published in English up to and including 31 January 2017. The search terms were 'necrotizing pneumonia' and 'children' in combination, in titles and abstracts, and the search was focused upon larger case series and publications from the last decade. The reference lists of articles identified by this search strategy were also searched and relevant articles retrieved. The search found eight retrospective reviews of 'all cause' NP involving 20–80 childhood cases [28, 30, 31, 33, 35–38]. In each of these, the diagnosis of NP was confirmed in one of three ways: radiographically, requiring solitary or multiple thin-walled cavities within areas of consolidation, while specifically excluding thick-walled, fluid or air-filled cavities with well-defined enhancing rims identifying pulmonary abscesses [28, 30, 31, 33, 36, 37]; by direct observation of lung necrosis during thoracoscopy [38]; or by inference from the report [35]. Similarly, another six retrospective reports describing NP in 10–57 children with proven *Streptococcus pneumoniae* (pneumococcal) necrotizing pneumonia (PNP) were identified where there was limited evidence of overlapping cases from the same institution and sufficient information on the radiographic criteria to differentiate these cases from those with empyema alone [25, 29, 32, 34, 39, 40]. However, two of these case series [29, 34] included abscess within their definition of NP. These 14 studies are summarized in Tables 1 and 2 and form the basis of our review.

Epidemiology

While the incidence of hospitalized childhood pneumonia has declined in countries that have introduced pneumococcal conjugate vaccines (PCVs) [41–43], population rates of complicated pneumonia have increased during the last two decades. Although still relatively uncommon and occurring in <1% of children with CAP [44], the incidence of 'all-cause' empyema has increased in the United States (US) [45], and in children aged 2–4 years it rose from 3.7 cases per 100,000 in 1996–1998 to 10.3 cases per 100,000 in 2005–2007 [46], with both pneumococci and *Staphylococcus aureus* the most common pathogens detected. In Utah, the incidence of pediatric pneumococcal empyema increased from 1 per 100,000 in 1993, to 5 per 100,000 in 1999, immediately prior to introducing the 7-valent PCV, before reaching 12.5 per 100,000 in 2007. This increase was due almost exclusively to non-vaccine serotypes [47]. Significant increases in complicated pneumonia have also been reported from the United Kingdom (UK) [48], Europe [49], Australia [44], and Israel [32], although for the latter study only the increase in NP cases was statistically significant, increasing from <0.5 per 100,000 in 2001–2003 to almost 2 per 100,000 in 2009–2010.

Single tertiary pediatric centers have also reported temporal increases in pediatric NP case numbers [18, 22, 28–32]. A French study found that NP contributed to 0.8% of all CAP cases and to 6% of those hospitalized with CAP aged <16 years, with rates of NP complicating hospitalized CAP doubling from 4.5% to 9% between 2006 and 2009 and 2009–2011, respectively [30]. Studies from the UK [18, 22] and the US [28] have reported similar increases in NP cases from the 1990s and into the first decade of this century. Reports of increasing NP rates among children with culture-confirmed (blood, pleural fluid, lung tissue or bronchoalveolar lavage fluid) pneumococcal pneumonia also appeared from centers in Utah [29] and Taiwan [32], where the proportions of children with NP rose from 13% in 1997–2000 to 33% in 2001–2006, and from 45% in 2001 to 81% in 2009, respectively. Reasons for this changing epidemiology are complex, but likely reflect heightened awareness as well as temporal changes in organism and antibiotic prescribing patterns [50].

Cases of NP in children occur globally and have been reported from North America [4, 7, 9, 10, 19, 20, 26, 28, 29],

Table 1 Retrospective studies in children with necrotizing pneumonia and where participant numbers exceeded 20 subjects

Study	Subjects	Causes	Imaging results	WBC count and inflammatory markers	Management	Course	Comments
Wong et al. [36] Taiwan. Single tertiary center. Almost 5 yr. review July 1995–March 1999.	No. = 21 12 (57%) males. Mean (SD) age = 2.4 (1.3) yrs. No co-morbidities.	Pathogen detected in 9 (43%) cases. Blood culture +ve in 2 (9.5%) cases - *S. pneumoniae* 2 Hib 1 Pleural culture +ve in 5 (24%) cases - *S. pneumoniae* 2 *S. aureus* 2 Hib 1 Four-fold increase in *M. pneumoniae* serum antibody titres and negative bacterial cultures $n = 2$ (9.5%).	All had CT scans confirming NP diagnosis. PPE 20 (95%) - 6 (30%) loculated empyema BPF 8 (38%) Abscess 4 (19%).	NR.	Antibiotics and chest tube drainage only 9 (43%). Thoracoscopy (VATS) 10 (48%) - pulmonary segmental resection 2. Antibiotics alone 2 (9.5%).	Medically treated: - mean (SD) fever duration before hospitalization 6.8 (3.3) days - mean (SD) total fever duration 9.5 (3.5) days - mean (SD) hospital LOS 21.7 (5.5) days Plus surgery: - mean (SD) fever duration before hospitalization 14.9 (9.6) days - mean (SD) total fever duration 16.5 (8.5) days - mean (SD) hospital LOS 30.0 (8.0) days $*P < 0.05$.	Fever (95%), cough (52%) and respiratory distress (43%) were the most common presenting symptoms. The 10 children undergoing VATS had more severe disease than those medically treated and had failed conservative treatment. At 6 mths, 19/21 (90%) had normal chest radiographs, 2 had small residual pneumatoceles.
Hacimustafaoglu et al. [37] Turkey. Single tertiary center. 4 yr. review of prospective collected data.	No. = 36. Mean (SD) age = 3.8 (3.3) yrs. (Range 9 mths-14 yrs). No co-morbidities.	Pleural fluid *S. pyogenes* 1 *S. pneumoniae* 3. All had received antibiotics before admission to hospital.	CT scans required for diagnosing NP. Lungs involved - right 20 (55%) left 12 (33%) both 4 (11%). PPE 34 (94%) - septated 80% loculated 33% BPF 20 (55%).	Mean (SD) peripheral WBC count = 19.3 (8.7) × 10^9/L. Mean (SD) CRP = 136 (117) mg/L. Pleural fluid (mean (SD)) -glucose 1.3 (1.2) mmol/L. LDH 793 (682) IU/L.	Thoracotomy 24 (67%)	Mean (SD) symptom duration before presentation = 11.9 (8.5) days. Mean (SD) febrile days = 8.9 (4.3) after hospitalization. Mean (SD) hospital LOS = 26 (9) days. Mortality rate 5.5%.	Diagnosis of NP by CT scan made on average 6 days after admission and 17 days after symptom onset.
Sawicki et al. [28] United States. Single tertiary center. 15 yr. review January 1990–February 2005.	No. = 80. 45 (53%) males. Median (IQR) age = 3.6 (2.4–6.2) yrs. Most were healthy - 14 asthma 1 CNLD 1 cerebral palsy 2 PID. Cases increased from 3 per yr. in 1990–93 to 14 per yr. in 2003–4.	Pathogen detected, in 38 cases (48%), 19 from testing pleural fluid in 50 cases. *S. pneumoniae* 18 (13 by culture) MSSA 5 MRSA 3 *Fusobacterium* 1 *P. aeruginosa* 1 CONS 4 *S. anginosus* 6 group. 54 (68%) had received antibiotics before admission to hospital.	CT scans required for diagnosing NP. -PPE 69 (86%) -BPF 10 (13%).	Mean (SD) peripheral WBC count = 18.4 (8.9) × 10^9/L. Mean (SD) CRP = 133 (93) mg/L. Mean (SD) haemoglobin = 10.4 (1.6) g/L. Mean (SD) serum albumen = 20 (16) g/L. Pleural fluid (mean (SD) or median (IQR)) - pH 7.08 (0.33) -glucose 0.5 (0.1–3.6) mmol/L -LDH 2810 (1413–9530) IU/L -Cell count 9.6 (1.2–56) × 10^6/L -Pleural neutrophils 70 (23)%.	Procedures for PPE – 69 (86%). Chest tube drainage only 47 (68%). Chest drainage + surgery 16 (23%). Thoracentesis only 6 (9%).	Intensive care 25 (31%); 1 ECMO. Median (IQR) pleural drainage days = 6 (4.5–9.5). Median (IQR) febrile days = 6 (3–9). Median (IQR) hospital LOS = 12 (9–17) days. Median (IQR) antibiotic days = 28 (20–40). No deaths.	Fever (96%) and cough (84%) were main symptoms, at a mean onset of 9 days before presentation. 8 (10%) readmitted within 2wks of being discharged; 64 seen 6mths post discharge, all well, 12 had PFTS, 3 had mild obstructive and 1 mild restrictive defects. CXR and CT scans markedly improved and near normal at 6 mths.

Table 1 Retrospective studies in children with necrotizing pneumonia and where participant numbers exceeded 20 subjects *(Continued)*

Macedo et al. [38] Brazil. Single tertiary center. 6 yr. review July 2002–June 2008.	No. = 24. 12 (50%) males. Median age 2 yrs. (Range 1–9 yrs).	Pleural fluid culture -*S. pneumoniae* 6 -MSSA 3 -*P. aeruginosa* 1.	CXR, CT and US performed. PPE 24 (100%) PTX 11 (46%) BPF 16 (67%).	NR.	All underwent thoracoscopy. Prior chest drainage had been undertaken in 19 (79%) of the children.	Median chest drainage time = 18 days (Range 1–30 days). Median hospital LOS = 19 days. 7–49 days). No deaths reported.	Subjects were children undergoing thoracoscopy for a loculated empyema and/or PTX and in whom a diagnosis of NP was made when a cavity containing necrotic debris was found in the lung tissue. None underwent a thoracotomy.
Jester et al. [35] UK. Single tertiary center. 10 yr. review January 2000–May 2010.	No. = 20. 13 (65%) males. Median age 2.5 yrs. (Range 0.8–6.8 yrs). All were referred because of BPF complicating empyema.	Pleural fluid culture or PCR *S. pneumoniae* 10 (serotype 3, $n = 3$) *S. aureus* 1 All had received antibiotics for a median duration of 7 days (Range 2–13) prior to referral	All had pre-operative CT scans. Lobes involved - right - lower 10 (50%) upper 4 (20%) - left - lower 3 (15%) upper 3 (15%). BPF was found on presentation in 11 (55%), in 4 (20%) during thoracoscopy, and in 5 (25%) post-operatively.	NR.	All had a serratus anterior muscle digitation flap inserted.	Median post-operative fever was 2 days (Range 1–3 days). Median duration of chest tube drainage post-operatively was 7 days (Range 5–15 days). Median hospital LOS = 9 days (Range 7–28 days). No deaths reported.	All were referred because of persistent signs of empyema with clinical deterioration and diagnosis of NP complicated by BPF. The median follow-up was 4 yrs. (Range 2 mths-10 yrs). All had normal thoracic volumes on CXR without signs of scoliosis.
Lemaitre et al. [30] France. Single tertiary center. 5 yr. review May 2006–April 2011.	No. = 41. 22 (54%) males. Median age 1.2 yrs. (Range 1 mth- 16 yrs). 1 child had sickle cell anemia. The rate of NP complicating CAP doubled from 4.5% in 2006–2009 to 9% in 2009–2011.	Blood/pleural/BAL fluid cultures +ve in 21 (51%) cases. - MSSA 12 - MRSA 1 (All *S. aureus* strains PVL + ve) -*S. pneumoniae* 7 (serotypes 3, 7F, 19A) -*F. nucleatum* 1 (14 yr. old with sickle cell anemia). 18 (44%) had received antibiotics before hospital admission.	CXR and CT scans performed. CXR revealed necrosis on admission in 11 (27%) cases. CT scan performed on 23 (56%) children and detected NP in 12 not apparent on CXR. PPE 26 (63%) PTX 8 (20%)	Median peripheral WBC count = 20,000 × 10^6/L (Range 1700–44,300). Median CRP = 141 mg/L (Range 5–434).	Procedures for PPE – 26 (63%). - Thoracentesis 10-VATS 6	Median symptoms before presentation = 4 days (Range 1–10 days). Nursed in intensive care 7 (17%). Median febrile days in hospital = 7 days (Range 1–25 days). Median hospital LOS = 16 days (Range 7–43 days). Median antibiotic days = 42 days (Range 31–60 days). No deaths.	NP diagnosis made by a combination of clinical signs of lung infection and radiographic signs of NP with multiple thin-walled cavities within a region of homogenous alveolar consolidation. The *S. pneumoniae* serotypes identified in this series are not included in PCV7 available in France at the time of the study.
Krenke et al. [33] Poland. Single tertiary center. 5 yr. review April 2008–July 2013.	No. = 32. 14 (44%) males. Median age 4 yrs. (Range 1–10 yrs). Most were healthy - 2 asthma 1 obesity and hypertension 1 atrial septal defect.	Blood cultures +ve in 6 (19%) cases. Pleural fluid cultures +ve in 7 (23%) children. - *S. pneumoniae* 8 - MSSA 2 -*S. milleri* 1- CONS 1 -*S. maltophilia* 1. All had received antibiotics before admission to hospital.	CXR ± CT scans performed. Lungs involved - right 18 (56%) left 10 (31%) both 4 (13%). PPE 31 (97%) PTX 2 (6%) BPF 8 (25%).	Median (IQR) peripheral WBC count = 21.3 (15.2–24.1) × 10^9/L. Median (IQR) CRP = 182 (152–241) mg/L. Median (IQR) haemoglobin = 8.9 (8.4–9.9) g/L. Median (IQR) serum albumen = 25 (23.5–27.5) g/L. Pleural fluid (median (IQR)) - pH 7.3 (7.0–7.5) glucose 2.8 (1.8–3.1) mmol/L -LDH 8670 (2828–14,254) IU/L.	Procedures for PPE – 31 (97%). Thoracentesis only 2 (6%). Chest tube drainage 28 (90%), including urokinase in 25 (81%). VATS 1 (3%).	Median febrile days before presentation = 6 days (Range 1–10 days). Median febrile days in hospital = 9 days (Range 0–22 days). Median (IQR) chest drainage time = 8.6 (6–11.25) days. Median hospital LOS = 26 days (Range 13–44 days). Median (IQR) antibiotic days = 28 (22.5–32.5) days. No deaths.	Rate of NP amongst all CAP admissions was 32/882 (3.6%). Fever (94%), tachypnea (90%) and cough (77%) most common symptoms. 5 mths later all children had normal physical exams and CXRs showed complete or almost complete resolution of pleural and lung abnormalities.

Table 1 Retrospective studies in children with necrotizing pneumonia and where participant numbers exceeded 20 subjects *(Continued)*

Erlichman et al. [31] Israel. Three tertiary centers. 10 yr. review 2001–2010.	No. = 29. 19 (66%) males. Median age 3.1 yrs. Case rates increased from <0.5/100,000 in 2001–2003 to ~2/100,000 in 2009–2010.	Blood cultures +ve in 3/29 (10%) cases - *S. pneumoniae* 3. Pleural fluid cultures +ve in 9/26 (35%) cases - *S. pneumoniae* 8- *S. pyogenes* 1. All *S. pneumoniae* isolates typed were serotype 5. 17 (59%) had received antibiotics before admission to hospital.	CXR ± CT scans performed.	Median peripheral WBC Count = 14.7 × 10^9/L.	Chest tube drainage 21 (72%), including urokinase in 6 (21%). VATS 1 (3%).	Median febrile days before presentation = 5 days. Median febrile days in hospital = 6 days. Median chest drainage time = 7 days. Median hospital LOS = 14 days. Median (IQR) antibiotic days = 13 (7) days. No deaths.	NP diagnosed by multiple thin-walled cavities within lung consolidation on CXR or lung tissue liquefaction on CT scan. Jewish ethnicity over-represented by 25 (86%) cases.

BAL bronchoalveolar lavage, *BPF* bronchopleural fistula, *CAP* community-acquired pneumonia, *CNLD* chronic neonatal lung disease, *CONS* coagulase negative staphylococcus, *CRP* c-reactive protein, *CT* computed tomography, *CXR* chest xray, *ECMO* extracorporeal membrane oxygenation, *Hib Haemophilus influenzae* type b, *IQR* interquartile range, *IU* international units, *LDH* lactate dehydrogenase, *LOS* length of stay, *mmol* millimoles, *MRSA* methicillin-resistant *Staphylococcus aureus*, *MSSA* methicillin-resistant *Staphylococcus* aureus, *No* number, *NP* necrotizing pneumonia, *NR* not reported, *PCV7* 7-valent pneumococcal conjugate vaccine, *PID* primary immunodeficiency (1 had Schwachman-Diamond syndrome, 1 chronic granulomatous disease), *PFT* pulmonary function tests, *PPE* parapneumonic empyema, *PTX* pneumothorax, *PVL* Panton-Valentine leucocidin, *SD* standard deviation, *US* ultrasound, *VATS* video-assisted thoracoscopy, *WBC* white blood cell

Table 2 Retrospective studies in children with necrotizing pneumonia secondary to *Streptococcus pneumoniae* infection

Study	Subjects	*S. pneumoniae* serotypes	Imaging results	Management	Course	Comments
Hsieh et al. [39] Taiwan. Single tertiary center. 5 yr. review May 1998–July 2003.	No. = 15. 2 (13%) males. Median age 49 mths (Range 9–85 mths).	10 isolates available for serotyping. Serotype 14 (50%) 3 (30%) 6A (10%) 18C (10%). 11 isolates available for penicillin MICs. 7 (64%) had non-penicillin (MIC ≥1 mg/L) susceptibility.	CXR + CT scans performed. Lungs involved - right 10 (67%) left 5 (33%) multi-lobar 5 (33%). PPE 14 (93%) PTX 1 (7%)	Procedures for PPE 14 (93%). Chest tube drainage only 6 (43%). VATS 8 (57%).	Median febrile days before presentation = 4 days (Range 2–11 days). Median febrile days in hospital = 9 days (Range 4–30 days). Median hospital LOS = 18 days (Range 5–40 days). Mean (SD) antibiotic days for 14 survivors = 24 (8) days (Range 12–38 days). 1 died from HUS and pulmonary gangrene.	Diagnosis of NP made on a median of 6 days (range 1–12) after admission. 13 (87%) received cefotaxime or ceftriaxone 10 (67%) received vancomycin 7 (47%) received both vancomycin and a cephalosporin together as directed therapy.
Fretzayas et al. [40] Greece. Single tertiary center. 6 yr. review January 1999–December 2004.	No. = 10. 5 (50%) males. Mean age 3.1 yrs. Representing 1.3% of all cases of lobar pneumonia in children aged <14 yrs. and 20% of bacteraemic pneumonia cases.	All had +ve blood cultures, 5/7 pleural fluid cultures were also +ve. Serotyping NR.	All had CXR evidence of NP, which was then confirmed by chest CT scans. Epyema present in 7 patients. Chest US aided diagnosis in all 8 cases where it was used.	Empyema drained by thoracentesis or by indwelling continuous intercostal tube drainage. None underwent thoracotomy.	Toxic appearance, persistent fever and abnormal chest findings were seen for a mean 23 days. Hospital LOS 15–35 days. 4 patients examined 1 yr. later had normal spirometry.	NP should be considered in those with continuation of fever, persistently raised or increasing blood inflammatory indices and abnormal auscultatory findings for >5-days, despite antibiotics and especially if bacteremia and empyema are present.
Bender et al. [29] United States. Single tertiary center. 9 yr. review January 1997–March 2006.	No. = 33. 18 (55%) males. Mean age 40 mths. Co-morbidities 2 (6%). Cases increased over time: 5/39 (13%) confirmed PNP cases in 1997–2000 vs 28/85 (33%) in 2001–2006 (OR 3.34, 95%CI 1.11–12).	Blood and pleural fluid isolates. 28/33 (85%) were non-PCV7 vaccine serotypes - 2/5 (40%) 1997–2000- 27/28 (96%) 2001–06. Commonest serotypes - serotype 3 11 (33%) 19 4 (12%) 19A 4 (12%) 1 3 (9%). All penicillin susceptible.	CXR or CT scans performed. PPE 32 (97%).	Procedures for PPE 32 (93%). Chest tube drainage only 19 (59%). Chest tube + surgery 11 (34%).	Nursed in intensive care 18 (55%). Mean hospital LOS = 14 days. 1 (3%) death	May have included a small number of cases with lung abscess. Serotype 3 was most often associated with NP with 11/14 (79%) children with culture-confirmed pneumonia developing cavities. Compared with other serotypes, serotype 3 was more likely to be associated with PNP (OR = 14.7, 95% CI 3.4–86).
Hsieh et al. [32] Taiwan. Single tertiary center. 9 yr. review January 2001–March 2010.	No. = 50. 18 had BPF - 4 (22%) males - mean (SD) age 3.5 (2.7) yrs. co-morbidity 1 (6%) PCV7 available in Taiwan since 2005, but coverage <16% by 2009. None of the PNP cases had received PCV7. Proportions of cases increased between 2004 and 2009.	Blood and pleural fluid isolates (*n* = 50). Commonest serotypes - serotype 14 19 (38%) 19A 10 (20%) 3 7 (14%) 6B 8 (16%). Commonest STs - ST46 7/19 (37%) serotype 14 isolates CC320 (ST320, ST3164) 10/10 (100%) serotype 19A isolates. 6/18 (33%) with BPF had non-penicillin susceptibility and 3/18 (17%) had ceftriaxone. non-susceptibility	CXR or CT scan. Of 18 children with BPF, all had PPE. Bilateral lung involvement 10 (56%).	Procedures for BPF 18 children subset. 9 developed BPF after removal of chest drains. Chest tube + surgery 15 (83%), pulmonary resection in 12. None received fibrinolytics.	18 children with BPF. Median febrile days before presentation = 7 days (Range 4–14 days). Median day of BPF diagnosis = 10 days (Range 1–21 days). Nursed in intensive care 9 (50%). Median febrile days in hospital = 13 days (Range 1–34) days. Median hospital LOS = 32 days (Range 11–62 days). None died.	Study focused upon 18 children with BPF, a more critically ill subset. 6 (33%) had HUS. Multivariate analysis found acute respiratory failure (OR = 8.9, 95%CI 2.6–31) and serotype 19A (OR = 5.0, 95%CI 1.2–22) were independent risk factors for BPF. 11/12 resected lung segments had coagulative necrosis with pulmonary infarction.

Table 2 Retrospective studies in children with necrotizing pneumonia secondary to *Streptococcus pneumoniae* infection *(Continued)*

Janapatla et al. [25] Taiwan. Single tertiary center. 3 yr. review January 2006–December 2009 Two subsets: a. PNP b. PNP + HUS.	No = 12 PNP. 5 (42%) males. Mean (SD) age = 4.6 (2.4) yrs. (Range 1–8 yrs). PCV7 available in Taiwan since 2005, but coverage <16% by 2009. No. = 17 with PNP + HUS (+ 1 other had empyema). 4 (23%) males. Mean (SD) age = 5.3 (2.8) yrs. (Range 2–10 yrs).	Blood and pleural fluid isolates (n = 12). Commonest serotypes - serotype 14 9 (75%) 3 1 (8%) 19A 2 (17%) Commonest STs - ST876 and ST46 in 7/9 (78%) serotype 14 isolates. *S. pneumoniae* isolated from blood (n = 16) and pleural fluid (n = 2). Commonest serotypes - serotype 14 9 (50%) 3 5 (28%) 19F 2 (11%). Commonest STs - ST46 in 5/9 (56%) serotype 14 isolates ST 180 in 5/5 (100%) serotype 3 isolates.	All cases of NP confirmed by CT scan. Results NR. CXR or CT scan Results NR.	Chest tube + surgery, either VATS or lobectomy, for 10 (83%) children. Chest tube alone 2 (11%) children, including the 1 child with empyema alone Chest tube + surgery, either VATS or lobectomy, for 16 (89%) children	Mean (SD) hospital LOS = 26.2 (9.0) days (Range 16–39 days). Deaths, NR. Mean (SD) hospital LOS = 31.4 (9.0) days (Range 11–65 days). Deaths, NR.	The main focus of this study was on PNP with HUS rather than PNP alone. The 12 children with PNP and 42 with IPD without NP served as controls. 5/18 cases of PNP + HUS had serotype 3 isolates compared with 4/54 IPD + PNP only cases (RR = 3.75, 95%CI 1.1, 12.7). 16/18 HUS isolates carried the *nanC* gene compared with 22/54 control isolates (RR = 2.18, 95%CI 1.52–3.13). As 16/17 children with HUS had PNP, NanC could be a virulence factor for NP too.
Hsieh et al. [34] Taiwan. Six tertiary centers. 2 yr. review March 2010–April 2012.	No. = 57 with PNP. 26 (46%) males. Mean (SD) age: a. Mild necrosis (n = 13) 45.4 (16) mths b. Cavitation (n = 27) 49.6 (15.7) mths c. BPF (n = 17) 39.4 (16.1) mths. No co-morbidities.	Blood and pleural fluid positive testing by culture or PCR. Commonest serotypes in pleural fluid: Serotype - 19A (69%)- 3 (12.5%). 12 (21%) had respiratory viruses detected by PCR.	CXR or CT scan. Mild necrosis (non-enhanced areas on contrast CT scans) (n = 13; 23%). Cavitation (including pneumatoceles and abscess) (n = 27; 47%). BPF (n = 17; 30%).	NR.	Mean (SD) duration of fever and hospital LOS- Mild necrosis: 11.4 (6) and 15.2 (4.5) days; Cavitation: 13.9 (6.5) and 18.3 (6.4) days; BPF: 17.8 (7.6) and 32.8 (16.8) days. No deaths.	Pleural fluid pneumococcal load was significantly higher for serotypes 19A and 3 than other serotypes. Severity of necrosis was associated with pleural fluid pneumococcal load and IL-8 levels.

BPF bronchopleural fistula, *CC* clonal complex *CI* confidence interval, *CT* computed tomography, *CXR* chest xray, *HUS* haemolytic uremic syndrome, *IL* interleukin, *IPD* invasive pneumococcal disease, *LOS* length of stay, *MIC* minimum inhibitory concentration, *No* number, *NP* necrotizing pneumonia, *NR* not reported, *OR* odds ratio, *PCR* polymerase chain reaction, *PCV7* 7-valent pneumococcal conjugate vaccine, *PNP* pneumococcal necrotizing pneumonia, *PPE* parapneumonic empyema, *PTX* pneumothorax, *RR* risk ratio, *SD* standard deviation, *ST* sequence type, *US* ultrasound, *VATS* video-assisted thoracoscopy

Latin America [26, 38], UK [22, 35], Europe [5, 6, 14, 16, 30, 33, 40], Middle East [3, 12, 27, 31, 37], Asia [8, 11, 17, 21, 24, 25, 32, 36, 39], and Australia [23]. Tables 1 and 2 show that the typical child with either NP or PNP is aged between 2 and 5 years and, except for studies from Taiwan [32, 39], is equally likely to be male or female. Surprisingly, few children have underlying co-morbidities, with asthma the most common chronic disorder identified. While both retrospective [51, 52] and prospective [53–55] studies have identified risk factors associated with complicated pneumonia, only one included cases identified as NP [55]. In this particular study, just 6 of 203 (3%) hospitalized children with CAP had this complication and when analyzing for risk factors they were combined with 52 other children with empyema and another four with lung abscesses. Consequently, in contrast with CAP, it is not possible currently to clearly identify risk factors specifically associated with NP, although some may be biologically plausible. Whenever evaluated, pre-admission ibuprofen was identified as a significant independent risk factor associated with complicated pneumonia, even after adjusting for potential confounding from age, sex, and symptom duration, although confounding by indication could not be excluded [51, 52, 55]. As receiving non-steroidal anti-inflammatory agents might mask both pain and fever, it has been proposed that this might lead to delayed presentation and treatment rather than these agents impairing the child's immune response to infection, as suggested by other experts [55, 56].

Microbiology

The most common pathogens associated with NP in children are pneumococci and *S. aureus.* Of the 197 bacterial and fungal pathogens detected in single case reports and case series cited in this review [3, 6–8, 11, 13, 14, 16–24, 26–28, 30, 31, 33, 35–38], 116 (59%) were pneumococci and 45 (23%) were *S. aureus*, including 15 methicillin-resistant *S. aureus* (MRSA) strains. In addition, there were other pediatric cases series restricted to either PNP (n = 194 isolates; see Table 2) or *S. aureus* (n = 16 isolates) alone [15].

Pneumococci possess multiple virulence factors [57], including its polysaccharide capsule, cell surface proteins, the cell wall, and pneumolysin, a pore-forming toxin [58]. Of these, the most important is the polysaccharide capsule, of which there are at least 98 different serotypes, each capable of shielding the organism from the immune system [59]. Individual serotypes vary in their capacity to colonize, cause local or invasive disease, and express antibiotic resistance genes [57, 60]. Serotypes also vary geographically and change over time, perhaps in response to local ecological competitive pressures from other organisms co-habiting the nasopharyngeal space, as well as selection pressures from antibiotics and PCVs [61]. Indeed, most pneumococcal serotypes associated with PNP (Tables 1 and 2) were not included in the 7-valent PCV, notably serotypes 3, 5, 7F, and 19A, reflecting possible temporal shifts in circulating serotypes and/or vaccine-induced strain replacement disease. Of these, serotypes 3 and 19A were most closely associated with PNP. Serotype 3 has a very thick capsule, which strongly resists opsonophagocytosis and induces a marked inflammatory response, including an intense neutrophilic infiltration with suppurative necrosis [1, 62]. In contrast, serotype 19A strains have greater invasive potential, may have a growth advantage over other pneumococcal serotypes in normally sterile sites, and are often resistant to multiple antibiotics [34, 63].

S. aureus also has many virulence factors that help it to instigate colonization, evade host-immune responses, cause tissue injury, and disseminate to other organs. In establishing infection, *S. aureus* expresses surface proteins that mediate adherence and impair local defences, while later in the infection secreted exotoxins disrupt epithelial barriers and immune cell function responses, thereby facilitating tissue invasion [64]. Although it has long been recognized as an important cause of NP, interest in this pathogen was renewed by recent studies linking strains expressing the virulence factor, Panton-Valentine leukocidin (PVL), with severe forms of this disease in previously healthy children and adults [8, 15, 23, 30, 65]. In many cases these PVL-producing isolates were also MRSA strains. PVL is a pore-forming exotoxin, which activates and then destroys immune cells, such as neutrophils, potentially releasing damaging proteases into the surrounding tissues [66]. Of concern, a multi-center French study [65] involving 50 cases of NP caused by PVL-producing strains of *S. aureus* in children and adults aged 1 month to 78 years reported a 56% case fatality rate. Factors associated with mortality were hemoptysis, erythematous rash within 24 h of admission, and peripheral blood leukopenia $<3.0 \times 10^6$/L. However, this was a non-comparative study and it is therefore difficult to infer whether PVL contributed to pathogenicity. Indeed, whether PVL itself is responsible for the pathological changes seen in NP is controversial. In part, this is because PVL has a strong cell and species specificity, behaving differently in various cell culture and experimental models. For example, neutrophils from humans and rabbits are very sensitive to the effects of PVL in vitro, while those from monkeys and mice are highly resistant [67]. Moreover, while a systematic review and meta-analysis found a strong association between PVL-producing strains of *S. aureus* and skin and soft tissue infections, no such association was seen for invasive infections, including pneumonia [68]. However, this review was limited by including only one small study in children from China, which compared cases of MRSA CAP where there were no significant differences in proportions of PVL-positive (3/22) and -negative (3/33) strains progressing to NP, respectively [21]. Similarly, linking NP with MRSA is also contentious. Many of the observational studies reporting an association between invasive disease and MRSA are from the US, where the PVL-producing USA300 MRSA clone predominates, while in Europe, Australasia, and elsewhere, there are many different MRSA strains in circulation [69]. Furthermore, a recent case-control study of 133 French children and adults with PVL-positive strains of *S. aureus* NP found no evidence for increased clinical severity in those with MRSA infections [70]. Consequently, there are substantial gaps in our knowledge concerning the pathogenesis of *S. aureus* NP and it is likely other cytotoxins play an important role. Indeed, attention has been focused recently on other pore-forming toxins including alpha-hemolysin (or α-toxin), with its proposed mechanisms of action including activating the NLRP3 inflammasome, resulting in severe alveolar necrosis, and inducing platelet-neutrophil aggregation, which leads to further tissue destruction [71].

In addition to pneumococci and *S. aureus*, other respiratory bacterial and fungal pathogens reported occasionally in studies included in the present review are *Streptococcus pyogenes* (n = 5); members of the *S. anginosus* group (n = 7); *Haemophilus influenzae* (n = 2); *Pseudomonas aeruginosa* (n = 3); *Stenotrophomonas maltophilia* (n = 1); the anaerobic organism *Fusobacterium nucleatum* (n = 2); *Mycoplasma pneumoniae* (n = 12); *Legionella pneumophila* (n = 1); and *Aspergillus* species (n = 1). Unlike in adults, *Klebsiella pneumoniae* is not a common cause of NP in children, and in contrast with simple pulmonary abscesses, oral anaerobes are reported rarely [1]. However, it should also be acknowledged many case series may not have undertaken anaerobic cultures. Nevertheless, the adult experience is that anaerobes play a minor role [2].

Viruses, even those associated with outbreaks of severe adenovirus pneumonia, are rarely the sole cause of NP [72]. In contrast, the association of respiratory syncytial virus (RSV) and influenza virus infections with increased nasopharyngeal colonization by pneumococci and *S. aureus* and greater risk of secondary bacterial CAP with enhanced severity is well recognized [73–77]. However, few studies of NP in children have collected information on respiratory viruses. This is surprising given the consistent reports of influenza-like illnesses occurring immediately prior to NP caused by PVL-producing strains of *S. aureus* [53, 65]. There are single case reports of NP associated with either RSV or influenza A alone [10, 12], or in association with MRSA [6], or pneumococci [7], while studies systematically testing for respiratory viruses are limited. In one series of 57 children with PNP, 12 (21%) had respiratory viruses (rhinovirus, n = 5; influenza, n = 4; parainfluenza, n = 2; human coronavirus NL63, 1) detected in their upper airways by polymerase chain reaction (PCR) assays [34]. Another small study [25] reported that 6 of 18 children with PNP complicated by the hemolytic uremic syndrome (HUS) had positive viral cultures (influenza, n = 3; and one each of adenovirus plus enterovirus, parainfluenza, and human metapneumovirus). The mechanisms associated with viral–bacterial interactions within the respiratory tract are complex, multi-layered, and incompletely understood. While beyond the scope of this review, viruses can decrease bacterial clearance by disrupting the respiratory epithelial barrier, impairing mucociliary function, increasing bacterial adherence by upregulating adherence proteins, and modulating immune function by interfering with critical components of the innate immune system, downregulating macrophage phagocytosis, decreasing neutrophil intracellular killing, and inducing apoptosis [78, 79]. How such interactions predispose to CAP, including NP, are still unknown, but important to understand when devising public health prevention strategies and seeking to optimize individual patient management.

Pathology

Histopathological findings in autopsy and surgical lung specimens from adults and children with NP are characterized by necrosis of lung parenchyma, which was thought primarily to be a vascular process triggered by infection leading to vasculitis, activation of the coagulation system and thrombotic occlusion of intrapulmonary vessels accompanied by cavity formation [2, 80]. However, in all age groups intense suppuration is also seen; it is postulated that direct cytotoxic effects from bacterial toxins and secondarily induced intense cytokine-mediated inflammatory responses,(including interleukin-8 mediated neutrophil recruitment, activation and release of proteolytic enzymes) also contribute to tissue injury and destruction [1, 32, 34, 37]. The mixture of coagulation and liquefactive lung necrosis leads to one or more thin-walled cavities that can form pneumatoceles from the one-way passage of gas [5], or evolve into pulmonary abscesses [81]. PPE and empyema are also common and if necrotic regions extend to the pleura, BPF may form, resulting in persistent gas leaks from communication between the lung and pleural space, especially following surgical interventions [32]. Rarely, the ischemia secondary to simultaneous thromboses of multiple intrapulmonary vessels can result in pulmonary gangrene of an entire lobe late in the disease course—this is a phenomenon that is recognized more commonly in adults [2, 39].

Clinical features

Most children with NP are young, aged <5 years, and have been healthy previously (Tables 1 and 2). The clinical features are those of pneumonia with fever, cough, chest pain, tachypnea, and localizing chest signs that may include percussion dullness, decreased breath sounds, and/or bronchial breathing. Symptoms may have been present for several days before presentation (Table 1) and despite receiving appropriate therapy the children are often disproportionately sick with persistent fever, respiratory distress and clinical and/or radiographic signs of a non-responding or progressive pneumonia [40, 48, 79]. Most (63–100%) have an accompanying PPE or empyema, while BPF diagnosed by either a pneumothorax on chest radiograph or persistent (>24 h) gas leaks from chest tubes [22, 32] are also a frequent (17–67%) complication (Tables 1 and 2). A much rarer complication is HUS that leads to a microangipathic hemolytic anemia, thrombocytopenia, and acute renal failure within a few days of symptom onset. Taiwanese studies [25] report PNP to be associated with HUS, especially from serotype 3 and other pneumococcal strains possessing the neuraminidase gene, *nanC*, whose enzyme product cleaves sialic acid residues on the surfaces of red blood cells, platelets and endothelial cells.

NP is frequently associated with elevated inflammatory markers, including high peripheral white blood cell counts in PNP and C-reactive protein levels exceeding 100 mg/L, while mild-to-moderate anemia and hypoalbuminemia are also common (Table 1). Pleural fluid typically has the features of an empyema with either frank pus, visible organisms on Gram stain, or increased white blood cells (≥15.0 × 10^6/L, predominantly neutrophils), and is characterized by pH <7.20, protein >30 g/L, glucose levels <2.2 mmol/L, and lactate dehydrogenase concentrations often ≥1000 U/L, the latter reflecting lung parenchymal injury [82]. In contrast, pleural fluid in patients with *M. pneumonia*-associated NP have high protein content, normal glucose concentration and often a predominance of lymphocytes [17].

Diagnosis

The diagnosis of NP should always be considered in a child with pneumonia who remains unwell, despite at least 72 h of appropriate antibiotics. This is particularly important if there is evidence of BPF or if a PPE or loculated empyema is present, which has undergone drainage or has been surgically managed without improvement [35, 40, 80]. Extrapulmonary sites of infection, such as in the skin and soft tissues or musculoskeletal systems, should be sought. Occasionally children with NP can deteriorate rapidly following their initial presentation with features of severe sepsis, including septic shock, multi-organ failure, and hypoxic respiratory failure [23]. The onset of pulmonary hemorrhage, hemoptysis, an erythematous rash, and declining peripheral white blood cell counts are all ominous signs, and are associated most strongly, but not exclusively, with *S. aureus* infections [64]. When NP is being considered there are several radiographic and microbiologic studies that can help make the diagnosis and identify the causative organism respectively.

Radiographic diagnosis

The diagnosis of NP is generally made by chest imaging studies (Figs. 1 and 2).

A. Chest radiographs

Although chest radiographs will demonstrate the underlying pneumonia, accompanying PPE, and if there is a resulting mediastinal shift, this investigation is only diagnostic in 27–41% of children with NP where one or more small lucencies or pneumatoceles (Fig. 1a,b and d; and Fig. 2a, b) are seen at a median of 4–8 days following hospitalization [30, 83]. The poor sensitivity of chest radiographs results from the cavitory lesions being filled with fluid following liquefaction necrosis that has the same density as the adjacent consolidated lung. The lesions become more visible later in the course of NP when the necrotic fluid drains into communicating bronchi and is replaced by gas [83].

B. Computed tomography (CT)

Contrast-enhanced chest CT scans are more sensitive than chest radiographs and have become the standard imaging procedure for making the diagnosis of NP, evaluating the lung parenchyma changes not visible on plain chest radiographs, and determining whether any underlying congenital lung malformations exist [16, 80, 81]. The key diagnostic features are poor or absent vascularity, loss of pulmonary architecture, and finally cavity formation. Multiple small, gas- or fluid-filled, thin-walled cavities are usually seen initially, often involving just a single lobe. These are non-enhancing, indicating reduced perfusion (Fig. 2c), while loculated fluid or gas within the pleural cavity is also generally present. As the lung undergoes further liquefactive necrosis, the multiple small cavities may coalesce and form larger cavities, including gas-filled pneumatoceles that develop in the later stages of NP. Nevertheless, controversies over interpretation of radiographic findings remain. These include what defines a cavity in terms of its wall thickness, where, for example, lung abscesses evolving from NP have thick walls in addition to contrast enhancement and often a gas-fluid level [14, 84, 85], while differentiating between pleural and parenchymal spaces can be difficult when a PPE is adjacent to areas of liquefied lung. CT scans are also not without other limitations, including exposure to ionizing radiation, cost, feasibility in critically ill patients, and availability in poorly resourced settings.

C. Sonography

Ultrasonography is the primary imaging modality to evaluate the pleural space in children with complicated

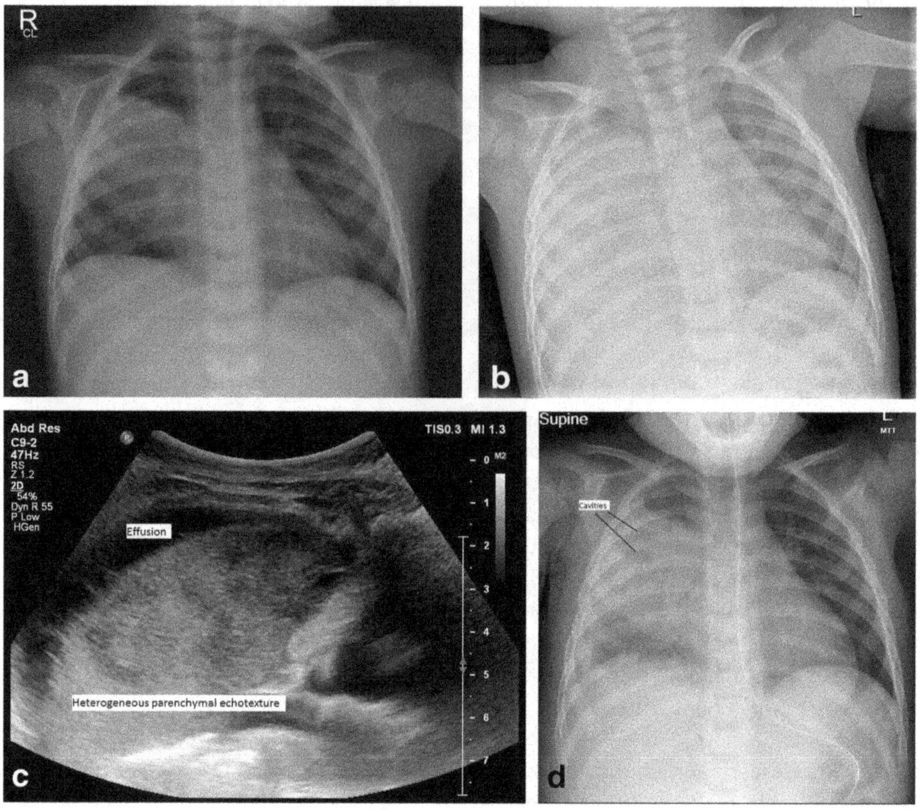

Fig. 1 A 2-year-old child presenting with 4 days of fever, cough, and intermittent grunting respirations. Pleural fluid tested positive for pneumococcal antigen. **a** Initial plain chest radiograph showing right mid-zone airspace opacity, consistent with pneumonia. **b** Plain chest radiograph 24 h later revealing a large right-sided pleural effusion. **c** Lung ultrasonographic image taken immediately afterwards depicting the pleural effusion and heterogeneous parenchymal echo texture, consistent with an underlying necrotizing pneumonia. **d** Plain chest radiograph 4 days later following thoracoscopy and removal of chest drains demonstrates right upper zone cavities within the region identified previously by ultrasonography

pneumonia [86]. It also identifies consolidated lung [87] and when combined with color Doppler to detect hypoperfused regions of the lung a retrospective study [88] found good correlation (r = 0.704) with CT scan results in 236 children with CAP, 80 of whom had evidence of NP. Lung ultrasonography has attractive features of portability, no radiation exposure, low cost, wide availability and no need for sedation in the young patient. It should therefore be considered when performing a CT scan is neither safe nor feasible, and where an early diagnosis of NP will influence patient management. Detecting hypoechoic lesions (Figs. 1c and 2d) or impaired regional perfusion using combined lung ultrasonography and color Doppler predicts the high likelihood of underlying NP and pneumatocele formation [88]. Nevertheless, this imaging technique is still operator-dependent and collateral circulation in areas of necrosis and ventilation-perfusion mismatch within consolidated lung may also affect sensitivity and specificity respectively.

Microbiologic diagnosis

Peripheral blood cultures, serological tests for pathogens, such as *M. pneumoniae*, and pleural fluid investigations, including Gram stain, culture and culture-independent tests (such as PCR or rapid antigen assays) are useful in establishing an etiologic cause. Of these, pleural fluid provides the greatest microbiologic yield (Tables 1 and 2), especially when using sensitive molecular diagnostic or rapid antigen techniques. Pleural fluid can be obtained at the time of inserting an intercostal tube to drain the pleural space, at the time of surgery, or even by intercostal needle aspiration if a PPE is present. Sputum cultures are generally not achievable and are unreliable as potential pathogens, such as pneumococci, are found frequently in healthy children. Similarly, while identifying viruses in respiratory secretions is important in gaining further understanding of the pathogenesis of NP, and possibly for infection control measures, positive results are unlikely to have a major influence on management (such as the discontinuation of antibiotics), as

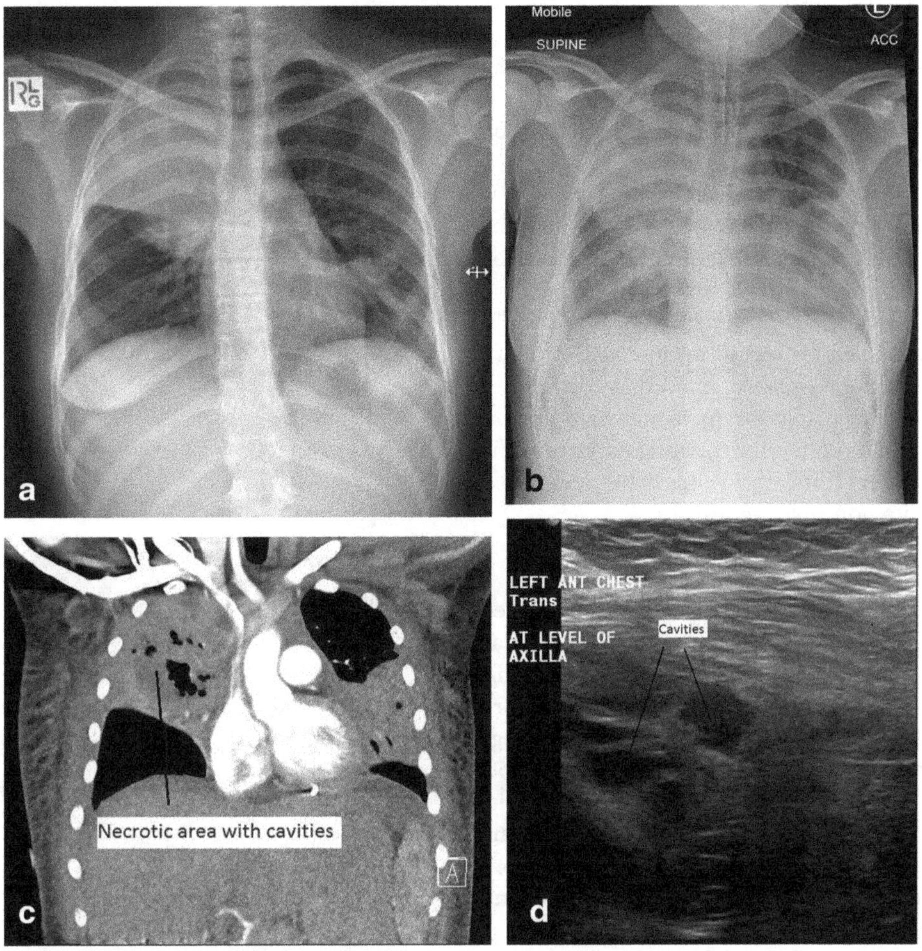

Fig. 2 A 14-year-old child presenting with 5 days of fever, cough, and sore throat. Over the next 24 h the patient developed progressive respiratory and multi-organ failure. *S. constellatus* (of the *S. anginosus* group) was cultured from pleural fluid collected on the second day of hospitalization. **a** Initial plain chest radiograph showing a dense right upper zone airspace opacity and lingula airspace changes, consistent with multi-focal pneumonia. The following images were performed 24 h later. **b** Plain chest radiograph with the child intubated and ventilated revealing cavitation in the right mid to upper zones, pleural effusion and more general airspace changes bilaterally. **c** Computed tomography (CT) scan, coronal view, demonstrating non-enhancing area (necrotic) thin-walled cavities within the right upper lobe and lingula. **d** Lung ultrasonographic image displaying thin-walled cavities in the lingula region of the left lung

detecting viruses does not mean they caused the underlying NP [89].

The studies of children with NP displayed in Table 1 show positive microbiology results in 8–55% of cases and demonstrate the challenges of making a microbiologic diagnosis. Many children (44–100%) had received antibiotics before hospitalization, which in one study [31] reduced positive culture results from 64% in those without antibiotics to 22% in those who had received them before hospitalization. Moreover, clinicians relied heavily upon traditional culture methods to identify the likely causative pathogen. The studies with the greatest microbiologic yields came from the US (48%), France (51%) and the UK (55%) [28, 30, 35]. However, the US study [28] included four cases with positive blood cultures for coagulase-negative staphylococci that are likely contaminants and of the 13 cases with positive pneumococcal cultures, an unknown number originated from sputum. Importantly, this study found that 5 of 50 pleural fluid samples produced positive pneumococcal antigen results, highlighting the usefulness of this test. In the French study [30], of the 13 children with *S. aureus* NP, 7 had positive blood cultures, 5 had positive pleural fluid cultures and 1 each had positive protected-brush specimen or bronchoalveolar lavage cultures for this organism, respectively. Of the 7 children with PNP, 2 had positive blood cultures, while all 7 had pneumococci cultured from their pleural fluid. In the same study, the importance of testing pleural fluid was shown when *F. nucleatum* was detected by 16S PCR testing [30]. The small, select UK surgical study also had a relatively high diagnostic yield from PCR and culture of pleural fluid, despite all having received antibiotics for several days previously [35].

Thus some of the diagnostic difficulties associated with prior antibiotics and low organism loads in sterile sites may be addressed by sensitive molecular techniques within the laboratory [90, 91]. PCR is being employed for detecting pneumococci in pleural fluid [34, 35], and while not yet an established test for blood specimens, this offers hope for the future [92]. Similarly, rapid diagnostic tests against a broad range of respiratory pathogens are undergoing development, although differentiating carriage from disease when sampling from non-sterile sites remains a major limitation with non-invasive tests [93].

Differential diagnosis

A broad range of disorders cause pulmonary cavities (Table 3). In children with NP, important differential diagnoses include other infections associated with lung cavities [84], secondarily infected congenital lung abnormalities and traumatic pseudocysts [94]. Underlying, unsuspected primary immunodeficiency is uncommon in patients with NP [28], but should be suspected in those with a history of recurrent severe or persistent infections, especially if caused by unusual or opportunistic pathogens or by catalase positive organisms when chronic granulomatous disease is being considered [Table 3]. Differentiating NP from a lung abscess is especially important, as the underlying causes and treatment can differ [15, 95]. A simple lung abscess often runs a more indolent course with fever and cough that may have been present for weeks, but this becomes complicated if investigations are delayed, as multiple thin-walled cavities in NP may coalesce to form one or more contrast-enhancing, thick-walled abscesses containing gas-fluid levels within areas of consolidated lung.

Table 3 Causes of pulmonary cavities in children

Primary infectious causes
Bacterial infections
- Necrotizing pneumonia
- Lung abscess
- Septic pulmonary emboli
Uncommon bacterial infections
- *Actinomyces* spp
- *Nocardia* spp
- *Burkholderia pseudomallei* (melioidosis)
Mycobacterial infections
- *Mycobacterium tuberculosis*
- Non-tuberculous mycobacteria spp
Fungal infections
- *Aspergillus*
- Mucormycoses
- Other – eg. *Cryptococcus* spp., *Pneumocystis jirovecii*
Helminthic infections
- *Echinococcus* spp
- Other – eg. *Paragonimus westermani*
Secondarily infected congenital lung malformations
- eg. bronchogenic cysts, congenital pulmonary adenomatoid malformation and bronchopulmonary sequestration
- or a congenital diaphragmatic hernia with an intercurrent respiratory illness
Other causes
Traumatic pseudocysts
Underlying immunodeficiency[a]
- eg. chronic granulomatous disease or hyper IgE syndrome with recurrent infections and pneumatoceles persisting >1 yr
Malignancy
- eg. primary germ cell tumor, lymphoproliferative disorders Langerhan cell histiocystosis
Vasculitis syndromes
- eg. Wegener granulomatosis, Churg-Strauss syndrome

[a]Uncommonly, the initial presentation of chronic granulomatous disease may be with necrotizing pneumonia in a previously well child. This should be considered when the isolated pathogen is one of the catalase +ve organisms associated with pulmonary disease in this disorder (eg. *S. aureus, Aspergillus, Pseudomonas, Burkholderia or Nocardia* species)

Management

Management of NP relies upon expert opinion, and results of retrospective observational studies from mainly single centers, as to date no randomized-controlled trials comparing different treatments have been performed. A multi-disciplinary team of pediatric respiratory physicians, intensivists, thoracic surgeons, and infectious diseases experts is often required. The overarching aims are to control and ultimately reverse the pathobiologic changes associated with NP. These include providing supplemental oxygen to relieve hypoxia, ensuring adequate analgesia to reduce pleuritic pain and improve ventilation, administering prolonged antibiotic therapy, and decreasing any mass effect or intrathoracic pressure by draining gas and/or intrapleural fluid [50, 80, 81, 86, 96]. Correcting fluid and electrolyte abnormalities and attention to nutrition, including managing hypoalbuminemia, is also important. Some children will require circulatory and ventilation support, while occasionally extracorporeal membrane oxygenation (ECMO) is used in those with refractory hypoxemic respiratory failure [19, 23, 28]. Severely ill children with suspected or proven *S. aureus* or

S. pyogenes infection—especially with bilateral lung involvement, pulmonary hemorrhage, or impaired circulation—may also benefit from high-dose intravenous (IV) immunoglobulin infusion (2 g/kg), which is repeated after 48 h if there is no improvement [66, 97].

Antibiotics

A prolonged course of IV antibiotics is the cornerstone of therapy. The initial choice of antibiotics in otherwise healthy, fully immunized children should be the same as for empyema and cover gram positive organisms, especially pneumococci, *S. aureus* and *S. pyogenes* [86], taking into account local epidemiologic and microbiologic data. Consequently, the recommended first-line treatment of IV penicillin or ampicillin for children hospitalized with severe but uncomplicated CAP [98, 99] will need broadening to include beta-lactam anti-staphylococcal antibiotics, such as oxacillin or flucloxacillin [28, 33]. Treatment can then be tailored according to microbiological results, although these may only be positive in 8–55% of cases (Table 1). When suspicion of MRSA is high (eg. local prevalence >10%, ethnicity, recent personal or household history of skin infections) or if it is confirmed by culture, antibiotics should be directed against this specific pathogen. Importantly, vancomycin penetrates poorly into lung parenchyma [100] and treatment failures can occur in up to 20% of MRSA pneumonia when used as monotherapy [101]. Thus, until MRSA is confirmed, a beta-lactam anti-staphylococcal antibiotic should be part of the treatment regimen. While high-level evidence is lacking, the addition of agents such as linezolid, clindamycin, or rifampicin capable of inhibiting protein synthesis (including toxin production) may result in better outcomes for those with *S. aureus* or *S. pyogenes* infections [21, 99]. When NP complicating an *M. pneumoniae* infection is suspected, a macrolide such as IV clarithromycin or azithromycin is added [24]. However, these agents should not invariably replace antibiotics active against pneumococci and *S. aureus*, given the high rates of mixed infection associated with *M. pneumoniae* pneumonia, frequent negative microbiology results in patients with NP, and increasing levels of macrolide resistance in respiratory bacterial pathogens [102]. Finally, the initial empiric antibiotic therapy may need to provide extended gram negative coverage by including a third or fourth generation cephalosporin if the child is unimmunized against *H. influenzae* type b (Hib), immunocompromized, or if the infection was hospital-acquired.

The optimal duration for antibiotic treatment of NP is unknown. The median length of antibiotic courses in case series listed in Table 1 range from 13 to 42 days, with 3 of the 5 studies providing these data reporting a median antibiotic course duration of 28 days [28, 33, 36]. Switching from IV to oral antibiotics is appropriate once the child is afebrile for at least 24 h and no longer showing signs of sepsis, their respiratory distress is resolving, enteral feeds are being tolerated, and inflammatory markers are declining [103]. At this point antibiotics are continued for at least another 10–14 days, a recommendation that aligns with consensus guidelines for PPE and empyema complicating pediatric CAP [86, 99].

Surgical management

While it is recommended that surgical intervention is kept to a minimum to avoid risking BPF [14, 28, 30, 33, 36, 38, 40], this is not always possible if a large pyopneumothorax, tension pneumatocele and/or loculated empyema are already present, especially if they persist or lead to mass effects causing hemodynamic instability and further compromise of ventilation. Moreover, necrotic lung may only be discovered at the time of surgery [8179]. Experienced pediatric surgeons are crucial for management, especially as surgical intervention has become less common in children with NP from Europe, the UK, and US (Table 1), and is particularly challenging because of risk of bleeding when ECMO is being used.

Surgery has two principal aims. The first is to manage concomitant pleural disease involving moderate to large PPE, multi-loculated empyema and persistent gas leak from BPF. This also provides an opportunity to collect pleural fluid for microbiologic testing. Chest tube drainage alone for large PPEs and pyopneumothorax may suffice, but for those with loculated empyema, chest tube insertion and installation of intrapleural fibrinolytics is an option preferred by some experts [50]. However, chest tube drainage >7 days and fibrinolytics may also be associated with increased risk of BPF developing [14, 28, 33, 35, 96] and can fail in 10–30% of empyema cases [104, 105]. Surgical intervention with either video-assisted thoracoscopic surgery or mini-thoracotomy to debride pyogenic material around the lung (decortication), breakdown loculations, and remove pus may be required when fever, signs of sepsis and/or respiratory distress continue, despite chest tube insertion with or without fibrinolytic therapy and repeat imaging shows persistent or increasing intrapleural collections [86]. However, if pleural disease is minimal, the aforementioned symptoms may be from the underlying NP and continuing IV antibiotics without surgery is recommended. BPF with pyopneumothorax may occur spontaneously in NP or be related to surgical intervention, including protracted chest tube placement, and cause significant morbidity [28, 33, 35]. If gas leak continues despite prolonged drainage, surgery may be required to seal the fistula with fibrin glue or insertion of a muscle flap [35].

The second aim of surgery is managing progressive lung parenchymal necrosis. This involves segmental or lobar resection or pneumonectomy and is rarely required in children. Indications for surgery include massive hemoptysis, large or multiple tension pneumatoceles, and pulmonary gangrene where cavities or subsequent abscesses exceed 50% of the involved lobe [2, 5, 106].

Course and outcome

Children with NP usually have a prolonged hospital stay. The median length of stay in cases listed in Table 1 ranged from 12 to 30 days. Not surprisingly, those undergoing surgery had a longer stay in hospital than those managed conservatively [36, 106].

Despite receiving appropriate antibiotic therapy and drainage of any accompanying PPE and empyema, children with NP often have intermittent fevers for several days. This can be part of the natural history of the infection, where poor penetration of antibiotics into hypoperfused regions of the lung and into cavitating lesions leads to delayed bacterial clearance, tissue necrosis, and ongoing inflammation [2]. Nevertheless, when the child remains toxic with persistent fevers, ongoing respiratory distress and supplemental oxygen requirement, accompanied by sustained elevations of inflammatory markers, further evaluations are required to determine whether primary source control within the thoracic cavity has been achieved, if other foci of infection exist (eg. osteomyelitis/septic arthritis, infective endocarditis/pericarditis, deep-seated abscesses or intravascular line infections) or venous thromboses have developed. In cases without a microbiologic diagnosis, incorrect antibiotic choices and the possibility of resistant organisms must also be considered.

Additional complications worth highlighting include HUS that may emerge during the course of PNP, particularly in Taiwanese children [25, 32], and the early or late-onset of life-threatening tension pneumatoceles and tension pneumothorax [4, 26]. Tension pneumatoceles arise from ball-valve mechanisms, trapping gas within the cavity, while a late tension pneumothorax may occur from an unrecognized small BPF leading to a low-grade leak and gradual accumulation of gas within the pleural cavity under pressure [26]. Both complications need urgent surgical intervention and thus experts advise that children with residual cavities should have repeat chest radiograph 2 weeks following discharge, or sooner if they develop signs of respiratory distress.

Unlike adults where case fatality rates for NP can range from approximately 40–50% [15, 65, 70, 101], deaths in children are uncommon despite them often being critically ill and requiring management in intensive care units. Although deaths are reported in single case reports and small case series, these articles are overrepresented by *S. aureus* infections and may be subject to publication bias [4, 15, 23, 72]. Of the 8 studies and 283 patients displayed in Table 1, only two deaths were reported, both from a single center (2/36; 5.5%) where 24 (67%) underwent thoracotomy [37]. Similarly, deaths were also uncommon in PNP (Table 2), where there were just two deaths, including 1 from HUS and pulmonary gangrene, amongst 72 patients from case series where fatalities were reported [29, 39]. In the largest case series published to date, most patients made a full clinical recovery within 2 months of hospitalization, although eight (10%) were readmitted within 2 weeks of discharge, mostly because of ongoing fever [28]. In this study, 12 children also had follow-up spirometry, eight had normal results, but mild obstructive defects were observed in 3 children and mild restriction in another, findings similar to those hospitalized with severe CAP [107]. In most cases, chest radiographs and CT scans normalized or improved markedly by 5–6 months [16, 28, 33, 35, 36, 83, 106].

Consequently, in addition to reviewing children and repeating their chest radiograph 2 weeks following discharge, the authors recommend further clinical reviews and chest radiographs at 6–8 weeks and 6 months as a minimum. In those old enough to perform spirometry, this investigation should be done at discharge and again at 6 months. Referral to a pediatric respiratory physician for further investigations is indicated when symptoms and radiographic abnormalities persist beyond the expected time frames of 2 months [28] and 6 months [16, 28, 33, 35, 36, 83, 106], respectively.

Prevention

Until there is a greater understanding of why NP occasionally complicates pneumonia, its prevention will depend upon reducing CAP and its severity. Efforts should focus upon children aged <5 years who have the highest incidence of CAP [108]. Indeed, since the year 2000, deaths from CAP in this age group have declined >50% globally, falling below one million in 2015 [109]. Decreases in CAP are attributed to a combination of improved housing, water supply and hygiene, better indoor air quality, reduced parental tobacco smoking, increased education, breastfeeding rates and nutrition, and greater healthcare access and vaccine uptake [110]. Vaccines contributing to this success globally are pertussis, measles, Hib, and pneumococcal conjugate vaccines [111].

Despite these advances, NP cases have increased in the last two decades [18, 22, 28–32]. In part, this may be from increased physician awareness and requesting chest CT scans in children with severe, refractory, or complicated pneumonia. Temporal changes in pathogens, including pneumococcal serotypes and *S. aureus*, may also be important. It is therefore encouraging that since replacing the 7-valent PCV in the US and France with a 13-valent formulation containing many of the serotypes associated with NP, rates of PPE/empyema in children fell rapidly by 37–53% [112, 113]. Whether this decline is also true for NP is unknown.

Nevertheless, replacement disease by non-vaccine pneumococcal serotypes remains a potential problem [108], and an effective vaccine against *S. aureus* continues to be elusive [114]. However, efforts continue to improve performance and acceptability of pertussis and influenza vaccine formulations [115, 116], and candidate vaccines against *S. pyogenes* and RSV are undergoing clinical trials [117, 118]. Maternal antenatal immunization with pertussis and influenza provide early protection in very young infants and are gaining wider acceptance [119, 120], while novel RSV vaccines administered during pregnancy and to older infants are also being evaluated [121]. Hopefully, these bundles of social, environmental, and medical interventions will further reduce pediatric CAP and its complications.

Conclusions

NP is an uncommon but increasingly recognized severe complication of pneumonia in previously healthy young children. The major pathogens are *S. pneumoniae* and *S. aureus* and the diagnosis should be considered when, despite appropriate antibiotics, the child remains febrile and unwell with persistent signs of respiratory distress and pneumonia. Most will have a PPE, empyema and/or BPF that has not improved despite chest drainage or surgical intervention. The diagnosis is confirmed by chest imaging, usually by a CT scan or sonography, while treatment requires prolonged IV antibiotics, which can be changed to oral medication for an additional 10–14 days, once the child is afebrile and clinically stable. Ideally, surgical intervention is kept to a minimum, but this is not always possible if there are mass effects from gas and fluid in the pleural cavity or pulmonary gangrene leading to massive hemoptysis, uncontrolled sepsis, or difficulties with assisted ventilation. Nevertheless, despite its severity, mortality in children is uncommon; the children improve clinically within a couple of months, radiographic changes are largely resolved after 5–6 months, and only a minority are left with mildly impaired lung function. Important targets for future research include identifying host–pathogen interactions leading to disease, improving the microbiologic diagnostic gap, optimizing medical and surgical management, and ultimately preventing this severe complication of pediatric pneumonia.

Abbreviations

BPF: Bronchopleural fistulae; CAP: Community-acquired pneumonia; CT: Computed tomography; ECMO: Extracorporeal membrane oxygenation; Hib: *Haemophilus influenzae* type b; HUS: Hemolytic uremic syndrome; IV: Intravenous; MRSA: Methicillin-resistant *Staphylococcus aureus*; NP: Necrotizing pneumonia; PCR: Polymerase chain reaction; PCV: Pneumococcal conjugate vaccine; PNP: Pneumococcal necrotizing pneumonia; PPE: Parapneumonic effusion; PVL: Panton-Valentine leucocidin; RSV: Respiratory syncytial virus; UK: United Kingdom; US: United States

Acknowledgements

Not applicable.

Funding

The authors received no support or funding for writing this manuscript.

Authors' contributions

All authors meet the ICMJE authorship criteria. IBM conceived and wrote the first draft of the manuscript. IBM, AFI and KG critically reviewed the manuscript for important intellectual content. IBM, AFI and KG approved the final version.

Competing interests

In the last 5-years, KG has been a member of Advisory Boards on pneumonia, otitis media and pneumococcal conjugate vaccines for GlaxoSmithKline (GSK) Biologicals, Rixensart, Belgium. IBM and AFI declare they have no competing interests.

Author details

[1]Department of Respiratory and Sleep Medicine, Lady Cilento Children's Hospital, South Brisbane, QLD, Australia. [2]School of Medicine and Menzies Health Institute Queensland, Gold Coast campus, Griffith University, Building G40, Southport Gold Coast, QLD, Australia. [3]Departments of Infectious Diseases and Paediatrics, Gold Coast Health, Southport Gold Coast, QLD, Australia.

References

1. Tsai Y-F, Ku Y-H. Necrotizing pneumonia: a rare complication of pneumonia requiring special consideration. Curr Opin Pulm Med. 2012;18:246–52.
2. Chatha N, Fortin D, Bosma KJ. Management of necrotizing pneumonia and pulmonary gangrene: a case series and review of the literature. Can Respir J. 2014;21:239–45.
3. Kerem E, Bar Ziv Y, Rudenski B, Katz S, Kleid D, Branski D. Bacteremic necrotizing pneumococcal pneumonia in children. Am J Respir Crit Care Med. 1994;149:242–4.
4. Al-Saleh S, Grasemann H, Cox P. Necrotizing pneumonia complicated by early and late pneumatoceles. Can Respir J. 2008;15:129–32.
5. Cicak B, Verona E, Mihatov-Stefanovic I. Necrotizing pneumonia in infants. Acta Clin Croat. 2010;49:321–6.
6. Obando I, Valderrabanos ES, Millan JA, Neth OW. Necrotising pneumonia due to influenza a (H1N1) and community-acquired methicillin-resistant *Staphylococcus aureus* clone USA300: successful management of the first documented paediatric case. Arch Dis Child. 2010;95:305–6.
7. Yazer J, Giacomantonio M, MacDonald N, Lopushinsky S. Severe necrotizing pneumonia in a child with pandemic (H1N1) influenza. Can Med J. 2011;183:215–9.
8. Chen J, Luo Y, Zhang S, Liang Z, Wang Y, Zhang T, et al. Community-acquired necrotizing pneumonia caused by methicillin-resistant *Staphylococcus aureus* producing Panton-valentine leucocidin in a Chinese teenager: case report and literature review. Int J Infect Dis. 2014;26:17–21.
9. Pawley B, Smith M, Nickels D. Core curriculum illustration: necrotizing pneumonia and empyema. Emerg Radiol. 2016;23:201–2.
10. Ramgopal S, Ivan Y, Medsinge A, Saladino RA. Pediatric necrotizing pneumonia and review of the literature. Pediatr Emerg Care. 2017;33:112–5.
11. Lu S, Tsai JD, Tsao TF, Liao PF, Sheu JN. Necrotizing pneumonia and acute purulent pericarditis caused by *Streptococcus pneumoniae* serotype 19A in a healthy 4-year old girl after one catch-up dose of 13-valent pneumococcal conjugate vaccine. Paediatr Int Child Health. 2016;36:235–9.
12. Ramoglu MG, Ucar T, Kendirli T, Eyileten Z, Atalay S. Necrotizing pneumonia caused by H1N1 virus in a child with total anomalous pulmonary venous connection after surgery. Acta Cardiol Sin. 2016;32:751–4.
13. McCarthy VP, Patamasucon P, Gaines T, Lucas MA. Necrotizing pneumonia in childhood. Pediatr Pulmonol. 1999;28:217–21.
14. Hoffer FA, Bloom DA, Colin AA, Fishman SJ. Lung abscess versus necrotizing pneumonia: implications for interventional therapy. Pediatr Radiol. 1999;29:87–91.
15. Gillet Y, Issartel B, Vanhems P, Fournet J-C, Lina G, Bes M, et al. Association between *Staphylococcus aureus* strains carrying gene for Panton-valentine leucocidin and highly lethal necrotising pneumonia in young immunocompetent patients. Lancet. 2002;359:753–9.

16. Hodina M, Hanquinet S, Cotting J, Schnyder P, Gudinchet E. Imaging of cavitary necrosis in complicated childhood pneumonia. Eur Radiol. 2002;12:391–6.
17. Wang RS, Wang SY, Hsieh KS, et al. Necrotizing pneumonitis caused by *Mycoplasma pneumoniae* in pediatric patients. Pediatr Infect Dis J. 2004;23:564–7.
18. Ramphul N, Eastham KM, Freeman R, Eltringham G, Kearns AM, Leeming JP, et al. Cavitatory lung disease complicating empyema in children. Pediatr Pulmonol. 2006;41:750–3.
19. Stroud MH, Okhuysen-Cawley R, Jaquiss R, Berlinski A, Fiser RT. Successful use of extracorporeal membrane oxygenation in severe necrotizing pneumonia caused by *Staphylococcus aureus*. Pediatr Crit Care Med. 2007;8:282–7.
20. Kalaskar AS, Heresi GP, Wanger A, Murphy JR, Wootton SH. Severe necrotizing pneumonia in children, Houston, Texas, USA. Emerg Infect Dis. 2009;15:1696–8.
21. Geng W, Yang Y, Wu D, Zhang W, Wang C, Shang Y, et al. Community-acquired, methicillin-resistant *Staphylococcus aureus* isolated from children with community-onset pneumonia in China. Pediatr Pulmonol. 2010;45:387–94.
22. McKee AJ, Ives A, Balfour-Lynn IM. Increased incidence of bronchopulmonary fistulas complicating pediatric pneumonia. Pediatr Pulmonol. 2011;46:717–21.
23. Schwartz KL, Nourse C. Panton-valentine leucocidin-associated *Staphylococcus aureus* necrotizing pneumonia in infants: a report of four cases and review of the literature. Eur J Pediatr. 2012;171:711–7.
24. Wang Y, Xu D, Li S, Chen Z. *Mycoplasma pneumoniae*-associated necrotizing pneumonitis in children. Pediatr Int. 2012;54:293–7.
25. Janapatla R-P, Hsu M-H, Hsieh Y-C, Lee H-Y, Lin T-Y, Chiu C-H. Necrotizing pneumonia caused by *nanC*-carrying serotypes is associated with pneumococcal haemolytic uraemic syndrome in children. Clin Microbiol Infect. 2013;19:480–6.
26. Demirel N, Quizon A, Belteton de Leon EL, Reiter J, Colin AA. On the nature of pleural involvement in necrotizing pneumonia: a report of two cases of life threatening late complications. Pediatr Pulmonol. 2014;49:E90–5.
27. Cakir E, Gedik AH, Ari E, Ozdemir A, Cakir FB, Uzuner S, et al. Nontuberculous pulmonary cavitary diseases of childhood. Pediatr Infect Dis J. 2015;34:320–2.
28. Sawicki GS, Lu FL, Valim C, Cleveland RH, Colin AA. Necrotising pneumonia is an increasingly detected complication of pneumonia in children. Eur Respir J. 2008;31:1285–91.
29. Bender JM, Ampofo K, Korgenski K, Daly J, Pavia AT, Mason EO, et al. Pneumococcal necrotizing pneumonia in Utah: does serotype matter? Clin Infect Dis. 2008;46:1346–52.
30. Lemaitre C, Angoulvant F, Gabor F, Makhoul J, Bonacorsi S, Naudin J, et al. Necrotizing pneumonia in children. Report of 41 cases between 2006 and 2011 in a French tertiary care center. Pediatr Infect Dis J. 2013;32:1146–9.
31. Erlichman I, Breuer O, Shoseyov D, Cohen-Cymberknoh M, Koplewitz B, Averbuch D, et al. Complicated acquired pneumonia in childhood: different types, clinical course, and outcome. Pediatr Pulmonol. 2017;52:247–54.
32. Hsieh YC, Wang C-W, Lai S-H, Lai J-Y, Wong K-S, Huang Y-C, et al. Necrotizing pneumococcal pneumonia with bronchopleural fistula among children in Taiwan. Pediatr Infect Dis J. 2011;30:740–4.
33. Krenke K, Sanocki M, Urbankowska E, Kraj G, Krawiec M, Urbankowski T, et al. Necrotizing pneumonia and its complications in children. Adv Exp Med Biol. 2015;12:9–17.
34. Hsieh Y-C, Chi H, Chang K-Y, Lai S-H, Mu J-J, Wong K-S, et al. Increase in fitness of *Streptococcus pneumoniae* is associated with the severity of necrotizing pneumonia. Pediatr Infect Dis J. 2015;34:499–505.
35. Jester I, Nijran A, Singh M, Parikh DH. Surgical management of bronchopleural fistula in pediatric empyema and necrotizing pneumonia: efficacy of the serratus anterior muscle digitation flap. J Pediatr Surg. 2012;47:1358–62.
36. Wong KS, Chiu CH, Yeow KM, Huang YC, Liu HP, Lin TY. Necrotising pneumonitis in children. Eur J Pediatr. 2000;159:684–8.
37. Hacimustafaoglu M, Celebi S, Sarimehmet H, Gurpinar A, Ercan I. Necrotizing pneumonia in children. Acta Paediatr. 2004;93:1172–7.
38. Macedo M, Meyer KF, Oliveira TCM. Necrotizing pneumonia in children submitted to thoracoscopy due to pleural empyema: incidence, treatment and clinical evolution. J Bras Pneumol. 2010;36:301–5.
39. Hsieh Y-C, Hsiao C-H, Tsao P-N, Wang J-Y, Hsueh P-R, Chiang B-L, et al. Necrotizing pneumococcal pneumonia in children: the role of pulmonary gangrene. Pediatr Pulmonol. 2006;41:623–9.
40. Fretzayas A, Moustaki M, Alexopoulou E, Nychtari G, Nicolaidou P, Priftis KN. Clinical notations on bacteraemic cavitating pneumococcal pneumonia in nonvaccinated immunocompetent children. J Trop Pediatr. 2009;55:257–61.
41. Griffin MR, Zhu Y, Moore MR, Whitney CG, Grijalva CG. U.S. hospitalizations for pneumonia after a decade of pneumococcal vaccination. N Engl J Med. 2013;369:155–63.
42. Jardine A, Menzies RI, McIntyre PB. Reduction in hospitalizations for pneumonia associated with the introduction of a pneumococcal conjugate vaccination schedule without a booster dose in Australia. Pediatr Infect Dis J. 2010;29:607–12.
43. Sgambatti S, Minamisava R, Bierrenbach AL, et al. Early impact of 10-valent pneumococcal conjugate vaccine in childhood pneumonia hospitalizations using primary data from an active population-based surveillance. Vaccine. 2016;34:663–70.
44. Strachan R, Jaffe A. Assessment of the burden of paediatric empyema in Australia. J Paediatr Child Health. 2009;45:431–6.
45. Grijalva CG, Zhu Y, Nuorti JP, Griffin MR. Emergence of parapneumonic empyema in the USA. Thorax. 2011;66:663–8.
46. Grijalva CG, Nuorti JP, Zhu Y, Griffin MR. Increasing incidence of empyema complicating childhood community-acquired pneumonia in the United States. Clin Infect Dis. 2010;50:805–13.
47. Byington CL, Hulten KG, Ampofo K, et al. Molecular epidemiology of pediatric pneumococcal empyema from 2001 to 2007 in Utah. J Clin Microbiol. 2010;48:520–5.
48. Spencer DA, Iqbal SM, Hasan A, Hamilton L. Empyema thoracis is still increasing in UK children. BMJ. 2006;332:1333. doi:10.1136/bmj.332.7553.1333.
49. Munoz-Almagro C, Jordan I, Gene A, Latorre C, Garcia-Garcia JJ, Palleres R. Emergence of invasive pneumococcal disease caused by nonvaccine serotypes in the era of 7-valent conjugate vaccine. Clin Infect Dis. 2008;46:489–95.
50. Spencer DA, Thomas MF. Necrotising pneumonia in children. Paediatr Respir Rev. 2014;15:240–5.
51. Byington CL, Spencer LY, Johnson TA, et al. An epidemiological investigation of a sustained high rate of pediatric parapneumonic empyema: risk factors and microbiological associations. Clin Infect Dis. 2002;34:434–40.
52. Francois P, Desrumaux A, Cans C, Pin I, Pavese P, Labarere J. Prevalence and risk factors of suppurative complications in children with pneumonia. Acta Paediatr. 2010;99:861–6.
53. Amorim P, Morcillo AM, Tresoldi AT, Fraga Ade M, Pereira RM, Baract EC. Factors associated with complications of community-acquired pneumonia in preschool children. J Bras Pneumonol. 2012;38:614–21.
54. Elemraid MA, Thomas MF, Blain AD, et al. Risk factors for the development of pleural empyema in children. Pediatr Pulmonol. 2015; 50:721–6.
55. Krenke K, Krawiec M, Kraj G, Peradzynska J, Krauze A, Kulus M. Risk factors for local complications in children with community-acquired pneumonia. Clin Respir J. 2016;00:000. doi:10.1111/crj12524.
56. Voiriot G, Dury S, Parrot A, Mayaud C, Fartoukh M. Nonsteroidal antiinflammatory drugs may affect the presentation and course of community-acquired pneumonia. Chest. 2011;139:387–94.
57. Shenoy AT, Orihuela CJ. Anatomical site-specific contributions of pneumococcal virulence determinants. Pneumonia. 2016;8:7.
58. Cillniz C, Amaro R, Torres A. Pneumococcal vaccination. Curr Opin Infect Dis. 2016;29:187–96.
59. Jauneikaite E, Tocheva AS, Jefferies JM, et al. Current methods for capsular typing of *Streptococcus pneumoniae*. J Microbiol Methods. 2015;113:41–9.
60. Woodhead M. Pneumococcal serotypes and respiratory failure: soil or seed? Eur Respir J. 2014;43:331–3.
61. Linares J, Ardunay C, Pallares R, Fenoll A. Changes in antimicrobial resistance, serotypes and genotypes in *Streptococcus pneumoniae* over a 30-year period. Clin Microbiol Infect. 2010;16:402–10.
62. Grabenstein JD, Musey LK. Differences in serious clinical outcomes of infection caused by specific pneumococcal serotypes among adults. Vaccine. 2014;32:2399–405.
63. Reinert RR, Jacobs MR, Kaplan SL. Pneumococcal disease caused by serotype 19A: review of the literature and implications for future vaccine development. Vaccine. 2010;28:4249–59.
64. Dayan GH, Mohamed N, Scully IL, et al. *Staphylococcus aureus*: the current state of disease, pathophysiology and strategies for prevention. Expert Rev Vaccines. 2016;11:1373–92.
65. Gillet Y, Vanhems P, Lina G, et al. Factors predicting mortality in necrotizing community-acquired pneumonia caused by *Staphylococcus aureus* containing Panton-valentine leucocidin. Clin Infect Dis. 2007;45:315–21.
66. Loffler B, Niemann S, Ehrhardt C, et al. Pathogenesis of *Staphylococucs aureus* necrotizing pneumonia: the role of PVL and an influenza coinfection.

Expert Rev Anti-Infect Ther. 2013;11:1041–51.
67. Loffler B, Hussain M, Grundmeler M, et al. *Staphylococcus aureus* Panton-Valentine leukocidin is a very potent cytotoxic factor for human neutrophils. PLoS Pathogens 2010;6(1):e1000715.
68. Shallcross LJ, Fragaszy E, Johnson AM, Hayward AC. The role of the Panton-valentine leucocidin toxin in staphylococcal disease: a systematic review and meta-analysis. Lancet Infect Dis. 2013;13:43–54.
69. Chua K, Laurent F, Coombs G, Grayson ML, Howden BP. Not community-associated methicillin-resistant *Staphylococcus aureus* (CA-MRSA)! A clinician's guide to community MRSA – its evolving antimicrobial resistance and implications for therapy. Clin Infect Dis. 2011;52:99–114.
70. Sicot N, Khanafer N, Meyssonnier V, et al. Methicillin resistance is not a predictor of severity in community-acquired *Staphylococcus aureus* necrotizing pneumonia – results of a prospective observational study. Clin Microbiol Infect. 2013;19:E142–8.
71. Tong SYC, Davis JS, Eichenberger E, Holland TL, Fowler VG. *Staphylococcus aureus* infections: epidemiology, pathophysiology, clinical manifestations, and management. Clin Microbiol Rev. 2015;28:603–61.
72. Vaideeswar P, Bavdekar SB, Jadhav SM, Balan R, Pandit SP. Necrotizing adenoviral pneumonia: manifestation of nosocomial infection in pediatric intensive care unit. Ind J Pediatr. 2008;75:1171–4.
73. De Lastours V, Malosh R, Ramaugu K, et al. Co-colonization by *Streptococcus pneumoniae* and *Staphylococcus aureus* in the throat during acute respiratory illnesses. Epidemiol Infect. 2016;144:3507–19.
74. Teo SM, Mok D, Pham K, et al. The infant nasopharyngeal microbiome impacts severity of lower respiratory infection and risk of asthma development. Cell Host Microbe. 2015;17:704–15.
75. Cevey-Macherel M, Galetto-Lacour A, Gervaix A, et al. Etiology of community-acquired pneumonia in hospitalized children based on WHO clinical guidelines. Eur J Pediatr. 2009;168:1429–36.
76. Elemraid MA, Sails AD, Eltringham GJA, et al. Aetiology of paediatric pneumonia after the introduction of pneumococcal conjugate vaccine. Eur Respir J. 2013;42:1595–603.
77. Yu KOA, Randolph AG, Agan AA, et al. *Staphylococcus aureus* α-toxin response distinguishes respiratory virus-methicillin-resistant *S. aureus* coinfection in children. J Infect Dis. 2016;214:1638–46.
78. Bosch AATM, Biesbroek G, Trzcinski K, Sanders EAM, Bogaert D. Viral and bacterial interactions in the upper respiratory tract. PLoS Pathog. 2013;9:e1003057.
79. Brealey JC, Sly PD, Young PR, Chappell KJ. Viral bacterial co-infection of the respiratory tract during early childhood. FEMS Microbiol Lett 2015;362.
80. Loizzi M, De Palma A, Pagliarulo V, Loizzi D, Sollitto F. Pulmonary infections of surgical interest in childhood. Thorac Surg Clin. 2012;22:387–401.
81. Thomas MF, Wort A, Spencer DA. Management and complications of pneumonia. Paediatr Child Health. 2014;25:172–8.
82. Ulloa-Gutierrez R. Pneumococcal necrotizing pneumonia and pleural fluid lactate dehydrogenase level. Clin Infect Dis. 2008;47:729–30.
83. Donnelly LF, Klosterman LA. Cavitatory necrosis complicating pneumonia in children: sequential findings on chest radiography. Am J Roentgenol. 1998;171:253–6.
84. Gadkowski LB, Stout JE. Cavitary pulmonary disease. Clin Microbiol Rev. 2008;21:305–33.
85. Agasthian T. Results of surgery for bronchiectasis and pulmonary abscesses. Thorac Surg Clin. 2012;22:333–44.
86. Islam S, Calkins CM, Goldin AB, et al. The diagnosis and management of empyema in children: a comprehensive review from the APSA outcomes and clinical trial committee. J Pediatr Surg. 2012;47:2101–10.
87. Shah VP, Tunik MG, Tsung JW. Prospective evaluation of point-of-care ultrasonography for the diagnosis of pneumonia in children and young adults. JAMA Pediatr. 2013;167:119–25.
88. Lai SH, Wong KS, Liao SL. Value of lung ultrasonography in the diagnosis and outcome prediction of pediatric community-acquired pneumonia with necrotizing change. PLoS One 2015;10(6):e0130082.
89. Sly PD, Zar HJ. The spectrum of lower respiratory tract illness in children after pneumococcal conjugate vaccination. Am J Respir Crit Care Med. 2017;195:13–5.
90. De Schutter I, Vergison A, Tuerlinckx D, et al. Pneumococcal aetiology and serotype distribution in paediatric community-acquired pneumonia. PLoS One. 2014;9:e89013.
91. Torrses A, Lee N, Cilloniz C, Vila J, Van der Eerden M. Laboratory diagnosis of pneumonia in the molecular age. Eur Respir J. 2016;48:1764–78.
92. Murdoch DR. How to best determine causative pathogens in pneumonia. Pneumonia. 2016;8:1. doi:10.1186/s41479-016-0004-z.
93. Gadsby NJ, Russell CD, McHugh MP, et al. Comprehensive molecular testing for respiratory pathogens in community-acquired pneumonia. Clin Infect Dis. 2016;62:817–23.
94. Odev K, Guler I, Altinok T, et al. Cystic and cavitary lung lesions in children: radiologic findings with pathologic correlation. J Clin Imaging Sci. 2013;3:60.
95. Wheeler JG, Jacobs RF. Complications of pneumonia. In: Cherry JD, Harrison GJ, Kaplan SL, Steinbach WJ, Hotez PJ, editors. Feigin and Cherry's textbook of Pediatric infectious diseases. 7th ed. Philadelphia: Elsevier Saunders; 2014. p. 306–22.
96. Pabary R, Balbour-Lynn IM. Complicated pneumonia in children. Breathe. 2013;9:211–22.
97. Kreienbuehl L, Charbonney E, Eggimann P. Community-acquired necrotizing pneumonia due to methicillin-sensitive *Staphylococcus aureus* secreting Panton-valentine leucocidin: a review of case reports. Ann Intensive Care. 2011;1:52.
98. Harris M, Clark J, Coote N, et al. British Thoracic Society guidelines for the management of community acquired pneumonia in children: update 2011. Thorax. 2011;66:ii1–23.
99. Bradley JS, Byington CL, Shah SS, et al. The management of community-acquired pneumonia in infants and children older than 3 months of age: clinical practice guidelines by the Pediatric Infectious Diseases Society and the Infectious Diseases Society of America. Clin Infect Dis. 2011;53:e25–76.
100. Le J, Lieberman JM. Management of community-associated methicillin-resistant *Staphylococcus aureus* infections in children. Pharmacotherapy. 2006;26:1758–70.
101. Li HT, Zhang TT, Huang J, Zhou YQ, Zhu JX, Wu BQ. Factors associated with the outcome of life threatening necrotizing pneumonia due to community-acquired *Staphylococcus aureus* in adult and adolescent patients. Respiration. 2011;81:448–60.
102. Korppi M, Heiskanen-Kosma T, Kleemola M. Incidence of community-acquired pneumonia in children caused by *Mycoplasma pneumoniae*: serological results of a prospective, population-based study in primary health care. Respirology. 2004;9:109–14.
103. McMullan BJ, Andresen D, Blyth CC, et al. Antibiotic duration and the timing of the switch from intravenous to oral route for bacterial infections in children: systematic review and guidelines. Lancet Infect Dis. 2016;16:e139–52.
104. Thomson AH, Hull J, Kumar MR, Wallis C, Balfour-Lynn IM. Randomised trial of intrapleural urokinase in the treatment of childhood empyema. Thorax. 2002;57:343–7.
105. Tuncozgur B, Ustunsoy H, Sivrikoz MC, et al. Intrapleural urokinase in the management of parapneumonic empyema: a randomized controlled trial. Int J Clin Pract. 2001;55:659–60.
106. Lai JY, Yang W, Ming YC. Surgical management of complicated necrotizing pneumonia in children. Pediatric Neonatol 2016 Oct 28. doi: 10.1016/j.pedneo.2016.06.002. [Epub ahead of print].
107. Grimwood K, Chang AB. Long-term effects of pneumonia in young children. Pneumonia. 2015;6:101–14.
108. Shaughnessy EE, Stalets EL, Shah SS. Community-acquired pneumonia in the post 13-valent pneumococcal conjugate vaccine era. Curr Opin Pediatr. 2016;28:786–93.
109. Lu L, Oza S, Hogan D, et al. Global, regional, and national causes of under 5 mortality in 2000-15: an updated systematic analysis with implications for the sustainable development goals. Lancet. 2016;388: 3027–35.
110. Izadnegahdar R, Cohen AL, Klugman KP, Qazi SA. Childhood pneumonia in developing countries. Lancet Respir Med. 2013;1:574–84.
111. Williams DJ, Shah SS. Community-acquired pneumonia in the conjugate vaccine era. J Pediatr Infect Dis Soc. 2012;1:314–28.
112. Simonsen L, Taylor RJ, Schuck-Paim C, Lustig R, Haber M, Klugman KP. Effect of 13-valent pneumococcal conjugate vaccine on admissions to hospital 2 years after its introduction in the USA: a time series analysis. Lancet Respir Med. 2014;2:387–94.
113. Angoulvant F, Levy C, Grimprel E, et al. Early impact of 13-valent pneumococcal conjugate vaccine on community-acquired pneumonia in children. Clin Infect Dis. 2014;58:918–24.
114. Dayan GH, Mohamed N, Scully IL, et al. *Staphylococcus aureus*: the current state of disease, pathophysiology and strategies for prevention. Expert Rev Vaccines. 2016;15:1373–92.

115. Kilgore PE, Salim AM, zervos MJ, Schmitt HJ. Pertussis: microbiology, disease, treatment, and prevention. Clin Microbiol Rev. 2016;29:449–86.
116. Pica N, Palese P. Toward a universal influenza virus vaccine: prospects and challenges. Annu Rev Med. 2013;64:189–202.
117. Good MF, Batzloff PM. Strategies in the development of vaccines to prevent infections with group a streptococcus. Hum Vaccin Immunother. 2013;9:1–5.
118. Modjarrad K, Giersing B, Kaslow DC, Smith PG, Moorthy VS. The WHO RSV vaccine consultation expert group. WHO report. WHO consultation on respiratory syncytial virus vaccine development report from a World Health Organization meeting held on 23-24 march 2015. Vaccine. 2016;34:190–7.
119. Amirthalingam G, Campbell H, Ribeiro S, Fry NK, Ramsay M, Miller E, et al. Sustained effectiveness of the maternal pertussis immunization program in England 3 years following introduction. Clin Infect Dis. 2016;63(Suppl 4):S236–43.
120. Munoz FM. Infant protection against influenza through maternal immunization. A call for more immunogenic vaccines. JAMA Pediatr. 2016;170:832–3.
121. Griffiths C, Drews SJ, Marchant DJ. Respiratory syncytial virus: infection, detection, and new options for prevention and treatment. Clin Microbiol Rev. 2017;30:277–318.

3

Pulmonary infections in the returned traveller

Ashleigh Trimble[1,2*], V. Moffat[3] and A. M. Collins[2,4]

Abstract

Pulmonary infections in the returned traveller are a common presentation. A wide variety of infections may present with pulmonary symptoms. It is important for clinicians to differentiate the cause of these symptoms. The risk of contracting certain travel-related pulmonary diseases depends on travel destination, length of stay, activities undertaken and co-morbidities. Some pathogens are found worldwide, whilst others are related to specific locations. This review article will discuss the approach to diagnosing and treating pulmonary infections in the returned traveller.

Keywords: Travel, Traveller, Pulmonary infections, Tropics, Respiratory infections

Background

International travel has steadily increased over the last few decades, and is no longer only for the wealthy and healthy. The number of travellers reached more than one billion for the first time in 2012 and continues to rise [1]. There are many risk factors that increase the likelihood of developing a travel-related illness and this review will focus on pulmonary-related infections (Table 1) [2–4]. Many illnesses are self-limiting and are a result of common pulmonary viruses that are prevalent worldwide [3, 5] but in certain circumstances travel-related pulmonary infections are serious and have potentially fatal implications, and can even cause epidemics.

Air travel has shown how efficiently pulmonary infections can be transmitted. Data suggests the risk of disease transmission to a symptom-free passenger within the aircraft cabin is associated with sitting within 2 rows of a contagious passenger for a flight time of more than 8 h. This association is mainly derived from investigations of in-flight transmission of tuberculosis (TB) [6]. Aircraft cabin ventilation appears to be a key factor enabling disease transmission. This was highlighted by the spread of severe acute respiratory syndrome (SARS) during a short-haul flight in 2002 [5]. With sea travel (especially cruising) becoming more popular, the ageing population of travellers with multiple pre-existing conditions is also a concern.

Clinicians should be aware of particular diseases that may present in the returned traveller and rank their diagnostic likelihood based on destination, length of stay and symptom duration (Tables 2 and 3).

Pneumonia is a frequent cause of fever amongst returned travellers [7]. Awareness of travel locations may be key to identifying the organism responsible, and polymerase chain reaction (PCR) testing is very important to look for atypical etiologies. Routinely, patients are started on antibiotics based on local guidelines for community-acquired pneumonia. It is unlikely these regimens will contain appropriate first-line therapy or be of sufficient duration to cover for pneumonias caused by *Coxiella burnettii* (Q fever) [8] or *Burkholderia pseudomallei* (melioidosis), which have been isolated in recent outbreaks that have occurred in Europe and South East Asia [9].

Pulmonary infections are diagnosed in up to 24% of returned travellers with fever, making it as common as travellers' diarrhea, with influenza being the most common vaccine-preventable infection acquired (vaccine protective against H1N1, H3N2 and two influenza B virus strains) [10, 11]. Pre-travel advice should be that travellers with co-morbidities should be vaccinated against both seasonal influenza virus and pneumococcus [12]. It should be noted that the influenza vaccine does not currently offer protection against the most recent strains causing epidemics (H5N1, H7N9) and

* Correspondence: a.trimble@nhs.net
[1]Crosshouse Hospital, Kilmarnock Road, Crosshouse KA2 0BE, UK
[2]Respiratory Infection Group, Liverpool School of Tropical Medicine, Pembroke Place, Liverpool L3 5QA, UK
Full list of author information is available at the end of the article

Table 1 Specific Risk factors

Risk activities	Common	Occasional
Bites		
Tick		Q fever
Mosquitos	Tropical eosinophilia *(Wuchereia bancrofti* and *Brugia malayi)*	Dirofilarisis
Animal	Avian influenza, Nipah virus, Hantaan virus, MERS	Q fever, tularemia, plague, SARS
Dust exposure (e.g., caves or deserts)	Coccidioimycosis, histoplasmosis	
Cruise ships/resorts	Legionella	
Rural/Farm	Q fever	
Soil	Strongyloidiasis, hookworm, ascariasis	Melioidosis
Fresh-water exposure	Schistosomiasis, leptospirosis	
Ingestion		
Undercooked/ raw food		Paragonimus, toxocariasis, hydatidosis
Sexual exposure	HIV	
Host factors		
Immunocompromised	Tuberculosis	

SARS severe acute respiratory syndrome, *MERS* Middle Eastern respiratory syndrome, *HIV* human immunodeficiency virus

the risk of acquiring the illness depends on season of travel and length of stay in affected areas [13].

In this review, we will discuss various pulmonary infections that are more common in returned travellers. A clear and thorough approach to a symptomatic returned traveller is an essential skill for the acute/general physician and general practitioner (Table 4). Particular attention should be given to infections that may spread by human-to-human transmission. Clinicians should be aware of where to source information should they suspect a travel-related infection or if they have concerns for public health. Infections related to travel are constantly evolving and it is important for clinicians to remain up to date with current disease outbreaks and management recommendations.

Table 2 Incubation periods of pulmonary infections

Incubation Period	Infection
Short (<10 days)	Viral: influenza, SARS, MERS, Nipah Bacterial: common organisms causing pneumonia (*Streptococcus pneumoniae, Haemophilus influenzae*), melioidosis, Legionellosis, plague, pertussis, diphtheria Fungal: histoplasmosis
Medium (10–21 days)	Viral: MERS, Nipah, hantavirus Bacterial: pertussis, melioidosis Fungal: histoplasmosis, coccidioidomycosis Eosinophilic: ascariasis, hookworm, strongyloides, toxocariasis
Long (>21 days)	Bacterial: Q fever, TB Eosinophilic: schistosomiasis, hydatidosis, dirofilariasis, paragonomiasis, *Wuchereia bancrofti, Brugia malayi*

SARS severe acute respiratory syndrome, *MERS* Middle Eastern respiratory syndrome, *TB* tuberculosis

Pulmonary infections caused by viruses and bacteria

Upper pulmonary infections are more common than lower pulmonary infections. In general, the types of pulmonary infections that affect travellers are similar to those in non-travellers, and exotic causes are rare [2, 13, 14]. An Australian study collected data over a 3-year period; it showed around 28% of Australian travellers returning from Asia developed an acute pulmonary infection within 72 h (defined as an illness episode involving the presence of at least two upper pulmonary symptoms; e.g., sore-throat, coryza). This translates to an incidence of 106.4 per 10,000 traveller days. PCR testing on these travellers was analyzed for influenza A and B virus, adenoviruses, respiratory syncytial virus (RSV), picornaviruses and para-influenza viruses 1, 2, and 3. Only 1% of these travellers acquired influenza A virus, with no data for the other detectable viruses included [15].

There is evidence that contracting a common upper pulmonary virus potentiates the risk of contracting a tropical disease as well. A study in 2008 [16] showed that during an epidemic of chikungunya in India, 87% of confirmed cases were also co-infected with RSV and another upper respiratory virus, 41% were co-infected with RSV alone and 9% were co-infected with influenza virus and adenovirus. It is likely that a parallel outbreak of pulmonary viral infections during this time resulted in higher morbidity and mortality during this epidemic.

Bacterial pathogens are generally not related directly to a particular travel destination. *Streptococcus pneumoniae, Mycoplasma pneumoniae, Haemophilus influenzae,* and *Chlamydophila pneumoniae* are the most common organisms known to cause pneumonia throughout the world and risk of infection is not directly related to travel. More specific illnesses caused by *C. burnettii* (Q fever), *Legionella pneumophila* (Legionella), *Bordetella Pertussis* (pertussis), *Corynebacterium diphtheriae* (diphtheria) and *Leptospira* (leptospirosis) are normally a result of an epidemic within a country [2, 10, 14]. This list may be very relevant to the treating clinician.

Travel to international mass gatherings is a proven risk factor for the spread of pulmonary infection. For example, during pilgrimage to Mecca, pneumonia caused by *S. pneumoniae* is the leading cause of hospitalization and intensive care unit admissions during the Hajj (nearly 40% of patients). Out of 300 participants less than 5% had been vaccinated despite 65% being eligible.

Table 3 Causes of pulmonary infections associated with specific geographical areas

Geographical Area	Common	Occasional	Rare but important
Sub-Saharan Africa	HIV-associated pulmonary infections, TB	Katayama syndrome, tropical pulmonary eosinophilia (*Wuchereia bancrofti*), Loeffler's syndrome (hookworm, strongyloides) hydatidosis	Histoplasmosis, pneumonic plague, paragonomiasis
North Africa, Middle East and Mediterranean		Q fever, tropical pulmonary eosinophilia (*Wuchereia bancrofti)* Loeffler's syndrome (hookworm, ascariasis, strongyloides) hydatidosis, toxocariasis	MERS
Eastern Europe and Scandinavia	Legionellosis	Pertussis, toxocariasis	Hantavirus, tularemia
South and Central Asia	diphtheria, TB, avian flu	Melioidosis, Loeffler's syndrome (hookworm, ascariasis, strongyloides) hydatidosis	Nipah virus
Southeast Asia	avian flu	Melioidosis, tropical pulmonary eosinophilia (*Brugia malayi*), Loeffler's syndrome (strongyloides, hookworm), leptospirosis, diphtheria	SARS, hantavirus, Nipah virus, dirofilariasis, Katayama syndrome, paragonomiasis
Northern Australia		Q fever	Melioidosis, dirofilarisis, pertussis
Latin America and Caribbean		Coccidioidomycosis histoplasmosis, leptospirosis, diphtheria, tropical pulmonary eosinophilia (*Wuchereia bancrofti*), Loeffler's syndrome (ascariasis, strongyloides), hydatidosis, toxocariasis	Hantavirus, dirofilariasis
North America	Legionellosis, pertussis, diphtheria	Coccidioidomycosis histoplasmosis, toxocariasis	Dirofilariasis, Q fever

HIV human immunodeficiency virus, *SARS* severe acute respiratory syndrome, *MERS* Middle Eastern respiratory syndrome, *TB* tuberculosis

Improved pre-travel vaccination advice could prevent diseases for many travellers [12].

Influenza

Particular attention should be paid to travellers returning from influenza-endemic areas, taking into account newly reported sub-types. The burden of influenza occurs in the winter months in temperate regions, in the Northern Hemisphere from November to April and the Southern Hemisphere from April to October. In the tropics, the virus circulates at a low level all year round [17]. Influenza is diagnosed from viral throat swabs using real time PCR (rt-PCR) that can differentiate particular influenza sub-types [18].

Avian influenza sub-type H5N1 virus has caused death in humans since 1997, predominately in Asia and North East Africa, with a current upsurge of cases in Egypt. From 2003 to October 2015, there have been a total of 844 laboratory-confirmed cases with mortality rates of more than 50% [19]. H7N9 is the most recently reported sub-type. It was first diagnosed in March 2013 in China and is characterized by rapidly progressive pneumonia, pulmonary failure and acute pulmonary distress syndrome (ARDS) [18]. As of October 2015, there have been 679 laboratory-confirmed cases, with 275 reported deaths [19].

Table 4 Checklist for taking a travel history

Questions	Examples
Country of travel and accommodation	Latent diseases, possible exposures
Occupation, hobbies, activities	Healthcare worker, business, visiting relatives, farmer, cave explorer, water exposure
Prophylaxis	Immunizations, prophylaxis, insect repellents
Treatment or procedures	Hospital treatment in country, tattoos
Diet	Seafood, raw food
Sex	Unprotected sex, paid sex, multiple partners
Animals	Birds, domestic animals, wildlife

Treatment of influenza remains a controversial topic but generally supportive management is adopted. Current recommendations are early administration of a neuraminidase inhibitor (e.g., oseltamivir) to the affected individual and their close contacts [18]. A recent meta-analysis of the H1N1 pandemic showed that hospitalized patients treated with a neuraminidase inhibitor had a lower mortality, and that this was further reduced by early instigation [20].

Prevention of avian influenza has proved difficult due to the antigenic diversity of the circulating viruses, which has hampered vaccine development [21]. Healthcare professionals should take post-exposure prophylaxis (e.g., oseltamivir) after a patient has been diagnosed with avian influenza and personal protective equipment is highly recommended.

Severe acute respiratory syndrome (SARS) and Middle Eastern respiratory syndrome (MERS)

Like influenza, other viral epidemics are gathering publicity, heightening awareness and recognition worldwide. MERS and SARS are zoonotic coronavirus infections with regular media coverage due to their symptom severity, associated mortality rates and anxiety regarding potential human-to-human transmission. Bats are thought to be the main intermediate host for both viruses, while there is compelling evidence that camels are also responsible for transmission of the MERS coronavirus [22, 23].

SARS was first reported as an atypical pneumonia to the World Health Organization (WHO) in November 2002 in China and subsequently spread worldwide. The first reported epidemic occurred in a Hong Kong hotel in February 2003. The virus was transmitted to 16 hotel guests who were staying on the same floor as an infected individual, and the virus spread through international air travel thereafter. WHO identified the coronavirus responsible through nasopharyngeal culture within 2 weeks of this event. More than 30 countries reported affected individuals, with more than 8,000 confirmed cases worldwide and a 9.6% mortality rate [24].

The pulmonary symptoms associated with SARS (typically, non-productive cough and subsequent dyspnea) did not present until several days after initial exposure to the virus. As SARS is caused by an airborne virus, the risk of transmission was greatest amongst those involved in the direct care of an infected individual. Since no medications effectively treated SARS, interrupting transmission was the key to controlling the outbreak. Simple public health measures, such as wearing surgical masks, offered the most effective protection against transmission and there were no further confirmed cases as of July 2003 [24].

The public health lessons learned during the SARS epidemic have proved invaluable in limiting the spread of MERS cases worldwide. MERS was first recognized in September 2012 and, as of October 2015, 1,611 cases have been reported with more than 570 related deaths [25]. To date, the largest cluster of cases to occur outside of the Middle East was reported in South Korea in May 2015. The index case was a businessman who developed pulmonary symptoms upon returning from a trip to the Middle East. A total of 185 cases were identified, with 36 deaths (19.5% mortality rate) [26]. This proved the migrating capabilities of the virus and potential for outbreaks worldwide. Any clinician who sees an individual returning from the Middle East presenting with fever and pulmonary symptoms within 14 days of travel should consider MERS as a diagnosis and prompt investigations (diagnosed by nasopharyngeal culture) and public health control methods should be initiated. No specific treatments or vaccine have been developed to date.

As with most infections, the groups with the poorest outcomes related to MERS infection are the young (<12 years), the elderly (>65 years), immunocompromised patients and those with multiple co-morbidities [22]. Clinically, presentation is similar to SARS but MERS has a longer incubation period and greater severity of pulmonary symptoms and an even higher mortality risk. All cases of MERS confirmed worldwide to date have had a direct or indirect link with the Middle East—predominately Saudi Arabia. It has proven to be less contagious than SARS so far, although it is expected that a more virulent virus will evolve.

The plague

Where SARS and MERS have attracted much media coverage, it should not be forgotten that the plague bacillus (*Yersinia pestis*) still affects a great number of people each year [27]. The pneumonic plague has seen endemic outbreaks in certain parts of Africa, with sporadic cases occurring worldwide.

Historically, there have been 3 pandemics involving the bubonic (swollen, painful lymph nodes) and pneumonic plague in the 6th century, the 14th century and the 19th century; however, it also re-emerged in the 1990s with a more limited distribution [27].

The pneumonic plague occurs as a complication of the bubonic plague and is the only form capable of transmission from human-to-human via pulmonary droplets. Clinical sequelae are a dry cough within 24 h of first exposure, which becomes productive before hemoptysis occurs with the sputum becoming increasingly more bloodied within the next 24–48 h—this is a sign of certain mortality. The major clinical clues in diagnosing the pneumonic plague are travel history, rapid onset of symptoms (sometimes hours from being asymptomatic to fever and cough/hemoptysis) and bilateral pneumonia [27, 28]. The patient is most contagious when hemoptysis develops; simple protective measures, such as wearing masks, help prevent transmission [28].

The last reported outbreak of the pneumonic plague was in Madagascar in September 2014. There were 263 reported cases, with a 26.9% mortality rate. The plague has been endemic on the island for the past 30 years—it is the most severely affected country in the world [29].

While developing countries are at most risk of outbreaks of the disease, sporadic cases can occur elsewhere. Four patients were diagnosed in July 2014 with pneumonic plague in Colorado, United States of America (USA). The index patient contracted the disease from his pet dog. No deaths occurred and all patients rapidly responded to antibiotic treatment; streptomycin, tetracyclines and sulphonamides are used as the standard antibiotics, with gentamicin and fluoroquinolones as alternatives [30]. All close contacts should be given prophylactic antibiotics and monitored for symptoms.

The plague bacillus has previously been used in biological warfare during the 20th century. *Yersinia Pestis* is an attractive agent due to easy accessibility, simple culture needs and transmission via aerosol [31]. It is important point to note that a plague outbreak can be easily controlled with simple public health measures and readily available antibiotics; however, if inappropriately managed the pneumonic plague is almost certainly fatal.

Hantaan and Nipah viruses

Two viral infections noted to be causing outbreaks throughout the world are the Hantaan (causing hantavirus cardiopulmonary syndrome [HPS]) and Nipah viruses. Both diseases were microscopically discovered in the 1990s and are zoonotic; they are transmitted to humans via rodents and via bats and pigs, respectively. Both have a range of clinical symptoms and may present with flu-like symptoms continuing onto encephalitis with Nipah virus or pulmonary failure and cardiogenic shock in Hantavirus-related infections [32, 33].

The first Nipah outbreak was in Malaysia in 1999; a total of 276 cases were diagnosed with a 38.4% mortality rate [34]. The outbreak spread into Singapore and it was discovered that the virus was transmitted to humans from pigs; this resulted in a cull of more than 1 million pigs to control the outbreak. Since then, outbreaks have occurred in Bangladesh and India with a mortality rate of around 75% [35]. Most cases presented with pulmonary symptoms (cough, dyspnea and bilateral opacities covering the majority of the lung fields on chest radiograph) and there was a higher human-to-human transmission rate in comparison to the Malaysian outbreak [36]. The Nipah virus was readily identified in the saliva of infected patients, allowing easy disease transmission.

There have only been outbreaks of the Nipah virus in South East Asia to date, but there is potential for this disease to occur in other countries. The intermediate host (fruit bats from the *Pteropodidae* family) has an extensive habitat distribution and is native to parts of Africa and northern Australia [37]. The treatment is limited to supportive care—control methods to prevent human-to-human transmission are very important to stop rapid spread. Studies have shown the antiviral drug ribavirin may reduce mortality from the infection [33].

At present, more than 21 Hantaviruses from the *Bunyaviridae* family have been identified as causing illness in humans. Signs of infection range from proteinuria to pulmonary edema and frank hemorrhagic illnesses [32]. HPS is most likely to occur in the Americas although there are sporadic case reports from Europe [38]. The disease is most likely to be transmitted in areas where sanitation is poor or in rural farming areas. Rodents shed the virus in their urine, droppings and saliva, and the virus is transmitted between humans via pulmonary droplets [32].

The first reported outbreak occurred in 1993 in the USA, although retrospectively it seems the Hantaviruses have been causing fatal pulmonary illnesses since the 1950s [39]. The cluster of around 30 cases in 1993 occurred in an area of southwest USA known as the 'Four Corners'. Clinicians identified a series of cases of a severe and acute pulmonary illness affecting young healthy adults where non-cardiogenic pulmonary edema developed rapidly. To date, more than 600 cases of HPS have been reported in the USA [40]. In 2012, the virus was discovered at Yosemite National Park where potentially hundreds of travellers were exposed to the infection. Ten cases of HPS were confirmed, 3 of which were fatal [41].

Treatment for Hantavirus remains supportive. Intravenous fluids should be used with caution, as aggressive fluid resuscitation is likely to accelerate the progression to pulmonary edema and failure due to capillary leakage [32]. Extracorporeal membrane oxygenation (ECMO) treatment has dramatically reduced mortality rates [42]. The benefits of ribavirin therapy remain undetermined due to small trial numbers [43]. To date, only one Hantavirus has evolved to transmit via human-to-human contact (the Andes virus, named after its geographical discovery location in 1996).

Accurate diagnosis requires a high degree of suspicion and should be considered in an individual presenting from a recent stay in North or South America with rapidly progressing pulmonary symptoms and/or signs [32]. The risk to a traveller in contracting any of the above outbreak diseases remains small given their limited geographical distribution at present. The risk of exposure may be increased by several factors (Table 1) such as activities undertaken, close contact with an infected individual, and not seeking appropriate pre-travel information or recommendations. As a clinician it is important to have up-to-date knowledge on current outbreaks occurring worldwide and their relevant geography as prompt recognition and diagnosis may prevent an epidemic.

Q fever

Q fever, caused by *C. burnettii*, is a worldwide zoonotic disease. Outbreaks in humans have been linked to abattoirs and carriage of *C. burnettii* by wind from farms of affected animals. Ticks can also act as a reservoir. It is not strictly a travel-related illness but it is most likely found in areas where contamination with animal waste is common. It presents as an acute febrile illness with non-specific signs such as atypical pneumonia [8]. Rural travelling is the greatest risk factor for acquiring the disease. Most recently, Q fever outbreaks have occurred in Hungary, where 70 cases were confirmed by micro-immunofluorescence testing and treated with 3 weeks of a tetracycline. No deaths occurred. Efforts to reduce the spread of Q fever after an outbreak include elimination of manure and disinfection of affected farms [8].

Legionella

Legionella (*L. pneumophila)* is a bacterium that can cause anything from a mild febrile illness to the potentially fatal form of pneumonia known as Legionnaires' disease. The bacterium is ubiquitous in the environment, and the same agent causes sporadic cases and outbreaks. Outbreaks are typically linked to contaminated water systems where conditions are ideal for rapid growth of the organism [44]. In 2014, the WHO confirmed 302 cases of Legionellosis in Lisbon, Portugal, that were related to a contaminated industrial cooling tower, with 5 deaths as a result of the disease [45]. Most cases are reported after travel to developed countries in Europe or North America. At risk individuals are those with comorbidities, the elderly, smokers and the immunosuppressed. It is caused by inhalation of aerosols containing the bacterium and accounts for 2–15% of hospital admissions for community-acquired pneumonia, with a summer or autumn peak [45]. Identification of affected individuals is by urinary PCR and treatment is with a macrolide antibiotic [46].

Pertussis and diphtheria

Pertussis and diphtheria are vaccine-preventable pulmonary infections; poor vaccine uptake has led to a recent increase in cases in developed countries. It is important, therefore, to take a full vaccination history in returned travellers who present with pulmonary symptoms [47].

Pertussis is a worldwide endemic-epidemic disease with outbreaks most likely during summer/autumn time. Pertussis is thought to still cause around 63,000 deaths per year in children under 5 years of age, although there is uncertainty over these estimates in view of the paucity of reliable surveillance data [48].

Recently, there has been an increase in the number of adolescent and young adults being diagnosed in some high-income countries, likely due to decreased vaccination uptake rates and a change in the vaccine itself. It is thought that the acellular vaccine currently used appears to have a short-lived immunity leading to increased infection rates [49]. Macrolide antibiotics are given to affected individuals to prevent further spread of pertussis [49].

Diphtheria presents as an acute infectious disease affecting the upper pulmonary tract caused by toxins produced by the bacterium. Characteristic features are membranous pharyngitis with fever, enlarged anterior cervical lymph nodes and edema of the soft tissues of the neck [50]. This manifestation may lead to airway obstruction. The bacterium has a short incubation period but untreated individuals may remain infectious for up to 4 weeks. Both pertussis and diphtheria are potentially fatal but easily preventable.

Leptospirosis

Leptospirosis is contracted either through direct contact with infected animal urine, or urine-contaminated water [10]. It can be found worldwide, but is predominantly found in tropical and subtropical countries (during rainy season). Those taking part in water sports are most at risk (an outbreak was reported among canyoning participants in Martinique, France) [51]. Increased cases are also found in rural parts of a country where drinking water can be easily contaminated with the bacteria; for example, where wells have been poorly constructed [52]. Lately, there has been an increase in the number of cases noted in Europe, with 97 cases identified in the Netherlands in 2014 (4.6-fold increase in comparison to previous years). Dutch tourists reported 33 cases of leptospirosis, and most of these tourists acquired the disease in Thailand [53].

The clinical course of leptospirosis is variable, with symptoms from myalgia to fever with cough and shortness of breath. Weil's disease is its severest form and may develop in 1–5% of cases. Patients progress from mild flu-like symptoms to signs of organ failure (jaundice and spontaneous bleeding) [54].

Where there is a high degree of clinical suspicion for leptospirosis, treatment should be instigated. Diagnosis is serological (via microscopic agglutination test [MAT] for antibodies or PCR urine antigen test) but it may take around 10 days after the onset of symptoms for these tests to become positive [10]. In early mild disease, penicillin and tetracycline antibiotics are effective [55]. Where the clinically more severe Weil's disease is manifest, patients may require organ support, and there is little evidence that antibiotic use is of any benefit at this stage [56]. In 2014, there were a total of 76 confirmed cases of leptospirosis in England and Wales, of which 22 were acquired overseas; the majority of these were related to recreational water exposure [57].

Tularemia

Recreational activities such as camping and visiting rural and agricultural areas lead to increased risk to exposure to the bacterium that causes tularemia [58]. Typically found in the Northern Hemisphere, the number of infected cases are underestimated and underreported [58]. Outbreaks have been reported on Martha's Vineyard (Massachusetts, USA), Sweden and Finland in the last 15 years [58].

Francisella tularensis is the bacterium responsible for what is a potentially fatal multi-systemic disease. Reservoirs of transmission are via ticks, biting flies, aerosol, water exposure and food [58]. There are 4 identified subtypes and clinical presentation depends on biotype, method of transmission and port of entry. There are 6 major clinical presentations: ulceroglandular, glandular, oculoglandular, oropharyngeal, pneumonic and typhoidal [58]. Pulmonary features may consist of lobar pneumonia, pulmonary effusions, infiltrates and hilar lymphadenopathy. Mortality in untreated pneumonic tularemia can be up to 60% [59].

Early diagnosis and treatment is key to prognosis, but isolation of the bacterium is hazardous and time consuming and most laboratories do not accept samples for culture [60]. Agglutination and enzyme-linked immunosorbent assay (ELISA) tests are the diagnostic tests of choice [58]. Aminoglycosides are bactericidal against *F. tularensis* and WHO recommend a 10-day course [61].

As an aside, *F. tularensis* subspecies tularensis (Type A) is one of the most infectious pathogens known to man, and these properties have led to tularemia being identified as a potential weapon of bioterrorism [60].

Melioidosis

In South East Asia and northern Australia, a particular Gram-negative organism called *B. pseudomallei* is responsible for an endemic of melioidosis disease [62]. Most commonly, the initial presentation is with low-grade fever and atypical pneumonia, rapidly progressing to multi-organ dysfunction. The mortality rate is very high, ranging from 14 to 40% in general and up to 80% with inappropriate antimicrobial therapy [9]. Difficulties in culturing the bacterium responsible mean that under-reporting is likely. The bacterium resides in soil and water with transmission occurring mainly from percutaneous inoculation and inhalation. Exposure is most likely to occur during the wet seasons in affected areas or after natural catastrophes such as tsunamis.

Sporadic cases of the infection are now being reported worldwide and manifestations of latent forms of the disease are appearing some tens of years after initial exposure [63]. As the number of international travellers continues to rise, particularly to more rural parts of South East Asia and northern Australia, this could lead to an increase in the number of travel-related melioidosis cases in the future.

Early recognition of melioidosis is essential as the bacterium is resistant to nearly all drugs given for community-acquired pneumonia [63]. Current treatment recommendations are ceftazidime or a carbapenem, followed by eradication therapy with trimethoprim and sulfamethoxazole for at least 3 months. There has been recent interest in vaccine development due to both public health and bioweapon concerns [64]. Mouse model vaccination has proved successful but to date there has been no testing on humans [64].

Tuberculosis (TB)

TB is a commonly found disease in certain parts of the world. The risk of TB as a travel-related disease has not been well established. A study from Italy in 2005 concluded that over half of returned travellers with pneumonia or TB presented with a febrile illness but no pulmonary symptoms [65]. TB can be transmitted on airplanes; a flight from Baltimore to Honolulu showed 4 of 15 passengers had a positive tuberculin skin test after sitting in close proximity to a passenger with pulmonary TB [6]. An overall probability of infection is 1 in 1,000 when a symptomatic source is present in close proximity [6].

Risk is linked to longer-term travel to areas of higher prevalence and proximity to affected individuals. Those most at risk would be healthcare workers or individuals visiting relatives [66]. TB risk in long-term travellers (of greater than 3 months) is the same as the local population in high endemic areas. A Dutch study showed there was substantial risk to long-term travellers with an overall incidence rate of 3.5 per 1,000 person-months travelled; however, no-one in this study had received a Bacillus Calmette–Guérin (BCG) vaccine prior to travelling, therefore incidence amongst those who have been vaccinated is likely to be lower [66].

In recent years, multidrug-resistant TB (MDR-TB) and extensively drug-resistant TB (XDR-TB) have become increasingly important public health problems in many countries (Eastern Europe, parts of Asia and Southern Africa) [67]. The potential risk of transmission of particularly dangerous forms of TB requires renewed vigilance. Since 2006, WHO have been informed of several incidences of patients travelling (short-haul) by air with MDR-TB and XDR-TB. In these cases, only close family members have been later diagnosed with the disease, but a potential risk to other travellers is possible given the infectious nature of these strains of TB [67]. WHO have since published guidelines for TB and air travel to prevent the spread of the disease [67].

The main advice to clinicians is that the number of TB infections is increasing, as are MDR-TB and XDR-TB disease. The risks to most travellers in contracting TB are small but increase depending on vaccination status, length of travel, mode of travel and travel destination. If pulmonary symptoms persist, despite negative standard microscopy, culture and sensitivity testing, TB should be added to the differential diagnosis list and should be investigated appropriately.

Pulmonary infections caused by fungi

Fungal infections in the absence of immunosuppression generally occur in the Americas, where the exact destination of the traveller plays an important role in distinguishing the fungus responsible.

Histoplasmosis and coccidioidomycosis

Histoplasmosis should be considered in travellers returning from the Midwest and central states of North America, throughout Latin America and Central and

Western Africa [68–70]. In 2013, approximately 300 cases were reported in the South West region of China, the first to be reported in Asia [68].

Coccidioidomycosis (Valley fever) has long been recognized as a travel-related mycosis. Endemic areas are in Southern California, Arizona and Central and South America [69]. In returned travellers when common causes for flu-like illness, non-productive cough and pleuritic chest pain have been ruled out but symptoms continue to persist, an underlying fungal infection should be considered as a differential diagnosis.

Histoplasma capsulatum is endemic in North and Latin America, while *H. dubiosii* is mainly found in Central and Western Africa [70]. The organism grows in soils enriched with bat and bird droppings, and human infection generally occurs after dust inhalation of disturbed soil. The incubation period is relatively short, and symptoms develop within 2 weeks of exposure [69]. Reticulonodular shadowing on chest radiograph is common, often with mediastinal lymphadenopathy. Detection of the histoplasma antibody in urine or serum is the most sensitive and widely used diagnostic method [70]. Detection of coccidioidomycosis (*Coccidioides immitis)* is similar but radiologically a cavitating pneumonia may be seen [69].

In healthy individuals, fungal infections are generally self-limiting. In those who are immunocompromised, and/or go on to develop severe infection with systemic complications, antifungals have been proven to be effective [70]. In contrast to histoplasmosis, coccidioidomycosis infection generally leads to acquired immunity therefore recurrence is unlikely [69].

Pulmonary infections caused by helminths

Pulmonary symptoms such as wheeze, breathlessness and hemoptysis and an eosinophilia in a returned traveller should prompt investigations for helminths. These infections may present as Loeffler's syndrome (a result of larval migration through the lungs) or tropical pulmonary eosinophilia (hypersensitivity to lymphatic filarial worms). Specific to schistosomiasis infections, Katayama syndrome should be suspected in travellers returning from Africa or South East Asia with fresh water exposure presenting with fever, eosinophilia, dry cough and urticarial rash. Other rare pulmonary presentation of helminths infections (such as paragonimus, toxocariasis and dirofilariasis) should be considered depending on travel destination and incubation period [71]. Treatment of these infections is generally straightforward once the causative helminths have been identified.

In 20% of hydatidosis (echinococcosis tapeworm) there are pulmonary infiltrations. The majority of cases are asymptomatic but following a leaking hydatid cyst in the liver, patients may present with pleuritic chest pain, breathlessness and cough; a 'water lily' sign may be seen on chest radiograph [72]. Surgery (aspiration) and anti-parasitic drugs are required to fully treat the infection.

Conclusion

The clinical spectrum of pulmonary infections in the returned traveller is vast. History taking is paramount (exact dates, contacts, length of stay, place of travel and timings of onset of symptoms) and a high degree of suspicion early on in the patient's management is vital. Most cases of pulmonary infections in travellers are mild and self-limiting but travel-specific pulmonary infections have high mortality rates if interventions are not prompt.

The main modes of transmission for pulmonary infections are by droplets or direct contact, hence the importance of implementing protective barriers and involving public health colleagues early to prevent further transmission. Advice is always available from online resources and specialist centers—as a clinician it is important to familiarize yourself with guidelines and protocols on travel-related infections. The WHO and Centers for Disease Control and Prevention (CDC) are continually updating guidelines on travel-related infections.

Search strategy

We identified references for this review by searches in different databases (PubMed, Ovid MEDLINE, Embase and Cochrane) and references from relevant articles. The following MeSH headings were used: "pulmonary", "respiratory", "tropical disease" 'travellers", "travel", "returning traveller".

The references were all further assessed by reading the title and abstract. Only articles published in English were included. We further assessed the references of all selected publications. The final reference list was generated on the basis of relevance to the topics covered in this review.

Funding

The authors have no support or funding to report.

Authors' contributions

All authors met ICMJE authorship criteria. AT, AC conceived and designed the research plan. AT, VM contributed to the acquisition, analysis and interpretation of the data. AT, VM, AC contributed equally to the writing of the first draft of the manuscript and writing of the manuscript. AT, VM, AC critically reviewed the manuscript for important intellectual content and agreed with the manuscript results and conclusions. All authors read and approved the final manuscript.

Competing interests

The authors declare that they have no competing interests.

Provenance

Commissioned; externally peer reviewed.

Text box

Where to look for help

British Infection Association (BIA), for United Kingdom recommendations and guidelines: www.britishinfection.org/

Centers for Disease Control and Prevention (CDC): www.cdc.gov/

National Travel Health Network and Centre: www.nathnac.org/

ProMED-mail (electronic reporting system for infectious diseases outbreaks): www.promedmail.org/

Travax, United Kingdom NHS National Services Scotland website: http://www.travax.nhs.uk

World Health Organization outbreak data: www.who.int/csr/don/en/

Author details

[1]Crosshouse Hospital, Kilmarnock Road, Crosshouse KA2 0BE, UK. [2]Respiratory Infection Group, Liverpool School of Tropical Medicine, Pembroke Place, Liverpool L3 5QA, UK. [3]Aintree Hospital, Longmoor Lane, Liverpool L9 7AL, UK. [4]Respiratory Research Group, Royal Liverpool and Broadgreen University Hospital Trust, Prescot Street, Liverpool L7 8XP, UK.

References

1. UNWTO. Annual Report 2013. UNWTO; 2013. Available from: http://www2.unwto.org/publication/unwto-annual-report-2013. Accessed 1 Nov 2015.
2. Korzeniewski K, Nitsch-Osuch A, Lass A, Guzek A. Respiratory infections in travelers returning from the tropics. Adv Exp Med Biol. 2015;849:75–82. PMID:25381557, http://dx.doi.org/10.1007/5584_2014_89.
3. Hearn P, Johnston V. Assessment of returning travellers with fever. Medicine. 2014;42:66–72. doi:10.1016/j.mpmed.2013.11.009.
4. Gherardin A, Sisson J. Assessing fever in the returned traveller. Australian Prescriber An independent review. 2012;35(1):10.
5. Jennings LC, Priest PC, Psutka RA, Duncan AR, Anderson T, Mahagamasekera P, et al. Respiratory viruses in airline travellers with influenza symptoms: results of an airport screening study. J Clin Virol. 2015;67:8–13. PMID: 25959149, http://dx.doi.org/10.1016/j.jcv.2015.03.011.
6. Mangili A, Gendreau MA. Transmission of infectious diseases during commercial air travel. Lancet. 2005;365:989–96. PMID:15767002, doi:10.1016/S0140-6736(05)71089-8.
7. Ansart S, Pajot O, Grivois JP, Zeller V, Klement E, Perez L, et al. Pneumonia among travelers returning from abroad. J Travel Med. 2004;11:87–91. PMID: 15109472, http://dx.doi.org/10.2310/7060.2004.17055.
8. Gyuranecz M, Sulyok K, Balla E, Mag T, Balazs A, Simor Z, et al. Q fever epidemic in Hungary, april to july 2013. Euro Surveill. 2014;19. PMID: 25108535, http://dx.doi.org/10.2807/1560-7917.ES2014.19.30.20863.
9. Saïdani N, Griffiths K, Million M, Gautret P, Dubourg G, Parola P, et al. Melioidosis as a travel-associated infection: case report and review of the literature. Travel Med Infect Dis. 2015;13:367–81. PMID:26385170, http://dx.doi.org/10.1016/j.tmaid.2015.08.007.
10. Johnston V, Stockley JM, Dockrell D, Warrell D, Bailey R, Pasvol G, British Infection Society and the Hospital for Tropical Diseases, et al. Fever in returned travellers presenting in the United Kingdom: recommendations for investigation and initial management. J Infect. 2009;59:1–18. PMID: 19595360, http://dx.doi.org/10.1016/j.jinf.2009.05.005.
11. Cadorna-Carlos JB, Nolan T, Borja-Tabora CF, Santos J, Montalban MC, de Looze FJ, et al. Safety, immunogenicity, and lot-to-lot consistency of a quadrivalent inactivated influenza vaccine in children, adolescents, and adults: a randomized, controlled, phase III trial. Vaccine. 2015;33:2485–92. PMID:25843270, http://dx.doi.org/10.1016/j.vaccine.2015.03.065.
12. Sridhar S, Belhouchat K, Drali T, Benkouiten S, Parola P, Brouqui P, et al. French Hajj pilgrims' experience with pneumococcal infection and vaccination: a knowledge, attitudes and practice (KAP) evaluation. Travel Med Infect Dis. 2015;13:251–5. PMID:25725996, http://dx.doi.org/10.1016/j.tmaid.2015.02.002.
13. Leder K, Sundararajan V, Weld L, Pandey P, Brown G, Torresi J, Groupa GSS. Respiratory tract infections in travelers: a review of the GeoSentinel surveillance network. Clin Infect Dis. 2003;36:399–406. PMID:12567296, http://dx.doi.org/10.1086/346155.
14. O'Brien DP, Leder K, Matchett E, Brown GV, Torresi J. Illness in returned travelers and immigrants/refugees: the 6-year experience of two Australian infectious diseases units. J Travel Med. 2006;13:145–52. PMID:16706945, http://dx.doi.org/10.1111/j.1708-8305.2006.00033.x.
15. Ratnam I, Black J, Leder K, Biggs BA, Gordon I, Matchett E, et al. Incidence and risk factors for acute respiratory illnesses and influenza virus infections in Australian travellers to Asia. J Clin Virol. 2013;57:54–8. PMID:23380660, http://dx.doi.org/10.1016/j.jcv.2013.01.008.
16. Sankari T, Hoti SL, Govindaraj V, Das PK. Chikungunya and respiratory viral infections. Lancet Infect Dis. 2008;8:3–4. PMID:18156080, doi:10.1016/S1473-3099(07)70295-5.
17. Harper SA, Fukuda K, Uyeki TM, Cox NJ, Bridges CB, Centers for Disease Control and Prevention (CDC) Advisory Committee on Immunization Practices (ACIP). Prevention and control of influenza: recommendations of the Advisory Committee on Immunization Practices (ACIP). MMWR Recomm Rep. 2004;53(RR-6):1–40. PMID:15163927.
18. Li Q, Zhou L, Zhou M, Chen Z, Li F, Wu H, et al. Epidemiology of human infections with avian influenza A(H7N9) virus in China. N Engl J Med. 2014; 370:520–32. PMID:23614499, http://dx.doi.org/10.1056/NEJMoa1304617.
19. Influenza at the human-animal interface: World Health Organization. Available from: http://www.who.int/influenza/human_animal_interface/about/en/. Accessed 10 May 2016.
20. Muthuri SG, Venkatesan S, Myles PR, Leonardi-Bee J, Al Khuwaitir TS, Al Mamun A, PRIDE Consortium Investigators, et al. Effectiveness of neuraminidase inhibitors in reducing mortality in patients admitted to hospital with influenza A H1N1pdm09 virus infection: a meta-analysis of individual participant data. Lancet Respir Med. 2014;2:395–404. PMID: 24815805, doi:10.1016/S2213-2600(14)70041-4.
21. Hala IA, Nagwa FE. Human pandemic threat by H5N1 (avian influenza). Afr J Microbiol Res. 2014;8:406–10. http://dx.doi.org/10.5897/AJMR10.303.
22. Al-Tawfiq JA, Zumla A, Memish ZA. Travel implications of emerging coronaviruses: SARS and MERS-CoV. Travel Med Infect Dis. 2014;12:422–8. PMID:25047726, http://dx.doi.org/10.1016/j.tmaid.2014.06.007.
23. Hui DS, Memish ZA, Zumla A. Severe acute respiratory syndrome vs. the Middle East respiratory syndrome. Curr Opin Pulm Med. 2014;20:233–41. PMID:24626235, http://dx.doi.org/10.1097/MCP.0000000000000046.
24. Parashar UD, Anderson LJ. Severe acute respiratory syndrome: review and lessons of the 2003 outbreak. Int J Epidemiol. 2004;33:628–34. PMID: 15155694, http://dx.doi.org/10.1093/ije/dyh198.
25. WHO. Middle East respiratory syndrome coronavirus (MERS-CoV): World Health Organization; 2015. [Updated 2015-12-05 00:11:04]. Available from: http://www.who.int/emergencies/mers-cov/en/. Accessed 1 Nov 2015.
26. WPRO. Middle East respiratory syndrome coronavirus (MERS-CoV): WPRO | WHO Western Pacific Region; 2015 [updated 2015-09-13 08:54:51. Available from: http://www.wpro.who.int/outbreaks_emergencies/wpro_coronavirus/en/. Accessed 1 Nov 2015.
27. Stenseth NC, Atshabar BB, Begon M, Belmain SR, Bertherat E, Carniel E, et al. Plague: past, present, and future. PLoS Med. 2008;5, e3. PMID:18198939, http://dx.doi.org/10.1371/journal.pmed.0050003.
28. Kool JL. Risk of person-to-person transmission of pneumonic plague. Clin Infect Dis. 2005;40:1166–72. PMID:15791518, http://dx.doi.org/10.1086/428617.
29. WHO. Plague in Madagascar: World Health Organization; 2015. [updated 2015-06-21 07:05:15.] Available from: http://www.who.int/csr/disease/plague/madagascar-outbreak/en/. Accessed 10 Nov 2015.
30. Runfola JK, House J, Miller L, Colton L, Hite D, Hawley A, Centers for Disease Control and Prevention (CDC), et al. Outbreak of human pneumonic plague with dog-to-human and possible human-to-human transmission–Colorado, june-july 2014. MMWR Morb Mortal Wkly Rep. 2015;64:429–34. PMID: 25928467.
31. Prentice MB, Rahalison L. Plague. Lancet. 2007;369:1196–207. PMID: 17416264, doi:10.1016/S0140-6736(07)60566-2.
32. Jonsson CB, Figueiredo LT, Vapalahti O. A global perspective on hantavirus ecology, epidemiology, and disease. Clin Microbiol Rev. 2010;23:412–41. PMID:20375360, http://dx.doi.org/10.1128/CMR.00062-09.
33. Chong HT, Kamarulzaman A, Tan CT, Goh KJ, Thayaparan T, Kunjapan SR, et al. Treatment of acute Nipah encephalitis with ribavirin. Ann Neurol. 2001;49:810–3. PMID:11409437, http://dx.doi.org/10.1002/ana.1062.

34. Chua KB, Lam SK, Goh KJ, Hooi PS, Ksiazek TG, Kamarulzaman A, et al. The presence of Nipah virus in respiratory secretions and urine of patients during an outbreak of Nipah virus encephalitis in Malaysia. J Infect. 2001;42: 40–3. PMID:11243752, http://dx.doi.org/10.1053/jinf.2000.0782.
35. SEARO. Nipah virus outbreaks in the WHO South-East Asia Region: SEARO | WHO South-East Asia Region; 2013. [updated 2013-02-11 12:10:49]. Available from: http://www.searo.who.int/entity/emerging_diseases/links/nipah_virus_outbreaks_sear/en/. Accessed 20 Nov 2015.
36. Luby SP, Gurley ES, Hossain MJ. Transmission of human infection with Nipah virus. Clin Infect Dis. 2009;49:1743–8. PMID:19886791, http://dx.doi.org/10.1086/647951.
37. Global_NiphaandHendraRisk_20090510.png (2027Ã—1358): World Health Organization; 2015. Available from: http://www.searo.who.int/entity/emerging_diseases/links/information_regarding_nipah_virus/en/. Accessed 20 Nov 2015.
38. Gizzi M, Delaere B, Weynand B, Clement J, Maes P, Vergote V, et al. Another case of "European hantavirus pulmonary syndrome" with severe lung, prior to kidney, involvement, and diagnosed by viral inclusions in lung macrophages. Eur J Clin Microbiol Infect Dis. 2013;32:1341–5. PMID: 23670277, http://dx.doi.org/10.1007/s10096-013-1885-x.
39. Zaki SR, Khan AS, Goodman RA, Armstrong LR, Greer PW, Coffield LM, et al. Retrospective diagnosis of hantavirus pulmonary syndrome, 1978–1993: implications for emerging infectious diseases. Arch Pathol Lab Med. 1996; 120:134–9. PMID:8712893.
40. CDC - Reported Cases of HPS - Hantavirus: centre for disease control. 2015. Available from: http://www.cdc.gov/hantavirus/surveillance/index.html. Accessed 20 Nov 2015.
41. Hartline J, Mierek C, Knutson T, Kang C. Hantavirus infection in North America: a clinical review. Am J Emerg Med. 2013;31:978–82. PMID: 23680331, http://dx.doi.org/10.1016/j.ajem.2013.02.001.
42. Crowley MR, Katz RW, Kessler R, Simpson SQ, Levy H, Hallin GW, et al. Successful treatment of adults with severe Hantavirus pulmonary syndrome with extracorporeal membrane oxygenation. Crit Care Med. 1998;26:409–14. PMID:9468181, http://dx.doi.org/10.1097/00003246-199802000-00047.
43. Mertz GJ, Miedzinski L, Goade D, Pavia AT, Hjelle B, Hansbarger CO, Collaborative Antiviral Study Group, et al. Placebo-controlled, double-blind trial of intravenous ribavirin for the treatment of hantavirus cardiopulmonary syndrome in North America. Clin Infect Dis. 2004;39:1307–13. PMID:15494907, http://dx.doi.org/10.1086/425007.
44. Falkinham 3rd JO, Hilborn ED, Arduino MJ, Pruden A, Edwards MA. Epidemiology and ecology of opportunistic premise plumbing pathogens: Legionella pneumophila, Mycobacterium avium, and Pseudomonas aeruginosa. Environ Health Perspect. 2015;123:749–58. PMID:25793551.
45. Sakamoto R. Legionnaire's disease, weather and climate. Bull World Health Organ. 2015;93:435–6. PMID:26240466, http://dx.doi.org/10.2471/BLT.14.142299.
46. Managing legionella in hot and cold water systems: health and safety executive. 2015. Available from: http://www.hse.gov.uk/healthservices/legionella.htm. Accessed 22 Nov 2015.
47. Larson HJ, Cooper LZ, Eskola J, Katz SL, Ratzan S. Addressing the vaccine confidence gap. Lancet. 2011;378:526–35. PMID:21664679, doi:10.1016/S0140-6736(11)60678-8.
48. WHO. Pertussis vaccines: WHO position paper - september 2015. Wkly Epidemiol Rec. 2015;90:433–58. PMID:26320265.
49. Carbonetti NH. Bordetella pertussis: new concepts in pathogenesis and treatment. Curr Opin Infect Dis. 2016;29:287–94. PMID:26906206, doi:10.1097/QCO.0000000000000264.
50. Burkovski A. Diphtheria and its etiological agents. In: Burkovski A, editor. Corynebacterium diphtheriae and related toxigenic species. Erlangen: Springer Netherlands; 2014. p. 1–14. doi:10.1007/978-94-077-7624-1_1.
51. Hochedez P, Escher M, Decoussy H, Pasgrimaud L, Martinez R, Rosine J, et al. utbreak of leptospirosis among canyoning participants, Martinique, 2011. Euro Surveill. 2013;18:20472. PMID:23725775.
52. Wynwood SJ, Graham GC, Weier SL, Collet TA, McKay DB, Craig SB. Leptospirosis from water sources. Pathog Glob Health. 2014;108:334–8. PMID:25348115, doi:10.1179/2047773214Y.0000000156.
53. Pijnacker R, Goris MG, Te Wierik MJ, Broens EM, van der Giessen JW, de Rosa M, et al. Marked increase in leptospirosis infections in humans and dogs in the Netherlands, 2014. Euro Surveill. 2016;21. PMID:27168584, http://dx.doi.org/10.2807/1560-7917.ES.2016.21.17.30211.
54. Health Care Workers | Leptospirosis | CDC: Centre for Disease Control. 2015. Available from: http://www.cdc.gov/leptospirosis/health_care_workers/index.html. Accessed 22 Nov 2015.
55. Katz AR, Ansdell VE, Effler PV, Middleton CR, Sasaki DM. Assessment of the clinical presentation and treatment of 353 cases of laboratory-confirmed leptospirosis in Hawaii, 1974–1998. Clin Infect Dis. 2001;33:1834–41. PMID: 11692294, http://dx.doi.org/10.1086/324084.
56. Brett-Major DM, Coldren R. Antibiotics for leptospirosis. Cochrane Database Syst Rev. 2012;2, CD008264. PMID:22336839.
57. Common animal associated infections quarterly report (England and Wales-fourth quarter 2014): Public Health England; 2015. Available from: https://www.gov.uk/government/publications/common-animalassociated-infections-quarterly-reports-2015. Accessed 22 Nov 2015.
58. Ulu-Kilic A, Doganay M. An overview: tularemia and travel medicine. Travel Med Infect Dis. 2014;12(6 Pt A):609–16. PMID:25457302, http://dx.doi.org/10.1016/j.tmaid.2014.10.007.
59. Cowley SC. Editorial: proinflammatory cytokines in pneumonic tularemia: too much too late? J Leukoc Biol. 2009;86:469–70. PMID:19720615, http://dx.doi.org/10.1189/jlb.0309119.
60. Tärnvik A, Chu MC. New approaches to diagnosis and therapy of tularemia. Ann N Y Acad Sci. 2007;1105:378–404. PMID:17468229, http://dx.doi.org/10.1196/annals.1409.017.
61. Clinicians | Tularemia | CDC: Centre for Disease Control. 2015. Available from: http://www.cdc.gov/tularemia/clinicians/index.html. Accessed 10 Nov 2015.
62. Hoffmaster AR, Aucoin D, Baccam P, Baggett HC, Baird R, Bhengsri S, et al. Melioidosis diagnostic workshop, 2013. Emerg Infect Dis. 2015;21. PMID: 25626057.
63. Fisher DA, Harris PN. Melioidosis: refining management of a tropical time bomb. Lancet. 2014;383:762–4. PMID:24284288, doi:10.1016/S0140-6736(13)62143-1.
64. Limmathurotsakul D, Funnell SG, Torres AG, Morici LA, Brett PJ, Dunachie S et al. Steering group on melioidosis vaccine development. Consensus on the development of vaccines against naturally acquired melioidosis. Emerg Infect Dis. 2015;21. PMID:25992835, http://dx.doi.org/10.3201/eid2106.141480.
65. Matteelli A, Beltrame A, Saleri N, Bisoffi Z, Allegri R, Volonterio A, SIRL Study Group, et al. Respiratory syndrome and respiratory tract infections in foreign-born and national travelers hospitalized with fever in Italy. J Travel Med. 2005;12:190–6. PMID:16086893, http://dx.doi.org/10.2310/7060.2005.12404.
66. Cobelens FG, van Deutekom H, Draayer-Jansen IW, Schepp-Beelen AC, van Gerven PJ, van Kessel RP, et al. Risk of infection with Mycobacterium tuberculosis in travellers to areas of high tuberculosis endemicity. Lancet. 2000;356:461–5. PMID:10981889, doi:10.1016/S0140-6736(00)02554-X.
67. Martinez L, Blanc L, Nunn P, Raviglione M. Tuberculosis and air travel: WHO guidance in the era of drug-resistant TB. Travel Med Infect Dis. 2008;6:177–81. PMID:18571104, http://dx.doi.org/10.1016/j.tmaid.2007.10.004.
68. Pan B, Chen M, Pan W, Liao W. Histoplasmosis: a new endemic fungal infection in China? Review and analysis of cases. Mycoses. 2013;56:212–21. PMID:23216676, http://dx.doi.org/10.1111/myc.12029.
69. Panackal AA, Hajjeh RA, Cetron MS, Warnock DW. Fungal infections among returning travelers. Clin Infect Dis. 2002;35:1088–95. PMID:12384843, http://dx.doi.org/10.1086/344061.
70. Information for Health Professionals about Histoplasmosis | Types of Diseases | Histoplasmosis | Fungal Disease | CDC: Centre for Disease Control. 2015. Available from: http://www.cdc.gov/fungal/diseases/histoplasmosis/health-professionals.html. Accessed 10 Nov 2015.
71. Checkley AM, Chiodini PL, Dockrell DH, Bates I, Thwaites GE, Booth HL, British Infection Society and Hospital for Tropical Diseases, et al. Eosinophilia in returning travellers and migrants from the tropics: UK recommendations for investigation and initial management. J Infect. 2010;60:1–20. PMID: 19931558, http://dx.doi.org/10.1016/j.jinf.2009.11.003.
72. Kunst H, Mack D, Kon OM, Banerjee AK, Chiodini P, Grant A. Parasitic infections of the lung: a guide for the respiratory physician. Thorax. 2011;66: 528–36. PMID:20880867, http://dx.doi.org/10.1136/thx.2009.132217.

Childhood pneumonia and meningitis in the Eastern Highlands Province, Papua New Guinea in the era of conjugate vaccines: study methods and challenges

Christopher C. Blyth[1,2,3*], Rebecca Ford[4], Joycelyn Sapura[4], Tonny Kumani[4], Geraldine Masiria[4], John Kave[4], Lapule Yuasi[4], Andrew Greenhill[4,5], Ilomo Hwaihwanje[6], Amanda Lang[4], Deborah Lehmann[2,4], William Pomat[2,4] on behalf of the Papua New Guinea Pneumonia and Meningitis Etiology Study Team

Abstract

Background: Pneumonia and meningitis are common causes of severe childhood illness in Papua New Guinea (PNG). The etiology of both clinical conditions in PNG has not been recently assessed. Changes in lifestyle, provision and access to healthcare, antimicrobial utilization and resistance, and the national childhood vaccination schedule necessitate reassessment.

Methods: A prospective case-control study was undertaken, enrolling children <5 years of age to determine the contemporary etiology of clinically defined moderate or severe pneumonia or suspected meningitis. Cases were identified following presentation for inpatient or outpatient care in Goroka town, the major population centre in the Eastern Highlands Province. Following enrolment, routine diagnostic specimens including blood, nasopharyngeal swabs, urine and (if required) cerebrospinal fluid, were obtained. Cases residing within one hour's drive of Goroka were followed up, and recruitment of healthy contemporaneous controls was undertaken in the cases' communities.

Results: 998 cases and 978 controls were enrolled over 3 years. This included 784 cases (78.6%) with moderate pneumonia, 187 (18.7%) with severe pneumonia and 75 (7.5%) with suspected meningitis, of whom 48 (4.8%) had concurrent pneumonia. The median age of cases was 7.8 months (Interquartile range [IQR] 3.9–14.3), significantly lower than community controls, which was 20.8 months (IQR 8.2–36.4). Half the cases were admitted to hospital (500/998; 50.1%). Recruitment of cases and controls and successful collection of diagnostic specimens improved throughout the study, with blood volume increasing and rates of blood culture contamination decreasing. The overall case fatality rate was 18/998 (1.8%). Of cases eligible for follow-up, outcome data was available from 76.7%. Low but increasing coverage of Haemophilus influenzae type B conjugate vaccines on the national schedule was observed during the study period: three dose DTPw-HepB-Hib coverage in children >3 months increased from 14.9 to 43.0% and 29.0 to 47.7% in cases and controls (both $p < 0.001$). Despite inclusion in the national immunization program in 2014, 2015 PCV13 three-dose coverage in cases and controls >3 months was only 4.0 and 6.5%.

(Continued on next page)

* Correspondence: christopher.blyth@uwa.edu.au
[1]School of Paediatrics and Child Health, The University of Western Australia, Princess Margaret Hospital for Children, Roberts Road, Subiaco 6008, WA, Australia
[2]Wesfarmers Centre for Vaccines and Infectious Diseases, Telethon Kids Institute, University of Western Australia, PO Box 855, West Perth 6872, WA, Australia
Full list of author information is available at the end of the article

(Continued from previous page)

Conclusions: Recruitment of large numbers of pediatric pneumonia and meningitis cases and community controls in a third-world setting presents unique challenges. Successful enrolment of 998 cases and 978 controls with comprehensive clinical data, biological specimens and follow up was achieved. Increased vaccine coverage remains an ongoing health priority.

Keywords: Pneumonia, Meningitis, Papua New Guinea, *Streptococcus pneumoniae*, *Haemophilus influenzae*, Vaccination

Background

Pneumonia and meningitis are common childhood diseases, resulting in significant morbidity and mortality among young children [1]. It is estimated that acute lower respiratory tract infection results in approximately 2.7 million deaths per annum, with 50% occurring in children <5 years of age. Of childhood pneumonia deaths, 33 and 16% are attributable to *Streptococcus pneumoniae* and *Haemophilus influenzae*, respectively [1]. Meningitis is estimated to result in >300,000 deaths (all ages) globally, with 26 and 21% estimated to be caused by *S. pneumoniae* and *H. influenzae* [1].

Papua New Guinea (PNG) was previously identified as a high priority country for the achievement of the United Nations Millennium Development Goals because the baseline child mortality rate is among the highest in the Western Pacific Region (<5 year old mortality rate in 2015: 57 per 1000 live births [2]). Pneumonia and meningitis are the most common causes for childhood deaths reported to the National Health Information Systems [3, 4]. Studies conducted in the Asaro Valley, including Goroka town, the provincial capital of Eastern Highlands Province (EHP), have repeatedly demonstrated the importance of *S. pneumoniae* and *H. influenzae* in the etiology of pneumonia and meningitis [5–11]. There are a paucity of contemporary data examining the bacterial causes of pneumonia and meningitis: the only recent study used opportunistically collected cerebrospinal fluid (CSF) samples from children admitted to Goroka General Hospital (GGH; 1996–2005) [9]. The current contribution of respiratory viruses to pneumonia also remains uncertain; apart from a single study assessing respiratory viruses in infants enrolled in a neonatal pneumococcal conjugate vaccine trial [12], prospective studies have not been undertaken since 1985 [13].

Conjugate *H. influenzae* type B (Hib) vaccine and 13-valent *S. pneumoniae* vaccine (13vPCV) were introduced into the national vaccination schedule in 2008 and 2014, respectively. From 2014, PNG infants were recommended neonatal BCG and hepatitis B vaccines followed by diphtheria, tetanus, whole-cell pertussis, hepatitis B and Hib vaccine (DTPw-HepB-Hib), 13vPCV and oral polio vaccines at 1, 2 and 3 months of age. Routine measles vaccines were recommended at 6 and 9 months [14]. In 2015, the PNG National Department of Health launched a Special Integrated Routine EPI Strengthening Program (SIREP Plus), a multimodal program aimed at improving coverage of vaccines already provided free under the national immunization program as well as introducing measles-rubella (MR, recommended at 6, 9 and 18 months) and inactivated polio vaccine (IPV, at 3 months) to all PNG children, and PCV13 to provinces yet to introduce the vaccine. Despite the 2014 launch, PCV13 was not available for use in children in the PNG highlands until 2015.

Given these changes, determining vaccine coverage in the PNG highlands and assessing the contemporary etiology of pneumonia and meningitis is a research priority. Commencing in 2013, we conducted a prospective case-control study enrolling children with clinically-defined moderate or severe pneumonia or suspected meningitis (cases) and contemporaneous community controls. This article describes the study methodology, population, vaccine coverage, and some of the operational and logistical challenges encountered throughout this study.

Methods

We performed a prospective case-control study recruiting children with clinical pneumonia and/or suspected meningitis presenting either to the Eastern Highlands Provincial Hospital (EHPH, previously known as the Goroka General Hospital, GGH) or community healthcare clinics elsewhere in Goroka town and contemporaneous healthy community controls (January 2013 to January 2016). The date of commencement was chosen to ensure sufficient recruitment prior to the national introduction of the 13vPCV.

The study aims were to: (i) determine the etiology of pneumonia and meningitis in a setting with previously reported high rates of both diseases; (ii) identify the serotypes of *S. pneumoniae* causing invasive disease; (iii) determine the antimicrobial susceptibility profiles of isolated bacterial pathogens; (iv) examine the utility of molecular and other diagnostic assays in PNG children with pneumonia and meningitis and (v) explore clinical and laboratory variables associated with specific pathogens and severe diseases.

Study location

The study was conducted in the EHP of PNG, an area of 11,157 km^2, located at 6^{0}30'S 145^{0}40'E with a population of 579,825 (2011 census) [15]. Goroka, the provincial capital of EHP (population of 23,277) is located 1600 m above sea level, is only accessible by air from the national capital Port Moresby, and by a narrow mountainous highway to the nearest sea port, Lae. Sealed roads exist between major centres, but are often in poor condition. Feeder roads to villages are generally unsealed tracks and many villages and hamlets are only accessible on foot. Living standards vary significantly. In rural areas people live in hamlets in traditional thatched houses and are primarily subsistence farmers, but may obtain cash through sales of coffee and market produce. In the urban and peri-urban areas, many houses are built with strong and long-lasting materials such as an iron roof and cement walls and floors, although houses in the poorer settlements are more traditional and made of bush materials. Modern houses are connected to the town water and electricity supply (though interruptions are common) but this is less common in the settlements [16].

EHPH is the only tertiary healthcare facility in EHP and caters for all age groups. EHPH has a dedicated pediatric ward and children's outpatient facility staffed by pediatricians, junior medical officers and pediatric nurses. In addition, urban clinics located in and around Goroka offer outpatient nurse-led care to children and adults. EHPH is the only site for inpatient hospital care in Goroka and surrounding villages and the EHPH children's Outpatient Clinic, North Clinic and Lopi Clinic are the busiest outpatient facilities in the region.

Children presenting to the Children's Outpatient Clinic, EHPH or two smaller urban clinics (North Clinic, Lopi Clinic) were eligible for recruitment. In addition, children presenting to the PNG Institute of Medical Research (PNGIMR) research clinic (located at the PNGIMR facility in Goroka, next to EHPH) or already admitted to the EHPH children's ward were eligible for recruitment. Research was undertaken by PNGIMR staff.

Recruitment of children with pneumonia and/or meningitis

Unwell children <5 years of age meeting the inclusion criteria were eligible for enrolment (see definitions of moderate and severe pneumonia and clinical meningitis as described in the PNG clinical manual and used nationwide [Table 1] [1]). Children not eligible for enrolment included those with severe congenital abnormalities, those hospitalized in the preceding 14 days and those previously enrolled within 30 days. Prior receipt of antibiotics was not an exclusion criteria.

Table 1 Inclusion and exclusion criteria including clinical case definitions [14]

Criteria	Classification	Definitions
Inclusion Criteria (cases)	Moderate pneumonia	Presence of all three symptoms and signs: • cough • tachypnoea rate (≥60/min if <2 months, ≥40/min if ≥2 mo of age) • lower chest wall indrawing
	Severe pneumonia	Moderate pneumonia with one of the following added features: • pulse >160/min with hepatomegaly >2 cm below costal margin • cyanosed or restless • inability to breastfeed/drink or vomiting.
	Suspected meningitis	Defined by the presence of fever (>37.5 °C) and one of the following additional features: • seizures • impaired or altered consciousness • irritability • a bulging fontanelle • signs of meningeal irritation (e.g. neck stiffness, Kernig's sign).
Exclusion criteria (cases)		The following children were excluded from enrolment as cases: • age ≥ 5 years • severe congenital abnormality • hospitalisation in preceding 14 days • previous enrolment as either case or control in the study within 30 days • parent unable or unwilling to give consent
Exclusion criteria (controls)		The following children were excluded from enrolment as controls • age ≥ 5 years • symptoms or signs of active infection including cough, tachypnoea, lower chest wall indrawing, fever (>37.5 °C), altered consciousness, drowsy or "staring eyes", irritability, bulging fontanelle and neck stiffness or signs of meningeal irritation • severe congenital abnormality • hospitalization in preceding 14 days • previous enrolment in the study as a control[a] • exposed to antibiotics in the past 30 days • parent unable or unwilling to give consent

Abbreviations: *Mo* months

[a] Controls could be subsequently enrolled as cases if more than 30 days since previous enrolment

Eligible children were identified by clinically-trained research staff using a screening questionnaire. Upon determining eligibility and obtaining informed consent, research staff undertook a brief history and examination before laboratory specimens were obtained and treatment provided. Verbal consent and minimal data were obtained initially ensuring timely provision of appropriate medical care. This was followed by a more in-depth interview exploring risk factors for disease, recent antibiotic exposure, vaccination history and symptoms, examination including oximetry (recorded using LifeBox Pulse Oximeter, Acare Technology Co. Ltd, Taiwan), written consent and further specimen collection as required. In addition to parental interview, individual health records were examined for perinatal history, co-morbidities and vaccination status.

Children meeting the inclusion criteria yet deemed well enough for outpatient management were still eligible for enrolment. In addition to children enrolled through outpatient clinics, inpatients presenting after-hours were enrolled following parental consent. This was restricted during the first year of the study to those identified <48 hours following admission, but was extended to 96 h to enhance recruitment, particularly for children with suspected meningitis perceived to be too sick to undergo an early lumbar puncture.

All admitted cases were reassessed daily during their hospital stay by clinically trained research staff. Children deemed well enough to be managed as outpatients were discharged and reviewed within 48 h. Contact mobile phone numbers, if available, were collected from all parents prior to discharge. Review of all children residing within one hour (by vehicle and/or foot) from Goroka was attempted, 2 to 4 weeks post-discharge. At review, their health status was assessed and the presence of ongoing symptoms and/or signs confirmed.

Recruitment of controls

Healthy children <5 years of age were enrolled to assist in determining community vaccination coverage and for further nasopharyngeal bacterial colonization and viral studies. Children were eligible if they met the inclusion/exclusion criteria (Table 1) and were recruited during community follow-up visits for discharged cases. PNGIMR staff conducted community clinics to provide primary healthcare and vaccination, thereby facilitating further identification and recruitment of controls. Given the logistical challenges of recruiting matched controls, formal case-control matching was not undertaken although contemporaneous controls were recruited from the same communities as cases. In an attempt to reduce bias, the number of cases recruited and median age were regularly assessed and used to guide targeted control recruitment. Following informed consent, a brief history and examination was undertaken, individual health and immunization records were examined and two nasopharyngeal swabs were collected.

Specimen collection

Consent was sought to collect blood, nasopharyngeal specimens, urine and (if clinically indicated) CSF from all cases (Additional file 1: Table S1), and nasopharyngeal specimens from controls. Although recommended in cases of suspected meningitis, a decision to collect CSF was left to the treating pediatric staff. Using appropriate aseptic technique (iodine solution followed by 70% alcohol, ensuring adequate drying time prior to procedure), PNGIMR research staff collected up to 5 ml of whole blood for culture (inoculated directly into BD BACTEC™ PedsPlus bottles; BD, Franklin Lakes, New Jersey, United States [US]), PCR and antimicrobial activity. Blood volume was recorded by clinical staff prior to blood culture inoculation. Additional blood tests, if clinically indicated (e.g. malaria blood slides, haemoglobin, human immunodeficiency virus [HIV] serology) were also obtained. If obtainable, urine was collected for antimicrobial activity and storage. Two deep-flocked nasopharyngeal swabs (Copan Diagnostics, Murrieta, California, US) were collected on all children: the first placed immediately in 1 ml of skim milk tryptone glucose glycerol broth (STGGB) and the second in 1 ml of viral transport media (VTM). Following initial processing, STGGB samples were stored at −80 °C whilst EDTA, serum, urine and VTM samples were stored at −20 °C. Blood and CSF culture contamination rates were monitored throughout the study and a review of collection technique and additional staff training was undertaken regularly during periods of higher-than-expected contamination.

Laboratory processing

All laboratory testing was undertaken at the PNGIMR Bacteriology and Molecular Laboratories, Goroka. Blood cultures were incubated for up to 5 days at 35 °C using a BD BACTEC™ automated blood culture system (BD, Franklin Lakes, NJ) or when unavailable, a 35–37 °C incubator. Positive bottles (using the BACTEC system) were subcultured onto standard and selective media and incubated with/without 5% CO_2. During periods when the BACTEC system was unavailable, manual daily subculture from inoculated BACTEC™ bottles was undertaken using methods previously described [5]. All CSF underwent macroscopic examination, manual cell count and Gram stain. In the setting of CSF pleocytosis, CSF was cultured on standard media and incubated with/without 5% CO_2, bacterial antigen detection for *S.pneumoniae* and *H.influenzae* using latex agglutination was performed and further staining for acid-fast bacilli and yeast undertaken. CSF biochemistry (protein and glucose) was undertaken using Uristix® reagent urinalysis strips (Siemens, Victoria, Australia).

Bacterial isolates were identified using colony morphology and standard confirmatory tests (*S.pneumoniae*: optochin sensitivity, bile solubility, catalase; *H.influenzae*: differential growth on blood/chocolate agar, X&V disks). Serotyping was undertaken by the Quellung reaction using commercially obtained antisera (Staten Serum Institut, Denmark) and *H.influenzae* agglutinating sera (Remel, Dartford, United Kingdom). Antimicrobial susceptibility testing was conducted on all clinically relevant isolates by disc diffusion with suspected resistance confirmed by E-tests® (bioMérieux,

Durham, North Carolina, US) using Clinical and Laboratory Standards Institute (CLSI) breakpoints [17].

For real-time PCR on blood and CSF samples, DNA was extracted from 200 μl blood/CSF using commercially available kits (Qiagen DNease Blood & Tissue Kit, Valencia, California, US) and an in-house real-time PCR for *S.pneumoniae* (*lyt*A) and *H. influenzae (hpd)* performed [18, 19]. In general, replicate samples within 0.5 Cq of each other and with a Cq value ≤35 (but within the limit of detection as determined by the standards) were deemed to be positive.

Respiratory virus testing was undertaken using the dedicated VTM sample and an in-house multiplexed real-time quantitative PCR assay. DNA/RNA were extracted using commercially available kits (Qiagen DNease Blood & Tissue Kit, Valencia, California, US). Viral targets are described in Additional file 2: Table S2 [20–22]. Semi-quantitative bacterial culture of STGGB was performed using blood, chocolate, gentamicin-blood and bacitracin-chocolate agar plates, incubated with 5% CO_2. Bacterial isolates were identified and typed and susceptibility testing performed as described above.

Antibiotic activity was measured in blood, urine and/or CSF to better understand the yield of blood and CSF cultures. This was performed by placing a specimen-soaked filter paper disk on agar inoculated with a 0.5 MacFarland suspension of *Staphylococcus aureus* ATCC 25923. Following incubation at 37 °C overnight, a zone of inhibition was examined and measured.

Radiology

When a chest X-ray was requested as part of clinical care, digital copies were extracted and stored on a dedicated hard drive. These will be reviewed by international experts using standardised methods [23].

Ethics, data and study management and analysis

Ethical approval was obtained from the Institutional Review Board of PNGIMR (IRB no 1204), the Medical Research Advisory Committee of PNG (MRAC number 11.29) and the University of Western Australia (RA/4/1/7960). Clinical and laboratory data were collected on paper forms, subsequently checked by a second staff member and entered in a dedicated Filemakerpro database 11 (DB services, Indianapolis, IN, US). Monthly teleconferences and regular data checks were undertaken to ensure the accuracy of all data collected.

Analysis was undertaken using SPSS 20.0.0 (IBM Corp, New York, NY, US). Continuous variables were compared with the Student's *t* test, and categorical variables were compared with $\chi 2$ or Fisher's Exact test. A *p* value of ≤0.05 was considered significant.

Results

From January 2013 to January 2016, 1001 children with pneumonia or meningitis and 994 heathy children were consented to the study. Three cases and 16 controls were excluded from the analysis as they did not meet the inclusion criteria (cases: not meeting clinical case definitions [$n = 2$]; >5 years of age [$n = 1$]; controls: evidence of acute respiratory infection [$n = 5$]; >5 years of age [$n = 11$], Table 1). Thirty-four children were enrolled as cases more than once and 14 controls were subsequently enrolled as cases.

Pneumonia and meningitis cases

The median age of enrolled cases was 7.8 months (interquartile range [IQR] 3.9–14.3) and 562/998 cases were male (56.3%; Table 2). Parents infrequently reported chronic health concerns (12/984; 1.2%), the most frequent being chronic respiratory disease ($n = 6$) and seizures ($n = 4$). Ninety-six (9.6%) and 7 (0.7%) cases reported a history of pneumonia and meningitis, respectively.

Case enrolment during the study increased from 286 cases in 2013 to 421 in 2015 (Table 2). Despite the seasonal nature of pneumonia (peak activity during the southern hemisphere winter), cases were recruited year round: the average number of cases recruited per month was 36 (range 9–61; Fig. 1). A significant proportion of cases were recruited following admission to EHPH (404/998; 40.5%) with the remainder recruited from the EHPH outpatient clinic (313; 31.4%), community (201; 20.1%) or PNGIMR research clinics (75; 7.5%). The proportion of children recruited prior to admission to hospital (i.e. from EHPH outpatients or community clinics, as opposed to the EHPH children's ward) increased over the duration of the study. This shift in recruitment was part of a dedicated focus to enhance recruitment of children prior to antibiotic delivery (2013: 30.8% recruited prior to admission to EHPH, 2014: 58.1%, 2015: 80.1%; $p < 0.0001$).

The most frequent diagnosis was moderate pneumonia ($n = 784$, 78.6%), followed by severe pneumonia ($n = 187$, 18.7%) and suspected meningitis (with or without pneumonia; $n = 75$, 7.5%). Nasopharyngeal samples were collected on all cases with blood obtainable from 987 children (98.9%; Table 2). The volume of blood collected per patient increased throughout the study period: mean volume in 2013, 1.36 ml; 2014, 1.49 ml; 2015, 1.95 ml; difference in means; 0.12 ml, (95% confidence interval [CI]: 0.016–0.224; p <0.03) and 0.46 ml (95%CI: 0.32–0.61; $p < 0.0001$), respectively. In addition, the number of children with dedicated EDTA samples increased over time: 2013, 89/286 (31.1%); 2014, 150/291 (51.5%) and 2015, 273/421 (64.8%), $p < 0.001$. The rate of contaminated blood cultures decreased during the study: 2013, 63/281

Table 2 Cases and controls: demographics, recruitment, diagnosis, diagnostic specimens and follow up

	Cases: *n* (%) (*n* = 998)	Controls: *n* (%) (*n* = 978)
Demographics		
Median age (months; IQR)	7.8 months (3.9–14.3)	20.8 months (8.2–36.4)
Male sex (%)	562 (56.3%)	520 (53.2%)
Recruitment year		
2013	286 (28.6%)	172 (17.6%)
2014	291 (29.1%)	288 (29.4%)
2015[a]	421 (42.2%)	518 (53.0%)
Recruitment site		
Children's ward, EHPH	404 (40.5%)	NA
Outpatient clinics, EHPH	313 (31.4%)	
North Clinic	194 (19.4%)	
Lopi Clinic	7 (0.7%)	
PNGIMR Research Clinic	75 (7.5%)	
Unknown	5 (0.5%)	
Diagnosis		
Moderate pneumonia	784 (78.6%)	NA
• Without suspected meningitis	753	
• With suspected meningitis	31	
Severe pneumonia	187 (18.7%)	
• Without suspected meningitis	170	
• With suspected meningitis	17	
Suspected Meningitis (without pneumonia)	27 (2.7%)	
Diagnostic specimens collected		
Blood culture	987 (98.9%)	NA
EDTA blood	512 (51.3%)	NA
Serum	363 (36.4%)	NA
CSF	31 (3.12%)	NA
Nasopharyngeal swab	998 (100%)	978 (100%)
Urine	42 (4.2%)	NA
Successful follow up (of eligible children) by year		
2013	156/223[b] (69.9%)	NA
2014	162/209[b] (77.5%)	
2015[a]	251/310[b] (81.0%)	

Abbreviations: *IQR* interquartile range, *EHPH* Eastern Highlands Provincial Hospital, *NA* not applicable
[a] inclusive of the first 3 weeks of January 2016
[b] denominator is children residing within 1 h by vehicle from Goroka

(22.4%); 2014, 41/285 (14.4%) and 2015, 48/421 (11.4%), $p < 0.001$. Collection of blood prior to antibiotics was also more frequently achieved over the course of the study: 2013, 139/275 (50.5%); 2014, 198/282 (70.2%) and 2015, 246/415 (83.4%), $p < 0.001$.

Both CSF and urine samples were infrequently collected during the study. In children with a clinical diagnosis of suspected meningitis ($n = 75$), only 29 underwent a CSF examination. Of the remainder, 24 cases were deemed by EHPH medical staff not to have clinical evidence of meningitis, seven cases had contraindication to lumbar puncture and eight had a lumbar puncture without CSF being obtained. In a further seven cases with suspected meningitis, it is uncertain why sampling was not performed. A further 2 CSF samples were taken from children not meeting the clinical definition of meningitis.

Half the patients were admitted to hospital (500/998; 50.1%) with the remainder managed as outpatients. Less than 25% of children had an X-ray performed. The median length of hospital stay was 2 days (IQR 2–5).

Eighteen deaths were identified (overall case fatality rate (CRF): 18/998, 1.8% overall; pneumonia, 1.5%; meningitis, 8.0%). The in-hospital CFR was 14/500 (2.8% overall: pneumonia, 2.3%; meningitis 8.7%). Follow-up was attempted in children residing within 1 h by vehicle from Goroka ($n = 742$). Outcome data was obtained on 569 children (76.7%). During the period of the study, the proportion of eligible children that were successfully followed up increased from 69.9% (2013) to 81.0% (2015), $p < 0.02$.

Controls

The median age of enrolled controls was 20.8 months (IQR 8.2–36.4) and 522/983 enrolled controls were male (53.2%; Table 2). Successful recruitment of controls increased during the study period, particularly following the institution of dedicated clinics in 2014 and 2015. Despite ongoing attempts to recruit younger controls, controls remained significantly older than cases throughout the study; median ages cases vs. controls: 6.6 vs. 14.3 months (2013), 9.3 vs. 22.7 months (2014) and 8.4 vs. 21.0 months (2015).

Vaccination coverage

Child health books that included vaccination status were assessable in 991 cases (99.3%) and 976 controls (99.8%). Coverage for one dose of DTPw-HepB-Hib in children >1 month of age was 65.5% in cases and 71.9% in controls ($p < 0.01$, Fig. 2), falling for three doses in children >3 months of age to 31.6% in cases and 43.3% in controls ($p < 0.001$). The significant difference in vaccine coverage between cases and controls remained when restricted to children < 12 months of age at enrolment. The overall median age of the first, second and third dose of DTPw-HepB-Hib was 1.4 months (IQR 1.1–3.0), 3.1 months (IQR 2.1–6.1) and 4.7 months (IQR 3.1–8.0). During the study, vaccine coverage significantly improved: three dose DTPw-HepB-Hib coverage in children >3 months of age increased from 14.9 to 43.0% in cases and 29.0 to 47.7% in controls ($p < 0.001$ in both).

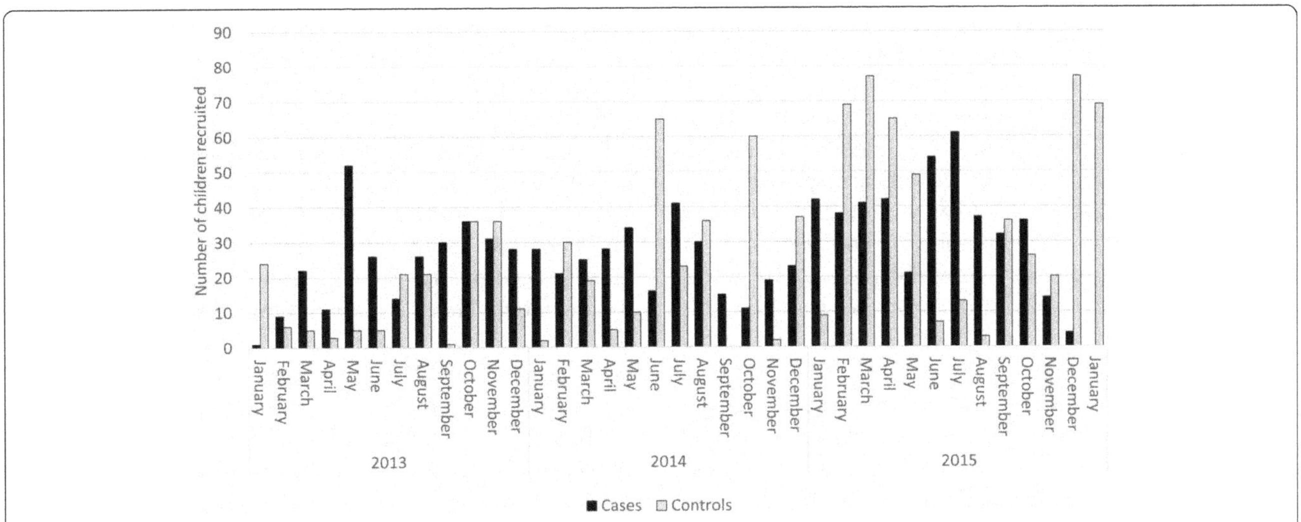

Fig. 1 Enrolment of cases and controls by month: January 2013 to January 2016

Despite the launch of the PCV13 program in 2014, the vaccine was not available in the EHP until 2015. The 2015 coverage of PCV13 was low in both cases and controls with only 25.4 and 24.4% of cases and controls >1 month receiving one dose, and 4.0 and 6.5% of cases and controls >3 months receiving three doses (no significant difference between cases and controls).

Discussion

The ongoing burden of childhood disease in PNG necessitates a contemporary reassessment of pneumonia and meningitis etiology and outcomes. Given the lack of access to and (if present) underutilisation of the microbiological laboratory in PNG, targeted projects using routine and contemporary diagnostics are required to assess the current pathogen-specific burden of disease. These data are essential to assess potential benefits of childhood vaccination and to identify potential changes in etiology.

Undertaking such studies, particularly in locations such as the highlands of PNG, pose unique challenges in study design, recruitment, specimen handling and laboratory practice. A number of these challenges are unique to both PNG and to other isolated highland communities, while others are frequent with any large prospective study. This paper outlines the methods and challenges observed in recruiting nearly 2000 children over 3 years.

Based on existing EHPH service data, the study proposed to recruit >1000 children with clinical pneumonia and meningitis over 2 years. Prior to commencement, concern was raised by the community about the invasive

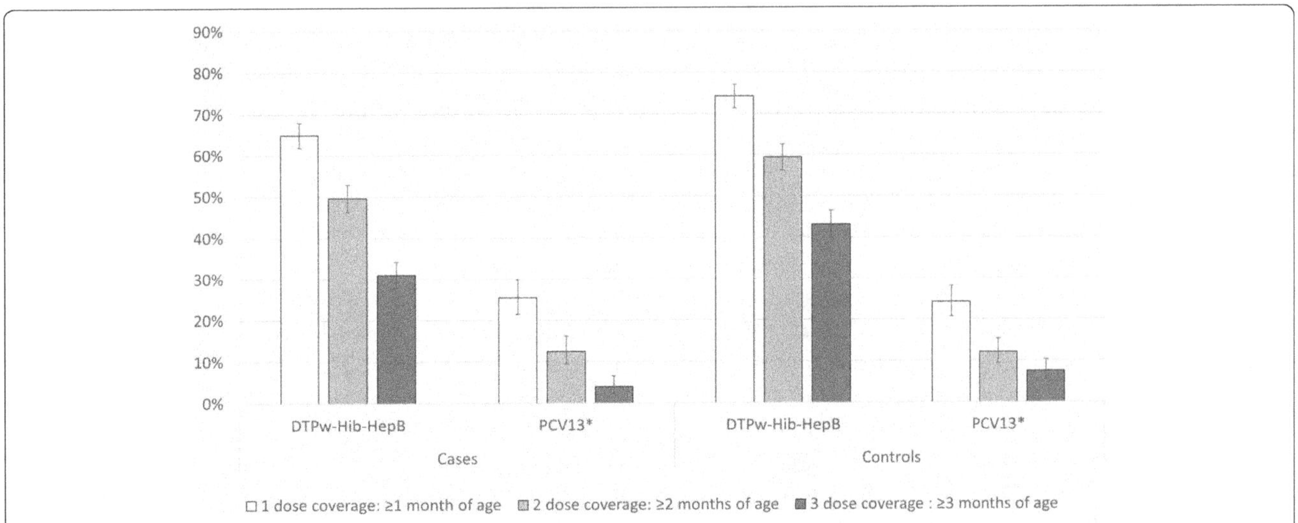

Fig. 2 Vaccine coverage by case-control status and age (*PCV13 data for 2015 only)

nature of the specimens proposed. PNGIMR has a long history of community engagement developed over many successful research studies. Regular visits to communities to discuss this study, explaining the routine nature of specimen collection in other healthcare settings and the collaborative nature of healthcare provided by PNGIMR and hospital staff was essential in the early phase of the study. The provision of non-monetary incentives such as transport from hospital to home for study participants and future access to the PNGIMR clinic are also likely to have assisted with recruitment, which improved throughout the study.

Barriers to recruitment included frequent and sometimes prolonged industrial action leading to closure of health facilities. As a result, lower numbers of children were admitted to the ward and at times, PNGIMR staff needed to focus on providing healthcare rather than the research project. Outbreaks of vaccine preventable diseases (e.g. an outbreak of measles in April to June 2015) required additional healthcare resources to be diverted away from research activities. Hospital senior and junior medical staff changed several times during the 3-year study period and a lack of familiarity with the study required regular re-engagement by the research team with the EHPH paediatric staff. Significant variation in practice, especially with CSF collection and utilisation of radiology were noted throughout the study. As both procedures were not mandated, rather recommended based on clinical need, it is likely that physician preference contributed to variable utilisation. Provision of a dedicated study doctor may have assisted with the variation in practice observed.

Compared with previous pneumonia studies conducted at EHPH [8], a number of differences should be noted: a lower proportion of enrolled children had severe pneumonia (19% of the pneumonia cohort in this study vs 46% in Barker et al. [8]). A higher number were deemed well enough to manage as outpatient following initial treatment (50% vs 0% in Barker et al. [8]). Forty per cent of children were enrolled from the ward following initial management by EHPH staff, albeit in decreasing numbers over the duration of the study. A significant number of children had been administered antibiotics even prior to their first interview at EHPH (data not shown). It is expected that these factors will reduce the rate of detection of bacteraemia and invasive bacterial isolates from the current cohort. The in-hospital mortality rate (2.8%) is significantly lower than Barker et al. (8%) [8] and the rate reported nationally (5.2%) by the Paediatric Hospital Reporting (PHR) system, yet comparable to 2013 PHR data collected from EHPH (2.4%) [4]. These severity of illness and mortality data are encouraging and suggest that, compared with past studies, improvements in access to health services, earlier recognition of childhood pneumonia with earlier institution of antimicrobial therapy and supportive care are leading to better outcomes for children with pneumonia.

Recruitment of controls was challenging, particularly in the early phases of the study. Despite regular visits to rural and peri-urban communities, well children (particularly those < 6 months of age) were often absent, frequently accompanying their parents to the fields early in the morning. There was an attempt to overcome this by scheduling PNGIMR community clinics and establishing age specified targets. Following institution of these clinics, larger numbers of controls were recruited, yet recruitment of younger controls remained an ongoing challenge. Given the uneven balance between cases and controls, assessment of biological samples (e.g. nasopharyngeal samples) will be undertaken in cases and controls matched post-enrolment by month of illness, age and village.

PNG has a long history of utilization of a hand-held child health record. Documentation of vaccination status is routinely recorded in the health book (on the reverse of front cover and in the continuous clinical records). The health record was assessable in more than 99% of cases and controls. The variable nature of recording required additional training and care to ensure accuracy of the data collected by the research team. This may have resulted in underestimation of the vaccine coverage early in the study. Replacement of lost hand-held records or an older child having more than one book may result in underestimation of vaccine uptake (data not presented). Despite this, the record provides a unique opportunity to assess uptake of vaccination status in a country where access to electronic or manually collected vaccine distribution data remains a challenge. Vaccine coverage in the highlands remains lower than the reported national average [2]: the reasons for this are likely to be multifactorial and may include reduced access to health services given the remoteness of highland villages, problems with consistent immunization supply and parental education with ongoing mistrust of infant immunization. Increased vaccine coverage is encouraging and suggests that targeted programs including the Special Integrated Routine EPI Strengthening Program (SIREP) is having an impact in the PNG highlands.

Undertaking a study dependent on key infrastructure in isolated locations poses unique challenges. For much of the study the BD BACTEC™ Instrumented Blood Culture System was not working, despite multiple attempts by the laboratory staff and the manufacturer to repair the machine both in Goroka and Port Moresby. The laboratory was reliant on manual subculture of blood cultures increasing the time and risk of contamination of critical specimens. Higher rates of contamination are likely to impact on the ability to detect significant bacteraemia. For significant periods of time, the hospital X-ray facility required repairs, meaning that physician-requested X-rays were not available. These key challenges must be considered when designing studies in third-world settings, particularly in locations outside the nation's capital city with difficult access by road or by air.

Achieving a follow up rate of >75% in an environment where formal town maps and permanent phone connections are largely non-existent is a testament to both study participants and staff. This was achieved by meticulous documentation of village, hamlet and house location and use of PNGIMR drivers to return children and their parents to their homes. This was also enhanced by the provision of ongoing healthcare clinics in larger villages and access for study participants to the PNGIMR clinic. Despite these incentives, numerous attempts were often required for follow up.

Conclusions

In summary, recruitment of large numbers of pediatric pneumonia and meningitis cases and community controls in a third-world setting with limited health services, health and other infrastructures presents unique challenges. The study successfully enrolled 998 cases and 978 controls, obtained comprehensive clinical data and biological specimens, and was able to follow up >75% following discharge. Furthermore, staff documented increasing coverage of pneumococcal and Hib conjugate vaccines in PNG children. Key aspects to overcoming the challenges of conducting research in third-world settings include a pragmatic and flexible study design and strong collaborative relationships with healthcare providers. Prior to commencing research, the infrastructure needs of the study (and alternative plans should key equipment be unavailable) must be considered. Ongoing community engagement is paramount to optimize recruitment and translation. In addition, the provision of ongoing training for both research and clinical staff ensures staff retention and facilitates translation of research findings into changes in clinical practice.

Abbreviations

13vPCV: 13-valent Pneumococcal conjugate vaccine; CSF: Cerebrospinal fluid; EHP: Eastern Highlands Province; EHPH: Eastern Highlands Provincial Hospital; GGH: Goroka General Hospital; HIV: Human immunodeficiency virus; PCR: Polymerase chain reaction; PHR: Paediatric Hospital Reporting; PNG: Papua New Guinea; PNGIMR: Papua New Guinea Institute of Medical Research; STGGB: Skim milk tryptone glucose glycerol broth; VTM: Viral transport media

Acknowledgement

The investigators would like to thank the study participants and the Eastern Highlands Province Hospital and urban clinic staff, without whom this study would not have been possible.

Members of the Papua New Guinea Pneumonia and Meningitis Etiology Study Team include: Yazid Abdad, Celestine Aho, Christopher Blyth, Trevor Duke, Rebecca Ford, Andrew Greenhill, Paul Horwood, Ilomo Hwaihwanje, John Kave, Wendy Kirarock, Lea-Ann Kirkham, Tonny Kumani, Sarah Javati, Dorcas Joseph, Joe Jude, Amanda Lang, Deborah Lehmann, Geraldine Masiria, Barry Nagepu, Tilda Orami, William Pomat, Peter Richmond, Joycelyn Sapura, Peter Siba, Johanna Wapling, Mition Yoannes, and Lapule Yuasi.

Funding

The study was co-funded by an investigator-initiated Pfizer Global Research Grant (WS1801400) and PNGIMR funds provided through the Internal Competitive Research Award Scheme (ICRAS). The sponsor had no role in the design of the study, collection, analysis, interpretation of the data and in writing the manuscript. CCB is supported by an Australian National Health and Medical Research Council Career Development Fellowship (APP1111596).

Authors' contributions

CB, AG, DL and WP conceived and designed the study, sought funding and supervised the study. JS, TK, GM and JK recruited cases and controls and undertook community engagement necessary to conduct this study. RF, LY, AG and AL performed microbiological studies on specimens collected. CB analysed data for this manuscript and wrote the draft manuscript. All authors have reviewed the manuscript prior to submission. All authors read and approved the final manuscript.

Competing interests

DL has previously been a member of the GSK Australia Pneumococcal-Haemophilus influenzae-Protein D conjugate vaccine ("Phid-CV") Advisory Panel, has received support from Pfizer Australia and GSK Australia to attend conferences, has received an honorarium from Merck Vaccines to attend a conference/seminar. WP has received support from Pfizer Australia to attend conferences. No other authors have competing interests.

Author details

[1]School of Paediatrics and Child Health, The University of Western Australia, Princess Margaret Hospital for Children, Roberts Road, Subiaco 6008, WA, Australia. [2]Wesfarmers Centre for Vaccines and Infectious Diseases, Telethon Kids Institute, University of Western Australia, PO Box 855, West Perth 6872, WA, Australia. [3]Department of Infectious Diseases and PathWest Department of Microbiology, Princess Margaret Hospital for Children, Roberts Road, Subiaco 6008, WA, Australia. [4]Papua New Guinea Institute of Medical Research, PO Box 60, Goroka 441, Eastern Highlands Province, Papua New Guinea. [5]School of Applied and Biomedical Sciences, Federation University Australia, Gippsland Campus, Northways Road, Churchill 3842, VIC, Australia. [6]Eastern Highlands Provincial Hospital, PO Box 392, Goroka 441, Eastern Highlands Province, Papua New Guinea.

References

1. GBD Mortality and Causes of Death Collaborators. Global, regional, and national age-sex specific all-cause and cause-specific mortality for 240 causes of death, 1990–2013: a systematic analysis for the Global Burden of Disease Study 2013. Lancet. 2015;385(9963):117–71.
2. GAVI: Papua New Guinea. In. http://www.gavi.org/country/papua-new-guinea/ (Accessed 8 Dec 2016): GAVI publications; 2016.
3. PNG Ministry of Health: Papua New Guinea Child Health Plan 2008-2015. 2008 http://www.rhtu.org.pg/wp-content/uploads/2013/06/PNG_Child_Health_Plan_2008-2015.pdf. Accessed 24 Feb 2017.

4. Child Health Advisory Committee: Child Morbidity and Mortality, Annual Report 2013. Edited by PNG National Department of Health and the PNG Paediatric Society; 2013. http://pngpaediatricsociety.org/wp-content/uploads/2013/05/2013-Annual-Child-Morbidity-and-Mortality-Report.pdf. Accessed 24 Feb 2017.
5. Gratten M, Montgomery J. The bacteriology of acute pneumonia and meningitis in children in Papua New Guinea: assumptions, facts and technical strategies. P N G Med J. 1991;34(3):185–98.
6. Lehmann D. Epidemiology of acute respiratory tract infections, especially those due to Haemophilus influenzae, in Papua New Guinean children. J Infect Dis. 1992;165 Suppl 1:S20–5.
7. Lehmann D, Michael A, Omena M, Clegg A, Lupiwa T, Sanders RC, Marjen B, Wai'in P, Rongap A, Saleu G, et al. Bacterial and viral etiology of severe infection in children less than 3 months old in the highlands of Papua New Guinea. Pediatr Infect Dis J. 1999;18(10 Suppl):S42–9.
8. Barker J, Gratten M, Riley I, Lehmann D, Montgomery J, Kajoi M, Gratten H, Smith D, Marshall TF, Alpers MP. Pneumonia in children in the Eastern Highlands of Papua New Guinea: a bacteriologic study of patients selected by standard clinical criteria. J Infect Dis. 1989;159(2):348–52.
9. Greenhill AR, Phuanukoonnon S, Michael A, Yoannes M, Orami T, Smith H, Murphy D, Blyth C, Reeder J, Siba P, et al. Streptococcus pneumoniae and Haemophilus influenzae in paediatric meningitis patients at Goroka General Hospital, Papua New Guinea: serotype distribution and antimicrobial susceptibility in the pre-vaccine era. BMC Infect Dis. 2015;15:485.
10. Lehmann D, Yeka W, Rongap T, Javati A, Saleu G, Clegg A, Michael A, Lupiwa T, Omena M, Alpers MP. Aetiology and clinical signs of bacterial meningitis in children admitted to Goroka Base Hospital, Papua New Guinea, 1989–1992. Ann Trop Paediatr. 1999;19(1):21–32.
11. Kirkham LAS, Smith-Vaughan HC, Greenhill AR. Improving aetiological diagnosis of bacterial pneumonia and meningitis in PNG. PNG Med J. 2010;53(3–4):139–46.
12. Chidlow GR, Laing IA, Harnett GB, Greenhill AR, Phuanukoonnon S, Siba PM, Pomat WS, Shellam GR, Smith DW, Lehmann D. Respiratory viral pathogens associated with lower respiratory tract disease among young children in the highlands of Papua New Guinea. J Clin Virol. 2012;54(3):235–9.
13. Phillips PA, Lehmann D, Spooner V, Barker J, Tulloch S, Sungu M, Canil KA, Pratt RD, Lupiwa T, Alpers MP. Viruses associated with acute lower respiratory tract infections in children from the eastern highlands of Papua New Guinea (1983–1985). Southeast Asian J Trop Med Public Health. 1990;21(3):373–82.
14. PNG Department of Health. Standard Treatment for Common Illness of Children in Papua New Guinea: a manual for nurses, community heatlh workers, health extension officers and doctors. 10th ed. Port Moresby: Papua New Guinea Department of Health and Paediatric Society of Papua New Guinea; 2016.
15. National Statistical Office PNG. National Population & Houseing Census 2011: "Count Me IN". In. Edited by National Statistical Office PNG. Port Moresby: PNG Government; 2011.
16. Phuanukoonnon S, Reeder JC, Pomat WS, Van den Biggelaar AH, Holt PG, Saleu G, Opa C, Michael A, Aho C, Yoannes M, et al. A neonatal pneumococcal conjugate vaccine trial in Papua New guinea: study population, methods and operational challenges. PNG Med J. 2010;53(3–4):191–206.
17. Clinical and Laboratory Standards Institute. Performance standards for antimicrobial susceptibility testing: approved standard, 23rd ed CLSI document M100-AS23. Wayne: Clinical and Laboratory Standards Institute; 2013.
18. Resti M, Moriondo M, Cortimiglia M, Indolfi G, Canessa C, Becciolini L, Bartolini E, Benedictis FM, de Martino M, Azzari C. Community-acquired bacteremic pneumococcal pneumonia in children: diagnosis and serotyping by real-time polymerase chain reaction using blood samples. Clin Infect Dis. 2010;51(9):1042–9.
19. Wang X, Mair R, Hatcher C, Theodore MJ, Edmond K, Wu HM, Harcourt BH, Carvalho MD, Pimenta F, Nymadawa P, et al. Detection of bacterial pathogens in Mongolia meningitis surveillance with a new real-time PCR assay to detect Haemophilus influenzae. Int J Med Microbiol. 2011;301(4):303–9.
20. Chidlow GR, Harnett GB, Shellam GR, Smith DW. An economical tandem multiplex real-time PCR technique for the detection of a comprehensive range of respiratory pathogens. Viruses. 2009;1(1):42–56.
21. Gunson RN, Collins TC, Carman WF. Real-time RT-PCR detection of 12 respiratory viral infections in four triplex reactions. J Clin Virol. 2005;33(4):341–4.
22. Klemenc J, Asad Ali S, Johnson M, Tollefson SJ, Talbot HK, Hartert TV, Edwards KM, Williams JV. Real-time reverse transcriptase PCR assay for improved detection of human metapneumovirus. J Clin Virol. 2012;54(4):371–5.
23. Cherian T, Mulholland EK, Carlin JB, Ostensen H, Amin R, de Campo M, Greenberg D, Lagos R, Lucero M, Madhi SA, et al. Standardized interpretation of paediatric chest radiographs for the diagnosis of pneumonia in epidemiological studies. Bull World Health Organ. 2005;83(5):353–9.

5

Encouraging rational antibiotic use in childhood pneumonia: a focus on Vietnam and the Western Pacific Region

Nguyen T. K. Phuong[1,6*], Tran T. Hoang[2], Pham H. Van[3], Lolyta Tu[4], Stephen M. Graham[5] and Ben J. Marais[6]

Abstract

Globally, pneumonia is considered to be the biggest killer of infants and young children (aged <5 years) outside the neonatal period, with the greatest disease burden in low- and middle-income countries. Optimal management of childhood pneumonia is challenging in settings where clinicians have limited information regarding the local pathogen and drug resistance profiles. This frequently results in unnecessary and poorly targeted antibiotic use. Restricting antibiotic use is a global priority, particularly in Asia and the Western Pacific Region where excessive use is driving high rates of antimicrobial resistance. The authors conducted a comprehensive literature review to explore the antibiotic resistance profile of bacteria associated with pneumonia in the Western Pacific Region, with a focus on Vietnam. Current management practices were also considered, along with the diagnostic dilemmas faced by doctors and other factors that increase unnecessary antibiotic use. This review offers some suggestions on how these issues may be addressed.

Background

Childhood pneumonia is a major contributor to under-5 mortality, especially in developing countries [1, 2]. In the Western Pacific Region, the highest burden of childhood pneumonia and pneumonia-related deaths occur in six countries: Cambodia, China, Laos, Papua New Guinea, the Philippines and Vietnam [3]. These countries report at least 0.2 pneumonia episodes per child year—more than 10 times the rates reported in developed countries from the same region such as Australia, New Zealand and Japan [4]. The management of childhood pneumonia is problematic in settings where a microbiological diagnosis is rarely pursued and the drug resistance profiles of common bacteria which cause respiratory disease are not readily available [5]. In many Asian countries this encourages excessive use of broad-spectrum antibiotics, irrespective of the child's disease severity. In the authors' experience, children are frequently hospitalized with pneumonia to administer intravenous antibiotics, despite relatively mild disease.

Unnecessary hospitalization for intravenous antibiotics increases healthcare cost, as well as treatment-related complications and the likelihood of nosocomial disease transmission. In order to encourage more rational use of intravenous antibiotics in children with community-acquired pneumonia, the authors performed a comprehensive review of common bacterial pathogens and their reported drug resistance profiles in the Western Pacific Region—Vietnam in particular. Factors that increase unnecessary antibiotic use (and measures that might reduce use) were also considered. PubMed, Google Scholar and Embase databases were searched using the following terms: antibacterial agents OR antibiotics OR drug therapy AND community acquired pneumonia OR acute respiratory tract infection AND child OR children OR childhood. Manuscript titles and abstracts were reviewed to identify original research papers that included children less than 5 years of age with pneumonia, with a geographic focus on Vietnam and the Western Pacific Region. In addition, the references of selected publications were reviewed, and co-authors suggested additional relevant papers. The term 'acute respiratory tract infection (ARTI)' describes all acute infections that involve the lungs or

* Correspondence: phuongty832000@gmail.com
[1]Respiratory Department, Da Nang Hospital for Women and Children, Da Nang, Vietnam
[6]Infectious Disease Team, The Children's Hospital at Westmead and Discipline of Paediatrics and Adolescent Medicine, University of Sydney, Sydney, NSW, Australia
Full list of author information is available at the end of the article

airways (upper and lower). The World Health Organization (WHO) defines 'pneumonia' as a child with tachypnoea, with or without signs of respiratory distress. Given the huge overlap in how these terms are applied in clinical practice, the authors considered 'pneumonia' and acute lower respiratory tract infection (LRTI) to be synonymous for the purpose of this review.

Common bacterial pathogens

Bacteria classically described to cause community-acquired pneumonia in children include *Streptococcus pneumoniae, Haemophilus influenzae* type b (Hib) and *Staphylococcus aureus* [6]. Table 1 presents an overview of pathogens commonly associated with acute LRTIs in children less than 5 years of age. With enhanced diagnostic tools, respiratory viruses and atypical bacteria such as *Mycoplasma pneumonia* are commonly detected in children with community-acquired pneumonia, particularly in studies from the Western Pacific Region [7–9]. This review focused on bacterial pathogens because they are the major cause of pneumonia-related mortality and the primary indication for antibiotic use. However, it is important to appreciate that accurate differentiation between viral and/or bacterial infection is a major challenge to clinicians and complicates management [10]. This review provides a brief overview of the most common bacterial pathogens and their reported drug resistance profiles from surveys conducted in the Western Pacific Region.

Table 1 Pathogens commonly associated with pneumonia or acute lower respiratory tract infection in children less than 5 years of age[e]

Age group	Bacteria	Viruses
<5 years	*Streptococcus pneumoniae*[a]	RSV
	Haemophilus influenzae[a]	Rhinovirus
	Mycoplasma pneumoniae[b]	Influenza virus (A and B)
	Staphylococcus aureus	Parainfluenza virus
	Klebsiella pneumoniae	Human metapneumovirus
	Streptococcus pyogenes	Adenovirus
	Bordetella pertussis[c]	Human corona virus
	Mycobacterium tuberculosis[d]	
Neonates	Group B streptococcus	
	Listeria monocytogenes	
	Enteric (gram negative) bacteria	
	Chlamydia trachomatis	

RSV Respiratory Syncytial Virus, *Staphylococcus aureus* includes methicillin resistant strains (MRSA); *Haemophilus influenzae* includes type b and other encapsulated strains

[a]Disease greatly reduced in settings with universal access to conjugated vaccines; [b]Typically considered as "atypical bacteria" requiring macrolide therapy; [c]mainly in unvaccinated babies, in older children it can present as a chronic cough; [d]The risk of tuberculosis is dependent on the likelihood of *Mycobacteria tuberculosis* exposure/infection, which is a particular problem in areas with uncontrolled tuberculosis transmission

[e]Adapted from [3, 6]

Streptococcus pneumoniae

The development of resistance mutations against multiple antibiotics is well documented in *S. pneumoniae,* as well as the expansion of resistant clones under antibiotic pressure. Resistance has been recorded against penicillin, tetracycline, cotrimoxazole, chloramphenicol, fluoroquinolones and macrolides [5, 11, 12]. Although the correlation between *in vitro* and *in vivo* resistance remains contentious, it is generally assumed that penicillin (at adequate dosages) should still be effective against pneumococcal pneumonia (not meningitis) caused by strains with low or intermediate levels of resistance *in vitro* [13]. This is difficult to verify, as many factors that influence the outcome of pneumonia treatment—-such as underlying comorbid conditions, disease severity and supportive treatment—are poorly described in historical datasets and adequately powered head-to-head comparisons are rare [14–16]. Another important factor to take into consideration is the roll-out of pneumococcal conjugate vaccines. Routine administration of pneumococcal conjugate vaccine (PCV) in infancy has led to major reductions in pneumonia hospitalization and invasive pneumococcal disease in young children [17]. Given that the most common drug resistant strains were included in 7- and 13-valent pneumococcal conjugate vaccines, drug resistant pneumococcal disease has been greatly reduced in areas with high vaccine uptake [18], while reductions in strain carriage also reduced secondary pneumonia cases among older adults [17]. However, recent studies from Canada and the United Kingdom demonstrated substantial increases in multidrug resistant non-vaccine serotypes in both colonizing and invasive strains since introducing PCV13, with similar findings for colonizing strains after introducing PCV7 in Korean children [19–21].

High penicillin and macrolide resistance rates have been reported in published surveys, but many of these surveys included select patient populations and used minimal inhibitory concentration (MIC) breakpoints with variable stringency, and were also done prior to routine PCV delivery [5, 22, 23]. The use of variable MIC breakpoints in different studies is a major source of confusion and complicates study comparison. MIC breakpoints defined by the Clinical and Laboratory Standards Institute (CLSI) are widely used in the United States, while Europe has adopted the European Committee on Antimicrobial Susceptibility Testing (EUCAST) standards. They use broadly similar *in vitro* methods and specify MIC breakpoints by considering the pharmacokinetic–pharmacodynamic (PK-PD) properties of the drug, the clinical site of disease and the specific mechanism of drug resistance [24]. Studies have shown reasonable comparability between antibiotic susceptibility profiles using revised CLSI and EUCAST breakpoints

[25, 26], but some significant differences remain. Against *S. pneumoniae* and *H. influenzae*, cefuroxime and cefaclor breakpoints still produce divergent results [26]. Global surveillance efforts would be greatly enhanced if uniform surveillance criteria can be agreed upon and MIC breakpoint definitions harmonized.

A study conducted in 11 Asian countries reported a low (0.7%; 365/2184) prevalence of penicillin resistance in *S. pneumoniae* from non-meningeal isolates, [12] but it used an MIC breakpoint of ≥8 μg/ml as recommended by CLSI, which is much higher than the >0.06 μg/ml breakpoint proposed by EUCAST. A small case series of children with S. *pneumoniae* septicemia in China reported high drug resistance rates (96%; 24/25) [23], but MIC breakpoints were not specified. In Malaysia, 18% (5/28) of *S. pneumoniae* isolated from blood in children with community-acquired pneumonia was resistant to penicillin (using revised CLSI breakpoints) [27]. Since nasopharyngeal carriage may create a reservoir of resistant *S. pneumoniae* clones, it is important to monitor resistance in carriage specimens as well [28]. Nasopharyngeal *S. pneumoniae* carriage has been reported in 17% (102/614) of healthy Chinese children; 51% were resistant to macrolides by the E-test method [29]. In rural Vietnam, *S. pneumoniae* carriage has been detected in 50% of children, with higher rates in those less than 2 years of age (6–23 months). The resistance rate to amoxicillin and benzylpenicillin was low (4%; 17/421), based on revised CLSI breakpoints, but 95% were resistant to at least one antibiotic (cotrimoxazole 78%, erythromycin 70%, ciprofloxacin 28%) [30]. A more recent Vietnamese survey confirmed excellent penicillin susceptibility in *S. pneumoniae* isolates from respiratory specimens (penicillin 87% using revised CLSI breakpoints), although cephalosporin and macrolide susceptibility was poor (cefuroxime 19%, cefaclor 8%; azithromycin 4%) [31]. This supports the Vietnam national guidance to use high dose (90 mg/kg/day) amoxicillin as first-line treatment of community-acquired pneumonia in children [13].

Haemophilus influenzae

Although the prevalence of *H. influenzae* type b (Hib) has declined dramatically with widespread roll-out of conjugated Hib vaccine [32, 33], it remains prevalent in settings with poor vaccine uptake. B-lactamase production is commonly associated with Hib infection. In Vietnam, 41% of respiratory Hib isolates produced β-lactamase and 14% were β-lactamase non-producing ampicillin-resistant [31]. However, it is impossible to differentiate clinical infection from asymptomatic colonization using respiratory specimens from non-sterile sites. In China, Hib carriage decreased from 36% in 2000 to 19% in 2012, but β-lactamase-producing isolates increased from 4 to 31% over the same time period. Amoxicillin/clavulanic acid and 2nd or 3rd generation cephalosporins remained universally effective [34]. Despite the national Hib vaccine roll-out in Vietnam, Hib remains a common invasive pathogen [31], but this is expected to decrease as vaccine uptake improves. With increased vaccination uptake, the role of other encapsulated *H. influenzae* strains have increased [35]. A study in China found that 100% of *H. influenzae* strains identified in the sputum of children with pneumonia were non-typable; 1% (2/279) were β-lactamase-positive and 5% were β-lactamase non-producing ampicillin-resistant or intermediately resistant [36].

Staphylococcus aureus

S. aureus remains a common cause of community-acquired pneumonia. Pioneering lung puncture studies performed in Chile and Papua New Guinea identified *S. aureus* as a common pathogen in children with community-acquired pneumonia [37]. More recent studies found the pathogen predominantly in children at the severe end of the pneumonia disease spectrum, with increased frequency in severely malnourished children [38, 39]. *S. aureus* also poses particular problems following influenza or measles infection, and as a secondary infection in hospitalized children [38, 40, 41]. A major challenge has been the emergence of methicillin-resistant *S. aureus* (MRSA) and more recently, a decrease in vancomycin susceptibility [42, 43]. Among positive *S. aureus* blood cultures in Australian and New Zealand children, MRSA has been reported in 13% (142/1,073) with three times the average rate (incidence rate ratio, 3 [95%, CI: 2–4]), found among Aboriginal and Pacific Islander populations [44, 45]. A recent Malaysian survey reported MRSA in 8% (3/38) of children with community-acquired S. *aureus* bacteremia; 32% had skin or soft tissues infections and 32% had community-acquired pneumonia [27]. A study assessing the prevalence of heterogeneous vancomycin-intermediately-resistant *S. aureus* (hVISA*)* in Asian countries (including South Korea, Taiwan, Hong Kong, Thailand, the Philippines, Vietnam, India and Sri Lanka) reported that among 462 MRSA isolates, 3.5% were hVISA, with the highest prevalence in South Korea and Vietnam (7.0%) [46]. A more extensive report on antibiotic resistance in 15 hospitals throughout Vietnam found MRSA in 20% of children and adults with *S. aureus* bacteremia; vancomycin resistance rates were very low [47].

Atypical bacteria

Mycoplasma pneumoniae is highly prevalent in children diagnosed with pneumonia in the Western Pacific Region [4]. *M. pneumoniae* is inherently resistant to all β-lactams antibiotics and vancomycin, because it does not have a cell wall. With excessive macrolide use in recent years, reported macrolide resistance is near universal (90–100%) in parts of Asia [48]. Most countries report high rates of macrolide resistance (Japan 89% [49, 50], China 83–98% [5, 51, 52], South Korea 63% [53], Hong Kong 47% [54], Taiwan 23% [55]), although the methods for *M. pneumoniae* susceptibility testing are poorly standardized. *M. pneumoniae* remains susceptible to macrolides in Australia where it is less frequently used [56]. Resistance to tetracyclines and fluoroquinolones have not been reported in clinical isolates and may provide a treatment alternative in some children, although reduced *in vitro* susceptibility has been reported [48]. However, most *M. pneumoniae* cases recover either without antibiotic treatment or despite documented drug resistance, thus the clinical value of antibiotic treatment remains uncertain [57].

Treatment of ARTIs is a major driver of antibiotic use in children. It is important for clinicians to be familiar with the most common bacterial causes, their local drug resistance profiles and the likely impact of antibiotic therapy (both positive and negative) in order to develop a rational treatment approach. Because a timely and definitive bacteriological diagnosis is currently impossible, empiric antibiotic treatment is justified in any acutely ill child. However, there is a need to critically consider factors that promote unnecessary and irrational antibiotic use, especially in children who are not acutely ill.

Factors promoting irrational antibiotic use

Antibiotic use generates selective pressure that increases the prevalence of drug resistant strains; hence, strategies to improve rational antibiotic use are important to protect antibiotics as a precious resource. A study of antibiotic use in Vietnamese hospitals showed that a large proportion of in-patients received inappropriate antibiotic therapy [58]. The main factors that promote unnecessary antibiotic use in the Western Pacific Region, using Vietnam as an exemplar, are listed below.

Unrestricted antibiotic access

Given unrestricted access to over-the-counter antibiotics, treatment of any respiratory infection with antibiotics is a common practice in Vietnam, Malaysia, and South Korea [59]. In Vietnam, the *Pharmaceutical Law* passed in 2005 requires an antibiotic prescription, but 38% of caregivers still access antibiotics without any formal medical assessment [60]; even injectable antibiotics can be acquired at local shops without prescription [61]. In the Western Pacific Region, antibiotic use before presentation to a doctor is common; more than 40% in Mongolia [62] and more than 50% of children admitted with ARTIs in the Philippines [63]. A study in nine international sites—Colombia, Ghana, India, Mexico, Pakistan, South Africa (2 sites), Vietnam and Zambia—-found that the use of antibiotics in the 48 h prior to hospital admission was associated with treatment failure (OR: 1.8; 95% CI: 1.27–2.66) [64]. In addition, agricultural use of antibiotics remains essentially unregulated in most Asian countries, with high rates of colistin and cephalosporin use in the pig and poultry industries, resulting in increased rates of drug-resistant infections in human populations [65, 66].

Unrealistic expectations and limited awareness

Limited awareness among the general public (including politicians) is a challenge in all settings; the WHO recently launched a program to increase awareness about antimicrobial resistance and the need for more prudent antibiotic use [59]. In response, country-specific strategies to limit antimicrobial resistance have been launched in the United Kingdom, the United States and Australia [67–69], but few Asian countries have followed suit. Unrealistic public expectation is a major factor driving excessive antibiotic use [59, 70]. A study in rural Vietnam showed that just 13% of caregivers had correct knowledge about acute respiratory infections and 38% of caregivers self-managed common colds by buying antibiotics without prescription at the local pharmacy [60]. In Malaysia, 67% of people believed antibiotics to be effective against viral infections, with 47% using antibiotics during a common cold [61]. Moreover, antibiotic use is strongly influenced by cultural preferences and beliefs. Patients in Vietnam and China believe injectable antibiotics are more potent than oral options, and readily access injectable antibiotics without prescription [71]. A lack of adequate knowledge is also a problem among healthcare providers. A study in Vietnam demonstrated poor awareness about the risks and consequences of drug resistance among rural health-care providers when treating ARTIs; only 19% complied with recommended guidelines and 79% used antibiotics for common colds [72].

Physician-related factors

Table 2 provides an overview of physician-related factors that explains some of the excessive antibiotic use seen in Vietnam and parts of the Western Pacific Region. The difficulty in accurately differentiating viral from bacterial pneumonia is a major challenge in all settings. A study in Finland showed that of the routine blood tests, only the C-reactive protein (CRP) level differed significantly between bacterial and viral pneumonia patients [10]. Most children with dense lobar infiltrates on chest radiograph had laboratory evidence of a bacterial infection, but interstitial infiltrates were seen in both viral and bacterial pneumonia [10]. A recent randomized-controlled trial in Vietnam showed that point-of-care

Table 2 Physician related factors that contribute to excessive antibiotic use in the Western Pacific Region

Factor identified	Examples from the Western Pacific Region
Professional hierarchy	• Junior physicians adopt the prescription habits of senior physicians without rigorous discussion or review of the evidence [86]. • In Vietnam, inappropriate antibiotic use is a particular problem in obstetrics, gynecology and surgery wards where professional hierarchy is most pronounced [58]
No consideration of "societal risk"	• Doctors and patients often prefer newer and more expensive antibiotics, which are considered more "powerful" [62] • Physicians provide antibiotics to help individual patients; potential societal risks are not considered [86]; • In the absence of functional microbiology services, physicians have limited information on local drug-resistance profiles and the impact of excessive antibiotic use;
Perceived patient/ parent expectation	• Doctors strive for patient satisfaction and if patients request antibiotics it is usually prescribed [70, 87]; In Korea, 73% of doctors prescribe antibiotics for a common cold if requested by parents [88]; In Malaysia, 67% of patients believe that antibiotics help for viral infections [61] • Doctors have no time or motivation to explain the rationale for not using antibiotics
Fear of poor patient outcome or litigation	• Fear of poor patient outcomes is often listed as a key motivation for the use of broad-spectrum antibiotics by doctors [58, 59, 89] • Fear of litigation is not yet a major driver in the Western Pacific, but is likely to become a more prominent factor with increased development [90]
Inadequate microbiology services	• Near universal use of empiric broad spectrum antibiotics is common in places with poor microbiology services [70, 87]. • In Vietnam, antibiotic use was reduced in hospitals with functional microbiology laboratories [58]
Financial incentives to use antibiotics	• Doctors' prescribing habits is influenced by personal income generated and incentives provided by pharmaceutical companies [70, 86, 87]. In China, as in many other Western Pacific countries, drug prescriptions supplement a doctor's income [62]. • In South-Korea drug dispensing by health care workers was banned in 2000, resulting in major reductions in antibiotic use [62]

CRP testing reduced inappropriate antibiotic use for non-severe ARTIs [73]. A previous randomized-controlled trial in China investigated whether serum pro-calcitonin (PCT) could reduce unnecessary antibiotic use [74], but although the mean duration of antibiotic treatment was shorter in the PCT group, the antibiotic prescription rate was higher. It is hoped that rapid point-of-care testing for common respiratory viruses and biomarkers of severe bacterial infection will offer better bedside guidance in the near future, assisting more appropriate antibiotic use.

Because most child pneumonia deaths are caused by bacterial pathogens, current WHO guidelines recommend antibiotic use in all pneumonia cases, as defined by the presence of fast breathing. This approach may encourage the overuse of antibiotics, especially in children without danger signs who present with wheezing as a sign of reactive airway disease, which usually indicates a viral infection. Audible wheezing has been noted in 49% of Vietnamese children admitted with 'pneumonia' [75], which may identify a subgroup that does not require antibiotics [76]. WHO guidelines previously advised intravenous antibiotics in all children diagnosed with severe pneumonia (signs of respiratory distress), but oral amoxicillin was found to be effective in 92% (948/1,025) of children with a clinical diagnosis of severe pneumonia in Pakistan [77]. Subsequent trials demonstrated that home-based treatment can be applied to a wide variety of settings [74]. A multi-center study conducted in Bangladesh, Egypt, Ghana and Vietnam reported 9% (95% CI: 7–11%) treatment failure with 5 days of high dose oral amoxicillin (80–90 mg/kg/day), varying from 6% (95% CI: 3–10%) in Ghana to 13% (95% CI: 8–18%) in Vietnam [75]. A sizeable (but unknown) proportion of cases enrolled in these "clinical pneumonia" studies would have had viral infections. Therefore, it is not clear how much "treatment failure" actually resulted from inadequate antibiotic treatment for bacterial pneumonia; most children found to be "unresponsive to antibiotics" probably had viral pneumonia [78, 79]. Despite the available evidence, most doctors in Vietnam routinely hospitalize children with "clinical pneumonia" to administer intravenous antibiotics; unnecessary hospitalization increases both healthcare cost and the risk of nosocomial infection.

Proposed recommendations

Actions and recommendations to improve rational antibiotic use in both the community and hospital environment are summarized in Table 3. Unrestricted antibiotic access and self-medication are firmly entrenched in Vietnam and most other Asian countries [80]. Given the multiple vested interests that protect the status quo, strong regulation and effective law enforcement will be required to limit excessive antibiotic use. In addition to public education programs, better training of healthcare providers to critically review the need for antibiotic use is essential [59]. Only 31% of countries in the Western Pacific Region report high awareness of antimicrobial resistance among their healthcare providers [59]. An educational program in Indonesia, including face-to-face clinician visits and group discussions, significantly

Table 3 Actions and recommendations to improve rational antibiotic use

Actions	Suggested high-level recommendations[a]
In general	
Enhanced regulation	• Limit over-the-counter availability of antibiotics; establish strong national policies for appropriate antibiotic regulation; implement measures to ensure compliance • Improved national surveillance of antimicrobial resistance and adherence to treatment guidelines • Regulate agricultural use of antibiotics
Patient/public education	• Increase general awareness of adverse effects associated with excessive antibiotic use • Educate parents, caretakers, politicians and the general community about the benefits of restricted antibiotic use
Universal Hib and PCV	• Make Hib and PCV universally available free of charge • Maintain high uptake of other vaccines (e.g. pertussis and measles)
Within hospitals	
Provide information on local drug resistance patterns	• Maintain a network of functional microbiology laboratories, with adequate quality assurance and sharing of information
Establish functional antimicrobial stewardship programs	• Each hospital should have an antimicrobial stewardship program and a Drug and Therapeutics Committee with access to reliable and up-to-date data on antibiotic usage and drug resistance profiles • Each hospital should have regular/annual antibiotic use audits led by pharmacists or infectious disease control personnel
Provide clear guidance	• Develop national/regional consensus treatment guidelines that consider the international evidence base, as well as local disease etiology and drug resistance data
Eliminate perverse incentives	• Delink remuneration from antibiotic prescription • Ban incentives to doctors to provide antibiotics or use specific medical products
Educate medical students and trainees	• Include antimicrobial stewardship in the undergraduate medical, nursing and pharmacy curriculum • Highlight the growing drug resistance problem and need for prudent use

PCV pneumococcal conjugate vaccine, *Hib Haemophilus influenzae* type b
[a]In addition, a detailed assessment of pneumonia case management should be conducted to understand clinical decision-making and provide more pragmatic guidance to clinicians in the field. Exemplars of comprehensive national strategies to address antimicrobial resistance and limit excessive antibiotic use include the United Kingdom, the United States and Australia [67–69]

reduced the use of injectable drugs [81], but has not been replicated elsewhere.

In 2013, the WHO facilitated a meeting of Western Pacific Region countries in Manila to identify feasible antimicrobial resistance (AMR) strategies [59], but this has not yet translated into revised childhood pneumonia guidance or management practices. In Vietnam, the Vietnam Resistance (VINARES) project aims to strengthen laboratory surveillance and reduce irrational antibiotic use. The project covers 16 participating hospitals [82], but outside of the participating hospitals AMR surveillance remains weak. Laboratory capacity to assist microbiological diagnosis and guide clinical management is insufficient throughout the region [83]. Functional antibiotic stewardship programs have been established in some countries, but this should become standard practice and be adapted to the local context [44]. An antibiotic stewardship program in Chinese hospitals set targets for antibiotic prescriptions and penalized doctors who prescribed antibiotics inappropriately [84]. After 2 years, antibiotic prescriptions decreased by 58–68% in inpatients and 15–25% in outpatients [85]. An antimicrobial stewardship program is currently being implemented in Vietnam (through VINARES), but the scope of the program is limited and there is a need for similar programs, including regular audits of antibiotic use, in every hospital [82].

Conclusion

Optimal child pneumonia management presents an opportunity to reduce excessive antibiotic use in the Western Pacific Region. However, encouraging the rational use of antibiotics requires education of healthcare professionals, facilitation of cultural change, improved clinical guidance and the establishment of functional microbiology laboratories to monitor disease etiology and drug resistance patterns, together with the removal of inappropriate incentives and effective enforcement of national regulations to restrict antibiotic use in healthcare and agriculture.

Abbreviations

ARTI: Acute respiratory tract infection; AMR: Antimicrobial resistance; CRP: C-reactive protein; CLSI: Clinical and Laboratory Standards Institute; CI: Confidence interval; EUCAST: European Committee on Antimicrobial Susceptibility Testing; *H. influenzae*: *Haemophilus influenzae*; Hib: *Haemophilus influenzae* type b; hVISA: Heterogeneous vancomycin-intermediate S.*aureus*; MRSA: Methicillin resistant *staphylococcus aureus*; MIC: Minimal inhibitory concentration; M. *pneumoniae*: *Mycoplasma pneumonia*; PK-PD: Pharmacokinetic-pharmacodynamic; PCV: Pneumococcal conjugate vaccine; PCT: Procalcitonin; S. *aureus*: *Staphylococcus aureus*; S. *pneumoniae*: *Streptococcus pneumoniae*; VINARES: Vietnam resistance project; WHO: World Health Organization

Acknowledgements

Not applicable

Funding
Not applicable

Authors' contributions
NTKP and BJM conceptualized the manuscript and wrote the first draft. All authors gave constructive inputs from personal experience, suggested additional references to consider, and read and approved the final manuscript.

Competing interests
The authors declare that they have no competing interests.

Author details
[1]Respiratory Department, Da Nang Hospital for Women and Children, Da Nang, Vietnam. [2]Neonatal Department, Da Nang Hospital for Women and Children, Da Nang, Vietnam. [3]Microbiology Department, The University of Medicine and Pharmacy, Ho Chi Minh, Vietnam. [4]Antimicrobial Stewardship Team, The Children's Hospital at Westmead, Sydney, Australia. [5]Centre for International Child Health, University of Melbourne and Murdoch Children's Research Institute, Melbourne, Australia. [6]Infectious Disease Team, The Children's Hospital at Westmead and Discipline of Paediatrics and Adolescent Medicine, University of Sydney, Sydney, NSW, Australia.

References
1. Walker CLF, Rudan I, Liu L, Nair H, Theodoratou E, Bhutta ZA, O'Brien KL, Campbell H, Black RE. Global burden of childhood pneumonia and diarrhoea. Lancet. 2013;381(9875):1405–16.
2. WHO. World Health Statistics 2016: Monitoring health for the SDGs. 2016. http://www.who.int/gho/publications/world_health_statistics/2016/en/. Accessed 1 Feb 2017.
3. Naor B-Z, Carolyn M, John M, Emmalita M, Marianna T. Integrated Management of Childhood Illness (IMCI) implementation in the Western Pacific Region: information package. World Health Organ WPG. 2013. http://www.wpro.who.int/child_adolescent_health/documents/imci_info_package/en/. Accessed 5 Feb 2017.
4. Nguyen TKP, Tran TH, Robert CL, Graham SM, Marais BJ. Child pneumonia in the Western Pacific Region. Paediatr Respir Rev. 2017;21:102–10.
5. Felmingham D, Feldman C, Hryniewicz W, Klugman K, Kohno S, Low D, Mendes C, Rodloff A. Surveillance of resistance in bacteria causing community-acquired respiratory tract infections. Clin Microbiol Infect. 2002; 8(2):12–42.
6. McIntosh K. Community-acquired pneumonia in children. N Engl J Med. 2002;346(6):429–37.
7. Huong PLT, Hien PT, Lan NTP, Binh TQ, Tuan DM, Anh DD. First report on prevalence and risk factors of severe atypical pneumonia in Vietnamese children aged 1–15 years. BMC Public Health. 2014;14:1304.
8. Wu Z, Li Y, Gu J, Zheng H, Tong Y, Wu Q. Detection of viruses and atypical bacteria associated with acute respiratory infection of children in Hubei. China Respirology. 2014;19(2):218–24.
9. Yoshida L-M, Suzuki M, Thiem VD, Smith WP, Tsuzuki A, Huong VTT, Takahashi K, Miyakawa M, Anh NTH, Watanabe K. Population based cohort study for pediatric infectious diseases research in Vietnam. Trop Med health. 2014;42(2):S47–58.
10. Virkki R, Juven T, Rikalainen H, Svedström E, Mertsola J, Ruuskanen O. Differentiation of bacterial and viral pneumonia in children. Thorax. 2002; 57(5):438–41.
11. Fuller JD, Low DE. A review of Streptococcus pneumoniae infection treatment failures associated with fluoroquinolone resistance. Clin Infect Dis. 2005;41(1):118–21.
12. Kim SH, Song J-H, Chung DR, Thamlikitkul V, Yang Y, Wang H, Lu M, So TM-K, Hsueh P-R, Yasin RM. Changing trend of antimicrobial resistance and serotypes in Streptococcus pneumoniae in Asian countries: an ANSORP study. Antimicrob Agents Chemother. 2012;56(3):1418–26.
13. Peterson LR. Penicillins for treatment of pneumococcal pneumonia: does in vitro resistance really matter? Clin Infect Dis. 2006;42(2):224–33.
14. Metlay JP. Update on community-acquired pneumonia: impact of antibiotic resistance on clinical outcomes. Curr Opin Infect Dis. 2002;15(2):163–7.
15. Feldman C, Anderson R. Controversies in the treatment of pneumococcal community-acquired pneumonia. Future Microbiol. 2006;1(3):271–81.
16. Metlay JP, Singer DE. Outcomes in lower respiratory tract infections and the impact of antimicrobial drug resistance. Clin Microbiol Infect. 2002;8(2):1–11.
17. Oliwa JN, Marais BJ. Vaccines to prevent pneumonia in children–a developing country perspective (Epub ahead of print). Paediatr Respir Rev. 2017;22:23–30.
18. Dagan R. Antibiotic resistance and the potential impact of pneumococcal conjugate vaccines. Commun Dis Intell Q Rep. 2003;27(2003):S134–42.
19. Duvvuri VR, Deng X, Teatero S, Memari N, Athey T, Fittipaldi N, Gubbay JB. Population structure and drug resistance patterns of emerging non-PCV-13 Streptococcus pneumoniae serotypes 22 F, 15A, and 8 isolated from adults in Ontario, Canada. Infect Genet Evol. 2016;42:1–8.
20. Sheppard C, Fry N, Mushtaq S, Woodford N, Reynolds R, Janes R, Pike R, Hill R, Kimuli M, Staves P. Rise of multidrug-resistant non-vaccine serotype 15A Streptococcus pneumoniae in the United Kingdom, 2001 to 2014. Euro Surveill. 2016;21(50):30423.
21. Lee S, Kim J-H, Kim S-H, Park M, Bae S. Prevalent multidrug-resistant nonvaccine serotypes in pneumococcal carriage of healthy Korean children associated with the low coverage of the seven-valent pneumococcal conjugate vaccine. Osong Public Health Res Perspect. 2013;4(6):316–22.
22. Low DE, Pichichero ME, Schaad UB. Optimizing antibacterial therapy for community-acquired respiratory tract infections in children in an era of bacterial resistance. Clin Pediatr. 2004;43(2):135–51.
23. Su X-Y, Wen S-H, Lin L, Li C-C. Clinical characteristics of children with Streptococcus pneumoniae septicemia and drug sensitivity of Streptococcus pneumoniae. Zhongguo dang dai er ke za zhi (Chinese journal of contemporary pediatrics). 2013;15(11):995–9.
24. Marchese A, Esposito S, Barbieri R, Bassetti M, Debbia E. Does the adoption of EUCAST susceptibility breakpoints affect the selection of antimicrobials to treat acute community-acquired respiratory tract infections? BMC Infect Dis. 2012;12(1):181.
25. Kahlmeter G. The 2014 Garrod Lecture: EUCAST–are we heading towards international agreement? J Antimicrob Chemother. 2015;70(9):2427–39.
26. Kassim A, Omuse G, Premji Z, Revathi G. Comparison of Clinical Laboratory Standards Institute and European Committee on Antimicrobial Susceptibility Testing guidelines for the interpretation of antibiotic susceptibility at a University teaching hospital in Nairobi, Kenya: a cross-sectional study. Ann Clin Microbiol Antimicrob. 2016;15(1):21.
27. Kaur AA. Community-acquired bacteremia in Paediatrics: Epidemiology, aetiology and patterns of antimicrobial resistance in a Tertiary Care Centre, Malaysia. Med J Malaysia. 2016;71(3):117–21.
28. Samore MH, Magill MK, Alder SC, Severina E, Morrison-de Boer L, Lyon JL, Carroll K, Leary J, Stone MB, Bradford D. High rates of multiple antibiotic resistance instreptococcus pneumoniae from healthy children living in isolated rural communities: association with cephalosporin use and intrafamilial transmission. Pediatrics. 2001;108(4):856–65.
29. Hu J, Sun X, Huang Z, Wagner AL, Carlson B, Yang J, Tang S, Li Y, Boulton ML, Yuan Z. Streptococcus pneumoniae and Haemophilus influenzae type b carriage in Chinese children aged 12–18 months in Shanghai, China: a cross-sectional study. BMC Infect Dis. 2016;16:149.
30. Hoa NQ, Trung NV, Larsson M, Eriksson B, Phuc HD, Chuc NT, Lundborg CS. Decreased Streptococcus pneumoniae susceptibility to oral antibiotics among children in rural Vietnam: a community study. BMC Infect Dis. 2010;10:85.
31. Van P, Binh P, Minh N, Morrissey I, Torumkuney D. Results from the Survey of Antibiotic Resistance (SOAR) 2009–11 in Vietnam. J Antimicrob Chemother. 2016;71(S1):i93–102.
32. Chen WJ, Moulton LH, Saha SK, Mahmud AA, Arifeen SE, Baqui AH. Estimation of the herd protection of Haemophilus influenzae type b conjugate vaccine against radiologically confirmed pneumonia in children under 2 years old in Dhaka, Bangladesh. Vaccine. 2014;32(8):944–8.
33. Flasche S, Takahashi K, Vu DT, Suzuki M, Nguyen TH-A, Le H, Hashizume M, Dang DA, Edmond K, Ariyoshi K. Early indication for a reduced burden of radiologically confirmed pneumonia in children following the introduction of routine vaccination against Haemophilus influenzae type b in Nha Trang, Vietnam. Vaccine. 2014;32(51):6963–70.

34. Zhu H, Wang A, Tong J, Yuan L, Gao W, Shi W, Yu S, Yao K, Yang Y. Nasopharyngeal carriage and antimicrobial susceptibility of Haemophilus influenzae among children younger than 5 years of age in Beijing, China. BMC Microbiol. 2015;15:6.
35. Van Eldere J, Slack MP, Ladhani S, Cripps AW. Non-typeable Haemophilus influenzae, an under-recognised pathogen. Lancet Infect Dis. 2014;14(12):1281–92.
36. Hu J, Wang X, Ai T, Xie X, Liu X, Liu H, Yang L, Li H, Yang T, Zhang T. Multicenter prospective epidemiological studies on Haemophilus influenzae infection among hospitalized children with lower respiratory tract infections. Zhonghua er ke za zhi (Chinese journal of pediatrics). 2016;54(2):119–25.
37. Mimica I, Donoso E, Howard JE, Ledermann GW. Lung puncture in the etiological diagnosis of pneumonia: a study of 543 infants and children. Amer J Dis Child. 1971;122(4):278–82.
38. Asghar R, Banajeh S, Egas J, Hibberd P, Iqbal I, Katep-Bwalya M, Kundi Z, Law P, MacLeod W, Maulen-Radovan I. Multicentre randomized controlled trial of chloramphenicol vs. ampicillin and gentamicin for the treatment of very severe pneumonia among children aged 2 to 59 months in low resource settings: a multicenter randomized trial (spear study). BMJ. 2008; 336:80–4.
39. Chisti MJ, Graham SM, Duke T, Ahmed T, Faruque ASG, Ashraf H, Bardhan PK, Shahid AS, Shahunja K, Salam MA. Post-discharge mortality in children with severe malnutrition and pneumonia in bangladesh. PLoS One. 2014; 9(9):e107663.
40. Hughes AJ, Ariffin N, Huat TL, Molok HA, Hashim S, Sarijo J, Latif NHA, Hanifah YA, Kamarulzaman A. Prevalence of nosocomial infection and antibiotic use at a university medical center in Malaysia. Infect Control Hosp Epidemiol. 2005;26(1):100–4.
41. Lee M, Chiu C, Chow V, Lam R, Lai R. Prevalence of hospital infection and antibiotic use at a university medical center in Hong Kong. J Hosp Infect. 2007;65(4):341–7.
42. Howden BP, Davies JK, Johnson PD, Stinear TP, Grayson ML. Reduced vancomycin susceptibility in Staphylococcus aureus, including vancomycin-intermediate and heterogeneous vancomycin-intermediate strains: resistance mechanisms, laboratory detection, and clinical implications. Clin Microbiol Rev. 2010;23(1):99–139.
43. Song J-H, Hsueh P-R, Chung DR, Ko KS, Kang C-I, Peck KR, Yeom J-S, Kim S-W, Chang H-H, Kim Y-S. Spread of methicillin-resistant Staphylococcus aureus between the community and the hospitals in Asian countries: an ANSORP study. J Antimicrob Chemother. 2011;66(5):1061–9.
44. NPS Medicinewise. Antimicrobial resistance - it's happening right now. 2014. http://www.nps.org.au/publications/health-professional/health-news-evidence/2014/antimicrobial-resistance. Accessed 5 Feb 2017.
45. McMullan BJ, Bowen A, Blyth CC, Van Hal S, Korman TM, Buttery J, Voss L, Roberts S, Cooper C, Tong SY. Epidemiology and Mortality of Staphylococcus aureus Bacteremia in Australian and New Zealand Children. JAMA Pediatr. 2016;170(10):979–86.
46. Chung DR, Lee C, Kang YR, Baek JY, Kim SH, Ha YE, Kang C-I, Peck KR, Lee NY, Song J-H. Genotype-specific prevalence of heterogeneous vancomycin-intermediate Staphylococcus aureus in Asian countries. Int J Antimicrob Agents. 2015;46(3):338–41.
47. Vietnam Ministry of Health. First report on antibiotics use and resistance in Vietnam. 2009. http://benhnhietdoi.vn/su-dung-khang-sinh/. Accessed 3 Feb 2017.
48. Pereyre S, Goret J, Bébéar C. Mycoplasma pneumoniae: current knowledge on macrolide resistance and treatment. Front Microbiol. 2016;7:974.
49. Bell DM. Promoting appropriate antimicrobial drug use: perspective from the Centers for Disease Control and Prevention. Clin Infect Dis. 2001;33(3): 245–50.
50. Matsuda K, Narita M, Sera N, Maeda E, Yoshitomi H, Ohya H, Araki Y, Kakuma T, Fukuoh A, Matsumoto K. Gene and cytokine profile analysis of macrolide-resistant Mycoplasma pneumoniae infection in Fukuoka, Japan. BMC Infect Dis. 2013;13:591.
51. Bao F, Qu J, Liu Z, Qin X, Cao B. The clinical characteristics, treatment and outcome of macrolide-resistant Mycoplasma pneumoniae pneumonia in children. Zhonghua jie he he hu xi za zhi (Chinese journal of tuberculosis and respiratory diseases). 2013;36(10):756–61.
52. Zhou Z, Li X, Chen X, Luo F, Pan C, Zheng X, Tan F. Macrolide-resistant Mycoplasma pneumoniae in adults in Zhejiang, China. Antimicrob Agents Chemother. 2015;59(2):1048–51.
53. Hong KB, Choi EH, Lee HJ, Lee SY, Cho EY, Choi JH, Kang HM, Lee J, Ahn YM, Kang Y-H. Macrolide resistance of Mycoplasma pneumoniae, South Korea, 2000–2011. Emerg Infect Dis. 2013;19(8):1281–4.
54. Ho P-L, Law PY, Chan BW, Wong C-W, To KK, Chiu SS, Cheng VC, Yam W-C. Emergence of macrolide-resistant Mycoplasma pneumoniae in Hong Kong is linked to increasing macrolide resistance in multilocus variable-number tandem-repeat analysis type 4-5-7-2. J Clin Microbiol. 2015;53(11):3560–4.
55. Wu PS, Chang LY, Lin HC, Chi H, Hsieh YC, Huang YC, Liu CC, Huang YC, Huang LM. Epidemiology and clinical manifestations of children with macrolide-resistant Mycoplasma pneumoniae pneumonia in Taiwan. Pediatr Pulmonol. 2013;48(9):904–11.
56. Xue G, Wang Q, Yan C, Jeoffreys N, Wang L, Li S, Gilbert GL, Sun H. Molecular characterizations of PCR-positive Mycoplasma pneumoniae specimens collected from Australia and China. J Clin Microbiol. 2014;52(5):1478–82.
57. Spuesens EB, Sauteur PMM, Vink C, van Rossum AM. Mycoplasma pneumoniae infections–Does treatment help? J Infect. 2014;69(S1):S42–6.
58. Thu TA, Rahman M, Coffin S, Harun-Or-Rashid M, Sakamoto J, Hung NV. Antibiotic use in Vietnamese hospitals: a multicenter point-prevalence study. Am J Infect Control. 2012;40(9):840–4.
59. WHO. Antimicrobial resistance: global report on surveillance. 2014. http://www.who.int/drugresistance/documents/surveillancereport/en/. Accessed 19 Jan 2017.
60. Hoa NQ, Chuc NTK, Phuc HD, Larsson M, Eriksson B, Lundborg CS. Unnecessary antibiotic use for mild acute respiratory infections during 28-day follow-up of 823 children under five in rural Vietnam. Tran R Soc Trop Med Hyg. 2011;105(11):628–36.
61. Nordberg P, Stalsby-Lundborg C, Tomson G. Consumers and providers-Could they make better use of antibiotics? Int J Risk Saf Med. 2005;17(3):117–25.
62. WHO. Antimicrobial Resistance in the Western Pacific region: A review of surveillance and Health system response. 2015. http://www.wpro.who.int/entity/drug_resistance/documents/amr_wpr.pdf. Accessed 9 Feb 2017.
63. Capeding MR, Bravo L, Santos J, Kilgore PE, Kim SA, Balter I, Hubler R, Ye J, Moscariello M. Prospective surveillance study of invasive pneumococcal disease among urban children in the Philippines. Pediatr Infect Dis. 2013; 32(10):383–9.
64. Addo-Yobo E, Chisaka N, Hassan M, Hibberd P, Lozano JM, Jeena P, MacLeod WB, Maulen I, Patel A, Qazi S. Oral amoxicillin versus injectable penicillin for severe pneumonia in children aged 3 to 59 months: a randomised multicentre equivalency study. Lancet. 2004;364(9440):1141–8.
65. Nguyen NT, Nguyen HM, Nguyen CV, Nguyen TV, Nguyen MT, Thai HQ, Ho MH, Thwaites G, Ngo HT, Baker S. The use of colistin and other critical antimicrobials on pig and chicken farms in southern Vietnam and their association with resistance in commensal Escherichia coli. Appl Environ Microbiol. 2016;82(13):3727–35.
66. Liu Y-Y, Wang Y, Walsh TR, Yi L-X, Zhang R, Spencer J, Doi Y, Tian G, Dong B, Huang X. Emergence of plasmid-mediated colistin resistance mechanism MCR-1 in animals and human beings in China: a microbiological and molecular biological study. Lancet Infect Dis. 2016;16(2):161–8.
67. Davies S, Gibbens N. UK five year antimicrobial resistance strategy 2013 to 2018. Lodon: UK Goverment. 2013. https://www.gov.uk/government/uploads/system/uploads/attachment_data/file/244058/20130902_UK_5_year_AMR_strategy.pdf. Accessed 9 Feb 2017.
68. CDC. Antibiotic resistance threats in the United States, 2013: Centres for Disease Control and Prevention, US Department of Health and Human Services. 2013. https://www.cdc.gov/drugresistance/threat-report-2013/index.html. Accessed 9 Feb 2017.
69. The Department of Health. Antimicrobial resistance. Australia Government (AMR). 2016. http://www.health.gov.au/internet/main/publishingnsf/Content/ohp-amr.htm. Accessed 9 Feb 2017.
70. Hulscher ME, van der Meer JW, Grol RP. Antibiotic use: how to improve it? Int J Med Microbiol. 2010;300(6):351–6.
71. Mills A, Brugha R, Hanson K, McPake B. What can be done about the private health sector in low-income countries? Bull World Health Organ. 2002;80(4): 325–30.
72. Hoa NQ, Larson M, Chuc NTK, Eriksson B, Trung NV, Stålsby CL. Antibiotics and paediatric acute respiratory infections in rural Vietnam: health-care providers' knowledge, practical competence and reported practice. Trop Med Int Health. 2009;14(5):546–55.
73. Do NT, Ta NT, Tran NT, Than HM, Vu BT, Hoang LB, van Doorn HR, Vu DT, Cals JW, Chandna A. Point-of-care C-reactive protein testing to reduce inappropriate use of antibiotics for non-severe acute respiratory infections in Vietnamese primary health care: a randomised controlled trial. Lancet Global Health. 2016;4(9):633–41.

74. Dai B, Yuan X, Liu J. Value of serum procalcitonin for the guidance of antibiotic therapy in children with lower respiratory tract infection. Zhongguo dang dai er ke za zhi (Chinese journal of contemporary pediatrics). 2015;17(12):1292–6.
75. Addo-Yobo E, Anh DD, El-Sayed HF, Fox LM, Fox MP, MacLeod W, Saha S, Tuan TA, Thea DM, Qazi S. Outpatient treatment of children with severe pneumonia with oral amoxicillin in four countries: the MASS study. Trop Med Int Health. 2011;16(8):995–1006.
76. Singh V, Aneja S. Pneumonia–management in the developing world. Paediatr Respir Rev. 2011;12(1):52–9.
77. Hazir T, Fox LM, Nisar YB, Fox MP, Ashraf YP, MacLeod WB, Ramzan A, Maqbool S, Masood T, Hussain W. Ambulatory short-course high-dose oral amoxicillin for treatment of severe pneumonia in children: a randomised equivalency trial. Lancet. 2008;371(9606):49–56.
78. Hazir T, Nisar YB, Abbasi S, Ashraf YP, Khurshid J, Tariq P, Asghar R, Murtaza A, Masood T, Maqbool S. Comparison of oral amoxicillin with placebo for the treatment of World Health Organization–defined nonsevere pneumonia in children aged 2–59 months: a multicenter, double-blind, randomized, placebo-controlled trial in Pakistan. Clin Infect Dis. 2011;52(3):293–300.
79. Jehan F, Nisar MI, Kerai S, Brown N, Balouch B, Hyder Z, Ambler G, Ginsburg AS, Zaidi AK. A double blind community-based randomized trial of amoxicillin versus placebo for fast breathing pneumonia in children aged 2–59 months in Karachi, Pakistan (RETAPP). BMC Infect Dis. 2016;16:13.
80. Van der Geest S, Hardon A. Self-medication in developing countries. J Soc Adm Pharm. 1990;7(4):199–204.
81. Hadiyono JEP, Suryawati S, Danu SS, Santoso B. Interactional group discussion: results of a controlled trial using a behavioral intervention to reduce the use of injections in public health facilities. Soc Sci Med. 1996; 42(8):1177–83.
82. Wertheim HF, Chandna A, Vu PD, Van Pham C, Nguyen PDT, Lam YM, Van Nguyen CV, Larsson M, Rydell U, Nilsson LE. Providing impetus, tools, and guidance to strengthen national capacity for antimicrobial stewardship in Vietnam. PLoS Med. 2013;10(5):e1001429.
83. Lee Y, Wakabayashi M. Key informant interview on antimicrobial resistance (AMR) in some countries in the western pacific region. Global Health. 2013;9:34.
84. Yin X, Song F, Gong Y, Tu X, Wang Y, Cao S, Liu J, Lu Z. A systematic review of antibiotic utilization in China. J Antimicrob Chemother. 2013;68(11):2445–52.
85. Xiao Y, Zhang J, Zheng B, Zhao L, Li S, Li L. Changes in Chinese policies to promote the rational use of antibiotics. PLoS Med. 2013;10(11):e1001556.
86. Hulscher ME, Grol RP, van der Meer JW. Antibiotic prescribing in hospitals: a social and behavioural scientific approach. Lancet Infect Dis. 2010;10(3):167–75.
87. Laxminarayan R, Duse A, Wattal C, Zaidi AK, Wertheim HF, Sumpradit N, Vlieghe E, Hara GL, Gould IM, Goossens H. Antibiotic resistance - the need for global solutions. Lancet Infect Dis. 2013;13(12):1057–98.
88. Cho H-J, Hong S-J, Park S. Knowledge and beliefs of primary care physicians, pharmacists, and parents on antibiotic use for the pediatric common cold. Soc Sci Med. 2004;58(3):623–9.
89. Murni IK, Duke T, Kinney S, Daley AJ, Soenarto Y. Reducing hospital-acquired infections and improving the rational use of antibiotics in a developing country: an effectiveness study. Arch Dis Child. 2015;100(5):454–9.
90. Fox C. Resisting antibiotic resistance: legal strategies to maintain man's dominion over microbes. Hous J Health L & Pol'y. 2011;12:35–62.

6

Global burden of childhood tuberculosis

Helen E. Jenkins

Abstract

In 2015, the World Health Organization (WHO) declared tuberculosis (TB) to be responsible for more deaths than any other single infectious disease. The burden of TB among children has frequently been dismissed as relatively low with resulting deaths contributing very little to global under-five all-cause mortality, although without rigorous estimates of these statistics the burden of childhood TB was, in reality, unknown. Recent work in the area has resulted in a WHO estimate of 1 million new cases of childhood TB in 2014 resulting in 136,000 deaths. Around 3% of these cases likely have multidrug-resistant TB and at least 40,000 are in HIV-infected children. TB is now thought to be a major or contributory cause of many deaths in children under five years old, despite not being recorded as such, and is likely in the top ten causes of global mortality in this age group. In particular, recent work has shown that TB is an underlying cause of a substantial proportion of pneumonia deaths in TB-endemic countries. Childhood TB should be given higher priority: we need to identify children at greatest risk of TB disease and death and make more use of tools such as active case-finding and preventive therapy. TB is a preventable and treatable disease from which no child should die.

Keywords: Incidence, Mortality, Estimation, Drug resistance

Background

In 1963, Edith Lincoln and Edward Sewell wrote in their seminal book 'Tuberculosis in Children': "At the present time the death rate from tuberculosis is markedly reduced in some areas and it is possible to look forward to the day when tuberculosis will no longer be a public health problem [1]." More than 50 years later, in 2015, the World Health Organization (WHO) declared tuberculosis (TB) to be the number one killer among infectious diseases [2].

The underlying reasons for this resurgence are complex. They include HIV, the oldest known sample of which was taken just three years before the publication of 'Tuberculosis in Children', although it was not identified as HIV until many decades later [3]. Another contributory factor, drug resistance, was already known about in 1963, although few could have foretold the devastating impact it would have on TB control. But what has the impact been on children? What proportion of the estimated 9.6 million new TB cases in 2015 [2] occurred in children? How many were HIV-infected or infected with drug-resistant TB? And how many died? We simply don't know many of these basic statistics, largely because the diagnosis of TB in children still relies heavily on the methods that Edith Lincoln was using in Bellevue Hospital more than half a century ago [1]. However, there is a growing understanding that many cases of TB disease in children are not reported as such [4].

Correspondence: jenkins.helen@gmail.com
Department of Biostatistics, Boston University School of Public Health, Boston, MA 02118, USA

While TB is the number one infectious cause of death among all age groups, pneumonia bears that title among children under five years old, with an estimated 935,000 deaths in 2013 [5]. *Mycobacterium tuberculosis*, the causative agent of tuberculosis, is also a recognized, although under-diagnosed, cause of pneumonia, especially in TB-endemic areas and among HIV-infected children [6]. A recent review found that between 1% and 23% of pneumonia cases also had TB disease [7]. The true extent to which tuberculosis is an underlying cause of morbidity and mortality attributed to other causes is unknown, largely due to problems with the diagnosis of TB in children [4]. However, with increasing attention on childhood TB in recent years [8], there have been considerable steps taken to use mathematical and statistical tools to help us understand the true burden of childhood TB.

Here, I summarize our current knowledge about the burden of childhood TB, with specific reference to incidence and mortality, as well as the impact of HIV and drug resistance on this vulnerable and often neglected population.

Why is it important to understand the burden of childhood TB?

Firstly, we must consider what we mean by the word "burden". Burden is a non-specific term measuring the impact of a health problem in terms of financial cost, mortality, morbidity or other indicators and here we will focus primarily on morbidity and mortality due to varying forms of TB. The reasons behind the need to understand disease burdens are broadly similar across diseases: without robust estimates of the true burden of disease, we cannot identify gaps in identification of cases, estimate the resources required to reduce this burden, begin to plan the types of interventions that might be effective or measure the impact of these interventions. The specific reasons for understanding the burden of childhood TB have been covered previously [9] but include the need to raise advocacy for childhood TB, which has been traditionally much neglected [10]; a need for increased research into improved diagnostics and treatment regimens specifically for children; demonstration of the importance of TB in the context of overall childhood morbidity and mortality; and also because childhood TB is a surveillance indicator for recent transmission within a community [11].

The END TB Strategy from WHO has the specific aims of reducing global TB incidence and mortality by 90% and 95% respectively by the year 2035 [12]. However, without good estimates of incidence and mortality it will be impossible to know if these targets have been met. Children make up 26% of the global population and 43% of the population in low-income countries [13]. Therefore, to monitor our progress towards the END TB goals, we need robust estimates of incidence and mortality in children.

Incidence of childhood TB disease

In 2011, the WHO produced their first estimate of global childhood (<15 years) TB annual incidence of 490,000 [14], assuming equal case detection rates in children and adults. Earlier estimates had included 663,990 [15] (1990), 884,019 [16] (2000) and 1,039,000 [15] (2000). In 2014, three new pediatric TB incidence estimates were put forward. Jenkins et al. published an estimate of approximately 1 million [17] (Table 1). This was produced by scaling up age-disaggregated smear positive notifications reported to the WHO, in such a way as to account for the substantial difference that exists between adults and children in terms of the proportion of all TB cases expected to be smear positive [18, 19]. In the second method, Dodd et al. used a mathematical model that estimated the incidence of TB infection in children using WHO TB prevalence data and demographic information [20]. Their model then estimated childhood TB disease incidence by incorporating the age-dependent risk of progression from infection to disease, accounting for HIV infection and Bacille Calmette-Guerin vaccination. They estimated that there were 651,000 incidence cases of childhood TB in the 22 high-burden countries (HBCs) [20] in 2010. This was later updated to produce a global estimate of around 850,000 [21] in 2014 (Table 1). A third independent group, the Institute of Health Metrics and Evaluation (IHME), estimated that there were 150,000 incident pediatric TB cases in 2013 [22] (among HIV-negative

Table 1 Annual estimates of the childhood tuberculosis (TB) burden among children aged 0-14 years

Measure	TB disease	Fraction of all pediatric TB cases	Latent TB infection
TB incidence	999,792 (95% CI: 937,877 – 1,055,414)[a]		
	847,000 (IQR: 558,000 – 1,280,000)[b]	N/A	67 million (IQR: 52.3 million – 85.7 million)[b]
	1,000,000 (UI: 900,000–1,100,000)[c]		
	150,000[d]		
INH-R TB	120,872 (95% CI: 96,628–149,059)[c]	12.1% (95% CI: 9.8%–14.8%)[c]	
	84,000[be]	9.9%[b]	6.8 million[b]
MDR-TB	31,948 (95% CI: 25,594–38,663)[a]	3.2%[a]	
	24,800 (IQR: 16,100–37,400)[b]	2.9% (IQR: 2.7%–3.1%)[b]	2.0 million (IQR: 1.6 million–2.6 million)[b]
Mortality	136,000 (range: 115,000–157,000)[c]	13.6%[c]	N/A
	60,000[d]		

INH-R Isoniazid resistant, *MDR* Multidrug-resistant, *CI* Confidence Interval, *IQR* Interquartile range, *UI* Uncertainty Interval
[a]Jenkins et al. 2014 [17]; [b]Dodd et al. 2016 [21]; [c]WHO 2015 [2]; [d]Murray et al. 2014 (Note: there are no uncertainty ranges around these estimates); Yuen et al. 2015 [35]
[e]Note that Dodd et al. 2016 produced an estimate of INH-R TB mono-resistance of 58,300 (IQR: 38,300 – 87,000) cases. The figure presented of 84,000 represents all forms of INH-R (i.e. mono-resistance plus MDR-TB) but because this was not formally estimated in Dodd et al. 2016, there is no IQR around this result

cases only). Notably, this was lower than the number of cases notified by countries to the WHO.

Following a meeting of the WHO Global Task Force on TB Impact Measurement in 2015 [23], it was recommended that the WHO combine the methods of Jenkins et al. [17] and Dodd et al. [20] to produce their pediatric TB incidence estimates [23]. The method of Murray et al. was excluded due to lack of information about the uncertainty of the estimate [24]. The new WHO combined estimate was 1 million incident child TB cases in 2014 [2] (Table 1).

Given that only 359,000 pediatric TB cases were notified to the WHO in 2014, this implies that two-thirds of all children that developed active TB disease in 2014 were not notified. The assumption is that these children were not diagnosed and therefore did not receive treatment. The morbidity and mortality implications of so many children not receiving treatment are profound and very worrying. Estimation of how many of these "invisible" children exist has been an essential part of raising advocacy for these children and demonstrating the need for improved diagnostics [25] and methods to find these children (e.g. active case-finding [26]). TB is both preventable and treatable but we need to identify these children in the first place.

Of particular concern are children under the age of five years. These children are less likely to be diagnosed with TB, given that they have the disease, but more likely to suffer serious sequelae such as TB meningitis [27]. So far, Dodd et al. are the only group to specifically estimate TB incidence in children under five, although WHO under-five estimates may be published in their annual TB report later in 2016. Dodd et al. estimated that 51.4% of all pediatric cases of TB disease in 2014 occurred in children under five years of age [21] (Table 2). Applying this to the WHO pediatric TB incidence estimate would indicate that 514,000 children under five years of age developed TB disease in 2014, which is nearly four and half times the number notified to the WHO for that year [28].

Table 2 Annual estimated burden of childhood tuberculosis (TB) among children aged 0–4 years[a]

Measure	Estimate (Interquartile range)	Fraction of all pediatric TB (0–14 years of age)
TB incidence	435,000 (278,000–651,000)	51.4%
Isoniazid-resistant TB	42,200[b]	50.2%
Multidrug-resistant TB	12,700 (8,020–19,000)	51.2%

[a]All estimates are from Dodd et al. 2016 [21]

[b]Note that Dodd et al. 2016 produced an estimate of INH-R TB mono-resistance of 29,500 (IQR: 18,800 - 44,300) cases. The figure presented of 42,200 represents all forms of INH-R (i.e. mono-resistance plus MDR-TB) but because this was not formally estimated in Dodd et al. 2016, there is no IQR around this result

Drug-resistant TB disease

Drug-resistant TB is under-diagnosed among all age groups due to the resources and costs required for diagnosis and limited access to testing facilities in many parts of the world [29]. Difficulties with obtaining bacteriologically positive sputum from children with TB only serve to amplify these issues [30]. It is believed that the majority of cases of pediatric drug-resistant TB are undiagnosed as such and therefore inappropriately treated [11], if they receive any treatment at all. With so much under-diagnosis of pediatric drug-resistant TB, how do we know how many children globally develop active TB disease annually due to a drug-resistant strain?

Until 2014, no estimate of the global burden of multidrug-resistant (strains resistant to the drugs isoniazid and rifampicin, the backbone of TB therapy) TB (MDR-TB) existed. A systematic review of the literature published before 12 January 2012 identified 97 reports that included 8,382 children with drug-susceptibility results for isoniazid and rifampicin [17]. Of these, 348 children tested positive for MDR-TB. In 2012, authors from the WHO reported results from an analysis of their full database of the Global Project on Anti-tuberculosis Drug Resistance Surveillance [31] on MDR-TB reporting between 1994 and 2011. They found that of 6,070 children tested for MDR-TB, 456 were positive. A 2012 review of the literature published before 31 October 2011 on treatment outcomes among children with MDR-TB identified 315 children with MDR-TB [32]. These three studies taken together indicate that, even assuming no overlapping of study populations, just 1,119 children with MDR-TB have been documented in the published literature.

In 2014, the first global estimate of the annual incidence of pediatric MDR-TB was published [17]. This work reviewed the literature for studies that included both children and adults tested for MDR-TB in the same setting and quantified the relationship between the percentage of new (treatment-naïve) adult TB cases with MDR-TB and the percentage observed in children. The authors then used WHO national estimates of the percentage of new TB cases with MDR-TB by country to estimate the percentage of childhood TB cases that had MDR-TB for every country worldwide. They then multiplied these percentages by their aforementioned pediatric TB estimates to obtain the global estimated number of pediatric MDR-TB cases in 2010 of 32,000 [17] (Table 1), i.e. 3.2% of total childhood TB incidence.

Although outcomes for children with MDR-TB who receive appropriate treatment can be excellent [32, 33], the vast majority of these 32,000 annual new cases are never correctly diagnosed with MDR-TB, much less receive appropriate treatment. It is sobering to think that the 1,119 children ever reported in the literature represent just 3.5% of the total incident cases that occur in one year.

The burden of other forms of drug-resistant TB also requires quantification. Isoniazid preventive therapy (IPT) is one of our most effective, but under-used, tools against pediatric TB [34]. However, its effectiveness could be undermined by isoniazid-resistant (INH-R) latent TB infection (LTBI). A recent review by Yuen et al. estimated that 12.1% of children with TB globally had INH-R TB disease (including mono-resistance and combined with other forms of resistance), representing 121,000 cases of disease [35] (Table 1). This percentage was highest in the former Soviet Union countries. Assuming that the percentage of TB cases with isoniazid resistance in children with active disease is reflected in those with LTBI, isoniazid preventive therapy will be ineffective in 12.1% of children with TB. It therefore crucial to understand which children might be at highest risk of INHR-TB so that other preventive methods can be used, such a regimen containing rifapentine or rifampicin [36].

Finally, Dodd et al. recently published an extension of their mathematical model to estimate the number of children with several different forms of drug-resistant TB [21]. Noting that their estimates worked from a lower baseline of overall TB incidence than those of Jenkins et al., they estimated that 24,800 had MDR-TB (i.e. 2.9% of all TB incidence) (Table 1) and 58,300 had mono-INH-R TB (i.e. 6.9% of all TB incidence). For comparison with the results from Yuen et al., the total INH-R TB resistance estimate from Dodd et al. was 84,000 cases constituting approximately 9.9% of all pediatric TB cases [21]. In addition, they estimated that 1,160 children had extensively drug-resistant TB (TB that is MDR-TB plus resistance to a fluoroquinolone and an injectable drug).

TB incidence among HIV-infected children

Despite the known importance of HIV co-infection in TB infected and diseased individuals [37], there are no estimates of the global burden of TB specifically in HIV-infected children. Dodd et al. estimated that 5.0% (IQR: 2.4%, 10.1%) of TB incidence in the 22 HBCs occurs in HIV-infected children [20]. This translates to 32,500 HIV-infected children developing active TB disease in the HBCs in 2010. A back-of-the-envelope calculation would suggest that globally in 2014 between 40,000 and 50,000 HIV-infected children developed TB disease.

We currently have two effective ways to prevent TB disease in TB-infected children: isoniazid prophylaxis [38] and anti-retroviral treatment (Dodd et al. in preparation). Many of these 40,000–50,000 annual cases could be prevented with more rigorous deployment of these preventive measures.

Childhood mortality due to TB

Globally, an estimated 6.3 million children under five years old died in 2013 [5] from all causes. But how many of these children are dying from TB? The first WHO estimates of TB mortality among children, released in 2015, found that 136,000 children under fifteen years old died in 2014 from TB [2] (Table 1). This estimate was based on data from vital registration systems and mortality surveys from 129 countries; an imputation method was used for the remaining countries without such data (largely from Africa). Vital registration death data have several limitations. For example, a cause might not be attributed [39] or if it is, it might be incorrect, especially if only one cause of death is allowed [40], despite multiple contributory causes. For example, studies have shown that TB may come close to bacterial pneumonia as a respiratory cause of death in children [41, 42]. In addition, in many countries there are few resources to carry out autopsies, and some deaths may not even be registered at all [43]. These limitations are likely to be amplified in high TB burden countries with few resources to carry out detailed autopsies. The IHME group also produced childhood TB mortality estimates of 60,000 TB-related deaths among HIV-negative children in 2014 [22].

An alternative method of estimating the number of children dying with TB is to multiply case fatality ratios (CFR; which could be defined in this context as the percentage of children that die within a year of a TB diagnosis) by the estimated incidence of pediatric TB. A recent systematic review and meta analysis has quantified CFRs among children with TB [44]. In particular, the authors searched the pre-chemotherapy literature to understand CFRs in children that do not receive TB treatment. The authors estimated that 21.9% (95% CI: 18.1%, 26.4%) of children from the pre-chemotherapy era studies died from TB, within a year of TB diagnosis. The case fatality ratio among children aged under 5 years old was substantially worse at 43.6% (95% CI: 36.8%, 50.6%) [44]. Children receiving treatment faired considerably better with less than 1% dying.

That nearly half of all children under five years of age that do not receive treatment will die should be a call to action. Mortality due to TB is likely a far more substantial problem than currently thought and we urgently need to find and treat these children to prevent unnecessary deaths. If we assume that all of the estimated children aged under five years with incident TB that were not notified to the WHO in 2014 did not receive treatment, our case fatality ratios would suggest that 173,000 of these children died. This is already substantially higher than the current childhood estimate of 136,000 and does not include children aged between 5 and 14 years old or account for any potential increased risk associated with HIV-infection.

Tuberculosis was not mentioned in a recent paper classifying the causes of global under-five mortality [5]. Assuming that 50% of the 136,000 deaths from TB, as per the WHO estimate, occur in children aged under five years, TB should have been classed as the ninth highest cause of death worldwide in children aged 1–59 months, above pertussis (Table in Liu et al. [5]). Our back-of-the-envelope estimate of 173,000 children would place TB at number six, ahead of meningitis, AIDS and measles.

The reality is that TB is causing disease in many more young children than we realize, resulting in undiagnosed, untreated TB and too many preventable deaths. TB is being misdiagnosed as other diseases and is also an underlying, undiagnosed cause of deaths that are attributed to other more easily diagnosed diseases, including pneumonia [4]. As Graham et al. [4] pointed out, if just 10% of the 935,000 currently attributed to pneumonia [5] were in fact due to TB, this would add a further 93,500 deaths to the WHO estimate of 136,000, increasing it by 69%. Full recognition of the contribution that TB is making to under-five mortality is a first and essential step in reducing that contribution.

Meningitis

The main cause of serious morbidity and mortality in children with TB is TB meningitis [27]. The successes of the roll-out of pneumococcal vaccines in recent years [45, 46] have resulted in TB meningitis becoming one of the most prevalent forms of bacterial meningitis [47, 48]. There are currently no estimates of the number of children that develop TB meningitis worldwide or that die from the disease, largely due to difficulties with diagnosis [49]. However, a recent study found that 19.3% (95% CI: 14.0%, 26.1%) of children with TB meningitis will die and that among the survivors 53.9% (95% CI: 42.6%, 64.9%) will experience neurological sequelae [50]. Given the high mortality and morbidity associated with this form of TB, we urgently need to understand how many children develop and die from this disease and where they are most prevalent. This is a major gap in our knowledge regarding the global burden of childhood TB.

Latent TB infection

One important way of preventing future morbidity and mortality due to TB is through active case-finding to identify probable cases of latent tuberculosis infection (LTBI) in children and target those children with preventive therapy [26]. However, we need robust estimates of how many children are likely to have LTBI and where these children are located so that we can maximize the effectiveness of our active case-finding. Dodd et al. estimated that 67 million children under fifteen years old were infected with TB in 2014 [21] (Table 1). The majority of these were located in the SouthEast Asia region (27 million) and the African region (20.9 million) [21]. In addition, Dodd et al. estimated the number of children latently infected with various forms of drug-resistant TB [21] (Tables 1 and 2). These estimates by Dodd et al. were generated assuming a constant annual rate of infection (ARI) and extrapolating backwards over 15 years. Houben and Dodd have recently produced an estimate of annual LTBI prevalence in children of 97 million [51]. In their method, the historical ARI was allowed to vary, based on changes in WHO estimates of TB disease prevalence and direct ARI estimates from tuberculin skin test surveys.

These are important statistics to know but it is unrealistic to think that all of these children can and should be given preventive therapy. Yuen et al. recently published estimates of how many children might be targeted for preventive therapy [52]. The authors estimated how many children live in a household with at least one adult diagnosed pulmonary TB case and, therefore, have been at risk of transmission and should be offered preventive therapy. The authors also estimated how many of these child contacts were likely to already have TB disease at the time that they are investigated. The result was an estimated 7.48 million children living with an adult diagnosed pulmonary TB case, of which, 2.41 million were under five years old. Of these 7.48 million, the authors estimated that approximately 660,000 would have TB disease upon investigation, with 239,000 aged under five years. National or sub-national targets such as these allow a national tuberculosis program to plan resources and interventions to identify and treat children at risk of or already experiencing TB disease.

Conclusions

Focus on and development of methods to estimate the global burden of childhood TB have advanced enormously in recent years; childhood TB is starting to get the recognition that it unfortunately deserves, although much more could be done. Approximately 1 million children develop TB disease each year and at least 14% die, probably considerably more. We are beginning to drill down and understand the burden among children infected with HIV, as well as the risk of drug-resistant forms of TB in children. The majority of these children are never diagnosed with or treated for their TB disease and TB is likely a far more important cause of under-five mortality than is currently believed. Now that we are beginning to appreciate the scale of the problem, we need a more accurate understanding of precisely which children are at greatest risk of morbidity and mortality so that they can be targeted with preventive treatment. No child should die from TB in the 21st century.

Abbreviations

ARI: Annual risk of infection; BCG: Bacille Calmette-Guerin vaccination; IHME: Institute of Health Metrics and Evaluation; INH-R TB: Isoniazid-resistant tuberculosis; IPT: Isoniazid preventive therapy; LTBI: Latent tuberculosis infection; MDR-TB: Multidrug-resistant tuberculosis; TB: Tuberculosis; WHO: World Health Organization

Acknowledgements

HEJ would like to thank Dr. Courtney Yuen, Dr. Pete Dodd, Dr. Rein Houben and Dr. James Seddon for helpful comments on an earlier version of this manuscript.

Funding

HEJ was funded by US National Institutes of Health US NIH K01AI102944. The content of the article is solely the responsibility of the authors and does not necessarily represent the views of the National Institute of Allergy and Infectious Disease or the Office of the Director, NIH. The funder had no role in the decision to publish this manuscript.

Authors' contributions

HEJ was invited to write this manuscript and was provided with the title by the series editor. HEJ conceived the structure and content of the manuscript. HEJ wrote the manuscript and was responsible for final approval and submission of the manuscript.

Competing interests

HEJ declares no competing interests.

References

1. Lincoln EW, Sewell EM. Tuberculosis in Children. New York: McGraw-Hill; 1963.
2. World Health Organization. Global Tuberculosis Report 2015. Geneva: World Health Organization; 2015.
3. Worobey M, Gemmel M, Teuwen DE, et al. Direct evidence of extensive diversity of HIV-1 in Kinshasa by 1960. Nature. 2008;455(7213):661–4.
4. Graham SM, Sismanidis C, Menzies HJ, Marais BJ, Detjen AK, Black RE. Importance of tuberculosis control to address child survival. Lancet. 2014; 383(9928):1605–7.
5. Liu L, Oza S, Hogan D, et al. Global, regional, and national causes of child mortality in 2000-13, with projections to inform post-2015 priorities: an updated systematic analysis. Lancet. 2015;385(9966):430–40.
6. Graham SM. Child pneumonia: current status, future prospects. Int J Tuberc Lung Dis. 2010;14(11):1357–61.
7. Oliwa JN, Karumbi JM, Marais BJ, Madhi SA, Graham SM. Tuberculosis as a cause or comorbidity of childhood pneumonia in tuberculosis-endemic areas: a systematic review. Lancet Respir Med. 2015;3(3):235–43.
8. Sandgren A, Cuevas LE, Dara M, et al. Childhood tuberculosis: progress requires an advocacy strategy now. Eur Respir J. 2012;40(2):294–7.
9. Seddon JA, Jenkins HE, Liu L, et al. Counting children with tuberculosis: why numbers matter. Int J Tuberc Lung Dis. 2015;19 Suppl 1:9–16.
10. Marais BJ, Schaaf HS. Childhood tuberculosis: an emerging and previously neglected problem. Infect Dis Clin North Am. 2010;24(3):727–49.
11. Becerra MC, Swaminathan S. Commentary: a targets framework: dismantling the invisibility trap for children with drug-resistant tuberculosis. J Public Health Policy. 2014;35(4):425–54.
12. World Health Organization. The WHO End TB Strategy. 2016. http://www.who.int/tb/post2015_strategy/en/. Accessed 8 Nov 2016.
13. World Bank. World development indicators 2014: population dynamics. 2015. http://wdi.worldbank.org/table/2.1. Accessed 8 Nov 2016.
14. World Health Organization. Global Tuberculosis Control 2011. Geneva: World Health Organization; 2011.
15. Dolin PJ, Raviglione MC, Kochi A. Global tuberculosis incidence and mortality during 1990-2000. Bull World Health Organ. 1994;72(2):213–20.
16. Nelson LJ, Wells CD. Global epidemiology of childhood tuberculosis. Int J Tuberc Lung Dis. 2004;8(5):636–47.
17. Jenkins HE, Tolman AW, Yuen CM, et al. Incidence of multidrug-resistant tuberculosis disease in children: systematic review and global estimates. Lancet. 2014;383(9928):1572–9.
18. Murray CJ, Styblo K, Rouillon A. Tuberculosis in developing countries: burden, intervention and cost. Bull Int Union Tuberc Lung Dis. 1990;65(1):6–24.
19. Kunkel A, Abel P, Nathavitharana RR, Marx FM, Jenkins HE, Cohen T. Smear positivity in paediatric and adult tuberculosis: systematic review and meta-analysis. BMC Infect Dis. 2016;16:282.
20. Dodd PJ, Gardiner E, Coghlan R, Seddon JA. Burden of childhood tuberculosis in 22 high-burden countries: a mathematical modelling study. Lancet Glob Health. 2014;2(8):e453–9.
21. Dodd PJ, Sismanidis C, Seddon JA. The global burden of drug-resistant tuberculosis in children: a mathematical model. Lancet Infect Dis. 2016; 16(10):1193–201.
22. Murray CJ, Ortblad KF, Guinovart C, et al. Global, regional, and national incidence and mortality for HIV, tuberculosis, and malaria during 1990-2013: a systematic analysis for the Global Burden of Disease Study 2013. Lancet. 2014;384(9947):1005–70.
23. World Health Organization. WHO Global Task Force on Impact Measurement. Report of the 3rd meeting of the TB estimates subgroup. 2015. http://www.who.int/tb/advisory_bodies/impact_measurement_taskforce/meetings/global_consultation_meeting_report.pdf?ua=1. Accessed 8 Nov 2016.
24. Sismanidis C, Glaziou P, Grzemska M, Floyd K, Raviglione M. Global epidemiology of paediatric tuberculosis. 2015. http://www.who.int/tb/advisory_bodies/impact_measurement_taskforce/meetings/global_consultation_doc08a_who_methods_children.pdf?ua=1. Accessed 8 Nov 2016.
25. Chiang SS, Swanson DS, Starke JR. New Diagnostics for Childhood Tuberculosis. Infect Dis Clin North Am. 2015;29(3):477–502.
26. Yuen CM, Amanullah F, Dharmadhikari A, et al. Turning off the tap: stopping tuberculosis transmission through active case-finding and prompt effective treatment. Lancet. 2015;386(10010):2334–43.
27. Marais BJ, Gie RP, Schaaf HS, et al. The natural history of childhood intra-thoracic tuberculosis: a critical review of literature from the pre-chemotherapy era. Int J Tuberc Lung Dis. 2004;8(4):392–402.
28. World Health Organization. TB case notifications. 2016. http://www.who.int/tb/country/data/download/en/. Accessed 22 May 2016.
29. Abubakar I, Zignol M, Falzon D, et al. Drug-resistant tuberculosis: time for visionary political leadership. Lancet Infect Dis. 2013;13(6):529–39.
30. Perez-Velez CM, Marais BJ. Tuberculosis in children. N Engl J Med. 2012; 367(4):348–61.
31. Zignol M, Sismanidis C, Falzon D, Glaziou P, Dara M, Floyd K. Multidrug-resistant tuberculosis in children: evidence from global surveillance. Eur Respir J. 2013;42(3):701–7.
32. Ettehad D, Schaaf HS, Seddon JA, Cooke GS, Ford N. Treatment outcomes for children with multidrug-resistant tuberculosis: a systematic review and meta-analysis. Lancet Infect Dis. 2012;12(6):449–56.
33. Gegia M, Jenkins HE, Kalandadze I, Furin J. Outcomes of children treated for tuberculosis with second-line medications in Georgia, 2009-2011. Int J Tuberc Lung Dis. 2013;17(5):624–9.
34. Ayieko J, Abuogi L, Simchowitz B, Bukusi EA, Smith AH, Reingold A. Efficacy of isoniazid prophylactic therapy in prevention of tuberculosis in children: a meta-analysis. BMC Infect Dis. 2014;14:91.
35. Yuen CM, Jenkins HE, Rodriguez CA, Keshavjee S, Becerra MC. Global and Regional Burden of Isoniazid-Resistant Tuberculosis. Pediatrics. 2015;136(1):e50–9.
36. World Health Organization. Guidelines on the management of latent tuberculosis infection. Geneva: World Health Organization; 2015.
37. Corbett EL, Watt CJ, Walker N, et al. The growing burden of tuberculosis: global trends and interactions with the HIV epidemic. Arch Intern Med. 2003;163(9):1009–21.
38. Zar HJ, Cotton MF, Strauss S, et al. Effect of isoniazid prophylaxis on mortality and incidence of tuberculosis in children with HIV: randomised controlled trial. BMJ. 2007;334(7585):136.
39. Gupta M, Rao C, Lakshmi PV, Prinja S, Kumar R. Estimating mortality using data from civil registration: a cross-sectional study in India. Bull World Health Organ. 2016;94(1):10–21.
40. Rao C, Osterberger B, Anh TD, MacDonald M, Chuc NT, Hill PS. Compiling mortality statistics from civil registration systems in Viet Nam: the long road

ahead. Bull World Health Organ. 2010;88(1):58–65.

41. Chintu C, Mudenda V, Lucas S, et al. Lung diseases at necropsy in African children dying from respiratory illnesses: a descriptive necropsy study. Lancet. 2002;360(9338):985–90.
42. Bates M, Mudenda V, Mwaba P, Zumla A. Deaths due to respiratory tract infections in Africa: a review of autopsy studies. Curr Opin Pulm Med. 2013; 19(3):229–37.
43. Vapattanawong P, Prasartkul P. Under-registration of deaths in Thailand in 2005-2006: results of cross-matching data from two sources. Bull World Health Organ. 2011;89(11):806–12.
44. Jenkins HE, Yuen CM, Rodriguez CA, et al. Mortality among children diagnosed with tuberculosis: Systematic review and meta-analysis. Lancet Infect Dis. 2016. In press.
45. Hausdorff WP, Hanage WP. Interim results of an ecological experiment - Conjugate vaccination against the pneumococcus and serotype replacement. Hum Vaccin Immunother. 2016;12(2):358–74.
46. Imohl M, Moller J, Reinert RR, Perniciaro S, van der Linden M, Aktas O. Pneumococcal meningitis and vaccine effects in the era of conjugate vaccination: results of 20 years of nationwide surveillance in Germany. BMC Infect Dis. 2015;15:61.
47. Wolzak NK, Cooke ML, Orth H, van Toorn R. The changing profile of pediatric meningitis at a referral centre in Cape Town, South Africa. J Trop Pediatr. 2012;58(6):491–5.
48. Donald PR, Cotton MF, Hendricks MK, Schaaf HS, de Villiers JN, Willemse TE. Pediatric meningitis in the Western Cape Province of South Africa. J Trop Pediatr. 1996;42(5):256–61.
49. Graham SM, Donald PR. Death and disability: the outcomes of tuberculous meningitis. Lancet Infect Dis. 2014;14(10):902–4.
50. Chiang SS, Khan FA, Milstein MB, et al. Treatment outcomes of childhood tuberculous meningitis: a systematic review and meta-analysis. Lancet Infect Dis. 2014;14(10):947–57.
51. Houben RMGJ, Dodd PJ. The global burden of latent tuberculosis infection - a re-estimation using mathematical modelling. PLoS Med. 2016;13(10):e1002152.
52. Yuen CM, Jenkins HE, Chang R, Mpunga J, Becerra MC. Two methods for setting child-focused tuberculosis care targets. Public Health Action. 2016; 6(2):83–96

7

Atypical bacterial pneumonia in the HIV-infected population

Breanne M. Head[1], Adriana Trajtman[1], Zulma V. Rueda[2], Lázaro Vélez[3] and Yoav Keynan[4,5,1*]

Abstract

Human immunodeficiency virus (HIV)-infected individuals are more susceptible to respiratory tract infections by other infectious agents (viruses, bacteria, parasites, and fungi) as their disease progresses to acquired immunodeficiency syndrome. Despite effective antiretroviral therapy, bacterial pneumonia (the most frequently occurring HIV-associated pulmonary illness) remains a common cause of morbidity and mortality in the HIV-infected population. Over the last few decades, studies have looked at the role of atypical bacterial pneumonia (i.e. pneumonia that causes an atypical clinical presentation or responds differently to typical therapeutics) in association with HIV infection. Due to the lack of available diagnostic strategies, the lack of consideration, and the declining immunity of the patient, HIV co-infections with atypical bacteria are currently believed to be underreported. Thus, following an extensive database search, this review aimed to highlight the current knowledge and gaps regarding atypical bacterial pneumonia in HIV. The authors discuss the prevalence of *Chlamydophila pneumoniae*, *Mycoplasma pneumoniae*, *Coxiella burnetii*, *Legionella* species and others in the HIV-infected population as well as their clinical presentation, methods of detection, and treatment. Further studies looking at the role of these microbes in association with HIV are required. Increased knowledge of these atypical bacteria will lead to a more rapid diagnosis of these infections, resulting in an improved quality of life for the HIV-infected population.

Keywords: Atypical, Bacteria, Pneumonia, HIV, Legionella, Chlamydophila, Mycoplasma, Coxiella, Tropheryma

Background

Bacterial pneumonia, the most frequent human immunodeficiency virus (HIV)-associated pulmonary illness, is a common cause of co-morbidity and mortality in the HIV population. Prior to the introduction of combination antiretroviral therapy (cART), bacterial pneumonia infection rates ranged from 3.9–20 cases per 100 person-years in HIV-positive individuals and were predominantly due to opportunistic pathogens such as *Streptococcus pneumoniae, Haemophilus influenzae, Staphylococcus aureus*, as well as acute *Mycobacterium tuberculosis* infections [1–8]. Although bacterial pneumonia rates have decreased since the introduction of cART, rates remain 10 times higher among HIV-infected individuals than in healthy individuals [2, 4, 5, 9, 10]. Additionally, HIV-associated pneumonia remains the most common cause of hospital admission with up to 90 cases per 1000 persons occurring yearly [5, 11–13].

Currently, the diagnosis of pneumonia is based on clinical features and X-ray. The etiological diagnosis, however, is based on empirical data, culture, serology, nucleic acid amplification techniques (NAAT), and bronchoscopy [5, 14]. When choosing any of these diagnostics, a number of points must be considered. Although very informative, empirical data (i.e. patient history, recent travel, intravenous [IV] drug exposure, prior infections, or antibiotic exposure) can only aid in narrowing the scope of infection and is not definitive [5]. In contrast, culture allows bacterial identification and is considered the preferred method in diagnostics. However, incubation periods can be lengthy (depending on the growth rate of the microorganism), not all microbes are cultivable, and the sensitivity of the assay decreases if the patient has had any pre-treatment with antibiotics [15]. Serological tests rely on the patient's ability to mount an effective antibody response; however, in the case of HIV, this response is greatly reduced.

* Correspondence: Yoav.Keynan@umanitoba.ca
[4]Department of Internal Medicine, University of Manitoba, Winnipeg, Canada
[5]Department of Community Health Sciences, University of Manitoba, Winnipeg, Canada
Full list of author information is available at the end of the article

Therefore, depending on the stage of HIV infection, serology may not be clinically useful [16]. Due to the low sensitivities of serology, NAAT (such as polymerase chain reaction [PCR]) is becoming the diagnostic tool of choice for rapid identification of atypical bacteria in respiratory samples of HIV-infected and uninfected individuals [14, 17, 18]. However, although NAAT is highly specific, sensitivity has been shown to vary depending on the patient sample being tested (e.g. nasopharyngeal sample vs. induced sputum) [19, 20]. Moreover, although the presence of NAAT is becoming more prominent in developed nations, it is still not readily available in developing countries. In the event that a definitive diagnosis cannot be reached, more invasive techniques (e.g. bronchoscopy) may be used for sample collection (bronchoalveolar lavage [BAL] or biopsy). Although very beneficial, bronchoscopy is currently underutilized in respect to HIV and advanced immunosuppression, despite it being recommended for patients with low CD4 cell counts (< 200 cells/μl). This underutilization is perhaps due to the fact that patients are too sick to undergo the BAL procedure, or due to the high volume of immunosuppressed patients admitted to hospital [5, 12, 21]. In addition, it can lead to complications such as bleeding and pneumothorax [5, 21].

Despite technological advancements, the etiology of HIV-associated pneumonia is identified less than 60% of the time, thus research looking into atypical pneumonia-causing agents is required [5, 9]. Limited information is available regarding atypical bacterial pneumonia (i.e. pneumonia that does not respond to beta-lactams, one of the antibiotics typically prescribed to pneumonia patients with co-morbidities), with even less information about these infections in HIV [22]. Due to the lack of consideration, the role that atypical bacteria play in disease severity and patient outcome in HIV-associated pneumonia is unknown. Consequently, this review will highlight the bacteria—namely *Chlamydophila pneumoniae, Mycoplasma pneumoniae, Coxiella burnetii, Legionella* species and others—that is responsible for causing atypical bacterial pneumonia in HIV. Specifically, the review explores the current knowledge regarding the prevalence of these microbes in the HIV-infected population, as well as their clinical presentation, methods of detection, and treatment.

Chlamydophila pneumoniae

Chlamydophila pneumoniae, an obligate intracellular pathogen that has caused pulmonary infections all over the world, remains a particular problem in the HIV-infected population [23–26]. Studies by Trinh et al. [27] have demonstrated that *C. pneumoniae* pneumonia rates are as high as 60% in cART-treated HIV-infected children. Likewise, in the adult population, coinfections with HIV have been reported to range from 3 to 39% [28–31]. In general, HIV-associated *C. pneumoniae* pneumonia rates have been shown to be inversely proportional to the patient's CD4 cell count, occurring at 6.8, 15.7, and 25.2% when CD4 counts are above 500, between 200 and 500, and below 200 cells/μl, respectively [30]. In other words, the rates increase with decreasing CD4, up to a quarter among individuals with advanced HIV and CD4 < 200. In a retrospective analysis [29] of 319 adult pneumonia-infected HIV seropositive individuals, *C. pneumoniae* was cited as a co-pathogen with other microorganisms in approximately 2.2% (n = 7) of cases.

Much of the research on HIV-associated *C. pneumoniae* pneumonia arises from the post-cART era with little information on the effect of this microorganism in untreated HIV. However, of those that have been reported, it was found that the risk of acquiring *C. pneumoniae* pneumonia was 5 times higher in untreated HIV than in the general population [30, 32, 33]. Regardless of these higher rates, the clinical course of disease is similar among both populations. Disease manifests as an acute respiratory infection (with focal pneumonia, pleural effusion, or bronchitis), although, as the degree of immunosuppression increases, more severe and diffuse interstitial pulmonary involvement and death can occur [29, 32, 34, 35]. Likewise, *C. pneumonia* infection has also been shown to cause chronic infections (e.g. arteriosclerosis or cardiovascular disease) [36].

Diagnosis of HIV-associated *C. pneumoniae* pneumonia is reliant on serology and NAAT. Microimmunofluorescence (MIF), a technique that indirectly measures the *C. pneumoniae*-specific antibody response, requires either single or convalescent serum samples to differentiate between a recent/current infection and a previous one [27, 30, 29, 34]. However, severely immunosuppressed HIV-infected adults (with CD4 counts <200 cells/μL) have been reported to be unable to mount an effective IgG response [25]. Conversely, HIV patients may have an asymptomatic *C. pneumoniae* infection while co-infected with another pneumonia-causing pathogen, which poses another limitation on the utility of this diagnostic test [25, 29]. Consequently, NAAT tests on respiratory specimens (BAL or nasophayngeal swab) are recommended as they have shown promise for *C. pneumonia* diagnosis in HIV [18, 27, 37]. In fact, the United States Food and Drug Administration has approved a BioFire FilmArray NAAT for the detection of both *C. pneumoniae* and *M. pneumoniae* [37].

Mycoplasma pneumoniae

Mycoplasma pneumoniae, the most common *Mycoplasma* respiratory pathogen, accounts for approximately 20% of all pneumonias in the United States (US) general population, and 11.3–21.0% (depending on the method of diagnosis) of all pneumonias in the US HIV-infected population, with higher rates correlated with the degree of immunosuppression [31, 38–40]. Indeed, in a study by Nadagir et al. [41], 18 of the 29 (62%) HIV-positive, *M. pneumoniae*-infected children had a CD4 cell count of <20 cells/μL. Additionally, a depleted CD4 associated with advanced HIV disease has been shown to enhance *M. pneumoniae* establishment in the lungs [40–43]. However, similarly to *C. pneumoniae*, the majority of the data on HIV-associated *M. pneumoniae* lung infections is from treated HIV patients, with minimal information on its effect in untreated HIV.

Clinical manifestations of *M. pneumoniae* pneumonia in HIV are similar to those seen in healthy individuals. Cough (reported in 100% of cases), anemia, arthralgia, dyspnea, and sore throat along with fever, rales, interstitial infiltrates, and lobar pneumonia are most commonly reported, making diagnosis nearly impossible based solely on clinical presentation [40–42, 38].

M. pneumoniae diagnosis relies on culture, serology, and NAAT [42, 44]. However, isolation requires up to 3 weeks incubation, limiting the practicality of this method in a clinical setting [40, 41, 38, 45]. Similarly, time is also a limiting factor for serology, as it is dependent on a convalescent serum sample [19]. Moreover, *M. pneumoniae* has been shown to persist within the host, with persistent IgM detectable years after infection [38, 41, 42, 45–50]. Furthermore, due to the fact that up to 20% of healthy individuals do not develop *M. pneumoniae*-specific IgM combined with the impaired immune response associated with HIV infection, immunosuppressed HIV-infected patients may never develop a detectable antibody response altogether, which means this technique is not reliable for diagnosis in this population [38, 51]. In fact, Shankar et al. [40] found that culture was more reliable for diagnosing *M. pneumoniae* infections in HIV-positive individuals since it was able to identify infections in 31% (n = 31) of their adult HIV population, while IgM enzyme-linked immunosorbent assay only identified 21% (n = 21), highlighting that relying solely on serology could lead to a false negative. Consequently, multiple laboratories have developed NAAT methods (e.g. the BioFire FilmArray NAAT, or real-time PCR) for the detection of *M. pneumoniae*, although the Center for Disease Control and Prevention has indicated that few of these developed methods are actually acceptable for diagnostic assessment [37, 44, 52]. Nonetheless, these amplification techniques have demonstrated higher sensitivities and specificities compared to other diagnostics and have emerged as the new standard for *M. pneumoniae* pneumonia detection in HIV [44].

Coxiella burnetii

Coxiella burnetii (Q fever) is an obligate intracellular bacterium capable of causing acute and chronic illnesses in both immunocompromised and immunocompetent individuals alike [53]. However, reports of HIV-associated Q fever pneumonia are currently limited. Of those that have been reported, majority of them are from the pre-cART era [25, 30, 53, 54]. Nevertheless, information from the pre-cART era allows us to make inferences as to how *C. burnetii* will affect untreated HIV-infected patients, and those that have previously been treated with cART but have already progressed to AIDS.

In the 1990s, Q fever pneumonia rates were 0.3% in the general population and 9.7% in the untreated HIV-seropositive adult population. During this time, HIV-infected individuals were reported to be 13 times more likely to contract Q fever than healthy individuals [54].

Like the other atypical pneumonias, the clinical course of *C. burnetii* pneumonia is similar in both HIV-positive and negative individuals [53]. Symptoms can last up to 10 days and are often non-specific (e.g. fever, headache, non-productive cough, myalgia); however, in 90% of cases involving HIV, lung nodules have been shown to occur.

Diagnosing HIV-associated Q fever pneumonia can be quite challenging due to the many clinical forms of the disease (e.g. acute or chronic pulmonary infection) and to the decreasing immunity associated with HIV [54]. Diagnosis is based on serology and NAAT, however the potential of false negatives seen in serology increases with HIV disease advancement [25, 30, 54]. Moreover, in Q fever endemic areas, single serum samples may result in false positives, thus convalescent serum samples may be required. NAAT, and, more specifically, PCR—a more promising alternative with high specificity—are not widely available [55, 56]. Due to the lack of knowledge regarding when to test for HIV-associated Q fever pneumonia, *C. burnetii* diagnostics in HIV-infected patients are infrequently attempted and are likely to be underrepresented [30, 54, 57].

Legionella pneumophila

The opportunistic intracellular pathogen *Legionella pneumophila* is a particular problem in immunosuppressed patients, and is estimated to be responsible for 20% of all adult HIV-associated pneumonias (compared to 15% in the general population), although surprisingly very few cases have actually been reported to date [15, 58–64]. Of the cases that have been recorded, many have shown that HIV-infected patients (particularly those with advanced immunosuppression) often present with a more severe clinical presentation compared to normal individuals [4, 58, 65].

In general, *L. pneumophila* pneumonia symptoms are non-specific with significantly higher rates of cough, dyspnea, bilateral pulmonary involvement, and hyponatremia in people with HIV [58, 62, 66, 67]. However, atypical manifestations involving the gastrointestinal tract or the central nervous system may also occur, making initial diagnosis quite challenging [62, 66, 67]. Recurrent lung cavitation has been shown to occur almost exclusively in immunosuppressed patients and often occurs shortly after initiation of therapy [58, 60, 68]. Complications due to respiratory failure and higher mortality rates have also been seen [67].

L. pneumophila infections may be underrepresented in the HIV population due to the fact that routine screening for *Legionella* is not usually performed and requires a special request from the clinician [4, 63]. Diagnosing HIV-associated *L. pneumophila* pneumonia has traditionally been reliant on culture and the urinary antigen test [62, 69]; however, culture requires specialized media, several days for growth, and still only has about 80% sensitivity [70]. For serology, depending on the severity of the patient's immunosuppression, measurable *L. pneumophila* antigen may not be detectable initially, resulting in a false negative for the urinary antigen test [62, 66]. In a case by Franzin et al. [62], a negative urinary antigen result postponed *L. pneumophila* diagnosis in a cART-adhering, HIV-infected adult male until cultures were obtained (several days later). Thus, definitive diagnosis of HIV-associated *L. pneumophila* pneumonia has been reliant on two methods, both known to have their own respective limitations [62, 69]. Consequently, NAAT has become the new standard in diagnostics. Real-time PCR methods, targeting the *Legionella* mip gene, are considered to be more specific, sensitive and rapid compared to traditional diagnostics (with approximately a 15% increased yield over culture) and have been adapted for use in multiple laboratories; however, in developing nations, these automated techniques are not readily available [17, 71, 72]. Lastly, HIV patients are often co-infected with more than one pathogen which could mask infection with *L. pneumophila*. Consequently, *L. pneumophila* may play a much larger role in HIV-associated pneumonia than is currently anticipated.

Non-pneumophila *Legionellas*

Pneumonia by other non-pneumophila *Legionella* species accounts for 10% of all legionellosis in the general population (with *Legionella micdadei* and *Legionella bozemanae* accounting for 90% of these cases) with limited information regarding these infections in HIV. However, of the information that has been gathered, it seems that cART-adhering HIV-infected individuals have higher rates of non-pneumophila pneumonia than healthy individuals [73–75].

In both treated and untreated HIV, *Legionella* non-pneumophila infections commonly manifest as fever, cough, dyspnea, diarrhea, pleuritic chest pain, and effusion, with documented instances of pulmonary cavities, nodules, and lung abscesses [73, 75–77]. Studies from the pre-cART era indicate that higher mortality rates are associated with infection in untreated HIV, although this may be due to the fact that these infections have only been reported in severely immunosuppressed patients and may not be due to the virulence of the microbes themselves [77–79].

Diagnosis of HIV-associated non-pneumophila *Legionella* pneumonia requires high clinical suspicion. Until a definitive diagnosis is reached, aggressive empirical therapy should be administered, especially in immunodeficient patients, in order to ensure a more positive outcome. Indeed, discontinuing empiric therapy in an immunocompromised adult HIV-infected individual despite a high suspicion of *Legionella* infection can lead to fatality [77].

Currently, culture is the best at diagnosing non-pneumophila pneumonia in HIV; however, sensitivities vary depending on the laboratory, with higher sensitivities having only been recorded in laboratories with a special interest in legionellosis [73, 75–77, 80, 81]. Urinary antigen, although useful for *L. pneumophila* serogroup 1 detection, is less sensitive for other serogroups and is practically useless for non-pneumophila species [77, 82]. NAAT methods, specifically PCR of lower respiratory tract specimens, have demonstrated high sensitivities (up to 100%) with *Legionella* species and may be a possible alternative for detecting non-pneumophila *Legionella* pneumonia in HIV-infected patients. However, although PCR assays can detect all of the various *Legionella* species with high specificity, they are currently not readily available for clinical use [17].

Little is known about non-pneumophila pneumonia and its prevalence in HIV, which may simply be due to the fact that *L. pneumophila* serogroup 1 is typically the only *Legionella* species that is often considered; the urinary antigen test targets *L. pneumophila* serogroup 1 and so do many serological assays [76]. The distribution of *Legionella* varies globally, therefore the usefulness of the urinary antigen test should be validated in each locale [83]. Moreover, HIV-associated legionellosis due to non-pneumophila is similar to *L. pneumophila*, which could prevent differentiation between these infections. To better determine the role of these pathogens in HIV infection, further development of more appropriate diagnostic techniques and increased clinical awareness are required.

Tropheryma whipplei

Tropheryma whipplei, although not usually considered one of the atypical bacteria, has been found in respiratory samples of treated HIV-infected individuals at higher prevalence rates than the general population [84–87]. Currently, it is unclear whether *T. whipplei* is a pneumonia-causing pathogen or merely a commensal organism, since it has been found in both symptomatic and asymptomatic cases alike [84, 88–90]. Although some studies report *T. whipplei* as a pathogen (and even attribute certain clinical manifestations to this bacterium), caution is required until more evidence is acquired about the role of this microbe in HIV-associated pneumonia.

Treatment of atypical bacterial pneumonia in HIV

Unlike typical bacterial pneumonia, atypical bacterial pneumonia does not respond to beta-lactams, aminoglycosides, and sulfa drugs; therefore, a 7–10 day course of macrolides (clarithromycin, erythromycin, or azithromycin), doxycycline and/or fluoroquinolones (levofloxacin or moxifloxacin) are required to treat these infections in HIV patients [29, 57, 62, 66, 91].

Conclusions

Bacterial pneumonia is an immense problem among immunocompromised HIV-infected individuals, contributing to the high morbidity and eventual death of these patients. Although a large proportion of pneumonia is attributable to typical bacterial infections, clinicians must be aware of other relevant pathogens, such as *C. pneumoniae, M. pneumoniae, C. burnetti, Legionella* species, and, possibly, *T. whipplei.*

Diagnosing HIV-associated atypical pneumonia remains a challenging task and becomes even more so when the patient is severely immunocompromised. Due to the lack of data, the lack of consideration, and the current subpar diagnostic methods, atypical bacterial pneumonia is often left undiagnosed in HIV-infected individuals. Studies using more invasive methods (e.g. bronchoscopy and BAL) may provide a more accurate depiction of pneumonia. Further studies, and the development of more appropriate diagnostic methods, are required to clarify the role and prevalence rates of atypical bacterial pneumonia in HIV.

Abbreviations

AIDS: Acquired immunodeficiency syndrome; BAL: Bronchoalveolar lavage; cART: Combination antiretroviral therapy; HIV: Human immunodeficiency virus; IFA: Immunofluorescence assay; MIF: Microimmunofluorescence; NAAT: Nucleic acid amplification techniques; PCR: Polymerase chain reaction

Acknowledgements

Not applicable.

Funding

This project is supported by funding from Colciencias (grant number: 111571249880). The funder had no role in the preparation of the manuscript nor the decision to publish.

Authors' contributions

BH conducted the literature search as well as drafted the review manuscript. BH also consulted with AT, ZR, LV and YK, for guidance, editing and to critically revise the intellectual content of the manuscript. All authors read and approved the final manuscript.

Competing interests

The authors declare that they have competing interests.

Author details

[1]Department of Medical Microbiology, University of Manitoba, Winnipeg, Canada. [2]Facultad de Medicina, Universidad Pontificia Bolivariana, Medellin, Colombia. [3]Grupo Investigador de Problemas en Enfermedades Infecciosas, Universidad de Antioquia UdeA, Medellin, Colombia. [4]Department of Internal Medicine, University of Manitoba, Winnipeg, Canada. [5]Department of Community Health Sciences, University of Manitoba, Winnipeg, Canada.

References

1. Kaplan JE, Benson C, Holmes KK, Brooks JT, Pau A, Masur H. Guidelines for prevention and treatment of opportunistic infections in HIV-infected adults and adolescents. MMWR. 2009;58:1–198.
2. Segal LN, Methé BA, Nolan A, Hoshino Y, Rom WN, Dawson R, et al. HIV-1 and bacterial pneumonia in the era of antiretroviral therapy. Proc Am Thorac Soc. 2011;8:282–7. doi:10.1513/pats.201006-044WR.
3. Cordero E, Pachón J, Rivero A, Girón JA, Gómez-mateos J, Collado A, et al. Community-acquired bacterial pneumonia in human immunodeficiency virus – infected patients. Am J Respir Crit Care Med. 2000;162:2063–8.
4. Pedro-Botet ML, Sopena N, García-Cruz A, Mateu L, García-Núñez M, Rey-Joly C, et al. *Streptococcus pneumoniae* and *Legionella pneumophila* pneumonia in HIV-infected patients. Scand J Infect Dis. 2007;39:122–8. doi:10.1080/00365540600951275.
5. Benito N, Moreno A, Miro JM, Torres A. Pulmonary infections in HIV-infected patients: an update in the 21st century. Eur Respir J. 2012;39:730–45. doi:10.1183/09031936.00200210.
6. Mangtania P, Mulhollanda K, Madhib SA, Edmonda K, O'Loughlina R, Hajjehc R. *Haemophilus influenzae* type b disease in HIV-infected children: a review of the disease epidemiology and effectiveness of Hib conjugate vaccines. Vaccine. 2010;28:1677–83.
7. Hidron AI, Kempker R, Moanna A, Rimland D. Methicillin-resistant *Staphylococcus aureus* in HIV-infected patients. Infect Drug Resist. 2010;3:73–86.
8. Auwaerter P. Johns Hopkins HIV Guide. Johns Hopkins Med 2016. https://www.hopkinsguides.com/hopkins/view/Johns_Hopkins_HIV_Guide/545087/all/Haemophilus_species. Accessed 5 June 2017.
9. Benito N, Rañó A, Moreno A, González J, Luna M, Agustí C, et al. Pulmonary infiltrates in HIV-infected patients in the HAART era in Spain. J Acquir Immune Defic Syndr. 2001;27:35–43.
10. Morris AM, Huang L, Bacchetti P, Turner J, Hopewell PC, Wallace JM, et al. Permanent declines in pulmonary function following pneumonia in human immunodeficiency virus-infected persons. Am J Respir Crit Care Med. 2000;162:612–6.
11. Thompson LH, Sochocki M, Friesen T, Bresler K, Keynan Y, Kasper K, et al. Medical ward admissions among HIV-positive patients in Winnipeg, Canada, 2003-10. Int J STD AIDS. 2012;23:287–8. doi:10.1258/ijsa.2011.011309.
12. Van Gaalen S, Rueda Z, Arroyave L, Kasper K, Keynan Y. Characteristics of pneumonia admissions in HIV-positive individuals: a single-centre, 10 -year cross-sectional retrospective analysis. J Assoc Med Microbiol Infect Dis Canada. 2016;1:SP08.
13. Lazarous DG, O'Donnell AE. Pulmonary infections in the HIV-infected patient in the era of highly active antiretroviral therapy: an update. Curr Infect Dis Rep. 2007;9:228–32.
14. Chalmers J. The modern diagnostic approach to community-acquired pneumonia in adults. Semin Respir Crit Care Med. 2016;37:876–85. doi:10.1055/s-0036-1592125.
15. Basnayake TL, Waterer GW. Rapid diagnostic tests for defining the cause of community-acquired pneumonia. Curr Opin Infect Dis. 2015;28:185–92. doi:10.1097/QCO.0000000000000148.

16. McMichael AJ, Borrow P, Tomaras GD, Goonetilleke N, Haynes BF. The immune response during acute HIV-1 infection: clues for vaccine development. Nat Rev Immunol. 2010;10:11–23. doi:10.1038/nri2674.The.
17. Phin N, Parry-Ford F, Harrison T, Stagg HR, Zhang N, Kumar K, et al. Epidemiology and clinical management of legionnaires' disease. Lancet Infect Dis. 2014;14:1011–21. doi:10.1016/S1473-3099(14)70713-3.
18. Prina E, Ranzani OT, Torres A. Community-acquired pneumonia. Lancet. 2015;386:1097–108. doi:10.1016/ S0140-6736(15)60733-4.
19. Herrera M, Aguilar YA, Rueda ZV, Muskus C, Vélez LA. Comparison of serological methods with PCR-based methods for the diagnosis of community-acquired pneumonia caused by atypical bacteria. J Negat Results Biomed. 2016;15:1–11. doi:10.1186/s12952-016-0047-y.
20. Weiss D, Boyd C, Rakeman JL, Greene SK, Fitzhenry R, McProud T, et al. A large community outbreak of legionnaires' disease associated with a cooling tower in new York City, 2015. Public Health Rep. 2017;132:241–50. doi:10.1177/0033354916689620.
21. UCLA Healthcare. Bronchoscopy with or without biopsy. UCLA Healthcare. 2003. https://www.uclahealth.org/lungcancer/workfiles/Bronchoscopy_consent.pdf. Accessed 5 June 2017.
22. Mandell LA, Wunderink RG, Anzueto A, Bartlett JG, Campbell GD, Dean NC, et al. Infectious diseases society of America/American Thoracic Society consensus guidelines on the management of community-acquired pneumonia in adults. Clin Infect Dis. 2007;44:S27–72. doi:10.1086/511159.
23. Montes M, Cilla G, Alcorta M, Pérez-Trallero E. High prevalence of *Chlamydia pneumoniae* infection in children and young adults in Spain. Pediatr Infect Dis J. 1992;11:972–3.
24. Koh WP, Taylor MB, Hughes K, Chew SK, Fong CW, Phoon MC, et al. Seroprevalence of IgG antibodies against *Chlamydia pneumoniae* in Chinese, Malays and Asian indians in Singapore. Int J Epidemiol. 2002;31:1001–7. doi:10.1093/ije/31.5.1001.
25. Comandini UV, Massetti AP, Marchese R, Zaccarelli M, Vullo V, Delia S. *Chlamydia pneumoniae* seroprevalence among HIV-1-infected and uninfected people with known HIV risk factor. AIDS. 1996;10:1543–7.
26. Trinh QD, Pham NT, Le Nguyen NT, Lam BQ, Le Phan KT, Truong KH, et al. Frequent *Chlamydophila pneumoniae* infection in vertically HIV-infected children in Vietnam. J Reprod Immunol. 2014;106:17. doi:10.1016/j.jri.2014.09.042.
27. Trinh QD, Pham NTK, Le Nguyen NT, Lam BQ, Le Phan KT, Truong KH, et al. Seroprevalence of *Chlamydophila pneumoniae* in HIV-infected children in Vietnam. J Infect Chemother. 2013;19:538–41. doi:10.1007/s10156-012-0483-7.
28. Tositti G, Rassu M, Fabris P, Giordani M, Cazzavillan S, Reatto P, et al. *Chlamydia pneumoniae* infection in HIV-positive patients: prevalence and relationship with lipid profile. HIV Med. 2005;6:27–32.
29. Comandini UV, Maggi P, Santopadre P, Monno R, Angarano G, Vullo V. *Chlamydia pneumoniae* respiratory infections among patients infected with the human immunodeficiency virus. Eur J Clin Microbiol Infect Dis. 1997;16:720–6.
30. Boschini A, Smacchia C, Fine M Di, Schiesari A, Ballarini P, Arlotti M, et al. Community-acquired pneumonia in a cohort of former injection drug users with and without human immunodeficiency virus infection : incidence, etiologies, and clinical aspects. Clin Infect Dis 1996;23:107–113.
31. Figueiredo-Mello C, Naucler P, Negra MD, Levin AS. Prospective etiological investigation of community-acquired pulmonary infections in hospitalized people living with HIV. Medicine (Baltimore). 2017;96:e5778. doi:10.1097/MD.0000000000005778.
32. Hammerschlag MR, Chirgwin K, Roblin PM, Gelling M, Dumornay W, Mandel L, et al. Persistent infection with *Chlamydia pneumoniae* following acute respiratory illness. Clin Infect Dis. 1992;14:178–82.
33. Blasi F, Cosentini R, Schoeller MC, Lupo A, Allegra L. *Chlamydia pneumoniae* seroprevalence in immunocompetent and immunocompromised populations in Milan. Thorax. 1993;48:1261–3. doi:10.1136/thx.48.12.1261.
34. Kuo CC, Jackson L, Cambell L, Grayston T. *Chlamydia pneumoniae*. Clin Microbiolgy Rev. 1995;8:451–61.
35. Miller R. HIV-associated respiratory diseases. Lancet. 1996;348:307–12.
36. Woolley IJ, Larsen M, Jones S, Gahan ME, Jasenko I, Johnsen SP, et al. *Chlamydia pneumoniae* in HIV-infected patients and controls assessed by a novel whole blood interferon-γ assay, serology and PCR. Clin Microbiol Infect. 2004;10:820–5.
37. Baron EJ, Miller JM, Weinstein MP, Richter SS, Gilligan PH, Thomson RB, et al. A guide to utilization of the microbiology laboratory for diagnosis of infectious diseases: 2013 recommendations by the Infectious Diseases Society of America (IDSA) and the American Society for Microbiology (ASM). Clin Infect Dis. 2013;57:485–8. doi:10.1093/cid/cit441.
38. Shankar EM, Kumarasamy N, Balakrishnan P, Vengatesan A, Kownhar H, Solomon S, et al. Seroprevalence of *Mycoplasma pneumoniae* in HIV-infected patients using a microparticle agglutination test. J Med Microbiol. 2006;55:759–63. doi:10.1099/jmm.0.46402-0.
39. Rao U, Shankar E, Kumarasamy N, Balakrishnan P, Solomon S. Pulmonary microbiology of HIV positive subjects with community-acquired pneumonia (CAP) with special emphasis on *Mycoplasma pneumoniae*. Int J Infect Dis. 2010;14:e401. doi:10.1016/j.ijid.2010.02.511.
40. Stevens CD, Miller LE. Serological and molecular detection of bacterial infections. In: DeChambeau DW, Bales E, editors. Clin. Immunol. Serol. A lab. Perspect. 4th ed., Philadelphia: F.A. Davis Company; 2017, p. 346–362.
41. Nadagir SD, Bahadur AK, Shepur TA. Prevalence of *Mycoplasma pneumoniae* among HIV infected children. Indian J Pediatr. 2011;78:430–4. doi:10.1007/s12098-010-0313-9.
42. Shankar EM, Kumarasamy N, Balakrishnan P, Saravanan S, Solomon S, Vengatesan A, et al. Detection of pulmonary *Mycoplasma pneumoniae* infections in HIV-infected subjects using culture and serology. Int J Infect Dis. 2007;11:232–8. doi:10.1016/j.ijid.2006.04.007.
43. Shankar EM, Kumarasamy N, Balakrishnan P, Solomon S, Devaleenol B, Rao UA. Incidence of *Mycoplasma pneumoniae* infection in HIV-infected patients with underlying upper and lower respiratory complaints and correlation with various immunological and haematological findings. Retrovirology. 2005;2:S97. doi:10.1186/1742-4690-2-S1-S97.
44. Ling CL, McHugh TD. Rapid Detection of Atypical Respiratory Bacterial Pathogens by Real-Time PCR. In: Wilks M, editor. PCR Detect. Microb. Pathog. 2nd ed., Springer Science; 2013, p. 125–33. doi:10.1007/978-1-62703-239-1_1.
45. Shankar EM, Kumarasamy N, Balakrishnan P, Solomon S, Lejith R, Vengatesan A, et al. Serosurveillance of acute *Mycoplasma pneumoniae* infection among HIV infected patients with pulmonary complaints in Chennai, southern India. J Inf Secur. 2006;53:325–30. doi:10.1016/j.jinf.2005.11.184.
46. Hammerschlag MR. *Mycoplasma pneumoniae* infections. Curr Opin Infect Dis. 2001;14:181–6. doi:10.1016/B978-032303506-4.10222-6.
47. Sillis M. The limitations of IgM assays in the serological diagnosis of *Mycoplasma pneumoniae* infections. J Med Microbiol. 1990;33:253–8.
48. Petitjean J, Vabret A, Gouarin S, Freymuth F. Evaluation of four commercial immunoglobulin G (IgG)- and IgM-specific enzyme immunoassays for diagnosis of *Mycoplasma pneumoniae* infections. J Clin Microbiol. 2002;40: 165–71. doi:10.1128/JCM.40.1.165.
49. Atkinson T, Duffy LB, Pendley D, Dai Y, Cassell GH. Reduced IgG antibody to *Mycoplasma pneumoniae* among subjects with asthma: results of a five year study. J Allergy Clin Microbiol. 2005;115:S171.
50. Waites KB, Talkington DF. *Mycoplasma pneumoniae* and its role as a human pathogen. Clin Microbiol Rev. 2004;17:697–728. doi:10.1128/CMR.17.4.697.
51. Twigg HL III, Spain BA, Soliman DM, Bowen LK, Heidler KM, Wilkes DS. Impaired IgG production in the lungs of HIV-infected individuals. Cell Immunol. 1996;170:127–33.
52. Bartlett JG. Diagnostic tests for agents of community-acquired pneumonia. Clin Infect Dis. 2011;52 doi:10.1093/cid/cir045.
53. Boschini A, Perri GD, Legnani D, Fabbri P, Ballarini P, Zucconi R, et al. Consecutive epidemics of Q fever in a residential facility for drug abusers: impact on persons with human immunodeficiency virus infection. Clin Infect Dis. 1999;28:866–72.
54. Raoult D, Levy P-Y, Tissot Dupont H, Chicheportiche C, Tamalet C, Gastaut J-A, et al. Q fever in HIV infection. AIDS. 1993:81–6.
55. Jaton K, Peter O, Raoult D, Tissot JD, Greub G. Development of a high throughput PCR to detect *Coxiella burnetii* and its application in a diagnostic laboratory over a 7-year period. New Microbes New Infect. 2013; 1:6–12. doi:10.1002/2052-2975.8.
56. Lamas CC, Rozental T, Bóia MN, Favacho AR, Kirsten AH, Da Silva AP, et al. Seroprevalence of *Coxiella burnetii* antibodies in human immunodeficiency virus-positive patients in Jacarepaguá, Rio de Janeiro, Brazil. Clin Microbiol Infect. 2009;15(2):140–1. doi:10.1111/j.1469-0691.2008.02144.x.
57. Madariaga MG, Pulvirenti J, Sekosan M, Paddock CD, Zaki SR. Q fever endocarditis in HIV-infected patient. Emerg Infect Dis. 2004;10:501–4.
58. Pedro-Botet ML, Sabrià M, Sopena N, García-Núñez M, Jesús Dominguez M, Reynaga E, et al. Legionnaires disease and HIV infection. Chest. 2003;124: 543–7. doi:10.1378/chest.124.2.543.
59. Bangsborg JM, Jensen BN, Friis-Moller A, Bruun B. Legionellosis in patients with HIV infection. Infection. 1990;18:342–6. doi:10.1007/BF01646400.
60. Blatt SP, Dolan MJ, Hendrix CW, Melcher GP. Legionnaires' disease in human immunodeficiency virus-infected patients: eight cases and review. Clin Infect Dis. 1994;18:227 32.

61. Rodero FG, Ortiz de la Tabla V, Martínez C, del AMr Masiá M, Chiner E, Calpe JL. Legionnaires' disease in patients infected with human immunodeficiency virus. Clin Infect Dis. 1995;21:712–3.
62. Franzin L, Dal Conte I, Cabodi D, Sinicco A. Culture proven *Legionella pneumophila* pneumonia in a HIV-infected patient: case report and review. J Inf Secur. 2002;45:199–201. doi:10.1016/S0163-4453(02)91030-3.
63. Marston BJ, Lipman HB, Breiman RF. Surveillance for legionnaires' disease: risk factors for morbidity and mortality. Arch Intern Med. 1994;154:2417–22. doi:10.1001/archinte.1994.00420210049006.
64. Wolter N, Carrim M, Cohen C, Tempia S, Walaza S, Sahr P, et al. Legionnaires' disease in South Africa, 2012–2014. Emerg Infect Dis. 2016;22: 131–3. doi:10.3201/eid2201.150972.
65. Pedro-botet ML, Sabria-Leal M, Sopena N, Manterola JM, Morera J, Blavia R, et al. Role of immunosuppression in the evolution of legionnaires' disease. Clin Infect Dis. 1998;26:14–9.
66. Sandkovsky U, Sandkovsky G, Suh J, Smith B, Sharp V, Polsky B. *Legionella pneumonia* and HIV: case reports and review of the literature. AIDS Patient Care STDs. 2008;22:473–81. doi:10.1089/apc.2007.0111.
67. Robbins NM, Kumar A, Blair BM. *Legionella pneumophila* infection presenting as headache, confusion and dysarthria in a human immunodeficiency virus-1 (HIV-1) positive patient: case report. BMC Infect Dis. 2012;12:1–6. doi:10.1186/1471-2334-12-225.
68. Edelstein PH, Edelstein MAC. In vitro activity of the ketolide HMR 3647 (RU 6647) for *Legionella* spp., its pharmacokinetics in guinea pigs, and use of the drug to treat guinea pigs with *Legionella pneumophila* pneumonia. Antimicrob Agents Chemother. 1999;43:90–5.
69. Edlestein PH. Legionnaires' disease. Clin Infect Dis. 1993;16:741–9.
70. Rathore MH. *Legionella* infection workup. Medscape 2016:1–2. http://emedicine.medscape.com/article/965492-workup. Accessed 4 June 2017.
71. Benitez AJ, Winchell JM. Clinical application of a multiplex real-time PCR assay for simultaneous detection of *Legionella* species, *Legionella pneumophila*, and *Legionella pneumophila* serogroup 1. J Clin Microbiol. 2013;51:348–51. doi:10.1128/JCM.02510-12.
72. Cross KE, Mercante JW, Benitez AJ, Brown EW, Diaz MH, Winchell JM. Simultaneous detection of *Legionella* species and *L. anisa*, *L. bozemanii*, *L. longbeachae* and *L. micdadei* using conserved primers and multiple probes in a multiplex real-time PCR assay. Diagn Microbiol Infect Dis. 2016;85: 295–301. doi:10.1016/j.diagmicrobio.2016.03.022.
73. Nzerue C, Gowda A. *Legionella micdadei* lung abscess in a patient with HIV-associated nephropathy. J Natl Med Assoc. 2001;93:220–3.
74. Taylor TH, Albrecht MA. *Legionella bozemanii* cavitary pneumonia poorly responsive to erythromycin: case report and review. Clin Infect Dis. 1995;20: 329–34. doi:10.1093/clinids/20.2.329.
75. Harris A, Lally M, Albrecht M. *Legionella bozemanii* pneumonia in three patients with AIDS. Clin Infect Dis. 1998;27:97–9.
76. Twigg HL III, Weinstock GM, Knox KS. Lung microbiome in HIV infection. Transl Res. 2016:1–11. doi:10.1016/j.trsl.2016.07.008.
77. Dumoff K, McGovern PC, Edelstein PH, Nachamkin I. *Legionella maceachernii* pneumonia in a patient with HIV infection. Diagn Microbiol Infect Dis. 2004; 50:141–5. doi:10.1016/j.diagmicrobio.2004.06.011.
78. Fang GD, Yu VL, Vickers RM. Disease due to the *Legionellaceae* (other than *Legionella pneumophila*). Historical, microbiological, clinical, and epidemiological review. Medicine (Baltimore). 1989;68:116–32. http://dx.doi.org/10.1097/00005792-198903000-00005.
79. Willkinson HW, Lanier Thacker W, Brenner DJ, Ryan KJ. Fatal *Legionella maceachernii* pneumonia. J Clin Microbiol. 1985;22:1055.
80. Sopena N, Sabrià-Leal M, Pedro-Botet ML, Padilla E, Dominguez J, Morera J, et al. Comparative study of the clinical presentation of *Legionella pneumonia* and other community-acquired pneumonias. Chest. 1998;113:1195–200. doi:10.1378/chest.113.5.1195.
81. Zuravleff JJ, Yu VL, Shonnard JW, Zuravleff JJ, Yu VL, Shonnard JW, et al. Diagnosis of legionnaires' disease. An update of laboratory methods with new emphasis on isolation by culture. JAMA J Am Med Assoc. 1983;250: 1981–5. doi:10.1001/jama.250.15.1981.
82. Yu VL, Plouffe JF, Pastoris MC, Stout JE, Schousboe M, Widmer A, et al. Distribution of *Legionella* species and serogroups isolated by culture in patients with sporadic community-acquired legionellosis: an international collaborative survey. J Infect Dis. 2002;186:127–8. doi:10.1097/00019048-200205000-00039.
83. Plouffe JF, Breiman RF, Fields BS, Herbert M, Inverso J, Knirsch C, et al. Azithromycin in the treatment of *Legionella pneumonia* requiring hospitalization. Clin Infect Dis. 2003;37:1475–80. doi:10.1086/379329.
84. Fenollar F, Ponge T, La Scola B, Lagier JC, Lefebvre M, Raoult D. First isolation of *Tropheryma whipplei* from bronchoalveolar fluid and clinical implications. J Inf Secur. 2012;65:275–8. doi:10.1016/j.jinf.2011.11.026.
85. Desnues B, Al Moussawi K, Fenollar F. New insights into Whipple's disease and *Tropheryma whipplei* infections. Microbes Infect. 2010;12:1102–10. doi:10.1016/j.micinf.2010.08.001.
86. Raoult D, Fenollar F, Birg M-L. Culture of *T. Whipplei* from the stool of a patient with Whipple's disease. N Engl J Med. 2006;355:1503–5. doi:10.1056/NEJMc061049.
87. Edouard S, Fenollar F, Raoult D. The rise of *Tropheryma whipplei*: a 12-year retrospective study of PCR diagnoses in our reference center. J Clin Microbiol. 2012;50:3917–20. doi:10.1128/JCM.01517-12.
88. Marth T, Moos V, Müller C, Biagi F, Schneider T. *Tropheryma whipplei* infection and whipple's disease. Lancet. 2016;16:e13–22. doi:10.1016/S1473-3099(15)00537-X.
89. Fenollar F, Laouira S, Lepidi H, Rolain J, Raoult D. Value of *Tropheryma whipplei* quantitative polymerase chain reaction assay for the diagnosis of Whipple disease: usefulness of saliva and stool specimens for first-line screening. Clin Infect Dis. 2008;47:659–67. doi:10.1086/590559.
90. Lozupone C, Cota-Gomez A, Palmer BE, Linderman DJ, Charlson ES, Sodergren E, et al. Widespread colonization of the lung by *Tropheryma whipplei* in HIV infection. Am J Respir Crit Care Med. 2013;187:110–1117. doi:10.1164/rccm.201211-2145OC.
91. Pereyre S, Goret J, Bébéar C. *Mycoplasma pneumoniae*: current knowledge on macrolide resistance and treatment. Front Microbiol. 2016;7:1–11. doi:10.3389/fmicb.2016.00974.

8

Pneumococcal conjugate vaccine implementation in middle-income countries

Serena Tricarico[1,2,3†], Hannah C. McNeil[1,2,3†], David W. Cleary[1,2], Michael G. Head[1,2,4], Victor Lim[5], Ivan Kok Seng Yap[5], Chong Chun Wie[5], Cheng Siang Tan[6], Mohd Nor Norazmi[7], Ismail Aziah[7], Eddy Seong Guan Cheah[8], Saul N. Faust[1,2,9,10], Johanna M.C. Jefferies[1,2,9], Paul J. Roderick[1], Michael Moore[1,2], Ho Ming Yuen[1,2], Marie-Louise Newell[1,4], Nuala McGrath[1,2,11], C. Patrick Doncaster[12], Alex R. Kraaijeveld[12], Jeremy S. Webb[12] and Stuart C. Clarke[1,2,3,4,5,13*]

Abstract

Background: Since 2000, the widespread adoption of pneumococcal conjugate vaccines (PCVs) has had a major impact in the prevention of pneumonia. Limited access to international financial support means some middle-income countries (MICs) are trailing in the widespread use of PCVs. We review the status of PCV implementation, and discuss any needs and gaps related to low levels of PCV implementation in MICs, with analysis of possible solutions to strengthen the PCV implementation process in MICs.

Main body: We searched PubMed, PubMed Central, Ovid MEDLINE, and SCOPUS databases using search terms related to pneumococcal immunization, governmental health policy or programmes, and MICs. Two authors independently reviewed the full text of the references, which were assessed for eligibility using pre-defined inclusion and exclusion criteria. The search terms identified 1,165 articles and the full texts of 21 were assessed for suitability, with eight articles included in the systematic review. MICs are implementing PCVs at a slower rate than donor-funded low-income countries and wealthier developed countries. A significant difference in the uptake of PCV in lower middle-income countries (LMICs) (71%) and upper middle-income countries (UMICs) (48%) is largely due to an unsuccessful process of "graduation" of MICs from GAVI assistance, an issue that arises as countries cross the income eligibility threshold and are no longer eligible to receive the same levels of financial assistance. A lack of country-specific data on disease burden, a lack of local expertise in economic evaluation, and the cost of PCV were identified as the leading causes of the slow uptake of PCVs in MICs. Potential solutions mentioned in the reviewed papers include the use of vaccine cost-effectiveness analysis and the provision of economic evidence to strengthen decision-making, the evaluation of the burden of disease, and post-introduction surveillance to monitor vaccine impact.

Conclusion: The global community needs to recognise the impediments to vaccine introduction into MICs. Improving PCV access could help decrease the incidence of pneumonia and reduce the selection pressure for pneumococcal antimicrobial resistance.

Keywords: Immunization, *Streptococcus pneumoniae*, Pneumonia, Pneumococcal vaccines, Middle-income countries, GAVI, Health policy

* Correspondence: S.C.Clarke@soton.ac.uk; s.c.clarke@southampton.ac.uk
†Equal contributors
[1]Faculty of Medicine, University of Southampton, Southampton, United Kingdom
[2]Institute for Life Sciences, University of Southampton, Southampton, United Kingdom
Full list of author information is available at the end of the article

Background

Pneumonia is the leading infectious cause of mortality among all age groups, especially among children. It accounts for 15% of all deaths of children under five years old worldwide, and killed an estimated 922,000 children in 2015 [1]. *Streptococcus pneumoniae* is the major cause of morbidity and mortality associated with childhood bacterial pneumonia and is responsible for at least 18% of severe episodes and 33% of pneumonia deaths in children worldwide [1, 2]. It is also responsible for other invasive infections such as meningitis, sepsis and peritonitis, as well as non-invasive diseases including acute otitis media [3] with a severe burden of associated morbidity.

Since 2000, the widespread adoption of pneumococcal conjugate vaccines (PCVs) has had a major impact on the prevention of pneumonia. PCVs are projected to prevent 1 million deaths among children worldwide by 2020, and 7 million by 2030 [4]. Two conjugate vaccines are currently available: the 10-valent (PCV10) and the 13-valent (PCV13), conferring protection against ten and 13 of the most prevalent and pathogenic serotypes, respectively [5]. The most recent estimate of serotypes implicated in the global burden of pneumococcal disease in children under five years of age attributed ≥70% of the disease burden to serotypes included in both the PCV10 and PCV13 vaccines [6]. The worldwide recommendation that PCVs be included in national immunization programmes (NIPs) for children aged less than two years was renewed by the World Health Organization (WHO) in 2012, with prioritization of PCV introduction given to countries with high child mortality rates [5].

However, five of the world's 7 billion people live in middle-income countries (MICs)[1] [7, 8], where the majority of vaccine preventable deaths occur [7]. As of 2014, just 31% of the global target population for PCV had been immunized, with only 14 more countries adding PCV to their NIP in 2014, after it was added by 103 countries in 2013 [9]. It is the authors' contention that in the dynamic and challenging vaccine environment, MICs may be struggling with PCV implementation without the international financial and technical support from which many low-income countries (LICs) benefit [10]. As a consequence, an opportunity to reduce a massive burden of mortality and morbidity is potentially being overlooked.

Given the number of countries where infant PCV immunization is still yet to be widely adopted, the authors undertook a systematic review into the status of PCV implementation in MICs. The review identifies potential impediments to PCV uptake and analyses possible solutions to improve PCV uptake in MICs that have yet to include PCVs in their NIP.

Methods

Search strategy

Literature on the implementation of the PCV in MICs was systematically reviewed, with contributions from peer-reviewed journals and institutional websites. The following databases were searched: PubMed, PubMed Central, Ovid MEDLINE 1946, and SCOPUS. The Cochrane Library (the Cochrane Database of Systematic Reviews and the Database of Abstracts of Reviews of Effects) and Zetoc were also scanned using search terms related to pneumococcal immunization, governmental health policy or programmes, and MICs. Websites of the World Health Organization (www.who.int), the United Nations International Children's Emergency Fund (www.unicef.org), the World Bank (data.worldbank.org), the Global Alliance for Vaccines and Immunization Alliance (GAVI; www.gavi.org), the Pan American Health Organization (www.paho.org), the Program for Appropriate Technology in Health (www.path.org), the International Health Partnership (www. internationalhealthpartnership.net), Centers for Disease Control and Prevention (www.cdc.gov), the John Hopkins School of Public Health (www.jhsph.edu) and Google (www.google.com) were searched for additional data. This review was conducted according to the PRISMA statement [11] with the search filtering process illustrated in Fig. 1.

The following search terms and structure were used and modified according to the syntax requirements of the database concerned: [*Streptococcus pneumoniae* OR pneumococcus OR pneumococcal OR pneumococci OR PCV OR pneumococcal conjugate vaccine] AND [(vaccin* adj3 policy) OR (vaccin* adj3 policies) OR (vaccin* adj3 implement*) OR (vaccin* adj3 progra*) OR (immun* adj3 progra*) OR (immun* adj3 implement*) OR (immun* adj3 policy) OR (immun* adj3 policies)] AND [middle income country OR middle income countries OR developing econom*] (example of Ovid MEDLINE 1946 search syntax), with the search of terms limited to title and abstract. We found that adding specific words such as child, childhood and pediatric to the search removed useful papers, so we kept the search as wide as possible with regard to age.

Inclusion and exclusion criteria

Two reviewers (ST and HM) performed the database search, reviewed the literature and extracted data. A continuous discussion was used as measure at all stages of the review to minimize bias and error and disagreements between the two reviewers were resolved by discussion.

SCC was regularly consulted to comment on the literature search, authoring and editorial process. The full texts of the references finally selected were assessed for eligibility using pre-defined inclusion and exclusion

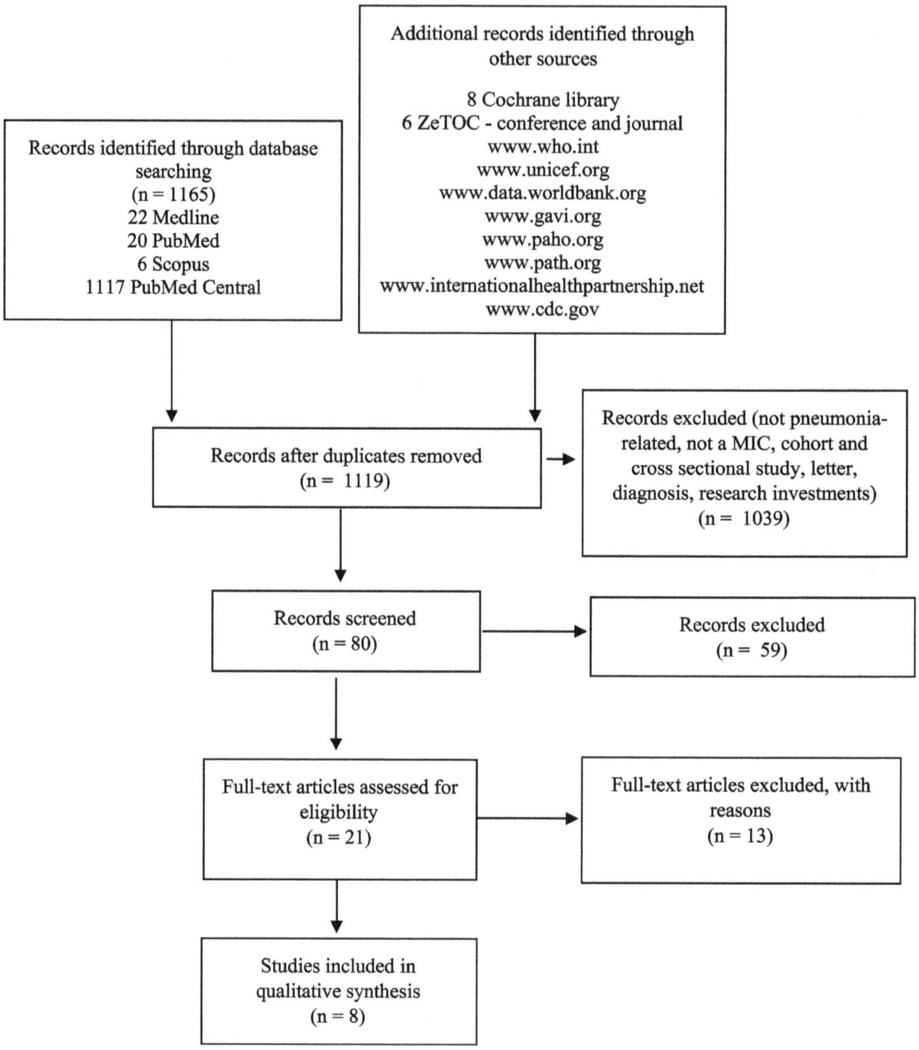

Fig. 1 Flowchart of study selection. The following search terms were used: [*Streptococcus pneumoniae* OR pneumococcus OR pneumococcal OR pneumococci OR PCV OR pneumococcal conjugate vaccine] AND [(vaccin* adj3 policy) OR (vaccin* adj3 policies) OR (vaccin* adj3 implement*) OR (vaccin* adj3 progra*) OR (immun* adj3 progra*) OR (immun* adj3 implement*) OR (immun* adj3 policy) OR (immun* adj3 policies)] AND [middle income country OR middle income countries OR developing econom *]

criteria. The search was limited to papers written in the English language, and published between 1990 and November 2015. A start date of 1990 was chosen because pneumococcal vaccines were introduced for the first time in NIP globally in the 1990s [12]. Articles reporting on active surveillance in relation to PCV policy guidance were included. Cross sectional or cohort studies, and articles relating to burden of disease, cost-effectiveness and other decision support tools and research investments (unless related to PCV policy implementation in MICs) were excluded. References were managed with the EndNote bibliographic database (Thomson Reuters, New York, United States).

Results

The search identified 1,165 articles, of which the full texts of 80 articles were screened. The full texts of 21 were assessed for suitability (Table 1). Finally, eight papers were included in the systematic review for the qualitative analysis because they met all of the inclusion criteria (Table 1). Although the database search was performed between the years 1990 and 2015, the full-text articles assessed for eligibility were all published in the last 11 years. Seven papers were published between 2004 and 2010, and 14 papers between 2011 and 2015.

Out of the 104 MICs, 43 (15/51 [29%] lower middle-income countries [LMICs] and 28/53 [52%] upper middle-income countries [UMICs]) had not introduced

Table 1 Summary table of studies reporting PCV implementation in MICs

Reference	Country	Issues	Solutions
Blau et al. [14]	Albania, Azerbaijan, Georgia, Croatia	Lack of local expertise in health economic and economic evaluation. Lack of available national data on disease burden and cost of treatment of disease preventable by new vaccines.	• to use cost-effectiveness analysis to strengthen decision making in immunization policy and to ensure the sustainability of vaccine introduction • to provide economic evidence to help decide if introducing new vaccine should be prioritized along with other public health programs • to maximise the commitment and support of existing advisory bodies in the country: National Immunization Technical Advisory Group (NITAG) or Interagency Coordination Committee (ICC) • to provide scientific recommendations to support final decisions of introducing PCV
Bonner et al. [16]	LICs and MICs (list of countries not specified)	The cost of PCV can be prohibitive, discouraging countries from including it in their EPI schedules.	• GAVI and its donors should respond to WHO recommendations and countries' needs and expand the vaccine subsidy window for vaccination in children up to age five • policy should be formulated to ensure that PCV is used in emergency contexts, including in extended age groups, as a rapid intervention to limit IPD-related morbidity and mortality • the global immunization community should address the obstacles to systematically using PCV as part of the health service package in emergencies
Gordon et al. [18]	LICs and LMICs (list of countries not specified)	Lack of economic expertise and an explicit desire to include economists in their NITAGs and interagency co-ordinating committees. The availability and consistency of financing was uniformly reported to be the greatest challenge.	
Levine et al. [20]	Global		• the need for post-introduction surveillance to monitor vaccine impact and any shifts in the serotype distribution
Moon et al. [17]	Developing countries (list of countries not specified)	No mechanism is in place ensuring that poorer countries get the lowest possible prices. This case underscores the difficulty in determining what is a "fair" price for MICs.	
Philippe et al. [13]	Global	Limited access to international support is resulting in LMICs beginning to lag behind the poorest countries in protecting their populations from vaccine-preventable diseases using newer vaccines and combination vaccines. Strong disease surveillance and programme monitoring systems are required.	• to seek more suitable formulations and presentations of new vaccines • surveillance of diseases targeted by new vaccines including enhanced laboratory networks and centres of excellence • supporting the establishment/strengthening of National Immunization Technical Advisory Committees • to ensure evidence-based decision at country level, which is particularly needed in view of the complexity of

Table 1 Summary table of studies reporting PCV implementation in MICs *(Continued)*

			the immunization programs and cost of new vaccines
Saxenian et al. [19]	GAVI graduating countries: Indonesia, Sri Lanka, Angola, Bolivia, Azerbaijan, Honduras, Georgia, Congo, Moldova, Armenia, Mongolia, Guyana, Bhutan, Kiribati	Countries had not carried out detailed financial projections of vaccine costs by funding source.	• Ministry of Health should ensure that vaccine procurement methods result in competitive prices for high quality products • need to build specialised market knowledge and skills • a well-functioning national regulatory agencies (NRA) • to maximise the commitment and support of existing advisory bodies in the country (NITAG)
Shen et al. [15]	Developing countries (list of countries not specified)	(1) policy, standards, and guidelines; (2) governance, organization and management; (3) human resources; (4) vaccine, cold chain, and logistics management; (5) service delivery; (6) communication and community partnerships; (7) data generation and use; (8) sustainable financing. An enabling environment, even in the poorest countries, depends on the political will of decision-makers.	• a strong routine immunization platform to benefit the overall health system by generating policy and skilled human resources • NITAGs is to guide the development of national immunization policies, guidelines, and standards • NRAs are necessary if countries are to self-procure and ensure a reliable supply of quality vaccines • to improving governance, organization, and management of routine immunization include • to invest to build the capacity and professional development of an appropriately trained health care • educating and mobilising the public to support immunization and to use immunization services is central to EPI • the generation of high-quality immunization data is important to informing programmatic decisions • sustainable financing

PCVs; 46 MICs (24 LMICs and 22 UMICs) introduced PCVs between 2000 and 2013; 13 MICs (10 LMICs and 3 UMICs) introduced PCVs between 2014 and 2015 and were supported by GAVI; 3 LMICs were approved for GAVI support in 2015 (Kyrgyzstan, Uzbekistan, and Myanmar); one graduating country[2] (Mongolia) was approved for PCV support in 2016 and another six graduating and graduated[2] countries have not yet applied but are eligible to do so (Bhutan, Cuba, Indonesia, Sri Lanka, Timor Leste, and Ukraine) (Table 2; Fig. 2).

A lack of country-specific data on disease burden is considered one of the leading causes of delay in PCV implementation, particularly in relation to the burden of pneumonia and other acute respiratory tract infections [13–15] (Table 1). The prohibitive cost of PCV is discouraging countries from including it in their NIPs [13, 15–18] and a lack of local expertise in economic evaluation [14, 18, 19] was also identified as a recurring problem (Table 1). Thus, the commonly suggested solutions to combatting the underuse of PCVs were the use of cost-effectiveness analysis and the provision of economic evidence to strengthen decision making in immunization policy [13–15, 18], the evaluation of the burden of disease with pre-assessments, and post-introduction surveillance to monitor vaccine impact and any shifts in the serotype distribution [13, 15, 18, 20] (Table 1). Maximizing the commitment and support of existing advisory bodies in MICs, national immunization technical advisory groups (NITAGs) or interagency coordination committees (ICCs) to provide scientific recommendations to support final decisions of introducing PCV [13–15, 18, 19] was also recommended, along with the expansion of the vaccine subsidy window by GAVI and its donors, in order to respond to WHO recommendations and countries' needs [16] (Table 1).

Discussion

This systematic review provides an update on the status of, and impediments to, PCV implementation in MICs. Although PCVs have been available since 2000, the literature assessing the problems MICs experience in implementing widespread PCV immunization has only been published since 2008. This review found that there

Table 2 PCV introduction status for LMICs and UMICs

LMIC/ UMIC	WHO REGION	Country name	PCV introduced Y/N	Year of introduction	PCV 1st dose coverage (%)							PCV 3rd dose coverage (%)							Ref
					2014	2013	2012	2011	2010	2009	2008	2014	2013	2012	2011	2010	2009	2008	
UMIC	EUR	Albania	Y	3/12/2011 (Exact)	99	99	99	99	-	-	-	99	99	99	99	-	-	-	a
UMIC	AFR	Algeria	N		-	-	-	-	-	-	-	-	-	-	-	-	-	-	b
UMIC	-	American Samoa	N		-	-	-	-	-	-	-	-	-	-	-	-	-	-	b
UMIC	AFR	Angola	Y	6/3/2013 (Exact)	84	44	-	-	-	-	-	61	9	-	-	-	-	-	b
LMIC	EUR	Armenia	Y	9/15/2014 (Exact)	-	-	-	-	-	-	-	-	-	-	-	-	-	-	b
UMIC	EUR	Azerbaijan	Y	12/1/2013 (Exact)	91	5	-	-	-	-	-	64	-	-	-	-	-	-	b
LMIC	SEAR	Bangladesh	Y	3/21/2015 (Exact)	-	-	-	-	-	-	-	-	-	-	-	-	-	-	c
UMIC	EUR	Belarus	Y	2014	99	-	-	-	-	-	-	86	-	-	-	-	-	-	b
UMIC	AMR	Belize	N		-	-	-	-	-	-	-	-	-	-	-	-	-	-	b
LMIC	SEAR	Bhutan	N		-	-	-	-	-	-	-	-	-	-	-	-	-	-	b
LMIC	AMR	Bolivia (Plurinational State of)	Y	1/30/2014 (Exact)	99	5	-	-	-	-	-	56	-	-	-	-	-	-	d
UMIC	EUR	Bosnia and Herzegovina	N		-	-	-	-	-	-	-	-	-	-	-	-	-	-	b
UMIC	AFR	Botswana	Y	7/3/2012 (Exact)	99	99	99	-	-	-	-	81	65	52	-	-	-	-	b
UMIC	AMR	Brazil	Y	2010	99	-	97	99	-	-	-	93	94	88	82	24	-	-	e
UMIC	EUR	Bulgaria	Y	2010	95	96	95	96	84	-	-	92	94	94	94	69	-	-	b
LMIC	AFR	Cabo Verde	N		-	-	-	-	-	-	-	-	-	-	-	-	-	-	b
LMIC	AFR	Cameroon	Y	7/1/2011 (Exact)	93	95	92	89	-	-	-	87	88	84	70	-	-	-	b
UMIC	WPR	China	N		-	-	-	-	-	-	-	-	-	-	-	-	-	-	b
UMIC	AMR	Colombia	Y	2011	91	89	94	81	99	99	-	89	87	84	46	71	-	-	e
LMIC	AFR	Congo (the)	Y	10/11/2012 (Exact)	90	90	50	-	-	-	-	85	85	10	-	-	-	-	b
UMIC	AMR	Costa Rica	Y	2007/2008	92	-	95	-	-	-	-	83	-	89	68	97	48	-	b,e
LMIC	AFR	Côte d'Ivoire	Y	9/30/2014 (Exact)	15	-	-	-	-	-	-	2	-	-	-	-	-	-	b
UMIC	AMR	Cuba	N		-	-	-	-	-	-	-	-	-	-	-	-	-	-	b
LMIC	EMR	Djibouti	Y	12/6/2012 (Exact)	93	87	-	-	-	-	-	78	82	-	-	-	-	-	b
UMIC	AMR	Dominica	N		-	-	-	-	-	-	-	-	-	-	-	-	-	-	b
UMIC	AMR	Dominican Republic (the)	Y	2013	94	88	-	2	33	-	-	27	-	-	1	3	-	-	b
UMIC	AMR	Ecuador	Y	2010	83	86	99	99	86	17	-	99	90	94	71	17	2	-	e
LMIC	EMR	Egypt	N		-	-	-	-	-	-	-	-	-	-	-	-	-	-	b
LMIC	AMR	El Salvador	Y	2010	92	91	93	-	77	-	-	-	92	94	98	69	-	-	e
UMIC	WPR	Fiji	Y	2013	91	90	-	-	-	-	-	92	87	-	-	-	-	-	b
UMIC	AFR	Gabon	N		-	-	-	-	-	-	-	-	-	-	-	-	-	-	b

Table 2 PCV introduction status for LMICs and UMICs *(Continued)*

LMIC	EUR	Georgia	Y	11/24/2014 (Exact)	10	-	-	-	-	-	-	-	-	-	-	-	-	-	b
LMIC	AFR	Ghana	Y	4/26/2012 (Exact)	99	93	87	-	-	-	-	98	89	56	-	-	-	-	b
UMIC	AMR	Grenada	N		-	-	-	-	-	-	-	-	-	-	-	-	-	-	b
LMIC	AMR	Guatemala	Y	2012	78	88	3	-	-	-	-	51	24	-	-	-	-	-	e
LMIC	AMR	Guyana	Y	1/10/2011 (Exact)	98	98	94	78	-	-	-	97	96	90	50	-	-	-	e
LMIC	AMR	Honduras	Y	4/1/2011 (Exact)	86	87	88	99	-	-	-	85	87	88	78	-	-	-	e
LMIC	SEAR	India	N		-	-	-	-	-	-	-	-	-	-	-	-	-	-	b
LMIC	SEAR	Indonesia	N		-	-	-	-	-	-	-	-	-	-	-	-	-	-	b
UMIC	EMR	Iran (Islamic Republic of)	N		-	-	-	-	-	-	-	-	-	-	-	-	-	-	b
UMIC	EMR	Iraq	N		-	-	-	-	-	-	-	-	-	-	-	-	-	-	b
UMIC	AMR	Jamaica	Y	2010	48	99	-	14	-	-	-	34	70	-	17	-	-	-	b
UMIC	EMR	Jordan	N		-	-	90	-	-	-	-	-	-	-	-	-	-	-	b
UMIC	EUR	Kazakhstan	Y	2012	70	62	51	-	-	-	-	58	52	39	-	-	-	-	b
LMIC	AFR	Kenya	Y	2/14/2011 (Exact)	88	88	88	99	-	-	-	81	84	82	85	-	-	-	b
LMIC	WPR	Kiribati	Y	2013	70	62	-	-	-	-	-	57	40	-	-	-	-	-	b
LMIC	-	Kosovo	N		-	-	-	-	-	-	-	-	-	-	-	-	-	-	b
LMIC	EUR	Kyrgyzstan	Y	GAVI approved 2015	-	-	-	-	-	-	-	-	-	-	-	-	-	-	b
LMIC	WPR	Lao People's Democratic Republic (the)	Y	10/2/2013 (Exact)	79	1	-	-	-	-	-	72	-	-	-	-	-	-	b
UMIC	EMR	Lebanon	Y	2015	-	-	-	-	-	-	-	-	-	-	-	-	-	-	b
LMIC	AFR	Lesotho	Y	7/10/2015 (Exact)	-	-	-	-	-	-	-	-	-	-	-	-	-	-	b
UMIC	EMR	Libya	Y	10/1/2013 Exact	98	-	-	-	-	-	-	97	-	-	-	-	-	-	b
UMIC	EUR	Macedonia (The former Yugoslav Republic of)	N		-	-	-	-	-	-	-	-	-	-	-	-	-	-	b
UMIC	WPR	Malaysia	N		-	-	-	-	-	-	-	-	-	-	-	-	-	-	b
UMIC	SEAR	Maldives	N		-	-	-	-	-	-	-	-	-	-	-	-	-	-	b
UMIC	WPR	Marshall Islands (the)	Y	2009	70	72	83	-	98	88	-	29	22	46	-	24	49	-	b
LMIC	AFR	Mauritania	Y	11/12/2013 (Exact)	88	23	-	-	-	-	-	84	20	-	-	-	-	-	b
UMIC	AFR	Mauritius	N		-	-	-	-	-	-	-	-	-	-	-	-	-	-	b
UMIC	AMR	Mexico	Y	2008/2009	-	88	-	99	97	93	99	94	84	99	98	92	46	14	b,e
LMIC	WPR	Micronesia (Federated States of)	Y	2008	88	92	92	89	80	-	-	56	61	60	63	70	-	-	b
LMIC	EUR	Moldova	Y	10/1/2013 (Exact)	83	17	-	-	-	-	-	72	1	-	-	-	-	-	b
UMIC	WPR	Mongolia	N		-	-	-	-	-	-	-	-	-	-	-	-	-	-	b
UMIC	EUR	Montenegro	N		-	-	-	-	-	-	-	-	-	-	-	-	-	-	b

Table 2 PCV introduction status for LMICs and UMICs *(Continued)*

LMIC	EMR	Morocco	Y	10/20/2010 (Exact)	99	99	86	91	16	-	-	80	80	72	23	1	-	-	b
LMIC	SEAR	Myanmar	Y	GAVI approved 2015	-	-	-	-	-	-	-	-	-	-	-	-	-	-	b
UMIC	AFR	Namibia	Y	11/11/2014 (Exact)	61	-	-	-	-	-	-	-	-	-	-	-	-	-	b
LMIC	AMR	Nicaragua	Y	12/12/2010 (Exact)	99	99	99	-	-	-	-	99	99	99	91	-	-	-	b
LMIC	AFR	Nigeria	Y	12/22/2014 (Exact)	2	-	-	-	-	-	-	-	-	-	-	-	-	-	b
LMIC	EMR	Pakistan	Y	10/9/2012 (Exact)	70	65	-	-	-	-	-	70	65	-	-	-	-	-	b
UMIC	WPR	Palau	Y	2008	99	99	86	95	87	81	90	93	93	82	61	45	18	7	b
UMIC	AMR	Panama	Y	2010	98	92	99	89	99	20	-	-	-	47	63	48	4	-	e
LMIC	WPR	Papua New Guinea	Y	11/12/2013 (Exact)	-	-	-	-	-	-	-	-	-	-	-	-	-	-	b
UMIC	AMR	Paraguay	Y	2012	78	73	99	-	-	-	-	71	73	81	-	-	-	-	e
UMIC	AMR	Peru	Y	2009	99	97	99	97	95	66	-	86	85	89	82	83	9	-	e
LMIC	WPR	Philippines (the)	Y	7/17/2013 (Exact)	42	-	-	-	-	-	-	35	-	-	-	-	-	-	b
UMIC	EUR	Romania	N		-	-	-	-	-	-	-	-	-	-	-	-	-	-	b
UMIC	AMR	Saint Lucia	N		-	-	-	-	-	-	-	-	-	-	-	-	-	-	b
UMIC	AMR	Saint Vincent and the Grenadines	N		-	-	-	-	-	-	-	-	-	-	-	-	-	-	b
LMIC	WPR	Samoa	N		-	-	-	-	-	-	-	-	-	-	-	-	-	-	b
LMIC	AFR	Sao Tome and Principe	Y	11/30/2012 (Exact)	98	99	64	-	-	-	-	95	97	-	-	-	-	-	b
LMIC	AFR	Senegal	Y	11/5/2013 (Exact)	94	-	-	-	-	-	-	81	-	-	-	-	-	-	b
UMIC	EUR	Serbia	N		-	-	-	-	-	-	-	-	-	-	-	-	-	-	b
LMIC	WPR	Solomon Islands	Y	2/17/2015 (Exact)	-	-	-	-	-	-	-	-	-	-	-	-	-	-	b
UMIC	AFR	South Africa	Y	4/1/2009 (Exact)	96	-	97	98	88	45	-	90	87	98	89	64	10	-	b
LMIC	SEAR	Sri Lanka	N		-	-	-	-	-	-	-	-	-	-	-	-	-	-	b
LMIC	EMR	Sudan (the)	Y	8/1/2013 (Exact)	99	70	-	-	-	-	-	97	30	-	-	-	-	-	b
UMIC	AMR	Suriname	N		-	-	-	-	-	-	-	-	-	-	-	-	-	-	b
LMIC	AFR	Swaziland	Y	4/23/2014 (Exact)	90	-	-	-	-	-	-	89	-	-	-	-	-	-	b
LMIC	EMR	Syrian Arab Republic (the)	N		-	-	-	-	-	-	-	-	-	-	-	-	-	-	b
LMIC	EUR	Tajikistan	Y	2015	-	-	-	-	-	-	-	-	-	-	-	-	-	-	b
UMIC	SEAR	Thailand	N		-	-	-	-	-	-	-	-	-	-	-	-	-	-	b
LMIC	SEAR	Timor-Leste	N		-	-	-	-	-	-	-	-	-	-	-	-	-	-	b
UMIC	WPR	Tonga	N		-	-	-	-	-	-	-	-	-	-	-	-	-	-	b
UMIC	EMR	Tunisia	N		-	-	-	-	-	-	-	-	-	-	-	-	-	-	b
UMIC	EUR	Turkey	Y	2008	96	97	97	98	-	-	-	96	97	97	96	93	97	-	b
UMIC	EUR	Turkmenistan	N		-	-	-	-	-	-	-	-	-	-	-	-	-	-	b

Table 2 PCV introduction status for LMICs and UMICs *(Continued)*

UMIC	WPR	Tuvalu	N		-	-	-	-	-	-	-	-	-	-	-	-	-	-	b
LMIC	EUR	Ukraine	N		-	-	-	-	-	-	-	-	-	-	-	-	-	-	b
LMIC	EUR	Uzbekistan	Y	GAVI approved 2015	-	-	-	-	-	-	-	-	-	-	-	-	-	-	b
LMIC	WPR	Vanuatu	N		-	-	-	-	-	-	-	-	-	-	-	-	-	-	b
LMIC	WPR	Viet Nam	N		-	-	-	-	-	-	-	-	-	-	-	-	-	-	b
LMIC	-	West Bank and Gaza	N		-	-	-	-	-	-	-	-	-	-	-	-	-	-	b
LMIC	EMR	Yemen	Y	1/29/2011 (Exact)	93	94	88	81	-	-	-	88	88	82	56	-	-	-	b
LMIC	AFR	Zambia	Y	5/10/2013 (Exact)	89	-	-	-	-	-	-	77	-	-	-	-	-	-	b

Sources: a, [12]; b, [46]; c, [47]; d, [48]; e, [49]

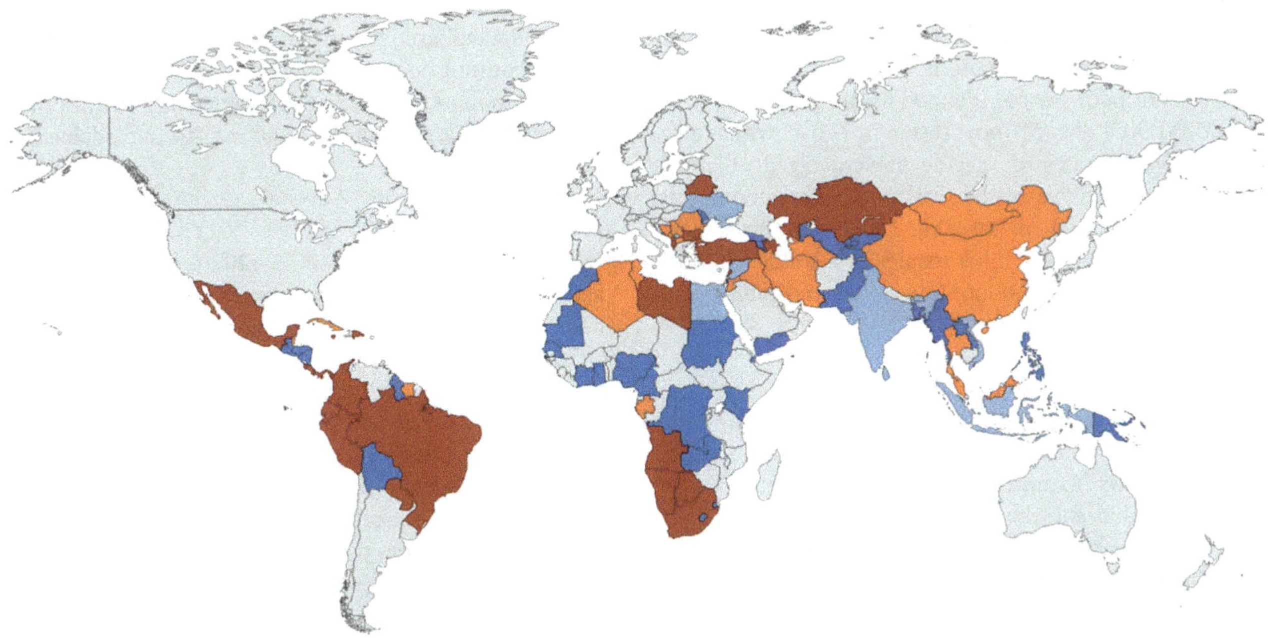

Fig. 2 World map highlighting LMICs that have introduced PCVs in their NIP (*dark blue*), LMICs that have not yet introduced PCV in their NIP (*light blue*), UMICs that introduced PCV in their NIP (*dark red*), UMICs that have not yet introduced PCV in their NIP (*light red*). Data source: WHO/IVB Database and WorldBank, as of February 2016

has been some progress since 2013, but most MICs have not yet added PCVs to their NIPs for infants.

The significant difference in the uptake of PCV in LMICs and UMICs, 71% and 48% respectively, is mainly due to an unsuccessful process of 'graduation'of MICs. Once a country crosses the income eligibility threshold for vaccine subsidy support by GAVI, the financial assistance phases out in a 'graduation' process. GAVI's graduation process is designed to ramp up domestic co-financing of vaccines; however, once GAVI support ends, the new UMICs may not be able to fully fund these vaccines.

Our review has found that a lack of country-specific data on disease burden is considered one of the leading causes of delay in PCV implementation in UMICs, together with a lack of local expertise in economic evaluation, and the cost of PCV. While WHO recommends that PCV be used, despite the lack of country-specific pneumococcal surveillance data [5], PCV is one of the most expensive vaccines that WHO recommends for inclusion in NIP. The cost can be prohibitive, discouraging many MICs from including it. PCV is sold at USD$3.30–$7 per dose (when purchased through GAVI); USD$14.12–$15.68 per dose to the Pan American Health Organization (PAHO) Revolving Fund [4, 21], and US$159.58 per dose to the private sector (pediatric PCV13) [22]. Therefore, in order to fully fund their immunization programmes, MICs should improve informed decision-making on vaccine introduction and other areas of immunization policy and enhance national funding of immunization through advocacy, technical assistance, and training.

The two most populated countries in the world, China and India, require an important mention. China (1.371 billion people) and India (1.311 billion people) [23] are still classified as LMICs and have not added PCV to their NIP. This means that, excluding the unmeasurable percentage of people who received PCV privately, almost 36.4% of the entire world population has not received PCV (See Additional file 1). The Indian government recently announced the possible introduction of PCV in a phased manner by 2017–18 [24, 25]. Mainland China has not yet included PCV in its publicly funded Expanded Program on Immunization (EPI), but it is available at immunization clinics for a fee [26]. However, Hong Kong did add PCV to its NIP in 2009. Without actions in these priority areas, a likely substantial reduction of child mortality and morbidity from pneumonia will not be reached.

Although substantial achievements have been made in preceding decades with other immunization programmes in MICs (e.g. diphtheria-tetanus-pertussis [DTP3], *Haemophilus influenzae* type b [Hib]) [27], PCV implementation is still lagging behind in these countries [28]. A similar delay in implementation has been observed for five other priority new or underused vaccines, namely rotavirus, human papilloma virus [HPV], inactivated poliovirus vaccine [IPV], Japanese encephalitis, and yellow fever vaccine. According to the latest WHO estimates, this leaves 20% of MICs unprotected from these important pathogens, [7]. The main issue is that the majority (73%) of the world's poor people (defined as people living at or below US$1.90 a day [8]) now reside in MICs, which also have the highest rates of vaccine preventable deaths [7]. MICs are home to five of the world's 7 billion people yet (with donors focused on assisting LICs) they have been slow to introduce PCVs. This results in a missed opportunity to dramatically reduce avoidable morbidity and mortality [7, 8].

Overview of PCV procurement opportunities

For the period 2010–2015, GAVI committed approximately US$1.9 billion through the pneumococcal Advance Market Commitment (AMC) to fund PCVs that are suitable for developing countries [29]. Those countries graduating or who have graduated from GAVI support and who have not yet been approved for PCV are able to apply for subsidized PCVs, with the terms and conditions of AMC set at a maximum of US$3.50 per dose [4]. Alongside this, the International Finance Facility for Immunization (IFFIm) provided US$41.58 million toward GAVI's PCV programme in 2011, with the aim to immunize more than 3 million children and prevent more than 1.5 million deaths by 2020 [30]. Prior to this, GAVI established the Accelerated Vaccine Introduction (AVI) initiative in 2008 with the core goal to broaden and speed up access to PCVs over the period 2009–2015 [31].

The WHO has actively developed different programmes to help MICs with PCV implementation. The WHO Integrated Global Action Plan for the Prevention and Control of Pneumonia and Diarrhoea (GAPPD) aims to reduce deaths from pneumonia to fewer than 3 children per 1,000 live births by 2025 [32]. The WHO Expanded Programme of Immunization has seen a dramatic increase in the implementation of new and under-utilized vaccines providing additional prevention of untimely deaths and disabilities, including from pneumococcal disease [33].

The PAHO Revolving Fund, also known as the Regional Revolving Fund for Strategic Public Health Supplies, helps Latin American countries negotiate a lower cost of PCV through bulk procurement, technical assistance on supply management, and assistance with planning, procurement systems, warehousing and distribution, and quality assurance [21]. PAHO's hospital-based surveillance network for bacterial pneumonia currently includes 10 MICs of which five are LMICs (Bolivia, El Salvador, Guatemala, Honduras, and Nicaragua) and five are UMICs (Brazil, Ecuador, Panama, Paraguay, and Peru) [21].

The WHO MIC Task Force has committed to investing approximately US$20 million per year for the 2016–2020 period to support activities included in the MIC Strategy [7]. It includes strengthened decision-making for timely and evidence-based immunization policy, increased political commitment and financial sustainability of NIPs, enhanced demand for and equitable delivery of immunization services, and improved access to affordable and timely supply.

The WHO Strategic Advisory Group of Experts on Immunization (SAGE) Global Vaccine Action Plan (GVAP) aims to make 2011–2020 the 'Decade of Vaccines' [34]. Its target was to introduce at least one under-utilized vaccine by 2015 into 90 LICs and MICs. So far, PCV has been the most frequently introduced vaccine. An estimated US$42 billion to US$51 billion will go towards expanding access to routine immunizations and introducing additional vaccines to routine immunization programmes.

The international non-profit organization Program for Appropriate Technology in Health (PATH) is collaborating with private- and public-sector partners to advance the development of PCVs in LICs [35]. In particular, their vaccine development portfolio includes projects to advance protein vaccines that can provide broad, affordable protection across the many varieties of the pneumococcus, as well as PCVs that are tailored to the health and cost needs of low-resource countries.

In 2015, Doctors Without Borders/Médecins Sans Frontières (MSF) launched a global campaign—'A Fair Shot'— calling on GlaxoSmithKline (GSK) and Pfizer to slash the price of PCV in developing countries, including MICs, to US$5 per child so that more children can be protected, and to disclose what they currently charge countries for the vaccine [36]. MSF believes that governments supporting GAVI must pressure companies to disclose the price they charge for the PCVs in all countries.

Solutions

With many initiatives aimed at improving access to vaccines predominantly being targeted only at LICs, MICs have a much slower rate of PCV uptake [7]. The inclusion of PCV in MIC NIPs is also less widespread than in developed countries. This is due to cost and poor knowledge of the burden of pneumococcal disease in MICs, as well as little logistical and technical support for MICs on how to formulate and implement a coherent policy on PCV immunization. MICs need assistance in integrating PCV immunization into their health systems. Greater political commitment is required towards commissioning epidemiological studies of pneumococcal disease and subsequent resource mobilization towards widespread PCV use at a national policy level. Carriage studies and disease surveillance of *S. pneumoniae*, including disease burden and cost-effectiveness analyses, will generate the data needed to define the economic saving of widespread PCV implementation and to monitor the ongoing impact of widespread PCV immunization at national level.

The first consequence of PCVs being licensed for use and yet not being added to the NIP is that there may be substantial use of PCV in the private sector. This creates a gap between richer and poorer classes with a consequent equity issue, especially since the poorest children tend to experience the highest disease burden. Disparities in access to vaccines are often poorly understood by decision makers, particularly in licensure or in implementation strategies for new vaccines. It is therefore important to apply pressure at national and regional level to ensure governments attempt to address these equity issues to help reduce child morbidity and mortality from pneumonia.

Since the cost per dose for PCVs is among the highest of the routine childhood immunizations, enhanced international advocacy on behalf of MICs for greater flexibility on pricing, and more rational procurement mechanisms for PCVs are critical actions. In particular, the lack of competition among manufacturers is a substantial barrier to reduction of vaccine cost. In fact, only two manufacturers, Pfizer and GSK, license and produce the two currently used PCVs—PCV13 and PCV10, respectively. Moreover, currently 60% of all GAVI-procured vaccines are manufactured in India. Through a recent partnership, GAVI and the Government of India will work together to create a more sustainable vaccine manufacturing base within India, ensuring valuable supplies for the children living in all 72 other GAVI-supported countries [25]. International donors should be encouraged to provide assistance to developing country manufacturers to produce vaccine nationally. Also, 'pooled procurement', which combines several buyers into a single entity that purchases vaccines on their behalf (generally at lower price per dose), would help vaccine procurement for PCV introduction in MIC [37]. Comprehensive multi-year strategic plans for immunization including PCV should be developed by all MICs, and NITAGs (or equivalent committee types) should be established—their role was found to be key in LMICs adoption of PCVs [38]. Alongside these, the World Bank Country Procurement Assessment Report is intended to be an analytical tool to evaluate the existing health system of a country, and may be useful in devising vaccine priorities.

In recent years, the anti-vaccination movement has become more vocal and even hostile [39, 40]. It is a matter of concern that some researchers from the anti-vaccine movements who can influence policy have advocated against the use of available technology due to perceived risks, often without scientific evidence. International organizations (e.g. WHO) and governments, particularly in LMICs, should ensure the implementation of evidence-based public practice. Only standard surveillance systems and research conducted by public health researchers can provide appropriate evidence for decision-making.

It is in the interests of the international community to be more aware of the immunization issues faced by many MICs. Uneven global uptake of PCVs will affect serotype dynamics and spread of antimicrobial resistance, which will have an impact beyond the borders of countries without widespread PCV immunization. Levels of resistance in *S. pneumoniae* are of international concern and were noted in a 2013 'Threat report' issued by the US Center for Disease Prevention and Control (CDC) [41] and there has been increasing resistance across Asia [42]. There have also been observed decreases in prevalence of *S. pneumoniae*-related resistance after implementation of PCV programmes [43, 44].

Donors and non-governmental organizations (NGOs) can contribute towards building capacity in public health surveillance by offering technical assistance in strategy and execution of widespread epidemiological surveillance towards informing immunization policies. This is crucial as the dynamics of pneumococcal epidemiology are complex and studies need to be well designed and the data properly analysed to optimize the quality of data that eventually feeds through to informing vaccine policy.

Additionally, MICs should be supported in identifying and initiating discussions with regional and local organizations with expertize in the planning, logistics and training required before implementing PCVs into a NIP. A successful example of this support model is the PAHO Revolving Fund (described earlier), which assists Latin American countries in managing the range of activities required for the implementation of PCVs.

To address and resolve the issue of poor implementation of PCVs in MICs, the authors suggest that MICs need to be considered as a whole group and collectively undertake a series of steps. MICs should undertake a mapping exercise of their procurement strategies and range of practices; build a central headquarters to collaborate with single countries; understand procurement challenges and opportunities; develop a structural framework for MICs to assess their own procurement systems; explore inter-country and pooled procurement mechanisms; and improve targeted collaborations between MICs and international funding organizations.

Limitations

A number of study constraints exist. First, there are a limited number of studies examining PCV policy. Second, the definition of MICs as a category is sometimes somewhat arbitrary, making analysis of the MIC data difficult. Gaps also exist in the available literature, which combined heterogeneous studies. The methodology used and the article types of the selected papers were also heterogeneous, so that very few quantitative data can be extracted from literature. The study examined grey literature for evidence of unpublished data or studies, but, given the complexity of grey literature, publication bias can be present. There are also many consultations, national and regional meetings and projects (e.g. The Pneumococcal Awareness Council of Experts [PACE] [45]) which are held to discuss new vaccine introductions, but whose proceedings are often not published.

Conclusions

The MICs are slowly implementing PCVs. The global community needs to recognise the barriers to PCV use in many MICs and respond to the situation by increasing scientific, financial, procurement and logistical support to broaden PCV access in MICs. MICs themselves need to strengthen decision making on pneumococcal immunization policy and to mobilize national political will and financing to reduce a significant, largely preventable disease burden, for the benefit of their populations and in the interests of wider international public health.

Endnotes

[1]As of 1 July 2015, middle-income countries (MICs) are defined as those with a Gross National Income (GNI) per capita (calculated using the World Bank Atlas method) of more than US$ 1,045, but less than US$ 12,736 ([50]. WorldBank. 2015 [Accessed 2015 November]. Available from: http://data.worldbank.org/news/new-country-classifications-2015). Of the 104 MICs, 51 are lower-middle-income (LMICs) and 53 upper-middle-income countries (UMICs), separated at a GNI per capita of US$ 4,125 ([50]. Ibid.). In the dynamic and challenging vaccine environment, MICs face increasing technical and economic issues to maintain levels of vaccine introduction and implementation comparable with lower-income countries (LICs) that benefit from international financial and technical support ([10]. Global Alliance on Vaccination and Immunization. 2015. Available from: http://www.gavi.org/support/nvs/pneumococcal/).

[2]In November 2013, the GAVI Board agreed to strengthen GAVI's approach to transition (formerly referred to as "graduation") to support countries in the accelerated transition phase. Each year, some countries enter the accelerated transition phase and start phasing out from GAVI support, as their GNI per capita on average over the previous three years increases beyond the eligibility threshold (set at US$1,580 in 2015) [51]. GAVI. 2016. Available from: http://www.gavi.org/support/apply/graduating-countries/.

Abbreviations

AMC: Advance market commitment; AVI: Accelerated vaccine introduction; CDC: Center for Disease Prevention and Control; DTP3: Diphtheria-tetanus-pertussis; GAPPD: Integrated Global Action Plan for the Prevention and Control of Pneumonia and Diarrhoea; GAVI: Global Alliance for Vaccines and Immunization Alliance; GSK: GlaxoSmithKline; GVAP: Global Vaccine Action Plan; Hib: *Haemophilus influenzae* type B; ICC: Interagency Coordination Committee; IFFIm: International Finance Facility for Immunization; LIC: Low-income country; LMIC: Lower middle-income country; MIC: Middle-income country; MSF: Médecins Sans Frontières/Doctors Without Borders; NGO: Non-governmental organization; NIP: National immunization programme; NITAG: National Immunization Technical Advisory Group; PAHO: Pan American Health Organization; PATH: Program for Appropriate Technology in Health; PCV: Pneumococcal conjugate vaccine; SAGE: Strategic Advisory Group of Experts on Immunization; UMIC: Upper middle-income country; WHO: World Health Organization

Acknowledgements

Not applicable.

Funding

This study was funded, in part, by a Newton Fund Institutional Links grant (172686537) to Stuart Clarke from the British Council. The funder had no role in drafting of the manuscript.

Authors' contributions

ST, HCM and SCC planned the systematic review. ST and HCM conducted the database search, extracted the data, discussed the results and wrote the main paper. MGH, DWC and SCC edited the manuscript. All authors and members of the MYCarriage study team (VL, IKSY, CCW, CST, MNN, AI, ESGC, SNF, JMCJ, PJR, MM, HMY, MLN, NMG, CPD, ARK, JSW) gave their approval of the final version of the manuscript. ST, HM and MH have nothing to disclose. DC reports grants from GSK during the conduct of the study. SCC reports grants from GSK, during the conduct of the study; grants from Pfizer, outside the submitted work.

Authors' information

Not applicable.

Competing interests

ST, HM and MH have nothing to disclose. DC reports grants from GSK during the conduct of the study. SCC reports a grant from GSK, during the conduct of the study, and an investigator-led grant from Pfizer, both of which are outside the submitted work. The authors declare that they have no competing interests.

Author details

[1]Faculty of Medicine, University of Southampton, Southampton, United Kingdom. [2]Institute for Life Sciences, University of Southampton, Southampton, United Kingdom. [3]University of Southampton Malaysia Campus, Johor, Malaysia. [4]Global Health Research Institute, University of Southampton, Southampton, United Kingdom. [5]International Medical University, Kuala Lumpur, Malaysia. [6]Faculty of Medicine and Health Sciences, Universiti Malaysia Sarawak, Kota Samarahan, Sarawak, Malaysia. [7]Universiti Sains Malaysia Health Campus, Kelantan, Malaysia. [8]Universiti Tunku Abdul Rahman, Kampar Campus, Kampar, Perak, Malaysia. [9]NIHR Southampton

Respiratory Biomedical Research Unit, University Hospital Southampton NHS Foundation Trust, Southampton, United Kingdom. [10]NIHR Wellcome Trust Clinical Research Facility, University Hospital Southampton NHS Foundation Trust, Southampton, United Kingdom. [11]Faculty of Social, Human and Mathematical Sciences, University of Southampton, Southampton, United Kingdom. [12]Centre for Biological Sciences, Faculty of Natural and Environmental Sciences, University of Southampton, Southampton, United Kingdom. [13]Postal address: Infectious Disease Epidemiology Group, Mailpoint 814, Level C, Sir Henry Wellcome Laboratories, South Block, University Hospital Southampton NHS Foundation Trust, Southampton, UKSO16 6YD.

References

1. WHO. 2015. Available from: http://www.who.int/mediacentre/factsheets/fs331/en/. Accessed Nov 2015.
2. Walker CLF, Rudan I, Liu L, Nair H, Theodoratou E, Bhutta ZA, O'Brien KL, Campbell H, Black RE. Global burden of childhood pneumonia and diarrhoea. Lancet. 2013;381(Suppl 9875):1405–16.
3. O'Brien KL, Wolfson LJ, Watt JP, Henkle E, Deloria-Knoll M, McCall N, Lee E, Mulholland K, Levine OS, Cherian T. Burden of disease caused by Streptococcus pneumoniae in children younger than 5 years: global estimates. Lancet. 2009;374(Suppl 9693):893–902.
4. GAVI. Advance Market Commitments. Advance Market Commitment for pneumococcal vaccine. Annual Report. 2015. www.gavi.org/library/gavi-documents/amc/2015-pneumococcal-amc-annual-report. Accessed Nov 2015.
5. WHO. Pneumococcal vaccines WHO position paper–2012–recommendations. Vaccine. 2012;30(Suppl 32):4717–8.
6. Johnson HL, Deloria-Knoll M, Levine OS, Stoszek SK, Freimanis Hance L, Reithinger R, Muenz LR, O'Brien KL. Systematic Evaluation of Serotypes Causing Invasive Pneumococcal Disease among Children Under Five: The Pneumococcal Global Serotype Project. PLoS Med. 2010;7(Suppl 10): e1000348.
7. WHO. Sustainable Access to Vaccines in Middle-Income Countries (MICs): A Shared Partner Strategy. Report of the WHO-Convened MIC Task Force. 2015; Suppl.
8. WorldBank. 2016. Available from: http://www.worldbank.org/en/country/mic/overview#1. Accessed Nov 2015.
9. WHO and UNICEF. Global Immunization Data. 2015 Suppl. http://www.who.int/immunization/newsroom/press/immunization_coverage_july_2016/en/. Accessed Jul 2016.
10. Global Alliance on Vaccination and Immunisation. 2015. Available from: http://www.gavi.org/support/nvs/pneumococcal/. Accessed Nov 2015.
11. Moher D, Liberati A, Tetzlaff J, Altman DG, Group TP. Preferred Reporting Items for Systematic Reviews and Meta-Analyses: The PRISMA Statement. PLoS Med. 2009;6(Suppl 7):e1000097.
12. International Vaccine Access Center (IVAC). VIMS Report: Global Vaccine Introduction. 2012. http://www.jhsph.edu/research/centers-and-institutes/ivac/view-hub/IVAC-VIMS_Report-2012-06.pdf. Accessed Nov 2015.
13. Duclos P, Okwo-Bele JM, Gacic-Dobo M, Cherian T. Global immunization: status, progress, challenges and future. BMC Int Health Human Rights. 2009;9(Suppl 1):S2.
14. Blau J, Hoestlandt C, DC A, Baxter L, Felix Garcia AG, Mounaud B, Mosina L. Strengthening national decision-making on immunization by building capacity for economic evaluation: Implementing ProVac in Europe. Vaccine. 2015;33(Suppl 1):A34–9.
15. Shen AK, Fields R, McQuestion M. The future of routine immunization in the developing world: challenges and opportunities. Glob Health Sci Pract. 2014;2 Suppl 4:381–94.
16. Bonner K, Welch E, Elder K, Cohn J. Impact of Pneumococcal Conjugate Vaccine Administration in Pediatric Older Age Groups in Low and Middle Income Countries: A Systematic Review. PLoS One. 2015;10(Suppl 8): e0135270.
17. Moon S, Jambert E, Childs M, von Schoen-Angerer T. A win-win solution?: A critical analysis of tiered pricing to improve access to medicines in developing countries. Glob Health. 2011;7(Suppl):39.
18. Gordon WS, Jones A, Wecker J. Introducing multiple vaccines in low- and lower-middle-income countries: issues, opportunities and challenges. Health Policy Plan. 2012;27(Suppl 2):ii17–26.
19. Saxenian H, Hecht R, Kaddar M, Schmitt S, Ryckman T, Cornejo S. Overcoming challenges to sustainable immunization financing: early experiences from GAVI graduating countries. Health Policy Plan. 2015;30(Suppl 2):197–205.
20. Levine OS, Knoll MD, Jones A, Walker DG, Risko N, Gilani Z. Global status of Haemophilus influenzae type b and pneumococcal conjugate vaccines: evidence, policies, and introductions. Curr Opin Infect Dis. 2010;23 (Suppl 3):236–41.
21. WHO/PAHO. 2015. Available from: http://www.paho.org/HQ/index.php?option=com_content&view=article&id=1864%3A2014-paho-revolving-fund&catid=839%3Arevolving-fund&Itemid=4135&lang=en. Accessed Nov 2015.
22. Centers for Disease Control and Prevention (CDC). CDC Vaccine Price List. 2016. Available from: http://www.cdc.gov/vaccines/programs/vfc/awardees/vaccine-management/price-list/#f5. Accessed Nov 2015.
23. World Bank. 2015 [26/10/2016]. Available from: http://databank.worldbank.org/data/reports.aspx?Code=SP.POP.TOTL&id=af3ce82b&report_name=Popular_indicators&populartype=series&ispopular=y. Accessed Nov 2015.
24. 2015 [26/10/2016]. Available from: http://www.livemint.com/Politics/OPypN8I71EHYpsh1JIUMIJ/Govt-may-introduce-Pneumococcal-Conjugate-Vaccine-by-201718.html. Accessed Nov 2015.
25. GAVI. 2016 [09/11/2016]. Available from: http://www.gavi.org/library/news/press-releases/2016/historic-partnership-between-gavi-and-india-to-save-millions-of-lives/. Accessed Nov 2015.
26. Hu J, Sun X, Huang Z, Wagner AL, Carlson B, Yang J, Tang S, Li Y, Boulton ML, Yuan Z. Streptococcus pneumoniae and Haemophilus influenzae type b carriage in Chinese children aged 12–18 months in Shanghai, China: a cross-sectional study. BMC Infect Dis. 2016;16(Suppl):149.
27. Kaddar M, Schmitt S, Makinen M, Milstien J. Global support for new vaccine implementation in middle-income countries. Vaccine. 2013; 31(Suppl):B81–96.
28. Richardson A, Morris DE, Clarke SC. Vaccination in Southeast Asia–reducing meningitis, sepsis and pneumonia with new and existing vaccines. Vaccine. 2014;32(Suppl 33):4119–23.
29. UNICEF. 2016. Available from: http://www.unicef.org/supply/index_60990.html. Accessed 2015 Nov.
30. IFFIm. 2016. Available from: http://www.iffim.org/Funding-GAVI/Results/Pneumococcal-vaccine/. Accessed Nov 2015.
31. AVI. Available from: http://www.gavi.org/results/evaluations/avi-project-review/. Accessed Nov 2015.
32. WHO, UNICEF. Ending preventable child deaths from pneumonia and diarrhoea by 2025. The integrated Global Action Plan for Pneumonia and Diarrhoea (GAPPD). 2013 Suppl.
33. WHO. 2013. Available from: http://www.who.int/immunization/programmes_systems/supply_chain/benefits_of_immunization/en/. Accessed Nov 2015.
34. WHO/SAGE. Global Vaccine Action Plan Secretariat Annual Report 2015. 2015. http://www.who.int/immunization/global_vaccine_action_plan/gvap_secretariat_report_2015.pdf. Accessed Nov 2015.
35. PATH. Available from: http://sites.path.org/vaccinedevelopment/pneumonia-and-pneumococcus/vaccine-development/. Accessed Nov 2015.
36. Médecins Sans Frontières. 2015. Available from: http://www.doctorswithoutborders.org/article/msf-kicks-global-campaign-reduce-price-pneumonia-vaccine-5-developing-countries. Accessed Nov 2015.
37. UNICEF, editor Developing a strategy to support new vaccine introduction in Middle Income Countries. SAGE meeting, 6–8 November; 2012.
38. Makinen M, Kaddar M, Molldrem V, Wilson L. New vaccine adoption in lower-middle-income countries. Health Policy Plan. 2012;27 Suppl 2:ii39–49.
39. Dube E, Vivion M, MacDonald NE. Vaccine hesitancy, vaccine refusal and the anti-vaccine movement: influence, impact and implications. Expert Rev Vaccines. 2015;14(Suppl 1):99–117.
40. Babu GR, Murthy GVS. "To Use or Not to Use"- Dilemma of Developing Countries in Introducing New Vaccines. J Glob Infect. 2011;3(Suppl 4):406–7.
41. Centers for Disease Control and Prevention (CDC). Antibiotic resistance threats in the United States. 2013.
42. Mamishi S, Moradkhani S, Mahmoudi S, Hosseinpour-Sadeghi R, Pourakbari B. Penicillin-Resistant trend of Streptococcus pneumoniae in Asia: A systematic review. Iran J Microbiol. 2014;6(Suppl 4):198–210.
43. dos Santos SR, Passadore LF, Takagi EH, Fujii CM, Yoshioka CRM, Gilio AE, Martinez MB. Serotype distribution of Streptococcus pneumoniae isolated from patients with invasive pneumococcal disease in Brazil before and after ten-pneumococcal conjugate vaccine implementation. Vaccine. 2013; 31(Suppl 51):6150–4.

44. Stephens DS, Zughaier SM, Whitney CG, Baughman WS, Barker L, Gay K, Jackson D, Orenstein WA, Arnold K, Schuchat A, Farley MM. Incidence of macrolide resistance in Streptococcus pneumoniae after introduction of the pneumococcal conjugate vaccine: population-based assessment. Lancet. 2005;365(Suppl 9462):855–63.
45. The Pneumococcal Awareness Council of Experts (PACE). 2016. [03/11/2016]. Available from: http://www.sabin.org/programs/vaccine-advocacy/pneumococcal-awareness-council-experts. Accessed Nov 2015.
46. International Vaccine Access Center (IVAC). VIMS Report: Global Vaccine Introduction. 2015.
47. GAVI. 2015. Available from: http://www.gavi.org/library/news/press-releases/2015/children-in-bangladesh-to-benefit-from-dual-vaccine-introduction/. Accessed Nov 2015.
48. UNICEF Supply Division. Pneumococcal Conjugate Vaccine: Supply & Demand Update. 2014. https://www.unicef.org/supply/files/PCV_Update_Note_July_2014.pdf. Accessed Nov 2015.
49. PAHO. Lessons Learned from the Introduction of the Pneumococcal Conjugate Vaccine (PCV) in Latin America and the Caribbean. 2012.
50. WorldBank. New Country Classifications. 2015. Available from: http://data.worldbank.org/news/new-country-classifications-2015. Accessed Nov 2015.
51. GAVI. Transition process. 2016. Available from: http://www.gavi.org/support/apply/graduating-countries/. Accessed Nov 2015.

9

Predictors of pneumococcal carriage and the effect of the 13-valent pneumococcal conjugate vaccination in the Western Australian Aboriginal population

Deirdre A. Collins[1,2*], Anke Hoskins[2], Thomas Snelling[2], Kalpani Senasinghe[2], Jacinta Bowman[3], Natalie A. Stemberger[3], Amanda J. Leach[4] and Deborah Lehmann[2]

Abstract

Background: The 7-valent pneumococcal conjugate vaccine (PCV7) was introduced to prevent invasive pneumococcal disease (IPD) in Western Australian (WA) Aboriginal people in 2001. PCV13 replaced PCV7 in July 2011, covering six additional pneumococcal serotypes; however, IPD rates remained high in Aboriginal people in WA. Upper respiratory tract pneumococcal carriage can precede IPD, and PCVs alter serotype distribution.

Methods: To assess the impact of PCV13 introduction, identify emerging serotypes, and assess risk factors for carriage, nasopharyngeal swabs and information on demographic characteristics, health, medication and living conditions from Aboriginal children and adults across WA from August 2008 to November 2014 were collected. Bacteria were cultured using selective media and pneumococcal isolates were serotyped by Quellung reaction. Risk factors were analysed by multivariable logistic regression.

Results: One thousand five hundred swabs pre- and 1385 swabs post-PCV13 introduction were collected. Pneumococcal carriage was detected in 66.8% of children <5 years old and 53.2% of 5–14 year-olds post-PCV13, compared with pre-PCV13 prevalence of 72.2% and 49.4%, respectively. The prevalence of PCV13-non-PCV7 serotypes decreased in children <5 years old from 13.5% pre-PCV13 to 5.8% post-PCV13 ($p < 0.01$), and from 8.4% to 6.1% in children 5–14 years old ($p > 0.05$). The most common serotypes post-PCV13 were 11A (prevalence 4.0%), 15B (3.5%), 16F (3.5%), and 19F (3.2%).

Risk of detection of pneumococcal carriage increased until age 12 months (odds ratio [OR] 4.19, 95% confidence interval [CI] 2.39–7.33), with nasal discharge (OR 2.49 [95% CI 2.00–3.09]), residence in a remote community (OR 2.21 [95% CI 1.67–2.92]) and household crowding (OR 1.36 [95% CI 1.11–1.67]). Recent antibiotic use was negatively associated with pneumococcal carriage (OR 0.48 [95% CI 0.33–0.69]). Complete resistance to penicillin was present among isolates of serotypes 19A (6.0%), 19F (2.3%) and non-serotypeable isolates (1.9%). Serotype 23F and newly emerged serotype 7B isolates showed high rates of resistance to cotrimoxazole, erythromycin and tetracycline (86.9%, 86.9%, 82.0%, respectively for 23F, 100.0%, 100.0% and 93.3% for 7B).

Conclusion: Since PCV13 replaced PCV7, carriage of PCV13-non-PCV7 serotypes decreased significantly among children <5 years old, those most likely to have received PCV13, and to a lesser extent in older people. Known risk factors for carriage including crowding and young age remain in the Aboriginal population.

Keywords: *Streptococcus pneumoniae*, Colonization, Pneumococcal disease, Aboriginal, Vaccination, Australia, PCV13

* Correspondence: deirdre.collins@ecu.edu.au
[1]School of Medical and Health Sciences, Edith Cowan University, Perth, WA, Australia
[2]Wesfarmers Centre of Vaccines & Infectious Diseases, Telethon Kids Institute, University of Western Australia, Perth, WA, Australia
Full list of author information is available at the end of the article

Background

Streptococcus pneumoniae is estimated to cause up to a million deaths from invasive pneumococcal disease (IPD) per year, worldwide [1]. While the greatest burden of IPD is concentrated in resource-poor countries, Australian Aboriginal people in central and western regions of Australia experience an almost five-fold greater incidence of IPD than non-Aboriginal Australians [2]. In addition to high rates of IPD, Aboriginal children also experience a high burden of other manifestations of pneumococcal disease, including pneumonia and otitis media (OM) [3].

Vaccination to prevent IPD is effective against targeted serotypes, but limited by the existence of at least 93 serotypes of *S. pneumoniae*, each differentiated by its polysaccharide capsule. The 7-valent pneumococcal conjugate vaccine (PCV7, covering serotypes 4, 6B, 9V, 14, 18C, 19F and 23F) was introduced for Australian Aboriginal children at 2, 4 and 6 months old in 2001 with a booster dose of 23-valent pneumococcal polysaccharide vaccine (23vPPV, covering PCV7 serotypes and 1, 2, 3, 5, 7F, 8, 9 N, 10A, 11A, 12F, 15B, 17F, 19A, 20, 22F, and 23F) scheduled at 18 months old. A catch-up schedule was in place for children <2 years old and for children <5 years old with predisposing medical conditions. All Australian children became eligible in 2005 for 3 primary doses of PCV7 with no scheduled booster. Following the introduction of PCV7, IPD rates initially fell in the Aboriginal population in Western Australia (WA) but subsequently increased in adults [2]. The observed increase was accompanied by a rise in IPD caused by non-PCV7 serotypes [4, 5].

On 1 July 2011, PCV7 was recalled and immediately replaced with PCV13 (covering the six additional serotypes 1, 3, 5, 6A, 7F and 19A). For Aboriginal children, a fourth dose of PCV13 at 18 months old replaced the 23vPPV booster over a transition period from September 2011 to October 2012 [6]. Following PCV13 introduction in Australia, IPD rates appeared to decrease; however, rates in IPD caused by non-PCV13 serotypes increased [4, 7].

Nasopharyngeal carriage of *S. pneumoniae* is generally asymptomatic but is an important precursor to pneumococcal disease. Pneumococcal carriage studies have been used to monitor the prevalence and distribution of *S. pneumoniae* serotypes in WA, and for surveillance of antibiotic resistant strains. Despite introduction of the PCV program, pneumococcal carriage rates remain high among Aboriginal people [8, 9], and have been observed to be higher in Aboriginal children than in non-Aboriginal children [10]. In WA, carriage rates were 71.9% and 34.6% among Aboriginal children <5 years old and people ≥5 years old, respectively, after introduction of PCV7 [9]. Most pneumococcal carriage serotypes in WA in the PCV7 era were non-PCV7 serotypes, the most common being 19A, 16F and 6C [9].

Given that the PCV vaccination program does not appear to have reduced overall IPD rates in the Aboriginal population in age groups other than children <5 years [4], it is important to identify risk factors for carriage of *S. pneumoniae* to help identify further opportunities for prevention of pneumococcal disease. Previously, household crowding and exposure to environmental tobacco smoke (ETS) have been identified as risk factors [11]. The authors have monitored pneumococcal carriage in Aboriginal people living in WA since 2008. This study describes the prevalence of overall carriage and that of individual serotypes in the WA Aboriginal population before and after the introduction of PCV13, along with epidemiological risk factors for carriage.

Methods

Study population

Aboriginal people make up about 3% of the total WA population (total 2.2 million people); 39% live in the Perth metropolitan area, the remainder in regional towns or scattered sparsely across remote areas of WA. The WA climate varies, from tropical in the north to inland deserts and warm temperate southwest coastal regions.

Sample and data collection and laboratory analysis

The surveillance study has been described previously [9]. In brief, nasopharyngeal swabs or nose blown samples [12] were collected opportunistically from Aboriginal people of all ages in communities across WA from August 2008 to November 2014. Participants were defined as having participated "pre-PCV13" introduction (from study start until 30 June 2011) or "post-PCV13" (from 1 July 2011 onwards). Demographic, environmental and health data including details on smoking behaviour and exposure, numbers of co-resident household members, recent medication and illness were collected by completing a questionnaire during face-to-face interviews. Swabs were cultured on selective media. *S. pneumoniae* isolates were confirmed by optochin susceptibility. Two pneumococcal isolates (or more, if morphologically distinct) per positive culture were subcultured and serotyped by the Quellung reaction using antisera from the Statens Serum Institut, Denmark [13]. Isolates that could not be serotyped by Quellung reaction were referred to as "non-serotypeable". Antimicrobial susceptibilities were tested by disc diffusion. E-test (bioMérieux Diagnostics, France) was performed where reduced antimicrobial susceptibility was determined by disc diffusion. Resistance to antimicrobials was classified according to the Clinical and Laboratory Standards Institute guidelines [14]. Breakpoints for intermediate and complete resistance to penicillin (collectively termed "non-susceptibility") were 4 μg/mL and 8 μg/mL, respectively.

The remoteness (metropolitan, regional or remote) of communities was classified using the Australian Statistical Geography Standard Remoteness Structure [15]. Household crowding was defined as ≥5 people sharing accommodation on the night prior to sample collection. Co-residence with a child was defined as sharing with at least one child <5 years old on the previous night. Respiratory symptoms were defined as any cough, sore throat, or blocked or runny nose as reported by the participant or guardian. Environmental tobacco smoke (ETS) exposure was considered present if it was reported that any co-resident was a smoker. The immunization status of children was determined from the Australian Childhood Immunization Register (ACIR), accessed using the participant's name and date of birth. Children were classified as vaccinated with PCV7 or PCV13 if they had received at least two doses of the relevant vaccine at least 2 weeks prior to specimen collection.

Statistical analysis

All descriptive and statistical analyses were performed using SPSS v22.0 (IBM Corp., Armonk, New York, United States of America [USA]) and Stata 11 (Stata Corporation, College Station, Texas, USA). Results of culture and serotyping were aggregated according to serotype to calculate the prevalence of individual serotypes among all study participants. Differences in crude proportions were compared using χ^2 test; statistical significance was considered if $p < 0.05$. A multivariable logistic regression model was used to identify independent risk factors for carriage of serotypeable pneumococci. Variables were included, if identified previously in the literature as risk factors for carriage, in a backwards stepwise model, eliminating variables using a cut-off value of $p > 0.05$. Vaccination status was excluded from the risk factor analysis due to poor recovery of vaccination records and low number of PCV13-vaccinated children (see Results section). The influence of age on carriage risk was modelled using a spline function with knots at age 1 year and at 20 years, based on previous findings of a peak in carriage at 12 months of age in this particular population [9]. The influence of calendar time was modelled as a linear continuous variable, with the influence of the PCV13 program on carriage explored using a simple marginal spline function with a single knot corresponding to 1 July 2011, the date of PCV13 introduction.

Ethical approval

Approval was granted by the Princess Margaret Hospital for Children Ethics Committee, the Western Australian Country Health Service Board Research Ethics Committee and the Western Australian Aboriginal Health Ethics Committee. Approval to approach communities in the Kimberley region was granted by the Kimberley Aboriginal Health Planning Forum. Consent was sought from adult participants and from the parents or guardians of child participants.

Results

Study population

In total 2885 nasopharyngeal samples (2824 nasopharyngeal swabs; 60 nose blown samples; 1 unknown) were collected: 1500 before the introduction of PCV13 on 1 July 2011, and 1385 afterwards. Most participants reported being healthy on the day of participation, while 31.5% had visible nasal discharge and 8.4% reported respiratory symptoms (Table 1). Most samples were collected among remote residents (78.2%). Crowding (61.7%) and co-residence with children (73.5%) were common across all age groups. Any ETS exposure was reported by 65.3% of participants; 22.9% reported exposure to indoor ETS, and 55.6% of adult respondents reported smoking themselves. Recent antibiotic use was reported by 7.6% of participants. Immunization status could be determined for only 628 (59.1%) participants <5 years old and 488 (51.5%) participants 5–14 years old. Among PCV7 age-eligible children whose immunization status was available, 504 (89.4%) of those <5 years old and 302 (74.6%) of those aged 5–14 years were vaccinated with PCV7 (Table 1). Among children eligible for PCV13 whose immunization status was known, 37 (59.7%) were vaccinated with at least two doses of PCV13 and 64 (98.5%) had received at least one dose. A combination of PCV7 and PCV13 (at least one dose of each) was received by 66 (6.8%) children.

Carriage prevalence

Compared to the pre-PCV13 period, carriage of any pneumococcal serotype was less common in the post-PCV13 period among adults (19.5% versus 9.9%, $p < 0.01$) and to a lesser extent among children <5 years old (72.2% versus 66.8%, $p = 0.054$) but not in children 5–14 years old (49.4% versus 53.2%, $p = 0.24$). Carriage of PCV13-non-PCV7 serotypes was less common post-PCV13 introduction among children <5 years old (13.5% versus 5.8%, $p < 0.01$; Table 1, Fig. 1). There was also a numerical reduction in carriage of vaccine serotypes in older age groups (Table 1). *S. pneumoniae* was recovered from 46.8% of nasopharyngeal swabs and 56.7% of nose-blown samples.

Culture identified 1357 pneumococcus-positive specimens (47.0%) giving 1590 distinct pneumococcal isolates, 1374 (86.4%) of which were serotypeable (Table 2). The most common of the 48 serotypes detected were 16F (prevalence 3.8%), 6C (3.6%), 11A (3.3%), 19F (3.0%),

Table 1 Descriptive characteristics of Aboriginal people in Western Australia enrolled before and after PCV13 introduction (1 July 2011), by age group (August 2008–November 2014)

	n (%)						
	<5 years		5–14 years		≥15 years		
	pre-PCV13	*post-PCV13*	*pre-PCV13*	*post-PCV13*	*pre-PCV13*	*post-PCV13*	Total
S. pneumoniae carriage							
Any serotype	406 (72.2)	334 (66.8)	235 (49.4)	251 (53.2)	90 (19.5)	41 (9.9)**	1357 (47.0)
PCV7 serotype	59 (10.5)	32 (6.4)*	35 (7.4)	28 (5.9)	9 (1.9)	5 (1.2)	168 (5.8)
PCV13-nonPCV7 serotype	76 (13.5)	29 (5.8)**	40 (8.4)	29 (6.1)	10 (2.2)	4 (1.0)	188 (6.5)
PCV13 serotype	133 (23.7)[a]	60 (12.0)[b]**	74 (15.5)[b]	57 (12.1)	19 (4.1)	9 (2.2)	352 (12.2)
Male	307 (54.6)	252 (50.6)	249 (52.3)	223 (47.2)	117 (25.3)	74 (17.9)	1222 (42.4)
Respiratory symptoms	65 (13.6)	66 (13.2)	14 (3.0)	20 (4.2)	26 (5.7)	44 (10.7)	235 (8.4)
Nasal discharge	294 (60.2)	234 (46.8)**	170 (36.2)	111 (23.5)**	31 (6.8)	43 (10.4)	883 (31.5)
Remoteness index							
Metropolitan	68 (12.1)	71 (14.2)	62 (13.0)	76 (16.1)	26 (5.6)	63 (15.3)	366 (12.7)
Regional	43 (7.7)	73 (14.6)	20 (4.2)	40 (8.5)	29 (6.3)	57 (13.8)	262 (9.1)
Remote	451 (80.2)	356 (71.2)	394 (82.8)	356 (75.4)	407 (88.1)	293 (70.9)	2257 (78.2)
≥5 people sharing (crowding)	308 (65.7)	280 (57.1)**	291 (66.1)	294 (66.4)	282 (66.4)	194 (47.8)**	1649 (61.7)
Sharing with ≥1 child <5 years	368 (78.6)	326 (66.5)**	336 (76.4)	303 (69.0)*	353 (83.6)	272 (67.3)**	1958 (73.5)
Antibiotic use in previous 2 weeks	46 (8.5)	60 (12.3)	13 (2.7)	35 (7.7)**	23 (5.0)	39 (9.5)*	216 (7.6)
Indoor environmental tobacco smoke exposure	103 (22.0)	103 (21.2)	91 (20.6)	96 (21.7)	131 (29.6)	91 (22.5)*	615 (22.9)
Any environmental tobacco smoke exposure	325 (67.6)	340 (69.7)	272 (59.4)	287 (64.3)	297 (66.6)	260 (63.9)	1781 (65.3)
Smoker	N/A	N/A	N/A	N/A	237 (59.1)	182 (52.1)	419 (55.6)
Season							
Summer	43 (7.7)	23 (4.6)	51 (10.7)	20 (4.2)	18 (3.9)	22 (5.3)	177 (6.1)
Autumn	108 (19.2)	94 (18.8)	103 (21.6)	82 (17.4)	91 (19.7)	93 (22.5)	571 (19.8)
Winter	275 (48.9)	242 (48.4)	204 (42.9)	183 (38.8)	169 (36.6)	190 (46.0)	1263 (43.8)
Spring	136 (24.2)	141 (28.2)	118 (24.8)	187 (39.6)	184 (39.8)	108 (26.2)	874 (30.3)
PCV7 vaccinated	360 (88.9)	144 (90.6)	168 (69.4)	134 (82.2)	N/A	N/A	806 (83.2)
PCV13 vaccinated[c]	N/A	37 (59.7)	N/A	N/A	N/A	N/A	37 (26.2)
Vaccination status unknown	151 (26.8)	283 (56.6)	165 (34.7)	295 (62.5)	N/A	N/A	894 (44.5)
H. influenzae	355 (63.2)	274 (54.8)**	170 (35.7)	186 (39.4)	40 (8.7)	24 (5.8)	1049 (36.4)
M. catarrhalis	353 (62.8)	356 (71.2)**	193 (40.5)	175 (37.1)	60 (13.0)	30 (7.3)**	1167 (40.5)
S. aureus	64 (11.4)	30 (6.0)**	73 (15.3)	77 (16.3)	46 (10.0)	35 (8.5)	325 (11.3)

Denominators for proportions varied due to missing data. Proportions were compared using χ^2

**p* < 0.05, ***p* < 0.01

[a]Two participants carried a PCV7 and PCV13-non-PCV7 serotype simultaneously

[b]One participant carried a PCV7 and PCV13-non-PCV7 serotype simultaneously

[c]Denominator is number of participants at time of enrolment pre/post PCV13. Includes participants vaccinated with PCV7 prior to introduction of PCV13

19A (2.9%) and 15B (2.6%). Several PCV13 serotypes decreased in frequency post-PCV13 introduction in children <5 years old: PCV7 type 23F (4.8% versus 1.8%, $p < 0.05$), PCV13-non-PCV7 types 6A (3.6% versus 1.4%, $p < 0.05$) and 19A (7.7% versus 3.2%, $p < 0.05$) (Fig. 2). Reductions in PCV13 types were also observed in participants ≥5 years old, to a lesser extent than that seen in children <5 years (15.5% to 12.1% in 5–14 years, $p = 0.12$; 4.1% to 2.2% in ≥15 years group, $p = 0.10$, Table 1).

Carriage of more than one serotype was identified in 131 (4.5%) specimens. Non-serotypeable isolates were detected in addition to a serotypeable isolate in 81 (2.8%) specimens. The prevalence of a non-serotypeable pneumococcus in the absence of serotypeable strains was lower post-PCV13 (4.7% versus 3.9%, $p = 0.06$).

Among 36 non-PCV13 serotypes identified, the prevalence of 11A (4.8% versus 8.4%, $p < 0.05$), 15B (2.1% versus 7.0%, $p < 0.01$) and 21 (0.9% versus 2.6%, $p < 0.05$) increased significantly among children <5 years old while

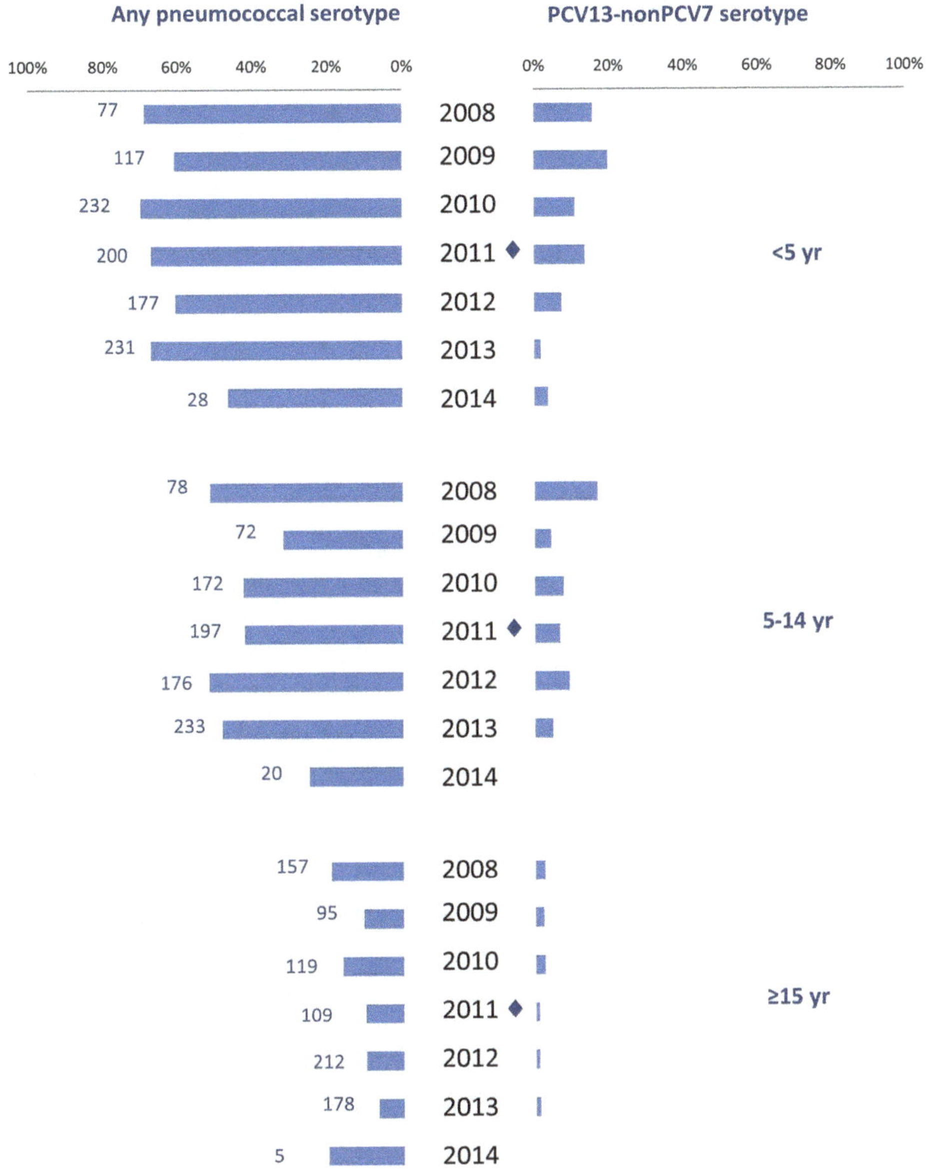

Fig. 1 Prevalence of any serotypeable pneumococcus or PCV13-nonPCV7 serotype only by year, by age group, among Aboriginal people in Western Australia, August 2008–November 2014. Numbers by bars represent number of participants per year. ♦PCV13 was introduced on 1 July 2011

7B and 29 were only detected post-PCV13 (2.0% and 1.8% respectively, both $p < 0.05$). Serotypes 6C and 23B were detected less frequently post-PCV13 introduction in children <5 years old (8.0% versus 3.4%, $p < 0.05$ and 5.0% versus 1.8%, $p < 0.05$; Fig. 2).

Antimicrobial susceptibility

Non-susceptibility to penicillin was present in 25.2% of isolates, including in 84.9% of serotype 19F isolates. Complete resistance to penicillin was uncommon, found among isolates of serotypes 19A (6.0%), 19F (2.3%) and non-serotypeable isolates (1.9%) only (Table 2). Serotype 23F isolates showed high rates of resistance to cotrimoxazole, erythromycin and tetracycline (86.9%, 86.9% and 82.0%, respectively). Multi-resistance to three or more antibiotics was recorded in 102 serotypeable isolates (7.4%) overall; mainly serotype 15A isolates (68.0%) and serotype 23F isolates (88.5%). Isolates of serotype 7B (n = 15), which were only detected post-PCV13, were all resistant to cotrimoxazole and erythromycin, non-susceptible to penicillin and 93.3% were resistant to tetracycline (Table 2). Overall, susceptibility of strains to antimicrobials did not change significantly after introduction of PCV13, apart from a decrease in cotrimoxazole resistance (26.1% to 21.3%, $p < 0.05$, Table 2). Multi-resistance was present in 17.6% of non-serotypeable isolates.

Table 2 Frequencies of serotypes and antibiotic resistance rates found among 1590 isolates of *Streptococcus pneumoniae* among Aboriginal people in Western Australia, August 2008–November 2014. PCV13 was introduced on July 1 2011

	Isolates		pen^{I} (%)		pen^{R} (%)		cotr^{R} (%)		ery^{R} (%)		tet^{R} (%)	
Serotype	Pre (*n*)	Post (*n*)	Pre	Post	Pre	Post	Pre	Post	Pre	Post	Pre	Post
16F	62	48	32.3	25.0	0.0	0.0	0.0	0.0	8.1	0.0	6.5	0.0
6C	73	30	0.0	0.0	0.0	0.0	64.4	43.3	4.1	3.3	0.0	0.0
11A	40	56	7.5	10.7	0.0	0.0	17.5	26.8	2.5	0.0	0.0	0.0
19F	41	45	90.2	75.6	0.0	4.4	0.0	4.4	0.0	6.7	0.0	4.4
19A	58	25	39.7	52.0	5.2	8.0	43.1	56.0	10.3	24.0	25.9	44.0
15B	27	49	14.8	2.0	0.0	0.0	7.4	18.4	11.1	8.2	0.0	0.0
23F	43	18	4.7	0.0	0.0	0.0	81.4	100.0	81.4	100.0	76.7	94.4
6A	37	18	2.7	0.0	0.0	0.0	8.1	11.1	59.5	50.0	2.7	0.0
10A	26	28	3.8	0.0	0.0	0.0	61.5	35.7	0.0	0.0	0.0	0.0
23B	32	18	18.8	38.9	0.0	0.0	0.0	11.1	0.0	0.0	0.0	0.0
15C	16	27	6.3	3.7	0.0	0.0	25.0	18.5	0.0	7.4	0.0	0.0
34	23	14	0.0	0.0	0.0	0.0	0.0	0.0	0.0	7.1	0.0	0.0
22F	21	16	0.0	0.0	0.0	0.0	0.0	0.0	71.4	50.0	0.0	0.0
35B	15	19	13.3	15.8	0.0	0.0	6.7	0.0	0.0	10.5	0.0	0.0
3	17	13	0.0	7.7	0.0	0.0	0.0	0.0	0.0	0.0	0.0	0.0
33F	21	9	4.8	0.0	0.0	0.0	4.8	11.1	0.0	22.2	0.0	11.1
7C	12	17	0.0	0.0	0.0	0.0	0.0	0.0	16.7	70.6	0.0	0.0
21	8	20	0.0	0.0	0.0	0.0	37.5	10.0	0.0	5.0	0.0	0.0
23A	13	15	0.0	6.7	0.0	0.0	0.0	0.0	0.0	0.0	0.0	0.0
38	10	18	0.0	0.0	0.0	0.0	0.0	0.0	0.0	0.0	0.0	22.2
15A	6	19	50.0	73.7	0.0	0.0	33.3	31.6	83.3	73.7	50.0	73.7
22A	14	7	7.1	0.0	0.0	0.0	0.0	0.0	0.0	0.0	0.0	0.0
31	12	12	0.0	0.0	0.0	0.0	0.0	0.0	16.7	0.0	0.0	0.0
17F	9	10	11.1	0.0	0.0	0.0	0.0	0.0	55.6	10.0	0.0	0.0
9 N	8	10	0.0	0.0	0.0	0.0	0.0	0.0	75.0	40.0	75.0	50.0
35F	10	8	0.0	0.0	0.0	0.0	0.0	0.0	0.0	0.0	0.0	0.0
8	6	11	0.0	0.0	0.0	0.0	0.0	0.0	0.0	0.0	0.0	0.0
7F	12	4	0.0	0.0	0.0	0.0	0.0	0.0	8.3	0.0	0.0	0.0
18A	7	9	0.0	0.0	0.0	0.0	0.0	0.0	0.0	0.0	0.0	0.0
7B	0	15	0.0	100.0	0.0	0.0	0.0	100.0	0.0	100.0	0.0	93.3
9 V	11	4	100.0	100.0	0.0	0.0	100.0	100.0	0.0	25.0	0.0	0.0
1	7	4	14.3	0.0	0.0	0.0	0.0	0.0	0.0	0.0	0.0	0.0
29	1	10	0.0	0.0	0.0	0.0	0.0	0.0	0.0	0.0	0.0	0.0
12F	7	3	0.0	0.0	0.0	0.0	0.0	0.0	0.0	0.0	0.0	0.0
10F	5	1	0.0	0.0	0.0	0.0	100.0	100.0	0.0	0.0	0.0	0.0
4	5	0	20.0	0.0	0.0	0.0	20.0	0.0	0.0	0.0	0.0	0.0
18C	3	2	0.0	0.0	0.0	0.0	100.0	100.0	0.0	0.0	0.0	0.0
13	1	3	0.0	33.3	0.0	0.0	0.0	0.0	0.0	33.3	0.0	0.0
20	2	2	0.0	0.0	0.0	0.0	0.0	0.0	0.0	0.0	0.0	0.0
33B	4	0	50.0	0.0	0.0	0.0	0.0	0.0	50.0	0.0	0.0	0.0
6B	3	0	0.0	0.0	0.0	0.0	0.0	0.0	33.3	0.0	0.0	0.0
33D	2	1	100.0	100.0	0.0	0.0	0.0	0.0	100.0	100.0	0.0	0.0

Table 2 Frequencies of serotypes and antibiotic resistance rates found among 1590 isolates of *Streptococcus pneumoniae* among Aboriginal people in Western Australia, August 2008–November 2014. PCV13 was introduced on July 1 2011 *(Continued)*

9A	1	0	0.0	0.0	0.0	0.0	0.0	0.0	0.0	0.0	0.0	0.0
11C	0	1	0.0	0.0	0.0	0.0	0.0	0.0	0.0	0.0	0.0	0.0
14	0	1	0.0	0.0	0.0	0.0	0.0	0.0	0.0	100.0	0.0	0.0
24F	0	1	0.0	0.0	0.0	0.0	0.0	0.0	0.0	0.0	0.0	0.0
25B	0	1	0.0	0.0	0.0	0.0	0.0	0.0	0.0	0.0	0.0	0.0
37	1	0	0.0	0.0	0.0	0.0	0.0	0.0	0.0	0.0	0.0	0.0
NT	126	90	76.2	63.3	0.0	0.0	46.0	38.9	34.1	23.3	9.5	11.1
TOTAL	858	732	25.5	23.4	0.3	0.5	26.1	21.3*	18.5	17.5	8.6	10.7

48 serotypes were identified among 1374 serotypeable isolates, 216 isolates were non-serotypeable (NT)
Cotr cotrimoxazole, *ery* erythromycin, *tet* tetracycline, *pen* penicillin; ^{R} resistant, ^{I} intermediate resistance
*$p < 0.05$

Risk factors for pneumococcal carriage

Carriage of any serotypeable pneumococcus was more common among males (OR 1.56 [95% CI 1.35–1.81]) and those who were carriers of *Haemophilus influenzae* (OR 10.29 [95% CI 8.60–12.30]) and *Moraxella catarrhalis* (OR 7.10 [95% CI 6.01–8.39]) compared with those who were not (Table 3). Pneumococcal carriage was detected more commonly among those reporting respiratory symptoms (OR 1.48 [95% CI 1.14–1.94]), in the presence of nasal discharge (OR 4.84 [95% CI 4.01–5.74]), among those living in a remote community (OR 1.86 [95% CI 1.41–2.35]) and those living in crowded households (OR 1.35 [95% CI 1.15–1.58]). Pneumococcal carriage was detected less commonly among those who

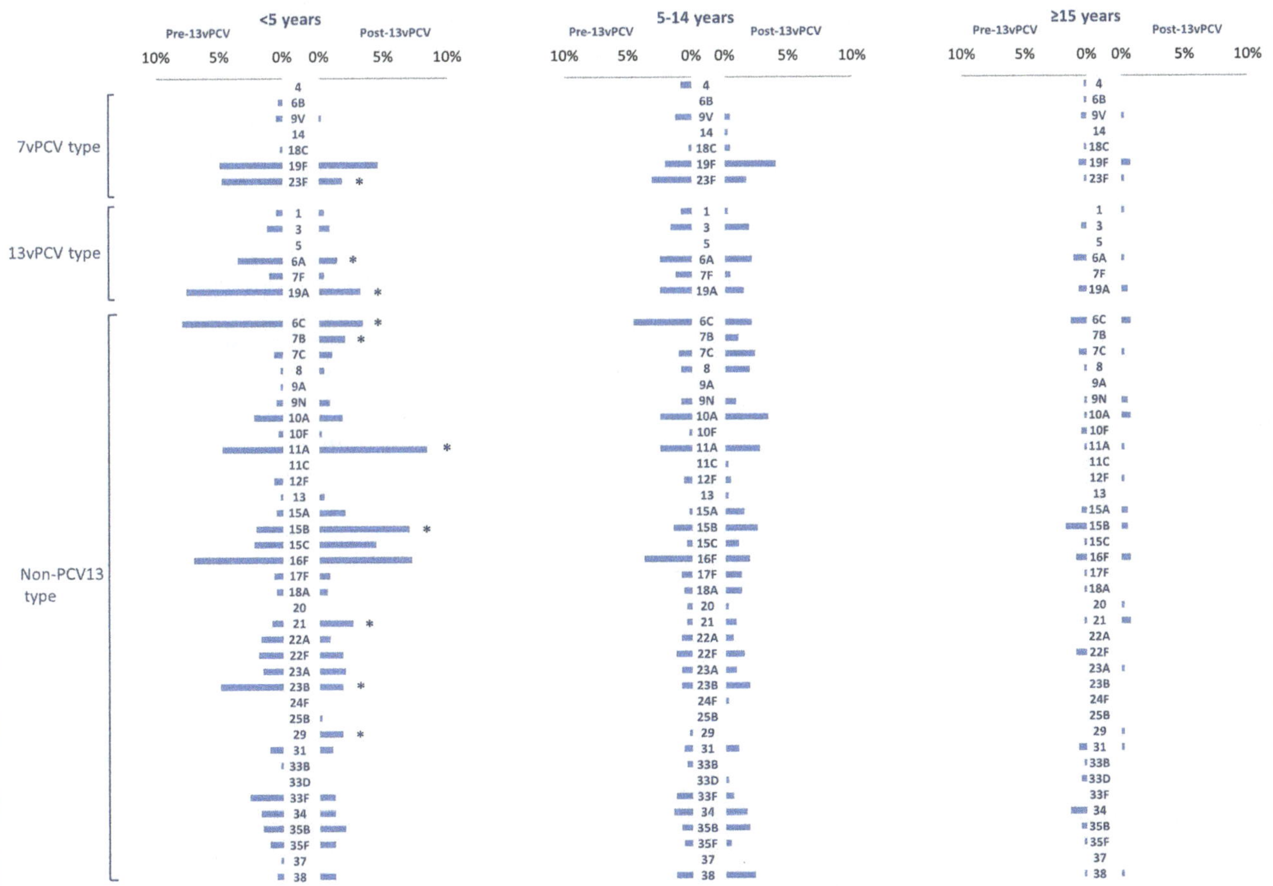

Fig. 2 Prevalence of serotypeable isolates by age group, pre- and post-PCV13 introduction (1 July 2011), among Aboriginal people in Western Australia, August 2008 to November 2014. *$p < 0.0$

Table 3 Univariable and multivariable analysis of risk factors for carriage of any serotypeable pneumococcus among Aboriginal people in Western Australia, August 2008–November 2014

	Odds Ratio (95% Confidence Interval)	
	Any pneumococcal serotype	
	Univariable	*Multivariable*
Male	*1.56 (1.35–1.81)*	0.81 (0.67–0.99)
Age increase by 12 months		
0–11 months	*4.60 (2.83–7.50)*	*4.19 (2.39–7.33)*
1 to 19 yr	*0.85 (0.84–0.87)*	*0.85 (0.84–0.87)*
20 + years	0.99 (0.98–1.01)	1.00 (0.99–1.02)
Annual increase		
Pre-PCV13	1.07 (0.98–1.18)	*0.86 (0.75–0.98)*
Post-PCV13	0.88 (0.75–1.05)	*1.37 (1.08–1.74)*
Respiratory symptoms	*1.48 (1.14–1.94)*	1.01 (0.72–1.43)
Nasal discharge	*4.84 (4.01–5.74)*	*2.49 (2.00–3.09)*
Recent antibiotic use	*0.73 (0.55–0.98)*	*0.48 (0.33–0.69)*
Remoteness		
Metropolitan	Ref	Ref
Regional	1.36 (0.97–1.89)	1.31 (0.88–1.96)
Remote	*1.86 (1.47–2.35)*	*2.21 (1.67–2.92)*
ETS	*1.24 (1.06–1.46)*	1.06 (0.87–1.29)
≥5 people sharing (crowding)	*1.35 (1.15–1.58)*	*1.36 (1.11–1.67)*
Sharing with ≥1 child <5 years	1.15 (0.96–1.37)	1.07 (0.85–1.34)
Season		
Spring	Ref	Ref
Summer	0.91 (0.66–1.27)	0.95 (0.62–1.45)
Autumn	0.86 (0.70–1.07)	1.35 (0.91–2.00)
Winter	*1.29 (1.08–1.53)*	1.11 (0.73–1.69)
H. influenzae	*10.29 (8.60–12.30)*	N/A
M. catarrhalis	*7.10 (6.01–8.39)*	N/A
S. aureus	*0.56 (0.44–0.72)*	N/A

Entries in italic considered statistically significant results

reported recent antibiotic use (OR 0.73 [95% CI 0.55–0.98]) and in *Staphylococcus aureus* carriers (OR 0.56 [95% CI 0.44–0.72]) than among those who were not (Table 3).

In the multivariable analysis, significant independent predictors of carriage of any serotypeable pneumococcus included the presence of nasal discharge (OR 2.49 [95% CI 2.00–3.09]), crowding (OR 1.36 [95% CI 1.11–1.67]) and remote versus urban residence (OR 2.21 [95% CI 1.67–2.92]). Recent receipt of antibiotics was associated with lower odds of detection of pneumococcal carriage (OR 0.48 [95% CI 0.33–0.69]). After modelling for the influence of age using the spline function, there was a significant risk of carriage of pneumococcus up to age 1 year (OR 4.19 [95% CI 2.39–7.33]), which then decreased from 1 year to 19 years (14.7% decline per year; OR 0.85 [95% CI 12.9–16.4], Table 3). Adjusting for other factors, there was no evidence that introduction of PCV13 was associated with an overall reduction in all pneumococcal serotypes (Fig. 1).

Discussion

The overall prevalence of carriage of pneumococci among WA Aboriginal children and adults remains high following the introduction of PCV13. For children, pneumococcal carriage has remained relatively stable over time, with carriage increasing in infants until around their first birthday and then slowly declining with increasing age to adulthood (Table 3).

IPD rates caused by non-PCV serotypes have increased since the introduction of PCV13 nationwide [4, 7]. In WA, the continuing high rates of carriage despite vaccination indicate an ongoing contribution of environmental factors to acquisition of pneumococcus.

The main factors associated with detection of pneumococcal carriage in our analysis were young age, presence of nasal discharge and household crowding. The age distribution of pneumococcal carriage—increasing each month of the first year and declining slowly thereafter—has been observed previously in Aboriginal children in WA [9] and correlates with the observed age distribution of OM which is hyper-endemic in this population [3, 16]. Nasal discharge was strongly associated with detection of pneumococcal carriage (Table 3). The authors speculate that pneumococcus plays a causative role in nasal discharge; however, it is also possible that nasal discharge merely improves detection of carriage. In either case, reinforcement of hygiene practices would be important for limiting transmission of pneumococcal strains.

The relationship between household crowding and pneumococcal carriage has been reaffirmed in this study. Previously crowding was linked with high carriage in a study conducted in communities surrounding Kalgoorlie in WA [17] and in other indigenous communities including Alaska Native people [18]. While not shown to be an independent risk factor in this analysis, ETS exposure was reported more frequently among those with pneumococcal carriage (univariable OR 1.24 [95% CI 1.06–1.46]) and this has previously been associated with both pneumococcal carriage [18] and OM in Aboriginal children [8, 19, 20]. These associations reinforce the need to promote healthy living conditions for Aboriginal people and the importance of smoking prevention programs.

Recent antibiotic use was strongly negatively associated with detection of pneumococcal carriage (Table 3). There was no appreciable change in rates of antibiotic resistance among carriage isolates over the study, apart from a decrease in resistance to cotrimoxazole in the post-PCV13 period (Table 2). Crude χ^2 tests of carriage of non-susceptible strains of pneumococcus or multi-resistant strains versus recent antibiotic use identified no significant differences between the groups (data not shown). Taken together, these findings suggest that recent antibiotic use may be protective against pneumococcal carriage.

After adjusting for age, date, gender, remoteness, and other factors, there was no evidence that the prevalence of carriage of all serotypeable pneumococci across all age groups decreased after introduction of PCV13 (Table 3). Among children <5 years old, those most likely to have been vaccinated with PCV13, the prevalence of carriage across all serotypes did not change significantly (Table 1) but there was evidence of a significant decrease in carriage of both PCV7 and PCV13 serotypes (Table 1, Fig. 2). A similar reduction in vaccine serotypes was previously reported in Alaska Native children [21]. It appears that non-vaccine strains are replacing vaccine-type strains after PCV13 introduction, rather than PCV13 reducing carriage overall. This study was unable to investigate possible herd immunity in more detail, particularly in infants <6 months old, due to low enrolment numbers in this age group. Carriage of PCV13 serotypes was also numerically reduced in the older age groups studied (Table 1), albeit to a lesser extent than in children <5 years old. Post-PCV13 vaccination coverage was estimated at ≥82% among 5–14 year olds (Table 1), and the Australian National Centre for Immunisation Research and Surveillance estimates PCV vaccination coverage in Aboriginal children in WA at >88% [22]. The numerical reduction in PCV serotypes in older study participants is consistent with an indirect effect of PCV13.

There were a number of strengths to this study, chiefly the large sample size, spread over a broad geographic region over several years. However there were also several limitations. The opportunistic nature of sampling meant the study did not achieve similar coverage of inhabitants in all communities, and certain seasons were favoured for visiting certain areas due to easier access by road/air compared to rainy seasons. This meant some regions/seasons may have been comparatively under-represented in some analyses. Immunization status for all children in this study could not be ascertained, due to an inability to identify ACIR records for some participants. This was primarily due to the method used to access immunization data: participants were identified by name and date of birth, as documented on records during interviews. It is common among Aboriginal communities for individuals to be identified by several different names and spellings can vary for the same person; thus the data could not always be matched to a record on the ACIR database.

Because most children <5 years old post-PCV13 appeared to have received at least one dose of PCV13, the reduction in PCV13-non-PCV7 serotypes may have been directly influenced by PCV13 vaccination. However, greater decreases in PCV13 serotype carriage were noted in Alaskan [23] and Massachusetts children [24] following PCV13 introduction. Due to the uncertainty in vaccination status for a large proportion of participants, and the small number of children confirmed as PCV13 vaccinated (n = 37, Table 2), vaccination status was not included as a variable in the risk factor analysis. Another limitation of the study was the lack of detailed information to allow accurate assessment of indirect effects within households. It would be highly informative to analyse carriage and possible transmission between household members, and to assess the impact of vaccination status of children on other household members. However, in the communities studied, movement of family members between houses and communities is often dynamic rather than static, so such an analysis is likely to be imprecise.

Despite observing reduced carriage of 6C and 19A in children, these serotypes remained among the most common serotypes carried following PCV13 introduction. The reduction in carriage of serotypes 6A, 23F and 19A is plausibly attributable to PCV13 as they are vaccine serotypes. The reduction in 6C in children <5 years old may be attributable to cross-protection from 6A which is covered by PCV13 [25]. The increase in non-vaccine types, most notably 11A, 7B and 15B warrants further monitoring. Increases in 11A and serogroup 15 have been reported from other regions and countries. IPD caused by serogroup 15 increased in Norway after PCV13 introduction [26]. Serotype 11A was identified as an emerging serotype in the Northern Territory Aboriginal population following PCV7 introduction [27], and carriage of 11A also increased in Sweden and Japan following PCV13 introduction [28, 29]. Moreover, high rates of antimicrobial resistance among serotypes 23F, 7B and 9 V are particularly concerning and warrant close surveillance (Table 2).

Conclusions

While PCV13 appears to have influenced the distribution of carriage serotypes among Aboriginal children in WA, the overall rate of pneumococcal carriage remains high across all age groups, with replacement of vaccine serotypes with emerging non-vaccine serotypes. The relevance of emerging carriage serotypes to IPD and more common pneumococcal manifestations of OM and pneumonia needs to be carefully assessed to properly understand the impact of conjugate vaccination.

Abbreviations

23vPPV: 23-valent pneumococcal polysaccharide vaccine; ACIR: Australian

Childhood Immunisation Register; CI: Confidence interval; ETS: Environmental tobacco smoke; IPD: Invasive pneumococcal disease; OM: Otitis media; OR: Odds ratio; PCV13: 13-valent pneumococcal conjugate vaccine; PCV7: 7-valent pneumococcal conjugate vaccine; WA: Western Australia

Acknowledgements
We thank the communities and the staff of Aboriginal Medical Services and Community Health Services who facilitated our study visits. We are grateful to all the study participants.

Funding
Funding for this study was provided by WA Department of Health through the Collaboration for Applied Research and Evaluation (CARE) and NHMRC Project Grant #545232. The funders had no role in study design, data collection and analysis, decision to publish, or preparation of the manuscript.

Authors' contributions
Conception, generation and design of the research plan: DL, AJL, AH. Data collection: AH, DC, JB, KS, NAS. Data analysis: DC, TS. Drafting of manuscript: DC, TS, DL. All authors performed critical review of the manuscript. All authors read and approved the final manuscript.

Competing interests
DL has previously been a member of the GSK Australia Pneumococcal-*Haemophilus influenzae*-Protein D conjugate vaccine ("PhiD-CV") Advisory Panel, has received support from Pfizer Australia and GSK Australia to attend conferences, has received an honorarium from Merck Vaccines to give a seminar at their offices in Pennsylvania and support to attend a conference, and is an investigator on an investigator-initiated research grant funded by Pfizer Australia. AJL has received research funding and support to attend conferences from GlaxoSmithKline and Pfizer Australia. A Hoskins has received support to attend conferences from Pfizer Australia. All other authors have no competing interests.

Author details
[1]School of Medical and Health Sciences, Edith Cowan University, Perth, WA, Australia. [2]Wesfarmers Centre of Vaccines & Infectious Diseases, Telethon Kids Institute, University of Western Australia, Perth, WA, Australia. [3]Division of Microbiology & Infectious Diseases, PathWest Laboratory Medicine WA, Perth, WA, Australia. [4]Menzies School of Health Research, Charles Darwin University, Darwin, Northern Territory, Australia.

References

1. World Health Organization. Pneumococcal vaccines WHO position paper - 2012. Wkly Epidemiol Rec. 2012;87:129–44.
2. Lehmann D, Willis J, Moore HC, Giele C, Murphy D, Keil AD, et al. The changing epidemiology of invasive pneumococcal disease in Aboriginal and non-Aboriginal Western Australians from 1997 through 2007 and emergence of non-vaccine serotypes. Clin Infect Dis. 2010;50:1477–86.
3. Lehmann D, Weeks S, Jacoby P, Elsbury D, Finucane J, Stokes A, et al. Absent otoacoustic emissions predict otitis media in young Aboriginal children: a birth cohort study in Aboriginal and non-Aboriginal children in an arid zone of Western Australia. BMC Pediatr. 2008;8:32.
4. de Kluyver R, Enhanced Invasive Pneumococcal Disease Surveillance Working Group. Invasive pneumococcal disease surveillance Australia, 1 January to 31 March 2015. Commun Dis Intell Q Rep. 2015;39:E308–11.
5. Giele CM, Keil AD, Lehmann D, Van Buynder PG. Invasive pneumococcal disease in Western Australia: emergence of serotype 19A. Med J Aust. 2009;190:166.
6. The Australian Immunisation Handbook. Canberra: Australian Government Department of Health; 2013.
7. Jayasinghe S, Menzies R, Chiu C, Toms C, Blyth CC, Krause V, et al. Long-term impact of a "3 + 0" schedule for 7- and 13-valent pneumococcal conjugate vaccines on invasive pneumococcal disease in Australia, 2002-2014. Clin Infect Dis. 2017;64:175–83.
8. Mackenzie GA, Leach AJ, Carapetis JR, Fisher J, Morris PS. Epidemiology of nasopharyngeal carriage of respiratory bacterial pathogens in children and adults: cross-sectional surveys in a population with high rates of pneumococcal disease. BMC Infect Dis. 2010;10:304.
9. Collins DA, Hoskins A, Bowman J, Jones J, Stemberger NA, Richmond PC, et al. High nasopharyngeal carriage of non-vaccine serotypes in Western Australian Aboriginal people following 10 years of pneumococcal conjugate vaccination. PLoS One. 2013;8:e82280.
10. Dunne EM, Carville K, Riley TV, Bowman J, Leach AJ, Cripps AW, et al. Aboriginal and non-Aboriginal children in Western Australia carry different serotypes of pneumococci with different antimicrobial susceptibility profiles. Pneumonia. 2016;8:1–9.
11. Jacoby P, Carville KS, Hall G, Riley TV, Bowman J, Leach AJ, et al. Crowding and other strong predictors of upper respiratory tract carriage of otitis media-related bacteria in Australian Aboriginal and non-Aboriginal children. Pediatr Infect Dis J. 2011;30:480–5.
12. Leach AJ, Stubbs E, Hare K, Beissbarth J, Morris PS. Comparison of nasal swabs with nose blowing for community-based pneumococcal surveillance of healthy children. J Clin Microbiol. 2008;46:2081–2.
13. Watson K, Carville K, Bowman J, Jacoby P, Riley TV, Leach AJ, et al. Upper respiratory tract bacterial carriage in Aboriginal and non-Aboriginal children in a semi-arid area of Western Australia. Pediatr Infect Dis J. 2006;25:782–90.
14. Clinical and Laboratory Standards Institute. Performance standards for antimicrobial susceptibility testing: seventh informational supplement M100-S17. Wayne, Pennsylvania, USA: CLSI; 2007.
15. Australian Bureau of Statistics. The Australian Statistical Geography Standard Remoteness Structure. Canberra: Australian Bureau of Statistics; 2011.
16. Leach AJ, Wigger C, Andrews R, Chatfield M, Smith-Vaughan H, Morris PS. Otitis media in children vaccinated during consecutive 7-valent or 10-valent pneumococcal conjugate vaccination schedules. BMC Pediatr. 2014;14:200.
17. Leach AJ, Wigger C, Beissbarth J, Woltring D, Andrews R, Chatfield MD, et al. General health, otitis media, nasopharyngeal carriage and middle ear microbiology in Northern Territory Aboriginal children vaccinated during consecutive periods of 10-valent or 13-valent pneumococcal conjugate vaccines. Int J Pediatr Otorhinolaryngol. 2016;86:224–32.
18. Reisman J, Rudolph K, Bruden D, Hurlburt D, Bruce MG, Hennessy T. Risk factors for pneumococcal colonization of the nasopharynx in Alaska Native adults and children. J Pediatric Infect Dis Soc. 2014;3:104–11.
19. Greenberg D, Givon-Lavi N, Broides A, Blancovich I, Peled N, Dagan R. The contribution of smoking and exposure to tobacco smoke to *Streptococcus pneumoniae* and *Haemophilus influenzae* carriage in children and their mothers. Clin Infect Dis. 2006;42:897–903.
20. Jacoby PA, Coates HL, Arumugaswamy A, Elsbury D, Stokes A, Monck R, et al. The effect of passive smoking on the risk of otitis media in Aboriginal and non-Aboriginal children in the Kalgoorlie-Boulder region of Western Australia. Med J Aust. 2008;188:599–603.
21. Bruce MG, Singleton R, Bulkow L, Rudolph K, Zulz T, Gounder P, et al. Impact of the 13-valent pneumococcal conjugate vaccine (PCV13) on invasive pneumococcal disease and carriage in Alaska. Vaccine. 2015;33:4813–9.
22. National Centre for Immunisation Research and Surveillance. Coverage estimates - Aboriginal and Torres Strait Islander children NSW: NCIRS; 2017 [updated 20 Apr 2017]. Available from: http://www.ncirs.edu.au/provider-resources/coverage-information/coverage-estimates-indigenous-children/.
23. Gounder PP, Bruce MG, Bruden DJ, Singleton RJ, Rudolph K, Hurlburt DA, et al. Effect of the 13-valent pneumococcal conjugate vaccine on nasopharyngeal colonization by *Streptococcus pneumoniae*-Alaska, 2008-2012. J Infect Dis. 2014;209:1251–8.
24. Loughlin AM, Hsu K, Silverio AL, Marchant CD, Pelton SI. Direct and indirect effects of PCV13 on nasopharyngeal carriage of PCV13 unique pneumococcal serotypes in Massachusetts' children. Pediatr Infect Dis J. 2014;33:504–10.
25. Cooper D, Yu X, Sidhu M, Nahm MH, Fernsten P, Jansen KU. The 13-valent pneumococcal conjugate vaccine (PCV13) elicits cross-functional

opsonophagocytic killing responses in humans to *Streptococcus pneumoniae* serotypes 6C and 7A. Vaccine. 2011;29:7207–11.

26. Steens A, Bergsaker MAR, Aaberge IS, Rønning K, Vestrheim DF. Prompt effect of replacing the 7-valent pneumococcal conjugate vaccine with the 13-valent vaccine on the epidemiology of invasive pneumococcal disease in Norway. Vaccine. 2013;31:6232–8.
27. Leach AJ, Morris PS, McCallum GB, Wilson CA, Stubbs L, Beissbarth J, et al. Emerging pneumococcal carriage serotypes in a high-risk population receiving universal 7-valent pneumococcal conjugate vaccine and 23-valent polysaccharide vaccine since 2001. BMC Infect Dis. 2009;9:121.
28. Galanis I, Lindstrand A, Darenberg J, Browall S, Nannapaneni P, Sjöström K, et al. Effects of PCV7 and PCV13 on invasive pneumococcal disease and carriage in Stockholm. Sweden Eur Respir J. 2016;47:1208–18.
29. Kawaguchiya M, Urushibara N, Aung M, Morimoto S, Ito M, Kudo K, et al. Emerging non-PCV13 serotypes of noninvasive *Streptococcus pneumoniae* with macrolide resistance genes in northern Japan. New Microbes New Infect. 2016;9:66–72.

10

Increased risk of pneumonia in residents living near poultry farms: does the upper respiratory tract microbiota play a role?

Lidwien A. M. Smit[1*], Gert Jan Boender[2], Wouter A. A. de Steenhuijsen Piters[3], Thomas J. Hagenaars[2], Elisabeth G. W. Huijskens[4,5], John W. A. Rossen[5,6], Marion Koopmans[7], Gonnie Nodelijk[2,8], Elisabeth A. M. Sanders[3,9], Joris Yzermans[10], Debby Bogaert[3] and Dick Heederik[1]

Abstract

Background: Air pollution has been shown to increase the susceptibility to community-acquired pneumonia (CAP). Previously, we observed an increased incidence of CAP in adults living within 1 km from poultry farms, potentially related to particulate matter and endotoxin emissions. We aim to confirm the increased risk of CAP near poultry farms by refined spatial analyses, and we hypothesize that the oropharyngeal microbiota composition in CAP patients may be associated with residential proximity to poultry farms.

Methods: A spatial kernel model was used to analyze the association between proximity to poultry farms and CAP diagnosis, obtained from electronic medical records of 92,548 GP patients. The oropharyngeal microbiota composition was determined in 126 hospitalized CAP patients using 16S-rRNA-based sequencing, and analyzed in relation to residential proximity to poultry farms.

Results: Kernel analysis confirmed a significantly increased risk of CAP when living near poultry farms, suggesting an excess risk up to 1.15 km, followed by a sharp decline. Overall, the oropharyngeal microbiota composition differed borderline significantly between patients living <1 km and ≥1 km from poultry farms (PERMANOVA $p = 0.075$). Results suggested a higher abundance of *Streptococcus pneumoniae* (mean relative abundance 34.9% vs. 22.5%, $p = 0.058$) in patients living near poultry farms, which was verified by unsupervised clustering analysis, showing overrepresentation of a *S. pneumoniae* cluster near poultry farms ($p = 0.049$).

Conclusion: Living near poultry farms is associated with an 11% increased risk of CAP, possibly resulting from changes in the upper respiratory tract microbiota composition in susceptible individuals. The abundance of *S. pneumoniae* near farms needs to be replicated in larger, independent studies.

Keywords: Air pollution, Environment, Microbiome, Pneumonia

Background

Community-acquired pneumonia (CAP) is among the leading causes of morbidity and mortality in adults worldwide, and the burden is markedly higher among the oldest adults [1–3]. Environmental risk factors, such as active and passive smoking, household air pollution due to biomass fuel use, and outdoor air pollution, have been shown to increase the susceptibility to lower respiratory tract infections, including CAP [1, 4–7].

In a rural population in the south of The Netherlands, we previously studied environmental risk factors of CAP using electronic GP medical records of 70,142 adult patients seen during 2009 [8]. In this study, we observed an increased risk of CAP in adults living at a distance of 1 km or less from a poultry farm [8]. Although poultry farms can be a source of zoonotic pathogens such as avian influenza or *Chlamydia psittaci*, a study of zoonotic infections in hospitalized CAP patients in a nearby

* Correspondence: L.A.Smit@uu.nl
[1]Institute for Risk Assessment Sciences (IRAS), Division Environmental Epidemiology, Utrecht University, PO Box 80178, 3508 TD Utrecht, The Netherlands
Full list of author information is available at the end of the article

area revealed very few cases caused by avian pathogens (e.g. *C. psittaci*: 1.7%) [9].

Recently, scientists have sounded the alarm over the large contribution of agriculture to particulate matter (PM) air pollution [10, 11]. Poultry farms in particular are known to emit large quantities of air pollutants such as PM and endotoxins [12–15]. Exposure levels in stables have been shown to cause airway inflammation, respiratory symptoms and airway obstruction in farmers [16, 17]. Despite ambient pollutant concentrations being considerably lower than levels in stables, there is growing evidence of respiratory health effects in susceptible individuals living near livestock farms as well [18]. Exposure to PM air pollution may predispose these individuals to respiratory infections through chronic airway inflammation and subsequent host–immune responses [4, 7], which might be amplified by exposure to environmental endotoxin [19].

With the advent of new molecular microbial identification methods, it has been proposed that respiratory infections might emerge from the disruption of the otherwise balanced upper respiratory tract (URT) bacterial ecosystem or 'microbiome' [20]. Spread of overgrown pathogens originating from the URT to the lower respiratory tract could perturb the lung microbial ecosystem and lead to respiratory tract infections, including pneumonia [21]. Indeed, recent studies have shown that CAP in adults was associated with dysbiosis of the oropharyngeal microbiota, characterized by increased abundance of pathogens such as *S. pneumoniae*, and the absence of facultative anaerobic commensals [22]. We hypothesized that environmental exposure from poultry farms may contribute to a shift in the oropharyngeal microbiome, and thereby facilitate the development of lower respiratory infections.

In the present study, refined spatial analyses are used to confirm the increased risk of CAP near poultry farms. Furthermore, the oropharyngeal microbiota composition in CAP patients is analyzed in relation to residential proximity to poultry farms.

Methods

Study design

The study was carried out in the province of Noord-Brabant, The Netherlands, a region with a high density of intensive livestock farms. Two cross-sectional analyses were performed: (i) the association between poultry farms, home address and GP-registered pneumonia [8] was re-analyzed using a spatial kernel model; and (ii) the oropharyngeal microbiota composition of hospitalized CAP patients was analyzed in relation to residential proximity to poultry farms.

Ethics

The study was carried out in accordance with Dutch legislation (the *Personal Data Protection Act*, and the *Medical Research Involving Human Subjects Act*) and with the Code of Conduct for Medical Research. All experimental protocols were approved by the Medical Ethical Committee of the University Medical Centre Utrecht (NL45307.041.13, GP-registered pneumonia; as part of the Farming and Neighbouring Residents' Health Study), and by the Medical Ethical Committee of the St. Elisabeth Hospital, Tilburg (hospitalized CAP patients). Ethical aspects of the study have been described earlier [8, 23–25]. In short, medical information and address records of GPs' patients were kept separated at all times by using a trusted third party. The need to obtain informed consent from individual patients was waived. Written informed consent was obtained from all hospitalized CAP patients.

Spatial kernel analysis

Briefly, the data on GP-diagnosed pneumonia and spatial location of home address of 92,548 GP patients (70,142 adults [18–70 year] and 22,406 children [0–17 years]) during the year 2009 [8] was re-analyzed by estimating the parameters of a spatial kernel model from this data. In this model it is assumed that each poultry farm independently generates a probability for individuals of experiencing GP-diagnosed pneumonia within this year. This probability is modelled through a function dependent on the distance between farm and home address (i.e. the spatial kernel). The parameterization of the spatial kernel utilizes three parameters and offers sufficient flexibility for identifying any distance dependency from the data, from short-range to long-range patterns and from very sharp to more gradual dependencies on distance. In addition, a constant background probability is assumed to allow for quantification of the part of CAP incidence that is not associated with proximity to poultry farms. The background probability and the three parameters of the kernel are all estimated from the data by maximum likelihood (ML). The method is described previously [26, 27], and more details are provided in Additional file 1.

Oropharyngeal microbiota composition

The microbiota composition of 126 patients hospitalized with CAP in the same region was analyzed, in relation to residential distance to poultry farms (Fig. 1). Characteristics, bacterial and viral etiology, and in-/exclusion criteria of the study population of hospitalized CAP patients have been described earlier [22, 25]. Oropharyngeal samples were taken before hospitalization at the emergency ward. Storage of samples, isolation of bacterial DNA, and 16S-rRNA-based sequencing of the V5–V7 region was performed as previously described [22]. Patients who received antibiotics during the two weeks before sampling, and patients with a positive qPCR result

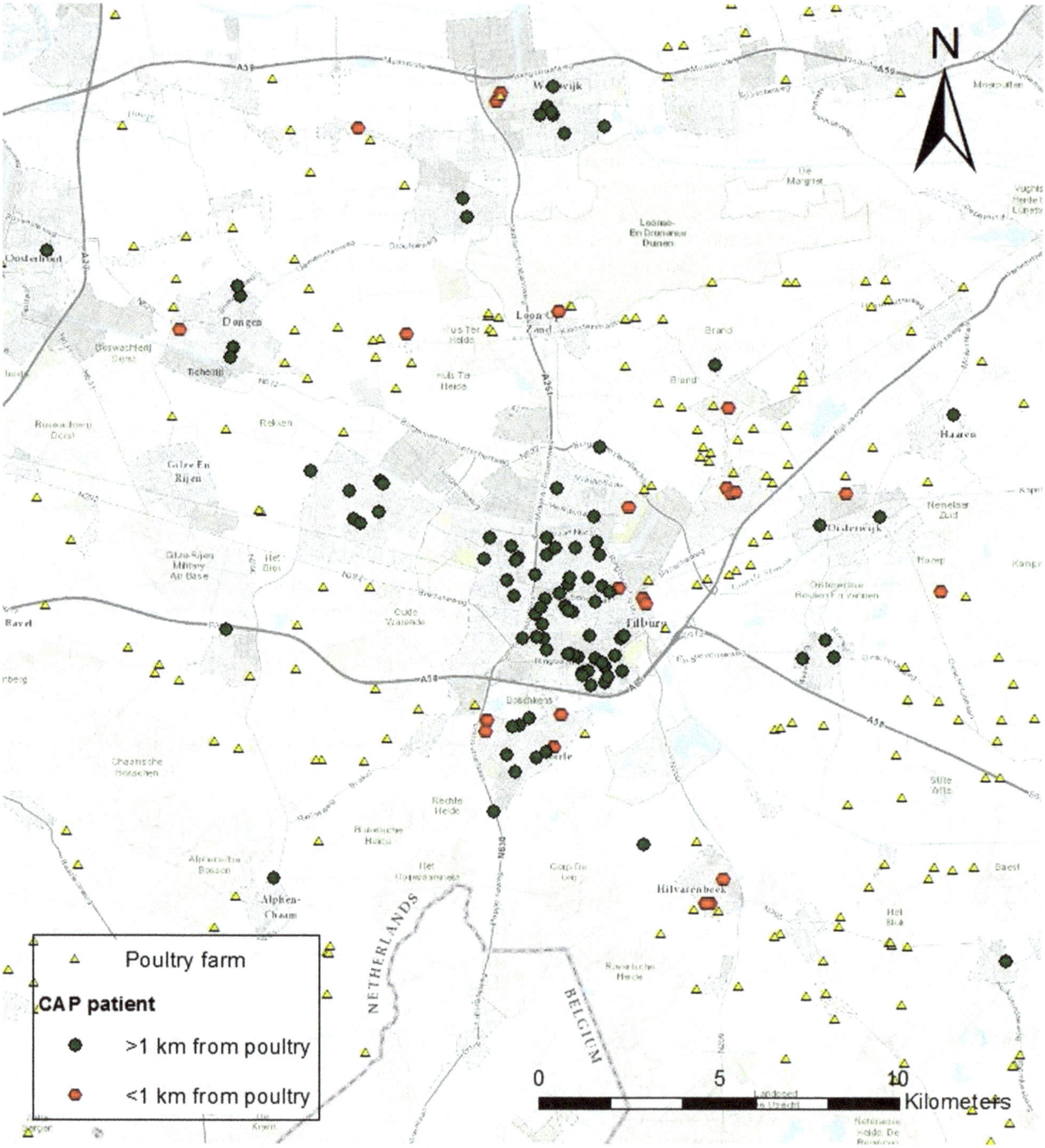

Fig. 1 Geographic distribution of 126 adult CAP patients and poultry farms around Tilburg, The Netherlands

for *C. burnetii* were excluded from microbiota composition analysis. The present analysis was performed on 126 patients from whom microbiota data and address records were available. The presence of animal farms around the home address was assessed using a geographic information system (ARCGIS 9.3.1., Esri, Redlands, California, United States), as described earlier [9].

Statistical analysis

Statistical analyses of oropharyngeal microbiota data were performed in R version 3.2.2. The study visualized the association between the vicinity of poultry farms and the overall bacterial community composition by non-metric multidimensional scaling (nMDS) of the Bray-Curtis dissimilarity metric and assessed its statistical significance by permutation analysis of variance [28].

Differentially abundant bacterial community members that might be related to changes in the overall microbiota composition were detected by Mann-Whitney U-tests, comparing patients living <1 km versus ≥1 km from poultry farms. The 1 km radius was chosen based on the original findings [8]. Sensitivity analyses were performed using a 1.15 km radius, based on the spatial kernel analysis results. The false discovery rate was controlled for by using the Benjamini-Hochberg technique [29]. Additionally, unsupervised hierarchical clustering was used to group patients based on similarity of microbial composition, which was visualized in a dendrogram [30]. The optimal number of clusters was based on clustering indices [22], and only clusters including >3 patients were considered for subsequent analyses. Fisher's exact tests were exploited to compare the proportion of patients living <1 km from a poultry farm over all patients in the cluster of interest versus that proportion in the other clusters.

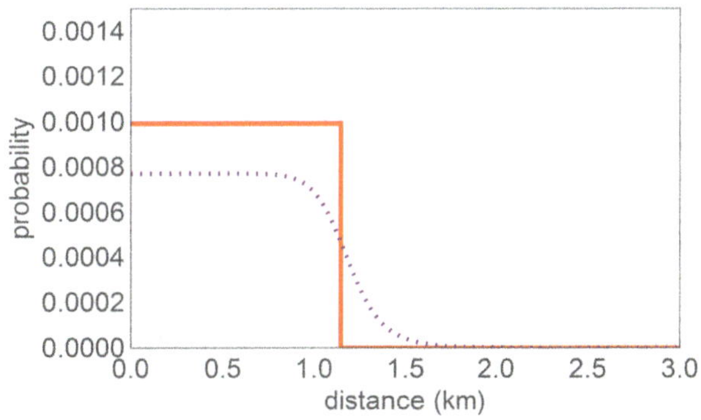

Fig. 2 Spatial kernel estimated from morbidity data: probability for an individual of experiencing GP-diagnosed pneumonia in 2009 as attributed to an individual poultry farm, as a function of the distance from the individual's residential location to that of the poultry farm. Red, full line: Maximum-Likelihood estimate (= fitted model). Grey, dotted line: Kernel for the lower confidence bound for the sharpness of the distance dependence and the corresponding profile-likelihood values for the other two parameters

Results

Spatial kernel analysis

The data was analyzed using spatial kernel models to characterize the association between living in the vicinity of poultry farms and CAP. In total, 993 patients (702/70,142 adults and 221/22,406 children) were diagnosed with CAP in 2009. Two alternative models were used: a distance-independent model with one estimable parameter (namely a constant per-individual probability of GP-reported pneumonia), and a model with a distance-dependent risk component (three additional estimable parameters) added to a constant background risk. Estimation of the distance-dependent risk component (spatial kernel) yields the results displayed in Fig. 2. The distance dependence of the fitted distance-dependent risk component (full line) is sharp, displaying a stepwise decline to zero at a distance of approximately 1.15 km. The excess CAP risk is approximately equal to 0.001 (per person year) per poultry farm within 1.15 km, which compares to a total background risk of 0.009 per person year (0.001/0.009 = ~11% increase in risk). Comparison with the distance-independent model shows that the distance-dependent component significantly contributes to the model fit ($p = 0.0067$, likelihood-ratio test, see Additional file 1). The sharp bound at 1.15 km of the distance-dependent risk model is largely maintained, even in the model including the 95% lower confidence bound value for the parameter determining the sharpness of the distance dependence (dashed line). For this lower confidence bound it was calculated (see Additional file 1) that 81% of the total CAP incidence attributed to proximity to individual poultry farms occurs within a 1.15 km distance from farms, and 95% within 1.35 km. To investigate potential age effects, kernel estimation was repeated for the partial datasets of 70,142 adults, and 22,406 children. No significant differences were observed between the parameter values estimated for these partial datasets, implying that both subpopulations show similar excess risks at close proximity from poultry farms (see Additional file 1).

Oropharyngeal microbiota analysis

The oropharyngeal microbiota composition of 100 adult hospitalized CAP patients living <1 km and 26 patients living ≥1 km to one or more poultry farms was studied to explore the hypothesis that the association between CAP and living near poultry farms is mediated through a direct effect on microbial community composition, including pathogen colonization within the respiratory tract (Fig. 1).

Table 1 shows characteristics of the 26 CAP patients who lived within 1 km of one or more poultry farms, and 100 patients who lived at ≥1 km. Sex, age, smoking, chronic obstructive pulmonary disease (COPD), immunocompromized status, and pneumonia severity did not differ between the two groups ($p > 0.25$). All subjects were included in the same winter season, between November 2008 and February 2009. Bacterial and viral etiology also did not differ between the two groups (see Additional file 1: Table S3).

The association between living within a 1 km radius from a poultry farm and the overall oropharyngeal microbiota composition was borderline significant (Fig. 3, PERMANOVA $p = 0.075$). This overall difference in bacterial community composition was related to a higher abundance of *S. pneumoniae* (mean relative abundance 34.9% versus 22.5%, Mann-Whitney *U*-test $p = 0.058$, $q = 0.541$) and a lower abundance of *Lactobacillus* (1.4%

Table 1 Characteristics of 126 CAP patients, by the presence of a poultry farm within 1 km of the home address

	Poultry farm at ≥1 km	Poultry farm at <1 km	p-value[a]
n	100	26	
Male sex, n (%)	61 (61.0)	15 (57.7)	0.76
Age, mean ± SD, yrs	70.3 ± 15.3	66.5 ± 13.6	0.26
CAP at age ≥60 year, n (%)	80 (80.0)	19 (73.1)	0.44
Current smoking, n (%)	40 (40.0)	8 (30.8)	0.30
Month of admission, n (%)			
November 2008	17 (17.0)	6 (23.1)	0.71
December 2008	27 (27.0)	8 (30.8)	
January 2009	26 (26.0)	7 (26.9)	
February 2009	30 (30.0)	5 (19.2)	
Recent antibiotics usage[b]	0 (0.0)	0 (0.0)	NA
COPD, n (%)	40 (40.0)	10 (38.5)	0.89
ICS, n (%)	6 (6.0)	3 (11.5)	0.39
PSI, n (%)			
Mild	26 (26.0)	8 (30.7)	0.60
Moderate	45 (45.0)	13 (50.0)	
Severe	29 (29.0)	5 (19.2)	

[a]Chi-square test, Fisher's exact test, or t-test. [b]Use of antibiotics <2 weeks before admission
COPD chronic obstructive pulmonary disease, *NA* not available, *ICS* immunocompromized status, *PSI* pneumonia severity index

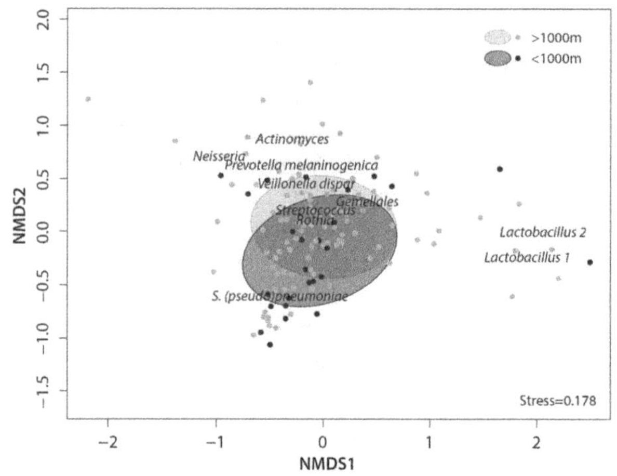

Fig. 3 Non-metric multidimensional scaling (nMDS) plot of the oropharyngeal microbiota based on Bray-Curtis dissimilarity metric. Each data point depicts the oropharyngeal bacterial communities of one patient. Data points and population standard deviation of data points (ellipses) are colored based on vicinity to poultry farm (dark gray, <1 km; light gray, ≥1 km). The stress-value indicates that the multi-dimensional structure of the data is well captured by the nMDS visualization.
The figure suggests an association between living close to a poultry farm and the abundance of *S. pneumoniae*, which was verified by both supervised and unsupervised learning methods

versus 3.8%, $p = 0.049$, $q = 0.541$) in patients living at <1 km compared to ≥1 km from a poultry farm.

These findings were verified using an unsupervised clustering approach, showing a total of seven microbiota clusters in our study cohort, six of which were characterized by either *Rothia*, *S. pneumoniae*, *Gemellales*, *Neisseria*, *Actinomyces* or *Lactobacillus* predominance. In addition, we identified one cluster without clear predominance of any species (Fig. 4). We observed an over-representation of individuals with the *S. pneumoniae* profile near poultry farms (12/36 versus 14/90 for the other clusters, Fisher's exact $p = 0.049$). All remaining individual clusters, including *Rothia* (9/60 in close proximity versus 17/66 in the remaining clusters, $p = 0.186$) and *Gemellales* (3/9 in close proximity versus 23/117 in the remaining clusters, $p = 0.390$) showed no statistically significant associations with residential proximity to poultry farms. These findings suggest an association between living in close vicinity to poultry farms and enrichment for *S. pneumoniae* in particular.

We performed a sensitivity analysis, in which we compared the microbiota profiles of 98 CAP patients living <1.15 km and 28 patients living ≥1.15 km to one or more poultry farms, based on the spatial kernel analysis results. In patients who—compared to the primary analysis—were now considered "exposed" (living between 1.0 and 1.15 km from a poultry farm), the relative abundance of *S. pneumoniae* was below the 10th percentile, which attenuated the difference in the microbiota composition between the two groups (overall microbiota comparison: PERMANOVA $p = 0.23$, mean relative abundance of *S. pneumoniae*: Mann-Whitney *U*-test $p = 0.14$, over-representation of the *S. pneumoniae* cluster near poultry farms: Fisher's exact $p = 0.095$).

Discussion

In this study, we found that living near poultry farms is associated with an ~11% increase in risk of CAP for each poultry farm within a distance of 1.15 km. Furthermore, the results suggested an association between living close to a poultry farm and the abundance of *S. pneumoniae* in adult patients hospitalized with CAP. To the best of our knowledge, this study is the first to show an association between the residential environment and the respiratory microbiota composition in adults. Because of the lack of a healthy control group and the relatively small sample size, results should be interpreted with caution. The abundance of *S. pneumoniae* in relation to living in the vicinity of poultry/livestock farms needs to be reassessed in future studies.

Kernel analysis confirmed the excess risk of CAP in the vicinity of poultry farms, as identified earlier using regression analysis [8]. In addition, it indicated that the excess risk has a sharp bound at around 1.15 km. The

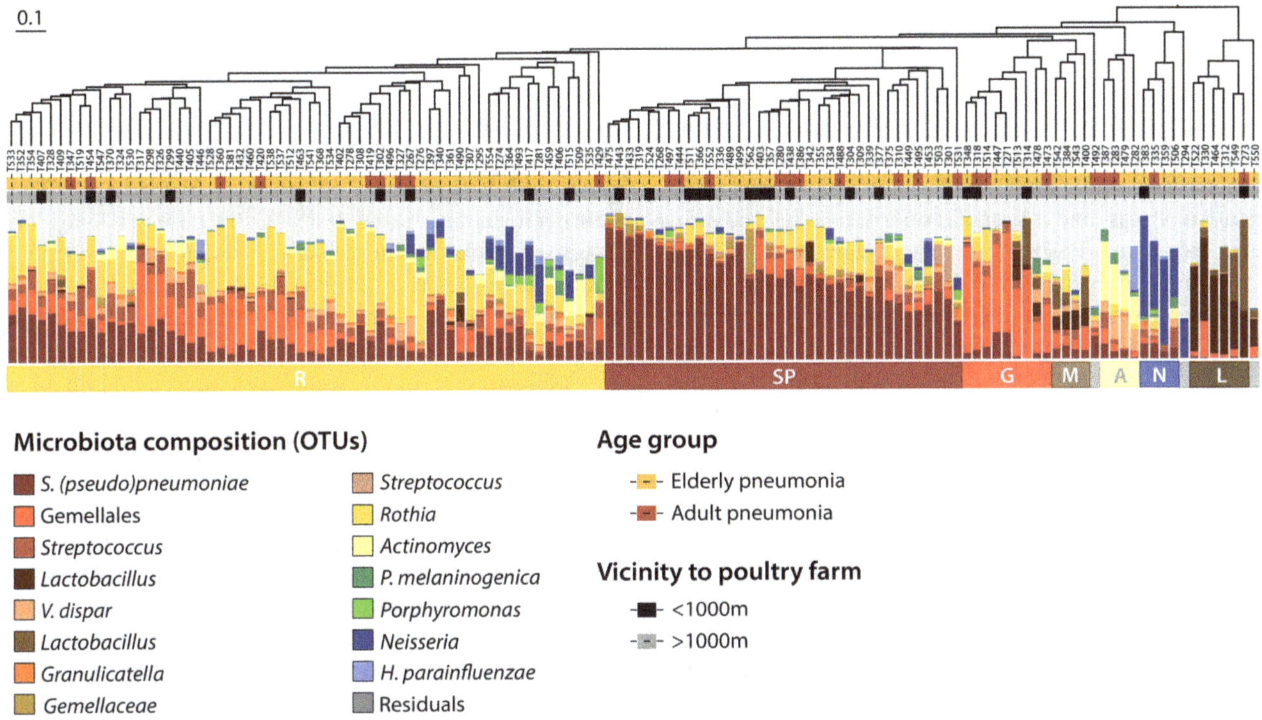

Fig. 4 Hierarchical clustering of patients based on oropharyngeal microbiome composition. Patients were hierarchically clustered based on their oropharyngeal bacterial communities using the Bray-Curtis dissimilarity measure, which was visualized in the dendrogram. Adjacent to the branches of the dendrogram information on age (yellow; elderly, red; adults) and proximity to poultry farms (dark gray, <1 km; light gray, ≥1 km) is shown. In addition, the relative abundance of the 15 highest ranking operational taxonomic units (OTUs) is shown per patient in vertical stacked bar plots. The colored horizontal bars represent the three major clusters we discerned based on clustering indices which were enriched for *Rothia* (R), *S. pneumoniae* (SP) and *Gemellales* (G). Furthermore, four smaller clusters were observed, distinguished by predominance of *Actinomyces* (A), *Neisseria* (N) and *Lactobacillus* (L). In the fourth cluster no predominance for any OTU was observed (mixed; M)

advantage of the kernel analysis compared to earlier analyses is that instead of regressing CAP occurrence to distance-to-the-nearest-farm, it models the distance-dependent per-farm contribution to the risk of CAP. Thus, the kernel models can assess the incremental risk per every additional poultry farm as well as local accumulation of risk due to the presence of multiple farms in the vicinity of an individual's home. In the earlier analyses, we considered an individual exposed when poultry farms were present within a 1 km radius of the home address. The distance dependence of the fitted kernel model is remarkably sharp, suggesting that the risk is strongly localized, possibly as a result of movement patterns around the home. This suggestion is supported by considering the kernel corresponding to the lower confidence bound of the parameter determining the sharpness of the distance dependence. Even for that kernel parameter set, we calculated that as much as 81% (on average) of the CAP incidence attributed to proximity to individual poultry farms occurs within a 1.15 km distance. This roughly corresponds to the earlier assumed 1 km radius around the home address. It should be realized that all risk estimates make use of the distance between a poultry farm and the home address as a proxy of exposure. Activity patterns lead to exposure misclassification and this may have modified the shape of the kernel function to some extent.

We hypothesized that the association between residential proximity to poultry farms and CAP might be mediated through an effect of emissions from poultry farms on microbiota composition in the URT. Our finding that the abundance of *S. pneumoniae* was increased in CAP patients living close to a poultry farm underlines our hypothesis that exposure to farm-related air pollutants may result in alterations of the oropharyngeal microbiota composition. An imbalanced URT microbiome may lead to decreased colonization resistance and reduced containment of commensals that may become pathogens (pathobionts) such as *S. pneumoniae*, consequently increasing the risk of respiratory tract infections [20].

We speculate that PM and endotoxin emissions from intensive agricultural operations are central to our findings, putatively by modulating innate immune responses resulting in an imbalanced respiratory microbiome, which is supported by animal and *in vitro* experiments

[31, 32]. Alveolar macrophages remove inhaled PM by phagocytosis and release pro-inflammatory mediators, including reactive oxygen species. Their function is altered by particulate loading, which was shown to result in reduced phagocytosis of *S. pneumoniae* [33]. Furthermore, PM increases adhesion of *S. pneumoniae* to human airway epithelial cells, which is mediated by oxidative stress and upregulation of platelet-activating factor receptors (PAFR) [34, 35]. In aged rats, a single exposure to ambient PM reduced the ability to handle ongoing pneumococcal infections [36]. It was recently shown that the composition of the lung microbiota shifted towards endogenous opportunistic pathogens in a lipopolysaccharide (LPS) induced lung inflammation mouse model [32]. It has earlier been proposed that a perturbed respiratory microbiome may be involved in the association between cigarette smoking and respiratory tract infections. Both culture-based and culture-independent studies have shown that smoking can simultaneously deplete members of the normal commensal airway flora and enrich for potential pathogens [37]. Morris et al. [38] showed significant differences in the microbiome of the oral cavity of smokers compared with nonsmokers. We postulate similar mechanisms are responsible for the current observations. Smoking status (and other potential confounders such as COPD) were not associated with residential proximity to a poultry farm, thus it is unlikely that confounding has influenced the results.

In this study, bacterial community changes were observed on top of the previously described dysbiotic oropharyngeal microbiota composition in CAP patients compared to healthy adults, which was characterized by an increase of *S. pneumoniae, Rothia* and *Lactobacillus* [22]. Most strikingly, we showed an increased abundance of the most important human pathobiont causing pneumonia (i.e. *S. pneumoniae*) in oropharyngeal samples of patients living near poultry farms, which was a consistent finding across supervised and unsupervised learning methods. Our results are of great relevance for studies in individuals exposed to other sources of PM such as traffic and solid biomass fuel combustion, which are linked to acute respiratory infections as well [4, 5, 7], and may also be associated with an altered respiratory microbiota composition.

The observation of enhanced growth of a human pathobiont suggests an indirect effect of exposure to poultry farm emissions on pathogenesis of CAP. This is in contrast to a Finnish study [39], which observed that environmental biodiversity was associated with a higher generic diversity of skin gammaproteobacteria, presumably resulting from direct contact with environmental microbiota. Although there is some evidence that transmission of farm-related bacteria may take place through air—for example, in pig and veal calf farmers and their family members, nasal colonization by livestock-associated methicillin-resistant *Staphylococcus aureus* (LA-MRSA) occurs frequently [40]—we did not find evidence of zoonotic infections explaining the increased risk of CAP around poultry farms [9].

Around 40% of the CAP patients also had COPD. It has been demonstrated that COPD patients living near livestock farms are more likely to use inhaled corticosteroids and report respiratory symptoms than patients living further away from farms, suggesting an increased risk of exacerbations [18, 24]. Dickson et al. [41] proposed that exacerbations of COPD are occasions of respiratory dysbiosis: disorder and dysregulation of the microbial ecosystem of the respiratory tract, coupled with a dysregulated host immune response. A similar mechanism as proposed in the present study, hinging on farm-related air pollutants and dysbiosis of the respiratory tract, may play a role in individuals with COPD living near livestock farms. We intend to study a rural population of both COPD patients and control subjects in a larger-scale future study. Including control subjects will help to interpret results, because the microbiota changes within patient groups may be a cause or a consequence of disease, or merely coinciding with disease status [22].

Indeed, a limitation of our preliminary microbiota study is that we did not include healthy controls from the same study area. However, hospitalized patients living near a poultry farm and those living further away from poultry farms did not differ with regard to potential confounders such as age, smoking, COPD, or pneumonia severity. Residual confounding due to demographic differences between the two groups (e.g. household size), contact with children or other risk factors for pneumonia or pneumococcal colonization cannot be entirely dismissed. Because of the relatively small sample size, the results are sensitive to the effect of outliers. In addition, there may be false positive results due to multiple comparisons. This should therefore be regarded as a hypothesis-generating study, and results need to be confirmed in larger, preferably longitudinal, studies.

Conclusions

Kernel analysis demonstrated an excess risk of GP-diagnosed pneumonia in areas of approximately 1.15 km around poultry farms. Oropharyngeal microbiota of patients with CAP living within 1 km of a poultry farm showed an increased abundance of *S. pneumoniae*. Exposure to air pollutants such as PM and endotoxin may contribute to dysbiosis of URT microbiota in susceptible individuals, which may consequently result in respiratory infections. These preliminary observations need to be replicated in larger, independent studies.

Acknowledgements
The authors would like to thank Mei Ling Chu for her technical assistance.

Funding
This research has received funding from the Dutch Ministry of Economic Affairs (project code BO-20-009-030), the (former) Dutch Ministry of Economic Affairs, Agriculture and Innovation and the Dutch Ministry of Health, Welfare and Sport, the Wilhelmina Children's Hospital Fund, ZonMW (grant 91209010) and NWO-VENI (grant 91610121).

Authors' contributions
LAMS, GJB, TJH, DB and DH conceived and designed the study. LAMS, GJB, WAAdSP, TJH, DB and DH wrote the manuscript. LAMS provided the farm exposure data. GJB and TJH were responsible for the spatial kernel analysis. DB provided the microbiota data. WAAdSP and DB analyzed the microbiota data. EGWH provided the hospitalized patients' data. JY provided the general practioners' data. All authors contributed to interpretation of the results, and critically reviewed the manuscript. All authors read and approved the final manuscript.

Competing interests
EAMS has received grants for vaccination studies from pharmaceutical companies (GlaxoSmithKline and Pfizer). EAMS declares no conflict of interest related to the present study. The other authors declare no conflict of interest.

Author details
[1]Institute for Risk Assessment Sciences (IRAS), Division Environmental Epidemiology, Utrecht University, PO Box 80178, 3508 TD Utrecht, The Netherlands. [2]Central Veterinary Institute, Wageningen University and Research Centre, Lelystad, The Netherlands. [3]Department of Paediatric Immunology and Infectious Diseases, The Wilhelmina Children's Hospital/ University Medical Center Utrecht, Utrecht, The Netherlands. [4]Department of Medical Microbiology, Albert Schweitzer Hospital, Dordrecht, The Netherlands. [5]Laboratory of Medical Microbiology and Immunology, St. Elisabeth Hospital, Tilburg, The Netherlands. [6]Department of Medical Microbiology, University of Groningen, University Medical Center Groningen, Groningen, The Netherlands. [7]Department of Virology, Erasmus Medical Centre, Rotterdam, The Netherlands. [8]Current address: GD Animal Health, Deventer, The Netherlands. [9]National Institute for Public Health and the Environment, Bilthoven, The Netherlands. [10]NIVEL, Netherlands Institute for Health Services Research, Utrecht, The Netherlands.

References
1. Torres A, Peetermans WE, Viegi G, Blasi F. Risk factors for community-acquired pneumonia in adults in Europe: a literature review. Thorax. 2013; 68:1057–65.
2. GBD 2013 Mortality and Causes of Death Collaborators. Global, regional, and national age-sex specific all-cause and cause-specific mortality for 240 causes of death, 1990-2013: a systematic analysis for the Global Burden of Disease Study 2013. Lancet. 2015;385:117 71.
3. Jain S, Self WH, Wunderink RG, Fakhran S, Balk R, Bramley AM, Reed C, Grijalva CG, Anderson EJ, Courtney DM, Chappell JD, Qi C, Hart EM, Carroll F, Trabue C, Donnelly HK, Williams DJ, Zhu Y, Arnold SR, Ampofo K, Waterer GW, Levine M, Lindstrom S, Winchell JM, Katz JM, Erdman D, Schneider E, Hicks LA, McCullers JA, Pavia AT, Edwards KM, Finelli L, CDC EPIC Study Team. Community-Acquired Pneumonia Requiring Hospitalization among U. S. Adults. N Engl J Med. 2015;373:415–27.
4. Neupane B, Jerrett M, Burnett RT, Marrie T, Arain A, Loeb M. Long-term exposure to ambient air pollution and risk of hospitalization with community-acquired pneumonia in older adults. Am J Respir Crit Care Med. 2010;181:47–53.
5. Gordon SB, Bruce NG, Grigg J, Hibberd PL, Kurmi OP, Lam KB, Mortimer K, Asante KP, Balakrishnan K, Balmes J, Bar-Zeev N, Bates MN, Breysse PN, Buist S, Chen Z, Havens D, Jack D, Jindal S, Kan H, Mehta S, Moschovis P, Naeher L, Patel A, Perez-Padilla R, Pope D, Rylance J, Semple S, Martin II WJ. Respiratory risks from household air pollution in low and middle income countries. Lancet Respir Med. 2014;2:823–60.
6. Almirall J, Bolibar I, Serra-Prat M, Roig J, Hospital I, Carandell E, Agusti M, Ayuso P, Estela A, Torres A. Community-Acquired Pneumonia in Catalan Countries (PACAP) Study Group. New evidence of risk factors for community-acquired pneumonia: a population-based study. Eur Respir J. 2008;31:1274–84.
7. MacIntyre EA, Gehring U, Molter A, Fuertes E, Klumper C, Kramer U, Quass U, Hoffmann B, Gascon M, Brunekreef B, Koppelman GH, Beelen R, Hoek G, Birk M, de Jongste JC, Smit HA, Cyrys J, Gruzieva O, Korek M, Bergstrom A, Agius RM, de Vocht F, Simpson A, Porta D, Forastiere F, Badaloni C, Cesaroni G, Esplugues A, Fernandez-Somoano A, Lerxundi A, Sunyer J, Cirach M, Nieuwenhuijsen MJ, Pershagen G, Heinrich J. Air pollution and respiratory infections during early childhood: an analysis of 10 European birth cohorts within the ESCAPE Project. Environ Health Perspect. 2014;122:107–13.
8. Smit LA, van der Sman-de Beer F, Opstal-van Winden AW, Hooiveld M, Beekhuizen J, Wouters IM, Yzermans J, Heederik D. Q Fever and pneumonia in an area with a high livestock density: a large population-based study. PLoS One. 2012;7:e38843.
9. Huijskens EGW, Smit LAM, Rossen JWA, Heederik D, Koopmans M. Evaluation of patients with community-acquired pneumonia caused by zoonotic pathogens in an area with a high density of animal farms. Zoonoses Public Health. 2016;63:160–6.
10. Brunekreef B, Harrison RM, Kunzli N, Querol X, Sutton MA, Heederik DJ, Sigsgaard T. Reducing the health effect of particles from agriculture. Lancet Respir Med. 2015;3:831–2.
11. Lelieveld J, Evans JS, Fnais M, Giannadaki D, Pozzer A. The contribution of outdoor air pollution sources to premature mortality on a global scale. Nature. 2015;525:367–71.
12. Cambra-Lopez M, Aarnink AJ, Zhao Y, Calvet S, Torres AG. Airborne particulate matter from livestock production systems: a review of an air pollution problem. Environ Pollut. 2010;158:1–17.
13. Jonges M, van Leuken J, Wouters I, Koch G, Meijer A, Koopmans M. Wind-Mediated Spread of Low-Pathogenic Avian Influenza Virus into the Environment during Outbreaks at Commercial Poultry Farms. PLoS One. 2015;10:e0125401.
14. Seedorf J, Hartung J, Schröder M, Linkert KH, Phillips VR, Holden MR, Sneath RW, Short JL, White RP, Pedersen S, Takai H, Johnsen JO, Metz JHM, Groot Koerkamp PWG, Uenk GH, Wathes CM. Concentrations and Emissions of Airborne Endotoxins and Microorganisms in Livestock Buildings in Northern Europe. J Agric Eng Res. 1998;70:97–109.
15. Schulze A, van Strien R, Ehrenstein V, Schierl R, Kuchenhoff H, Radon K. Ambient endotoxin level in an area with intensive livestock production. Ann Agric Environ Med. 2006;13:87–91.
16. Schenker MB, Christiani D, Cormier Y, Dimich-Ward H, Doekes G, Dosman J, Douwes J, Dowling K, Enarson D, Green F, Heederik D, Husman K, Kennedy S, Kullman G, Lacasse Y, Lawson B, Malmberg P, May J, McCurdy S, Merchant J, Myers J, Nieuwenhuijsen M, Olenchock S, Saiki C, Schwartz D, Seiber J, Thorne P, Wagner G, White N, Xu XP, Chan-Yeung M. Respiratory health hazards in agriculture. Am J Respir Crit Care Med. 1998;158:S1–S76.
17. Smit LA, Heederik D, Doekes G, Blom C, van Zweden I, Wouters IM. Exposure-response analysis of allergy and respiratory symptoms in endotoxin-exposed adults. Eur Respir J. 2008;31:1241–8.
18. Borlée F, Yzermans CJ, van Dijk CE, Heederik D, Smit LAM. Increased respiratory symptoms in COPD patients living in the vicinity of livestock farms. Eur Respir J. 2015;46:1605–14.
19. Sandstrom T, Bjermer L, Rylander R. Lipopolysaccharide (LPS) inhalation in healthy subjects increases neutrophils, lymphocytes and fibronectin levels in bronchoalveolar lavage fluid. Eur Respir J. 1992;5:992–6.

20. de Steenhuijsen Piters WA, Sanders EA, Bogaert D. The role of the local microbial ecosystem in respiratory health and disease. Philos Trans R Soc Lond B Biol Sci. 2015;370(1675). doi:10.1098/rstb.2014.0294.
21. Dickson RP, Erb-Downward JR, Huffnagle GB. Towards an ecology of the lung: new conceptual models of pulmonary microbiology and pneumonia pathogenesis. Lancet Respir Med. 2014;2:238–46.
22. de Steenhuijsen Piters WA, Huijskens EG, Wyllie AL, Biesbroek G, van den Bergh MR, Veenhoven RH, Wang X, Trzcinski K, Bonten MJ, Rossen JW, Sanders EA, Bogaert D. Dysbiosis of upper respiratory tract microbiota in elderly pneumonia patients. ISME J. 2016;10:97–108.
23. Smit LAM, Hooiveld M, van der Sman-de Beer F, Opstal-van Winden AWJ, Beekhuizen J, Wouters IM, Yzermans CJ, Heederik D. Air pollution from livestock farms, and asthma, allergic rhinitis and COPD among neighbouring residents. Occup Environ Med. 2014;71:134–40.
24. van Dijk CE, Garcia-Aymerich J, Carsin AE, Smit LAM, Borlée F, Heederik DJ, Donker GA, Yzermans CJ, Zock JP. Risk of exacerbations in COPD and asthma patients living in the neighbourhood of livestock farms: observational study using longitudinal data. Int J Hyg Environ Health. 2016;219:278–87.
25. Huijskens EG, van Erkel AJ, Palmen FM, Buiting AG, Kluytmans JA, Rossen JW. Viral and bacterial aetiology of community-acquired pneumonia in adults. Influenza Other Respir Viruses. 2013;7:567–73.
26. Lindstrom T, Hakansson N, Wennergren U. The shape of the spatial kernel and its implications for biological invasions in patchy environments. Proc Biol Sci. 2011;278:1564–71.
27. Boender GJ, Hagenaars TJ, Bouma A, Nodelijk G, Elbers AR, de Jong MC, van Boven M. Risk maps for the spread of highly pathogenic avian influenza in poultry. PLoS Comput Biol. 2007;3:e71.
28. Oksanen J, Blanchet FG, Friendly M, Kindt R, Legendre P, McGlinn D, Minchin PR, O'Hara RB, Simpson GL, Solymos P, Stevens MHH, Szoecs E, Wagner H. vegan: Community Ecology Package. R package version 2.4-1. https://CRAN.R-project.org/package=vegan. 2016.
29. Benjamini Y, Hochberg Y. Controlling the False Discovery Rate: A Practical and Powerful Approach to Multiple Testing. J R Statist Soc B. 1995;57:289–300.
30. Letunic I, Bork P. Interactive Tree Of Life v2: online annotation and display of phylogenetic trees made easy. Nucleic Acids Res. 2011;39:W475–8.
31. Lee A, Kinney P, Chillrud S, Jack D. A Systematic Review of Innate Immunomodulatory Effects of Household Air Pollution Secondary to the Burning of Biomass Fuels. Ann Glob Health. 2015;81:368–74.
32. Poroyko V, Meng F, Meliton A, Afonyushkin T, Ulanov A, Semenyuk E, Latif O, Tesic V, Birukova AA, Birukov KG. Alterations of lung microbiota in a mouse model of LPS-induced lung injury. Am J Physiol Lung Cell Mol Physiol. 2015;309:L76–83.
33. Rylance J, Fullerton DG, Scriven J, Aljurayyan AN, Mzinza D, Barrett S, Wright AK, Wootton DG, Glennie SJ, Baple K, Knott A, Mortimer K, Russell DG, Heyderman RS, Gordon SB. Household air pollution causes dose-dependent inflammation and altered phagocytosis in human macrophages. Am J Respir Cell Mol Biol. 2015;52:584–93.
34. Mushtaq N, Ezzati M, Hall L, Dickson I, Kirwan M, Png KM, Mudway IS, Grigg J. Adhesion of Streptococcus pneumoniae to human airway epithelial cells exposed to urban particulate matter. J Allergy Clin Immunol. 2011;127:1236–42.
35. Grigg J, Walters H, Sohal SS, Wood-Baker R, Reid DW, Xu CB, Edvinsson L, Morissette MC, Stampfli MR, Kirwan M, Koh L, Suri R, Mushtaq N. Cigarette smoke and platelet-activating factor receptor dependent adhesion of Streptococcus pneumoniae to lower airway cells. Thorax. 2012;67:908–13.
36. Zelikoff JT, Chen LC, Cohen MD, Fang K, Gordon T, Li Y, Nadziejko C, Schlesinger RB. Effects of inhaled ambient particulate matter on pulmonary antimicrobial immune defense. Inhal Toxicol. 2003;15:131–50.
37. Charlson ES, Chen J, Custers-Allen R, Bittinger K, Li H, Sinha R, Hwang J, Bushman FD, Collman RG. Disordered microbial communities in the upper respiratory tract of cigarette smokers. PLoS One. 2010;5:e15216.
38. Morris A, Beck JM, Schloss PD, Campbell TB, Crothers K, Curtis JL, Flores SC, Fontenot AP, Ghedin E, Huang L, Jablonski K, Kleerup E, Lynch SV, Sodergren E, Twigg H, Young VB, Bassis CM, Venkataraman A, Schmidt TM, Weinstock GM. Lung HIV Microbiome Project. Comparison of the respiratory microbiome in healthy nonsmokers and smokers. Am J Respir Crit Care Med. 2013;187:1067–75.
39. Hanski I, von Hertzen L, Fyhrquist N, Koskinen K, Torppa K, Laatikainen T, Karisola P, Auvinen P, Paulin L, Makela MJ, Vartiainen E, Kosunen TU, Alenius H, Haahtela T. Environmental biodiversity, human microbiota, and allergy are interrelated. Proc Natl Acad Sci U S A. 2012;109:8334–9.
40. Bos ME, Verstappen KM, van Cleef BA, Dohmen W, Dorado-Garcia A, Graveland H, Duim B, Wagenaar JA, Kluytmans JA, Heederik DJ. Transmission through air as a possible route of exposure for MRSA. J Expo Sci Environ Epidemiol. 2016;26:263–9.
41. Dickson RP, Martinez FJ, Huffnagle GB. The role of the microbiome in exacerbations of chronic lung diseases. Lancet. 2014;384:691–702.

11

How and when to use common biomarkers in community-acquired pneumonia

Erica J. Shaddock[1,2]

Abstract

Community-acquired pneumonia (CAP) is a leading cause of death in both the developed and developing world. The very young and elderly are especially vulnerable. Even with appropriate early antibiotics we still have not improved the outcomes in these patients since the 1950s, with 30-day case fatality rates of between 10–12%. Interventions to improve outcomes include immunomodulatory agents such as macrolides and corticosteroids. Treating doctors identify CAP patients who are likely to have poor outcomes by using severity scores such as the pneumonia severity index and CURB-65, which allows these patients to be placed in ICU settings from the start of the admission. Another novel way to identify these patients is with the use of biomarkers. This review illustrates how various biomarkers have been shown to predict mortality, complications and response to treatment in CAP patients. The evidence using either procalcitonin or C-reactive protein to demonstrate response to treatment and hence that the antibiotics chosen are appropriate can play an important role in antibiotic stewardship.

Keywords: Biomarkers, Pneumonia, Procalcitonin, C-reactive protein

Background

The first description of pneumonia has been credited to Hippocrates, and in the 2500 years following his account we have accumulated vast knowledge and understanding of Osler's "Captain of the Men of Death". Community-acquired pneumonia (CAP) is, however, still a leading cause of death in the developed and developing world. Whilst treatment options and diagnostic techniques have improved, overall 30-day mortality for CAP is still 10–12.1% [1, 2], and researchers continue to try to find methods to improve outcomes. One of these approaches is the use of biomarkers and there is a growing body of evidence to suggest that biomarkers could help with this challenge. There are many excellent biomarker review articles available; this review hopes to add to the literature with some recent practical data [3–6].

Biological markers, more commonly called biomarkers, were (as recently as 1998) defined by the National Institutes of Health Biomarkers Definitions Working Group, as "a characteristic that is objectively measured and evaluated as an indicator of normal biological processes, pathogenic processes, or pharmacologic responses to a therapeutic intervention" [7]. Numerous biomarkers have been tested and validated for use in CAP. This review will be examining recent evidence and how biomarkers may be of use in daily practice.

Traditional biomarkers such as white cell count (WCC) and erythrocyte sedimentary rate (ESR) have become less relied upon due to their lower sensitivity and specificity compared to the more promising C-reactive protein (CRP) and procalcitonin (PCT), which are currently in widespread use. Other inflammatory mediators such as interleukin (IL)-1β, IL-6, tumor necrosis factor (TNF)-α, and IL-8, have also been found to be elevated in response to the infection. Unfortunately these pro-inflammatory cytokines have very short half-lives and lack specificity; therefore, they are not currently viewed as good prospective biomarkers [3].

Basic science

The biomarkers that have been the most thoroughly validated in CAP and that are accessible to most medical practitioners are CRP and PCT.

CRP is secreted from hepatic cells in response to elevated IL-6, IL-1β, and TNF-α. These cytokines are

Correspondence: ericashaddock@gmail.com
[1]Division of Pulmonology and Critical Care, Department of Internal Medicine, Area 552 Charlotte Maxeke Johannesburg Academic Hospital, Jubilee Road, Parktown, Johannesburg 2193, South Africa
[2]Faculty of Health Sciences, University of the Witwatersrand, Johannesburg, South Africa

potent pro-inflammatory agents that are released from various innate inflammatory cells when they encounter pathogen-associated molecular patterns (PAMPS) from invading organisms. Additional sources of CRP synthesis have been recently identified and include lymphocytes, monocytes, neurons, and atherosclerotic plaques [8]. CRP's name originates from its ability to precipitate C-polysaccharide of *Streptococcus pneumonia*, and it was one of the first acute phase proteins to be described. Due to the main production of CRP occurring in the liver, it is important to remember it is not a reliable marker for sepsis in patients with liver failure. CRP synthesis starts very rapidly after a single stimulus: serum concentrations rise within about 6 h and peak around 48 h. The plasma half-life of CRP is about 19 h, which is constant in health and disease. Therefore, the main determinant of plasma CRP concentration is the synthesis rate, which directly reflects the degree of the pathological process stimulating CRP production [8].

PCT is a 116 amino acid peptide, with a molecular weight of 14.5 kDa. It belongs to the calcitonin superfamily of peptides, and is a precursor to calcitonin production usually taking place in the C cells of the thyroid gland [9]. PCT synthesis is very interesting and occurs in a tissue-specific manner. If there is no infection, transcription of the *CALC-1* gene for PCT in the non-neuroendocrine tissue is suppressed, except in the C cells of the thyroid gland. A microbial infection induces a substantial increase of *CALC-1* gene expression in all parenchymal tissue and differentiated cell types in the body that produce PCT. We are currently uncertain of the exact function of PCT synthesised in the non-neuroendocrine tissues under microbial infection [9]. PCT is detectable within 2–4 h of infection, peaks within 6–24 h, and can be present for up to 7 days. The half-life is 22–26 h in plasma and it is cleared mainly through proteolysis with minimal renal excretion [10]. The response to antibiotics can also be monitored well with PCT; as a "rule of thumb", a decline of > 30% per day indicates improvement of systemic inflammation. This decrease is due to the natural plasma disappearance rate of PCT if no further inflammatory activation is occurring [11]. Interferon-gamma (IFN-γ), an important mediator in viral infections, down-regulates PCT production, making PCT a very useful test to help distinguish between viral and bacterial infections.

Diagnosis

Biomarkers are helpful in aiding with the initial diagnosis of CAP. In many patients, making the diagnosis of CAP is straightforward: a history is taken, followed by examination and then a chest X-ray to confirm the diagnosis. However, in some patients there might be co-morbidities or the picture might not be typical, which makes it more difficult for the clinician to make a confident diagnosis. As the world's population ages and the number of patients on therapeutic immunosuppression increases, the differential diagnoses for patients with dyspnea and cough increases. This diagnosis list includes cardiac failure, an acute exacerbation of chronic obstructive pulmonary disease, atypical pneumonia, pulmonary embolism or even interstitial lung disease. This is the place where biomarkers can aid in diagnosis. Müller et al. [12] demonstrated a significant improvement in diagnostic accuracy when adding PCT and CRP to standard clinical signs and symptoms. These biomarkers also performed better than standard makers of infection such as white cell count and raised temperature in different settings, including primary care and the emergency room, as well as in bacteriaemic and non-bacteraemic patients (Fig. 1 [12, 13]). The area under the curve (AUC) of clinical signs and symptoms alone was 0.79 (95% CI 0.75–0.83); with added PCT and highly sensitive CRP it was 0.92 (95% CI 0.89–0.94; $p < 0.001$) [12].

Response to treatment and antibiotic stewardship

Biomarkers can be monitored to evaluate response to treatment, which can impact length of antibiotic use and predict outcomes. A paper by Coelho et al. [14] adds a new dimension to the basic blood test C-reactive protein (CRP), showing its use to predict outcomes. In patients with severe CAP, they found that a CRP ratio comparing day 5 (D5) CRP against admission CRP predicted ICU outcome, using receiver operating characteristic (ROC) curves with a value of 0.73 (95% CI 0.64–0.82). This prospective observational cohort study classified CAP patients into the following groups: fast response—when D5 CRP was ≤ 0.4 of day 1 (D1) CRP concentration; slow response—when D5 CRP > 0.4 and D7 ≤ 0.8 of D1 CRP concentration; and non-response—when D7 CRP was > 0.8 of D1 CRP concentration. The group then performed comparisons between survivors and non-survivors using standard statistical analysis. When these groups were analysed for ICU survival, mortality was as follows: 4.6% in fast response patients, 17.3% in slow response, and 36.4% in non-response patients ($p < 0.001$). Hospital mortality showed a similar pattern. If clinicians were to use biomarkers in this fashion they could identify patients who are ready for discharge, those who have shown a fast response to treatment versus those patients who might not have adequate source control or resistant organisms; that is, those with slow or no response to treatment who require further interventions to improve outcomes.

Is it safe to base antibiotic decisions on biomarkers? A large multi-centred, prospective, randomised, controlled, non-inferiority trial [15, 16] with open intervention performed in Switzerland recruited 1359 patients, and was designed to examine whether a PCT algorithm can reduce antibiotic exposure without increasing the risk for

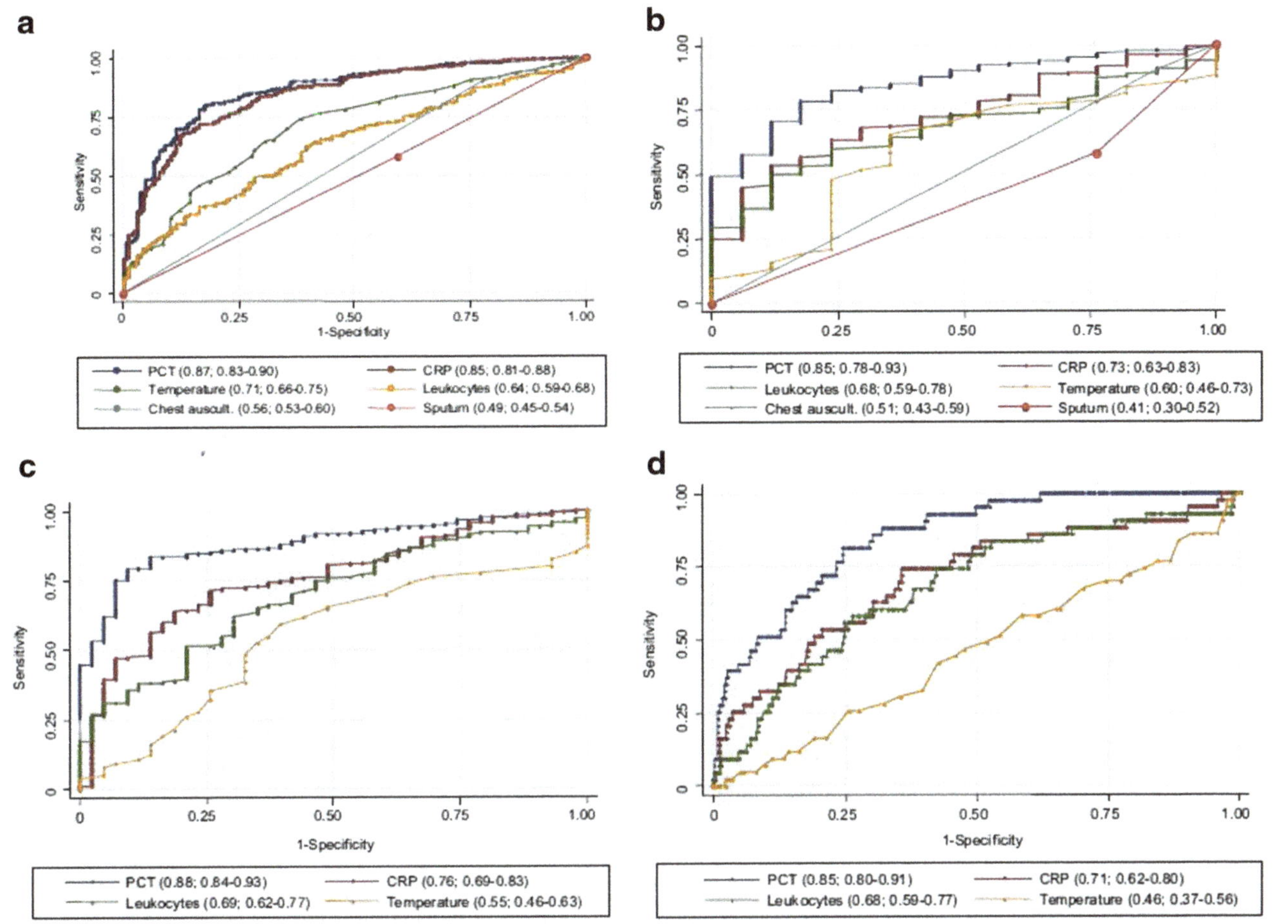

Fig. 1 Receiver operating characteristics curves (ROC) of different parameters for the diagnosis of pneumonia. **a** Diagnostic accuracy to predict CAP without chest radiography: Primary care approach. **b** Diagnostic accuracy to predict radiographically suspected CAP (control group ($n = 20$) includes other non-infectious diagnoses initially diagnosed as CAP): Emergency department approach. **c** Diagnostic accuracy to predict radiographically suspected CAP (control group ($n = 44$) includes other non-infectious diagnoses initially diagnosed as CAP ($n = 20$) plus patients without a clinically relevant bacterial aetiology of CAP ($n = 24$). **d** Diagnostic accuracy to predict bacteraemic CAP. Values show areas under the ROC curve with 95% CI. Chest auscult. = abnormal chest auscultation; CRP, C-reactive Protein; PCT, procalcitonin. Sourced from [12]

serious adverse outcomes (ProHOSP Study). Patients with lower respiratory tract infections (LRTI) presenting to the emergency departments were recruited, including patients with CAP, acute bronchitis and chronic obstructive pulmonary disease with acute exacerbations. The primary non-inferiority end point was a 30-day composite of overall adverse events including death from any cause, ICU admission for any reason, disease specific complications and recurrence of LRTI in need of antibiotics, with or without hospital readmission. Using predetermined PCT cut-offs (Fig. 2 [16],) the trial demonstrated an overall adverse outcome similar in the PCT-driven group versus the control group (15.4% [$n = 103$] vs. 18.9% [$n = 130$]; difference, -3.5%; 95% CI -7.6 to 0.4%). The odds ratio (OR) for the combined adverse outcome was 0.76 (95% CI 0.57–1.01). The secondary endpoint of mean duration of antibiotic exposure was lower in the PCT group versus the control group in all patients (5.7 vs. 8.7 days; relative change, -34.8%; 95% CI -40. to 28.7%) as well as in the subgroup analysis of patients with CAP ($n = 925$, 7.2 vs. 10.7 days, 32.4%; 95% CI -37.6 to -26.9%).

As mentioned previously, IFN-γ down-regulates PCT production, which could help distinguish between viral and bacterial infections. Algorithms based on PCT values have been validated to aid in deciding whether patients have bacterial CAP versus viral CAP and hence require antibiotics. The suggestions are identical to those used in the ProHOSP study above and are as follows: PCT <0.10 mcg/l: strongly discourage antibiotic use; PCT between 0.10-0.25 mcg/l: discourage antibiotic use; PCT between 0.25-0.50 mcg/l: encourage antibiotic use; PCT >0.50 mcg/l: strongly encourage antibiotic use [17]. This has been shown to be effective in studies evaluating LTRI to aid in diagnosis and decrease antibiotic prescription [17, 18]. A recent study [19], which evaluated 2259 adults with radiographic evidence of CAP requiring hospitalisation in the United States,

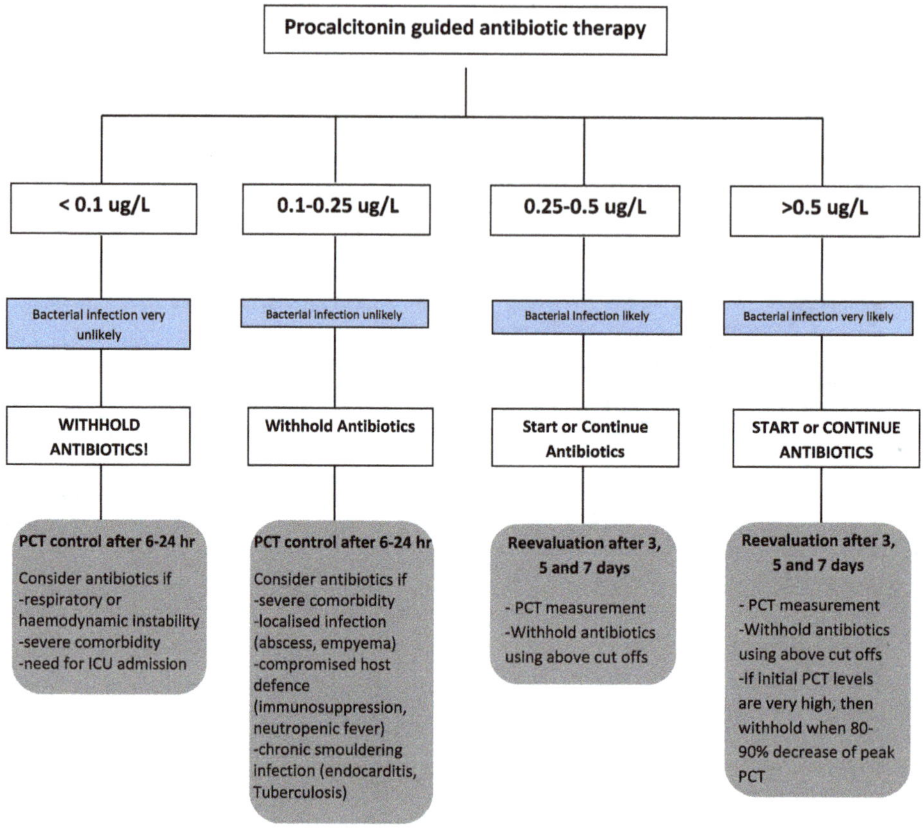

Fig. 2 Antibiotic stewardship based on procalcitonin (PCT) cut-off ranges. Re-evaluation of the clinical status and measurement of serum PCT levels is mandatory after 6–24 h in all persistently sick and hospitalized patients in who antibiotic are withheld. PCT, procalcitonin; ICU, intensive care unit. Adapted from [16]

demonstrated that in the 853(38%) patients on whom they were able to culture an organism, 530 (23%) had one or more viruses, 247 (11%) had bacteria, and bacterial and viral pathogens in were found in 59 (3%), The viral burden in CAP is often underappreciated and this study illustrates that PCT may be useful in helping with antibiotic decision making.

The Cochrane meta-analysis evaluating the use of PCT to initiate or discontinue antibiotics in LRTI analysed data from 14 trials with 4221 patients with acute respiratory infections (50% had CAP), including the Swiss cohort. They demonstrated a reduction in antibiotic exposure (from a median of 8 to 4 days) [20]. The reduction of antibiotics used did not impact on outcomes; there was no increase in mortality or treatment failure in any of the clinical settings it was investigated in (outpatient clinic, emergency department) or in patients with any type of acute respiratory infection, including CAP. This can be seen as a major gain for antibiotic stewardship programs.

Predicting complications, outcomes and mortality

There now is evidence that biomarkers can be also be used to predict complications, outcomes and mortality. A recent study performed in Uganda looking at the usefulness of PCT in HIV-infected individuals with lower respiratory tract infections to predict in-hospital mortality is particularly useful. Often HIV-infected and immunosuppressed patients are excluded from studies; therefore, one is never sure how to extrapolate the biomarker evidence into actual practice, especially if that practice is in a country with a high HIV prevalence. Tokmen and colleagues [21] performed a prospective, nested, case control study on data from the larger International HIV-associated Opportunistic Pneumonias (IHOP) study, investigating the mortality predictability of PCT in HIV-infected individuals with lower respiratory tract infections. This study is different from many of those undertaken before, as it looked at only HIV-infected individuals and at patients with symptoms for longer than 2 weeks, therefore looking to include patients with tuberculosis and Pneumocystis pneumonia (PCP). A cohort of 241 HIV-infected patients had PCT measurements performed. The cohort had advanced HIV disease with a median CD4 count of 47 cells/μL. Unfortunately, a final diagnosis could not be made in 22.8% of the group due to death or inability to follow up;

this resulted in a final group of 203 diagnoses in 186 patients. As predicted, tuberculosis was the most common diagnosis at 71.9% ($n = 146/203$), with bacterial pneumonia second at 12.3% ($n = 25/203$) and only 1% being PCP ($n = 2/203$). The median PCT level was 1.45 ng/ml. The authors decided to use a cut-off of 0.5 ng/ml for PCT assessment of mortality prediction. If patients had an elevated PCT (>0.5 ng/ml), it was associated with an increased predicted probability of mortality (1% mortality in those with PCT ≤ 0.5 ng/ml vs. 10% mortality in those with a PCT of > 0.5 ng/ml; $p = 0.004$). This cohort had a reported in-hospital mortality that was very low and this could be a confounding factor if the data were extrapolated to other institutions. They performed further data analysis and found that by combining elevated PCT plus tachypnoea plus hypoxaemia, the accuracy of in-hospital mortality prediction resulted in an AUC of 0.741 (95% CI 0.65–0.83). This was a marked improvement compared to tachypnoea and hypoxaemia without PCT, which had an AUC of 0.659 (95% CI 0.55–0.77; $p = 0.05$). It is exciting that the authors have shown that adding a biomarker to easily assessable clinical criteria can markedly improve the ability to predict in-hospital mortality.

Another study [22], from the large Swiss cohort previously mentioned, evaluated the performance of PCT as a prognostic indicator, alongside the already validated CAP scores, the PSI, and the CURB-65 score. The study of the prognostic potential of PCT was a predefined secondary end point of the large multicentre Procalcitonin Guided Antibiotic Therapy and Hospitalisation in Patients with Lower Respiratory Tract Infections (ProHOSP) study. A total of 925 patients were included in the analysis. The median age of patients enrolled was 73 years, with 41% being female. While this population group would be appropriate for the developed world, those who practice in the developing world where the population would be much younger should take this into consideration. Survivors had a much lower median PCT level on admission than non-survivors: 0.44 ug/l (IGR 0.15–2.63 ug/l) versus 0.83 ug/l (IQR 0.30–5.67 ug/l) ($p = 0.02$), as did patients without adverse outcomes versus those with adverse outcomes: 0.39 ug/l (IQR 0.14–2.2 ug/l) vs. 1.30 ug/l (IQR 0.38–7.47 ug/l); $p < 0.001$. This group did not find that PCT improved the AUC to predict morality (AUC 0.60), and was in fact lower than the clinical risk scores alone (AUC CURB-65 = 0.72; AUC PSI = 0.79). Even when PCT was added to the PSI and CURB-65 clinical scores, it did not significantly improve either for mortality prediction. However, for prediction of adverse events combining the PCT with either the CURB-65 or PSI improved the ability to predict these events better than the clinical scores alone (PSI plus PCT AUC = 0.71 [0.66–0.76], $p < 0.01$; CURB-65 plus PCT AUC = 0.70 [0.65–0.75], $p = 0.008$). This group also found that the follow up PCT levels measured on day 3, 5 and 7 were able to provide information about increased risk of mortality and adverse events in a very similar fashion to the Coelho group [17]. Those patients who did not show a clear decrease of PCT had worse outcomes.

Skouras and colleagues [23] used the biomarker CRP to evaluate its clinical utility as a predictor in parapneumonic effusions (PPE). It has been estimated that approximately 40% of CAP can be associated with a PPE, most of which are inconsequential [24]. Up to 7.2% of CAP patients can go on to develop complicated parapneumonic effusions (CPPE) or empyema [25]. This is a significant burden in CAP patients and having the ability to predict or be aware of patients who are likely to develop this complication would be very useful. This was a prospective study from two tertiary Greek hospitals and 54 patients were included. Whilst this a small sample size, there is very little evidence-based medicine in this field. The cohort was evaluated in 2 groups, those with uncomplicated PPE and those with CPPE. Admission serum and pleural CRPs were compared in these 2 groups, as well as residual pleural thickening 6 months after hospital discharge. Residual pleural thickening can result in restrictive pulmonary disease. This study did demonstrate that an elevated serum CRP of >150 mg/l had a sensitivity of 61% and specificity of 91%, with a ROC of 0.82, for predicting residual pleural thickening post-PPE. The higher CRP levels are a marker of a more exuberant inflammatory response, which could explain the greater risk for pleural thickening. This finding adds a useful and easy test to allow for identification of patients who are at risk for long-term complications from PPE. Serum CRP and pleural CRP were significantly higher in CPPE. ROC curves evaluating accuracy to identify CPPE were 0.73 for pleural CRP and 0.68 for serum CRP, compared to the ROC of the more traditionally used low pleural fluid pH (pH < 7.1) of 0.93. Therefore, by themselves these tests are clearly inferior to tests used in current clinical practice. However, when combined with the classical criteria using an 'AND' or 'OR' rule, the positive and negative predictive values for diagnosis of a CPPE were improved. The group concluded that the serum CRP has value as an independent predictor for the development of residual pleural thickening. They also showed that it could be used in combination with the more traditional biomarkers—pleural fluid LDH, glucose and pH—to help with treatment decisions in non-purulent PPE.

The future

The biomarker of the future will most likely be pro-adrenomedullin (pro-ADM). Adrenomedullin (ADM) is produced at times of physiologic stress and has vasodilatory, antimicrobial, and anti-inflammatory properties. As early as 1996, Hirata and colleagues showed that levels of ADM increased with disease severity in adults with sepsis [26]. However ADM is not an ideal biomarker as it is rapidly cleared from circulation due to its rapid binding to receptors and its half-life of 22 min, so midregional-proadrenomeddullin (MR-proADM), a more stable precursor molecule, is used in clinical practice.

There have been several studies that have shown that MR-proADM has better predictive power than even CRP and PCT. In a prospective cohort study of 491 patients with CAP, admission MR-proADM levels correlated with and improved clinical severity scores [27]. Studies by Christ-Crain et al. and Kruger et al. both demonstrated the improved mortality prediction of MR-proADM when added to the PSI [28, 29]. A systematic review, which included twelve studies, evaluated the prognostic value of MR-proADM in short and long term mortality in CAP. The authors demonstrated an increase in short-term mortality (OR = 6.8; 95% CI: 4.65–10.13; $p < 0.001$) and complications (OR = 5.0; 95% CI: 3.86–6.49; $p < 0.001$) with elevated MR-proADM. A further pooled analysis of 4 of the studies showed an improved discriminant ability for predicting mortality in CAP patients of 8% (95% CI: 2–14%) when MR-proADM was added to the CURB-65/CRB-65 score [30]. When this test becomes more commercially available, there will be another important tool for CAP outcome prediction.

Further fascinating work has recently been done to identify a novel biomarker in CAP by analysis of the blood genomic response in CAP patients. Global gene expression profiles of whole blood leukocytes were collected within 24 h after ICU admission from CAP and non-CAP patients and then compared with those of healthy individuals [31]. A 78-gene signature was defined for CAP and the FAIM3:PLAC8 gene expression ratio was derived with an AUC of 0.845 (95% CI, 0.764–0.917) and positive and negative predictive values of 83 and 81%, respectively, when looking at ability to diagnosis CAP. Interestingly FAIM3, encoding the FAS apoptotic inhibitory molecule 3, and PLAC8, encoding placenta-specific 8, are both negative regulators of apoptosis. The FAIM3: PLAC8 ratio outperformed plasma procalcitonin and IL-8 and IL-6 in discriminating between CAP and non-CAP patients. Studies looking at gene expression in CAP, such as the above by Scicluna and colleagues, are not only about biomarkers but also add information to the understanding of the pathophysiology of the immune response in CAP.

Another up and coming approach to the biomarker field is that of metabolomics. Metabolomics is the investigations of the biochemical molecules derived from cellular processes, and it is studied under specific conditions, including CAP [32]. An example of metabolomics application in CAP is kynurenine (Kyn). Kyn is a toxic metabolite formed during the degradation of tryptophan (Trp), and patients with CAP and sepsis show significantly higher Kyn levels and lower Trp levels compared to controls [33, 34]. A more familiar metabolomic example, which has been used in critical care for prognosis and severity, is lactate. In adults with pneumonia, the lactate level has been shown to be a better predictor of 28-day mortality than the CURB-65 score, and a combination of CURB-65 with lactate level improves the predictive value of CURB-65 score alone [35]. For further reading Nickler and colleagues have written an interesting review article looking at this growing field and its impact on our understanding of respiratory conditions [32].

Conclusion

Point-of-care tests are now available, making it possible to utilise knowledge about biomarkers, even in the emergency room and doctor's room setting. Clinicians can make real-time decisions about the care and the admission path of patients. Once there is a complete understanding of all the information that can be gained from these simple tests, there will be greater insight into the future management of patients with CAP. This is especially true with regards to predicting complications and outcomes and, most importantly, response to treatment and earlier discontinuation of antibiotics. Hopefully, in the future, the benefits of implementing what is known about biomarkers will be reflected in improved patient outcomes.

Abbreviations

ADM: Adrenomedullin; AUC: Area under the curve; CAP: Community acquired pneumonia; CPPE: Complicated parapneumonic effusion; CRB-65: Confusion, Respiratory rate, Blood pressure, age > 65; CRP: C-reactive protein; CURB-65: Confusion, Urea, Respiratory Rate, Blood pressure, age > 65; ESR: Erythrocyte sedimentary rate; FAIM3: FAS apoptotic inhibitory molecule 3; HIV: Human immunodeficiency virus; IFN-γ: Interferon gamma; IL: Interleukin; Kyn: Kynurenine; LRTI: Lower respiratory tract infection; MR-proADM: Midregional-proadrenomeddullin; OR: Odds ratio; PAMPS: Pathogen associated molecular pattern; PCP: Pneumocystis pneumonia; PCT: Procalcitonin; PLAC8: Placenta-specific 8; PPE: Parapneumonic effusion; pro-ADM: Pro-adrenomedullin; ROC: Receiver operating curve; TNF-α: Tumour necrosis factor alpha; Trp: Tryptophan; WCC: White cell count

Acknowledgements

Nil.

Funding

Nil.

Authors' contributions

The author met ICMJE authorship criteria. ES generated and designed the research plan. ES wrote the first draft of the manuscript and approved the final version of the manuscript.

Authors' information

Dr Erica Shaddock MBBCh (WITS), FCP (SA), Certificate in Pulmonology (CMSA), Certificate in Critical Care (CMSA). Senior Pulmonologist and Intensivist.

Competing interests

The author declares that she has no competing interests.

References

1. Johnstone J, Marrie TJ, Eurich DT, Majumdar SR. Effect of pneumococcal vaccination in hospitalized adults with community-acquired pneumonia. Arch Intern Med. 2007;167:1938–43. PMID:17923592, http://dx.doi.org/10.1001/archinte.167.18.1938.
2. Metersky ML, Waterer G, Nsa W, Bratzler DW. Predictors of in-hospital vs postdischarge mortality in pneumonia. Chest. 2012;142:476–81. PMID:22383662, http://dx.doi.org/10.1378/chest.11-2393.
3. Cheng CW, Chien MH, Su SC, Yang SF. New markers in pneumonia. Clin Chim Acta. 2013;419:19–25. PMID:23384502, http://dx.doi.org/10.1016/j.cca.2013.01.011.
4. Torres A, Ramirez P, Montull B, Menéndez R. Biomarkers and community-acquired pneumonia: tailoring management with biological data. Semin Respir Crit Care Med. 2012;33:266–71. PMID:22718212, http://dx.doi.org/10.1055/s-0032-1315638.
5. Lippi G, Meschi T, Cervellin G. Inflammatory biomarkers for the diagnosis, monitoring and follow-up of community-acquired pneumonia: clinical evidence and perspectives. Eur J Intern Med. 2011;22:460–5. PMID:21925053, http://dx.doi.org/10.1016/j.ejim.2011.02.023.
6. Seligman R, Ramos-Lima LF, Oliveira VA, Sanvicente C, Pacheco EF, Dalla Rosa K. Biomarkers in community-acquired pneumonia: a state-of-the-art review. Clinics (Sao Paulo). 2012;67:1321–5. PMID:23184211 http://dx.doi.org/10.6061/clinics/2012(11)17.
7. Biomarkers Definitions Working Group. Biomarkers and surrogate endpoints: preferred definitions and conceptual framework. Clin Pharmacol Ther. 2001; 69:89–95. PMID:11240971, http://dx.doi.org/10.1067/mcp.2001.113989.
8. Jialal I, Devaraj S, Venugopal SK. C-reactive protein: risk marker or mediator in atherothrombosis? Hypertension. 2004;44:6–11. PMID:15148294, http://dx.doi.org/10.1161/01.HYP.0000130484.20501.df.
9. Jin M, Khan AI. Procalcitonin: uses in the clinical laboratory for the diagnosis of Sepsis. Lab Med. 2010;41:173–7.
10. Davies J. Procalcitonin. J Clin Pathol. 2015;68:675–9. PMID:26124314, http://dx.doi.org/10.1136/jclinpath-2014-202807.
11. Meisner M. Update on procalcitonin measurements. Ann Lab Med. 2014;34: 263–73. PMID:24982830, http://dx.doi.org/10.3343/alm.2014.34.4.263.
12. Müller B, Harbarth S, Stolz D, Bingisser R, Mueller C, Leuppi J, et al. Diagnostic and prognostic accuracy of clinical and laboratory parameters in community-acquired pneumonia. BMC Infect Dis. 2007;7:10. PMID:17335562, http://dx.doi.org/10.1186/1471-2334-7-10.
13. Christ-Crain M, Opal SM. Clinical review: the role of biomarkers in the diagnosis and management of community-acquired pneumonia. Crit Care. 2010;14:203. PMID:20236471, http://dx.doi.org/10.1186/cc8155.
14. Coelho LM, Salluh JI, Soares M, Bozza FA, Verdeal JC, Castro-Faria-Neto HC, et al. Patterns of c-reactive protein RATIO response in severe community-acquired pneumonia: a cohort study. Crit Care. 2012;16:R53. PMID:22449513, http://dx.doi.org/10.1186/cc11291.
15. Schuetz P, Christ-Crain M, Thomann R, Falconnier C, Wolbers M, Widmer I, ProHOSP Study Group, et al. Effect of procalcitonin-based guidelines vs standard guidelines on antibiotic use in lower respiratory tract infections: the ProHOSP randomized controlled trial. JAMA. 2009;302:1059–66. PMID:19738090, http://dx.doi.org/10.1001/jama.2009.1297.
16. Schuetz P, Christ-Crain M, Wolbers M, Schild U, Thomann R, Falconnier C, ProHOSP study group, et al. Procalcitonin guided antibiotic therapy and hospitalization in patients with lower respiratory tract infections: a prospective, multicenter, randomized controlled trial. BMC Health Serv Res. 2007;7:102. http://dx.doi.org/10.1186/1472-6963-7-102. PMID:17615073.
17. Schuetz P, Chiappa V, Briel M, Greenwald JL. Procalcitonin algorithms for antibiotic therapy decisions: a systematic review of randomized controlled trials and recommendations for clinical algorithms. Arch Intern Med. 2011; 171:1322–31. PMID:21824946, http://dx.doi.org/10.1001/archinternmed.2011.318.
18. Briel M, Schuetz P, Mueller B, Young J, Schild U, Nusbaumer C, et al. Procalcitonin-guided antibiotic use vs a standard approach for acute respiratory tract infections in primary care. Arch Intern Med. 2008;168:2000–7. PMID:18852401, http://dx.doi.org/10.1001/archinte.168.18.2000.
19. Jain S, Self WH, Wunderink RG, Fakhran S, Balk R, Bramley AM, CDC EPIC Study Team, et al. Community-acquired pneumonia requiring hospitalization among U.S. adults. N Engl J Med. 2015;373:415–27. PMID:26172429, http://dx.doi.org/10.1056/NEJMoa1500245.
20. Schuetz P, Müller B, Christ-Crain M, Stolz D, Tamm M, Bouadma L, et al. Procalcitonin to initiate or discontinue antibiotics in acute respiratory tract infections. Cochrane Database Syst Rev. 2012;9:CD007498. PMID:22972110.
21. Tokman S, Barnett CF, Jarlsberg LG, Taub PR, den Boon S, Davis JL, International HIV-Associated Opportunistic Pneumonias (IHOP) Study Group, et al. Procalcitonin predicts mortality in HIV-infected Ugandan adults with lower respiratory tract infections. Respirology. 2014;19:382–8. PMID:24460728, http://dx.doi.org/10.1111/resp.12237.
22. Schuetz P, Suter-Widmer I, Chaudri A, Christ-Crain M, Zimmerli W, Mueller B, Procalcitonin-Guided Antibiotic Therapy and Hospitalisation in Patients with Lower Respiratory Tract Infections (ProHOSP) Study Group. Prognostic value of procalcitonin in community-acquired pneumonia. Eur Respir J. 2011;37: 384–92. PMID:20595156, http://dx.doi.org/10.1183/09031936.00035610.
23. Skouras V, Boultadakis E, Nikoulis D, Polychronopoulos V, Daniil Z, Kalomenidis I, et al. Prognostic value of C-reactive protein in parapneumonic effusions. Respirology. 2012;17:308–14. PMID:21995428, http://dx.doi.org/10.1111/j.1440-1843.2011.02078.x.
24. Light RW, Girard WM, Jenkinson SG, George RB. Parapneumonic effusions. Am J Med. 1980;69:507–12. PMID:7424940, http://dx.doi.org/10.1016/0002-9343(80)90460-X.
25. Chalmers JD, Singanayagam A, Murray MP, Scally C, Fawzi A, Hill AT. Risk factors for complicated parapneumonic effusion and empyema on presentation to hospital with community-acquired pneumonia. Thorax. 2009;64:592–7. PMID:19131449, http://dx.doi.org/10.1136/thx.2008.105080.
26. Hirata Y, Mitaka C, Sato K, et al. Increased circulating adrenomedullin, a novel vasodilatory peptide, in sepsis. J Clin Endocrinol Metab. 1996;81:1449–53.
27. España PP, Capelastegui A, Mar C, Bilbao A, Quintana JM, Diez R, et al. Performance of pro-adrenomedullin for identifying adverse outcomes in community-acquired pneumonia. J Infect. 2015;70:457–66. PMID:25499199, http://dx.doi.org/10.1016/j.jinf.2014.12.003.
28. Christ-Crain M, Morgenthaler NG, Stolz D, Müller C, Bingisser R, Harbarth S, et al. Pro-adrenomedullin to predict severity and outcome in community-acquired pneumonia. [ISRCTN04176397]. Crit Care. 2006;10:R96. PMID:16805922 http://dx.doi.org/10.1186/cc4955.
29. Krüger S, Ewig S, Giersdorf S, Hartmann O, Suttorp N, Welte T, Competence Network for the Study of Community Acquired Pneumonia (CAPNETZ) Study Group. Cardiovascular and inflammatory biomarkers to predict short- and long-term survival in community-acquired pneumonia: results from the German Competence Network, CAPNETZ. Am J Respir Crit Care Med. 2010; 182(11):1426e34.
30. Cavallazzi R, El-Kersh K, Abu-Atherah E, et al. Midregional proadrenomedullin for prognosis in community-acquired pneumonia: A systematic review. Resp Med. 2014;108:1569–158031.
31. Scicluna BP, Klein Klouwenberg PMC, van Vught LA, et al. A molecular biomarker to diagnose community-acquired pneumonia on intensive care unit admission. Am J Respir Crit Care Med. 2015;192:826–35.
32. Nickler M, Ottiger M, Steuer C, Huber A, Byron Anderson J, et al. Systematic review regarding metabolic profiling for improved pathophysiological understanding of disease and outcome prediction in respiratory infections. Respir Res. 2015;16:125. doi:10.1186/s12931-015-0283-6.
33. Suzuki Y, Suda T, Yokomura K, Suzuki M, Fujie M, Furuhashi K, et al. Serum activity of indoleamine 2,3-dioxygenase predicts prognosis of community acquired pneumonia. J Infect. 2011;63(3):215–22.
34. Darcy CJ, Davis JS, Woodberry T, McNeil YR, Stephens DP, Yeo TW, et al. An observational cohort study of the kynurenine to tryptophan ratio in sepsis: association with impaired immune and microvascular function. PLoS One. 2011;6(6):e21185.
35. Chen YX, Li CS. Lactate on emergency department arrival as a predictor of mortality and site-of-care in pneumonia patients: a cohort study. Thorax. 2015;70(5):404–10.

12

Risk factors for community-acquired pneumonia among adults in Kenya

Esther Muthumbi[1*], Brett S. Lowe[1,2], Cyprian Muyodi[3], Esther Getambu[3], Fergus Gleeson[4] and J. Anthony G. Scott[1,5]

Abstract

Background: Pneumonia is a leading cause of morbidity and mortality among adults worldwide; however, the risk factors for community-acquired pneumonia in Africa are not well characterized.

Methods: The authors recruited 281 cases of community-acquired pneumonia and 1202 hospital controls among patients aged ≥15 years who attended Kilifi District Hospital/Coast Provincial General Hospital in Kenya between 1994 and 6. Cases were admissions with an acute illness with ≥2 respiratory signs and evidence of consolidation on a chest radiograph. Controls were patients without signs of pneumonia, frequency matched by age, sex and hospital. Risk factors related to socio-demographic factors, drug use, clinical history, contact patterns and exposures to indoor air pollution were investigated by questionnaire, anthropometric measurements and laboratory assays. Associations were evaluated using a hierarchical logistic regression model.

Results: Pneumonia was associated with human immunodeficiency virus (HIV) infection (Odds Ratio [OR] 2.06, 95% CI 1.44–3.08), anemia (OR 1.91, 1.31–2.74), splenomegaly (OR 2.04, 95% CI 1.14–3.41), recent history of pneumonia (OR 4.65, 95% CI 1.66–12.5), history of pneumonia >2 years previously (OR 17.13, 95% CI 5.01–60.26), coryza in the 2 weeks preceding hospitalization (OR 2.09, 95% CI 1.44–3.03), current smoking (2.19, 95% CI 1.39–3.70), use of khat (OR 3.44, 95% CI 1.72–7.15), use of snuff (OR 2.67, 95% CI 1.35–5.49) and contact with several animal species. Presence of a Bacillus Calmette-Guerin (BCG) scar was associated with protection (OR 0.51, 95% CI 0.32–0.82). The risk factors varied significantly by sex.

Conclusion: Pneumonia in Kenyan adults was associated with global risk factors, such as HIV and smoking, but also with specific local factors like drug use and contact with animals. Intervention strategies should account for sex-specific differences in risk factors.

Keywords: Community acquired pneumonia, Adults, Africa, Risk factors, Air pollution

Background

Community-acquired pneumonia (CAP) is a common cause of morbidity and mortality worldwide. In Africa, CAP is associated with an in-hospital mortality of 6–15% among adults, as reported from hospital-based studies [1–3].

Studies from high-income countries have identified several risk factors for CAP including smoking [4–7], age > 65 years [4, 8, 9], immunosuppression by any cause [8], underlying lung diseases such as chronic obstructive pulmonary disease (COPD) [7–10], recent viral upper respiratory infections (URTI) [11–13] and the presence of co-morbidities [6]. In addition, low body-mass index (BMI), contact with children and poor dental hygiene were identified as risk factors for CAP in a systematic literature review and meta-analysis from studies in Europe [5].

Different environmental and socio-economic circumstances in sub-Saharan Africa are likely to give rise to different risks for pneumonia, including younger age at presentation, which has been observed [14]. There is a

* Correspondence: emuthumbi@kemri-wellcome.org
[1]KEMRI-Wellcome Trust Research Programme, Center for Geographical Medicine Research Coast, Kilifi, Kenya
Full list of author information is available at the end of the article

single published study of pneumonia risk factors in tropical Africa, which is confined to human immunodeficiency virus (HIV)-infected adults in Kenya. This identified additional risk factors as being single, widowed or divorced (i.e. not married), being of low socio-economic status and experiencing overcrowding in the home [15]. Here the authors present an analysis of a previously unpublished dataset from 1994 to 1996, exploring the risk factors for pneumonia among adults in Kenya.

Methods

Study design

This case–control study was conducted at Kilifi District Hospital (KDH), and Coast Provincial General Hospital (CPGH) in Kenya among patients who presented either to the outpatient clinic or the casualty department. Cases were adult patients aged ≥15 years who were admitted with CAP. CAP was defined as an acute illness (<14 days), characterized by at least two respiratory symptoms (cough, sputum, breathlessness, chest pain, hemoptysis or fever) and evidence of consolidation on a chest radiograph. The radiographs were read by a study physician and later confirmed, independently, by a consultant thoracic radiologist.

Controls were adults aged ≥15 years who presented to the outpatient clinics of the same hospitals who did not meet the clinical case definition of CAP. They were frequency matched on age, sex and hospital of presentation in a ratio of 4:1 with cases. Controls with diagnoses that were strongly associated with the exposures of interest (e.g. meningitis, septicemia, tuberculosis, Kaposi's sarcoma, sickle cell crisis, diabetic ketoacidosis or oropharyngeal candidiasis) were excluded.

A target sample size of 1500 (300 cases: 1200 controls) was sought for the study. The study was powered to detect relevant odds ratios using a range of prevalence estimates for a wide variety of exposures included in the study (Additional file 1).

Study procedures

Patients were questioned on clinical history, lifestyle habits and contact history using a standard questionnaire. Anthropometry and a physical examination were performed for all participants in a standardized manner. Venous blood was collected and tested for HIV-1 antibodies by enzyme-linked immunosorbent assay (ELISA), malaria parasites by microscopy, and sickle cell status. A full hemogram, glycosylated hemoglobin (HbA1C) test and blood grouping (ABO) were also performed.

Statistical analysis

Associations with case status were analyzed using logistic regression, adjusting for the matching variables (age, sex and route of presentation) in each model. Because this was the first study of risk factors for pneumonia in an unselected population in Africa, a wide range of potential exposures were explored. A hierarchical process was used to define the final model, whereby related exposures were first examined in intermediary models before the best representative exposures were selected for a final, multi-variable model. The intermediary models examined 5 categories of related variables (Table 1). Within each category, univariate analysis was performed and variables were selected with a likelihood ratio (LR) p-value of <0.1 to include in the intermediary multivariable model. Risk factors contributing significantly (LR test, p = <0.05) to the intermediary multivariable models were subsequently included in a final multivariable model. Backward stepwise analysis was used in each of the multivariable analyses. In addition, prompted by the presence of sex-specific exposures (e.g. pregnancy) and several instances of effect modification due to sex, two sex-restricted models were developed following a similar hierarchical process.

Some variables, e.g. BMI and presence of a scar following Bacillus Calmette-Guerin (BCG) vaccine, were introduced shortly after the study had begun, leading to some missing data (Additional file 1). However, this is unlikely to have caused bias unless there was a systematic difference in the

Table 1 Variable categories for the intermediary logistic regression models

Group name	Variables
Socio-demographic variables	Ethnic group, religion, recent immigration, years of education, monthly income, type of house and employment status
Contact variables	Number of children in the household, contact with children of different ages, with or without an URTI, number of adults in the household, size of house, hours of childcare, sharing a room with children when sleeping, contact with a case of pneumonia, recent travel beyond the immediate residential vicinity, use of public minibuses for transport (matatu), frequenting social places and contact with selected animals, working and living in different locations
Drug use	Quantified alcohol consumption and use of traditional brews (matingas, busaa, changaa, mnazi, muratina), quantified present and past cigarette smoking, use of ground tobacco (snuff), use of Khat (miraa).
Indoor air pollution	Exposure to cooking fuel smoke in the home, use of mosquito coils, ventilation in the cooking room, use of air conditioning, passive smoking and occupational exposure during welding
Clinical variables	Chronic bronchitis, recent history of viral URTI (<14 days), previous history of pulmonary TB, previous pneumonia, body mass index, mid upper-arm circumference, anemia, splenomegaly, malaria parasitemia, sickle cell status, HIV sero-positivity, ABO blood group, Glycosylated hemoglobin (HbA1c) and current pregnancy status.

HIV, human immunodeficiency virus; TB, tuberculosis; URTI, upper respiratory tract infection admissions across the time periods of the study; therefore, data imputation was not used.

All statistical analysis were performed using STATA V.13 (Stata Corp, College Station, Texas, United States [US]).

Results

Between March 1994 and May 1996, 301 cases and 1202 controls were recruited. After review of the chest radiographs by the radiologist, 20 of the original cases were excluded as non-CAP. Among the 281 remaining cases, 177 (63%) were male and 22 (7.8%) were aged ≥55 years. The matching achieved a similar distribution of age, sex and route of recruitment across cases and controls (Table 2). Among controls, malaria was the most common presenting diagnosis, accounting for 26% (316/1202, Additional file 1: Table S3).

The results of the univariate analysis for 72 variables, by category of exposure, are listed in the Additional file 1: Tables S4–S8. In Table 3 the results of the intermediary and final adjusted models are presented for 25 variables, with significant results at the intermediary model stage.

Clinical factors

Previous history of pneumonia was a major risk factor for current pneumonia. This risk was almost 20-fold higher among those whose history of pneumonia was more than 2 years ago (Table 3). History of previous URTI, HIV infection, splenomegaly and anemia were all associated with a 2-fold increase in risk of pneumonia; HIV was present in 30% (356/1202) of the controls. Malaria and presence of a BCG scar was associated with a reduced risk of pneumonia. The risk of pneumonia was reduced by 35% for every cm increase in mid-upper arm circumference (MUAC, Table 3, Additional file 1: Table S4). For most of the significant clinical variables, there was no evidence of confounding by variables in other categories as the effect sizes varied little between intermediary and final models. Of note from the univariate analyses, there was no association between pneumonia and sickle cell trait, Blood group A or history of previous tuberculosis (Additional file 1: Table S4).

Table 2 Distribution of matching variables across cases and controls

Matching variable	Categories	Cases	%	Controls	%
Sex	Male	177	63%	749	62%
	Female	104	37%	453	38%
Age group	15–24	65	23%	267	22%
	25–29	48	17%	265	22%
	30–34	63	22%	193	16%
	35–44	61	22%	255	21%
	45–54	22	8%	110	9%
Route of recruitment	CPGH Filter clinic	45	16%	214	18%
	CPGH Casualty	188	67%	785	65%
	Kilifi District Hospital	48	17%	203	17%

Socio-demographic factors

In the intermediate model, pneumonia was inversely associated with the number of years in education and with current employment. However, these associations did not remain significant in the final model. In the univariate analysis, there was no evidence of an association between pneumonia and ethnicity, religion or economic status measured either as amount of income or type of roofing (Additional file 1: Table S5).

Air pollution and related factors

Among a wide range of air-pollution variables, only two were significant in the univariate analyses; cooking in a room with only one ventilation exit (the door) was more common among cases; cooking for oneself was more common among controls (Additional file 1: Table S6). Pneumonia was not associated with indoor cooking, nor sleeping in the cooking room, nor with the type of fuel used for cooking.

Drug use and related factors

The prevalence of drug use differed by sex. Males accounted for 87% (268/307) of alcohol consumers and 97% (312/321) of current smokers. Females were the largest consumers of snuff (60% vs. 40% in males), but did not report consumption of *busaa* and *matingas* (traditional brews). Current smokers and ex-smokers had a 2-fold increased risk of pneumonia compared to never-smokers; recent ex-smokers had a 10-fold increase in risk (Table 3). There was no evidence of increased risk with an increase in smoking pack-years. Passive smoking and alcohol intake were not associated with pneumonia.

Contact patterns

Exposure to animals was reported in 43% (519/1202) of the controls. Significant associations in the intermediary model included exposure to monkeys, chickens, ducks and goats, of which only the latter two remained significant in the final model (Table 3). Adults frequenting cafés or working at a different location from home were at slightly increased risk of pneumonia; those using public minibuses (matatus) or visiting nightclubs had lower risks of pneumonia. In the univariate analysis, pneumonia was associated with the total number of other people in the home, and with the number of co-resident girls aged <5y. Contact with a child under the age of 5 years with coryza or sleeping in the same room as a child were not associated with pneumonia.

Table 3 Risk factors for pneumonia in intermediate and final regression models

	Observed results				Intermediate models		Final model		
Variable	Control	%	Case	%	aOR[a]	95% CI	aOR[b]	95% CI	*p*-value
Clinical									
HIV infection	356	30.3	147	52.3	2.13	(1.48, 3.07)	2.06	(1.44,3.08)	<0.001
History of coryza	283	23.5	120	43.2	2.3	(1.62,3.26)	2.09	(1.44,3.03)	<0.001
Splenomegaly	81	6.8	46	17.2	2.34	(1.44,3.81)	2.04	(1.17,3.41)	0.009
Anaemia	607	51.1	202	72.4	1.88	(1.31,2.68)	1.91	(1.31,2.74)	0.001
Malaria	155	13.2	9	3.2	0.17	(0.08,0.36)	0.12	(0.06,0.29)	<0.001
Presence of BCG scar	1030	88	207	81.5	0.58	(0.37,0.90)	0.51	(0.32,0.82)	0.005
History of previous pneumonia									
None	1180	98.3	248	89.21	1		1		<0.001
> 2 yrs. ago	4	0.3	17	6.1	20.39	(5.08, 81.79)	17.13	(5.01, 60.26)	
< 2 yrs. ago	16	1.3	13	4.7	5.26	(1.86, 14.84)	4.65	(1.66, 12.54)	
HbA1C									
< 4.0	677	60.2	141	52.4	0.7	(0.64, 1.69)	–		
4.0–5.6	397	35.3	118	43.4	1		–		
5.7–6.4	29	2.6	3	1.1	0.27	(0.07, 1.00)	–		
> 6.5	21	1.9	7	2.6	1.15	(0.35, 3.72)	–		
MUAC									
< 22	200	16.8	65	24.1	1		1		<0.001
22–23	179	15	86	31.9	1.45	(0.99, 2.13)	1.92	(1.19, 3.11)	
24–25	239	20.1	65	24.1	0.8	(0.53, 1.20)	1.02	(0.62, 1.67)	
26–27	292	24.5	34	12.6	0.34	(0.21, 0.53)	0.53	(0.30, 0.94)	
28+	281	23.6	20	7.4	0.21	(0.12, 0.35)	0.38	(0.20, 0.72)	
Socio-demographic									
Level of education									
None	221	18.4	72	25.9	1				
1–6 years	244	20.3	63	22.7	0.61	(0.40, 0.93)	–		
Primary	313	26	65	23.4	0.44	(0.28, 0.68)	–		
Secondary	310	25.8	64	23	0.41	(0.26, 0.65)	–		
Tertiary	114	9.5	14	5	0.26	(0.13, 0.51)	–		
Employment Status									
Unemployed	423	35.2	86	30.9	1				
Employed	715	59.5	187	67.3	1.47	(1.05, 2.05)	–		
In Education	64	5.3	5	1.8	0.43	(0.16, 1.14)	–		
Air pollution									
More than one ventilations in cooking room[c] (*n* = 1036)	812	78.4	171	70.1	0.61	(0.44, 0.85)	–		
Drugs									
Smoking									
None smoker	697	58	117	42.1	1				<0.001
Passive smoker	177	14.7	31	11.2	0.92	(0.59, 1.44)	0.86	(0.51, 1.57)	
Ex-smoker	88	7.3	31	11.2	2.9	(1.76, 4.77)	2.44	(1.38, 4.72)	
Recent ex-smoker	12	1	12	4.3	7.57	(3.19, 17.98)	10.4	(3.49, 35.38)	
Current smoker	228	19	87	31.3	2.24	(1.48, 3.40)	2.19	(1.39, 3.70)	

Table 3 Risk factors for pneumonia in intermediate and final regression models *(Continued)*

	Observed results				Intermediate models		Final model		
Variable	Control	%	Case	%	aOR[a]	95% CI	aOR[b]	95% CI	*p*-value
Smoking pack years									
0	885	80.3	153	65.1	1				
1–5	113	10.3	36	15.3	1.82	(1.11, 2.99)	–		
6–10	50	4.5	22	9.4	2.11	(1.11, 4.01)	–		
11–15	28	2.5	8	3.4	1.47	(0.60, 3.62)	–		
16–20	11	1	11	4.7	4.53	(1.73, 11.83)	–		
20+	15	1.4	5	2.1	2.16	(0.71, 6.58)	–		
Khat	42	3.5	31	11.2	2.42	(1.40, 4.18)	3.44	(1.72, 7.15)	<0.001
Snuff	48	4	23	8.3	2.79	(1.57, 4.99)	2.67	(1.35, 5.49)	0.005
Muratina	2	0.2	4	1.4	8.61	(1.42, 52.2)	–		
Alcohol	218	18.1	84	30.2	1.46	(1.01, 2.08)	–		
Contacts									
Work and lives in different locations	317	26.4	87	31.3	1.49	(1.08, 2.07)	1.66	(1.13, 2.57)	0.011
Visited a disco in the last 2 weeks	36	3	3	1.1	0.29	(0.08, 0.97)	0.16	(0.05, 0.81)	0.024
Visited a café in last 2 weeks	131	10.9	53	19.1	2.31	(1.57, 3.40)	1.82	(1.08, 2.85)	0.024
Used a matatu in last 2 weeks	947	78.9	199	71.6	0.59	(0.43, 0.81)	0.46	(0.31, 0.68)	<0.001
Exposure to ducks	12	1	9	3.2	3.03	(1.18, 7.78)	4.14	(1.28, 13.46)	0.018
Exposure to goats	219	18.2	76	27.3	1.56	(1.09, 2.23)	1.69	(1.16, 2.59)	0.007
Exposure to chickens	471	39.2	143	51.4	1.48	(1.08, 2.03)	–		
Exposure to monkeys	3	0.2	5	1.8	8.73	(1.92, 39.63)	–		

OR = Odds Ratio; aOR = adjusted odds ratio;
[a]first stage multivariable model adjusted results (within-category)
[b]second stage multivariable model adjusted results
[c]among those cooking indoors

Risk factors by sex

After restricting the analysis by sex, HIV infection, history of coryza, splenomegaly and anemia were independent risk factors shared by both sexes (Table 4). Decreasing MUAC, history of tuberculosis, smoking, use of khat and exposure to chickens were risk factors unique to males. Among females, use of snuff and exposure to ducks and sheep were unique risk factors. The presence of a BCG scar was a protective factor among males only.

Discussion

These results suggest that several of the risk factors for pneumonia are common to both developed and developing countries. These include smoking tobacco, exposure to animals, recent URTI and anemia. The results have also identified novel modifiable risk factors, such as the use of snuff (ground tobacco) and khat, which are particular to this population.

Smoking is a well-established risk factor for CAP [7, 16]. The risk was highest among recent ex-smokers; this was interpreted to mean that their decision to stop smoking was influenced by an ailing respiratory system—a form of reverse causality. Passive smoking was not associated with an increased risk of pneumonia. Passive cigarette smoke exposure is a known risk factor for lower respiratory tract infections (LRTIs) among children [16–18], but not among adults.

Use of snuff and khat are novel associations found among women and men, respectively. Snuff use is a risk factor for oral cancer [19], while khat, a natural amphetamine, is associated with a range of effects from tooth decay to psychosis [20–22]. Khat, *Catha edulis* Forsk, is a shrub whose leaves and twigs are chewed for their stimulant effect and there is no obvious biological explanation of this association. Overall, however, drug use appeared to be a major avoidable risk factor.

History of coryza (representing URTIs) was associated with pneumonia [11]. Viral URTIs suppress immune function leading to increased susceptibility to secondary infections. Influenza vaccine can reduce both primary pneumonia and secondary bacterial pneumonia [23–26], and may be useful to prevent CAP in adults.

Patients with a previous history of pneumonia were at a higher risk of CAP in the current study, especially those whose initial episode occurred more than 2 years previously; in previous studies the risk was higher for

Table 4 Risk factors for pneumonia by sex

	MALE			FEMALE		
Variable	aOR	95% CI	*p*-value	aOR	95% CI	*p*-value
Clinical						
HIV-infected	2.67	(1.51, 4.71)	0.001	3.06	(1.66, 5.64)	<0.001
History of coryza	2.36	(1.42, 3.92)	0.001	2.30	(1.26, 4.18)	0.006
Splenomegaly	2.24	(1.07, 4.72)	0.033	3.44	(1.55, 7.64)	0.002
Anemia	2.32	(1.34, 4.00)	0.003	3.25	(1.70, 6.20)	<0.001
Malaria	0.04	(0.01, 0.16)	<0.001	0.15	(0.05, 0.48)	0.001
Presence of BCG scar	0.33	(0.16, 0.69)	0.003			
Previous history of pneumonia						
Pneumonia >2 yrs. ago	8.35	(1.07, 65.25)	<0.001	26.57	(4.80, 147.21)	<0.001
Pneumonia <2 yrs. ago	17.99	(3.77, 85.73)		3.19	(0.63, 16.18)	
Previous history of TB infection						
TB >2 yrs. ago	4.38	(1.18, 16.31)	0.033	–		
TB <2 yrs. ago	7.51	(0.72, 77.95)		–		
MUAC						
< 22	1		<0.001	–		
22–23	2.60	(1.26, 5.36)		–		
24–25	0.94	(0.44, 2.00)				
26–27	0.47	(0.20, 1.10)		–		
28+	0.18	(0.07, 0.48)		–		
Drugs						
Smoking			0.001			
Passive smoker	2.12	(0.68, 6.68)		–		
Ex-smoker	3.00	(1.37, 6.54)		–		
Recent ex-smoker	13.06	(2.86, 59.58)		–		
Current smoker	2.79	(1.57, 4.98)		–		
Khat (miraa)	4.85	(2.07, 11.38)	<0.001	–		
Snuff	–			4.34	(1.87, 10.05)	0.001
Contact						
Exposure to chickens	2.47	(1.46, 4.17)	0.001			
Exposure to ducks	–			7.59	(1.47, 39.16)	0.015
Exposure to sheep	–			6.91	(1.02, 46.69)	0.047

HIV, human immunodeficiency virus; MUAC, middle upper arm circumference; TB, tuberculosis

more recent episodes [7]. Childhood pneumonia is associated with development of chronic lung disease and later hospitalizations with pneumonia [27–29] and in this study, 40% of cases were <30 years of age. In addition, patients with recent episodes of pneumonia are more likely to recognize the symptoms and the seriousness of the illness, and therefore more likely to seek early treatment, averting hospital admission. In Kenya, pneumococcal vaccines are rarely used in adults; however, post-hospitalization vaccination could potentially reduce the rate of recurrence with pneumonia [30].

The authors found that low social economic status (SES), measured directly by level of income and indirectly by proxy measures like the materials used for house construction, was not associated with pneumonia. However, higher education, increased use of *matatus* (minibuses for public transport) and frequent visits to a nightclub, which are all likely to be indicators of higher SES, were associated with a reduced risk of disease despite also implying more human contact and therefore, potentially, a greater risk of infection.

Indoor air pollution is a leading risk factor for respiratory diseases [31], including pneumonia, in children [32–34] though evidence in adults is weak [35]. In this study, exposure to air pollution, including biomass fuels, was not associated with an increased risk of pneumonia.

However, this study relied upon questionnaire methods to ascertain exposure to air pollution and this is likely to admit significant misclassification. More direct measurements of air quality would be useful to estimate the role of this risk factor [36].

As in other studies from developed countries [37, 38], HIV infection was associated with a 2-fold increase in risk of CAP. This effect size is likely to be an underestimate due to the use of hospital controls, despite attempts to exclude from the control population those with HIV-related diseases. The prevalence of HIV among controls was 30.3%; population-based estimates of HIV sero-prevalence at the same time were 7.5% [39]. Use of hospital controls also explains the seemingly protective effect of malaria infection. Infection with malaria parasites in the tropics is a common cause of presentation to hospitals with non-pneumonia syndromes. Interestingly, markers of chronic malaria infection, anemia and splenomegaly were strongly associated with pneumonia, suggesting that chronic or recurrent malaria may in fact be a risk factor for pneumonia, although splenomegaly may also be a marker of HIV or tuberculosis, both common in this population.

Evidence of BCG vaccination was associated with a 70% reduction in risk of pneumonia among men. The effect in women was smaller and non-significant. In the complementary study of pneumonia etiology conducted in the same cases, *Mycobacterium tuberculosis* was found in 9% [1]. Several vaccines have demonstrated non-specific protective and harmful effects, which differ by sex [40, 41]. For example, those who develop a BCG scar following vaccination are known to be less likely to get sepsis, with the beneficial effect occurring predominantly in girls [42]. These benefits have been observed to extend into adulthood [43]. The WHO suggests these heterologous effects of vaccines are intriguing, currently inexplicable and "warrant further research" [44].

The limitation of this study is that it is an analysis of historical data and therefore, due to changes in epidemiology in the ensuing years, the relative importance of some of the observations may have changed. First, several risk factors that were identified have changed in prevalence; for example, HIV-infection and malaria have both declined and smoking has increased. While this alters the public health importance of these factors and invalidates any attempt to calculate the current population-attributable fraction for pneumonia, it does not invalidate the etiological association.

Second, temporal changes may have modified the effect of risk factors; for example, the introduction of anti-retroviral therapy reduces the risk of pneumonia in HIV-infected individuals [45, 46]. Third, changes in urbanization and lifestyle habits may have introduced new risk factors for pneumonia, which are not captured by the dataset that has been analyzed. Nonetheless, historical data such as these can offer unique insights into the epidemiology of pneumonia and can stimulate and inform new studies.

The authors believe this is the only case–control study on the risk factors of CAP ever conducted in an unselected adult population in Africa. As the major risk factors were unknown at the outset, the study examined many different exposures simultaneously. Although this leads to a risk of false-positive associations, the purpose was to scan a broad range of potential risks that could be explored and confirmed in subsequent focused studies. As such, several key risk factors have been identified that are amenable to vaccination or to changes in lifestyle habits. Furthermore, in this setting the study has demonstrated that the risk factors for pneumonia among men and women were sufficiently different that they should be investigated and managed separately.

Conclusion

This study was designed as a hypothesis-generating study. It has identified a number of potential risk factors that suggest that interventions that induce changes in lifestyle habits (especially smoking and the use of other drugs) may have a beneficial impact on the incidence of pneumonia in this population—these are worth considering in confirmatory studies. Previous history of pneumonia was the strongest risk factor of all in this study, suggesting a target for post-discharge vaccination.

Acknowledgements

We would like to thank the nursing and clinical staff of Coast Provincial General Hospital and Kilifi District Hospital, and the patients and their families. This paper is published with the approval of the Director, Kenya Medical Research Institute.

Funding

The work was supported by the Wellcome Trust through fellowship support for JAS (098532).

Authors' contributions

EM conducted the data analysis and wrote the manuscript. BL, CM, EG coordinated the hospital and lab aspects of the study. FG read and interpreted the radiographs. JAS conceived the study, coordinated the data collection and has contributed to data analysis and manuscript writing. All authors read and approved the final manuscript.

Competing interests

The authors declare that they have no competing interests.

Author details

[1]KEMRI-Wellcome Trust Research Programme, Center for Geographical Medicine Research Coast, Kilifi, Kenya. [2]Centre for Tropical Medicine & Global Health, University of Oxford, Oxford, UK. [3]Coast Provincial General Hospital, Mombasa, Kenya. [4]Department of Radiology, Churchill Hospital, University of Oxford, Oxford, UK. [5]Department of Infectious Disease Epidemiology, London School of Hygiene & Tropical Medicine, London, UK.

References

1. Scott JA, Hall AJ, Muyodi C, Lowe B, Ross M, Chohan B, et al. Aetiology, outcome, and risk factors for mortality among adults with acute pneumonia in Kenya. Lancet. 2000;355(9211):1225–30.
2. Yone EW, Balkissou AD, Kengne AP, Kuaban C. Influence of HIV infection on the clinical presentation and outcome of adults with acute community-acquired pneumonia in Yaounde, Cameroon: a retrospective hospital-based study. BMC Pulm Med. 2012;12:46.
3. Sow O, Frechet M, Diallo AA, Soumah S, Conde MK, Diot P, et al. Community acquired pneumonia in adults: a study comparing clinical features and outcome in Africa (Republic of Guinea) and Europe (France). Thorax. 1996;51(4):385–8.
4. Farr BM, Bartlett CL, Wadsworth J, Miller DL. Risk factors for community-acquired pneumonia diagnosed upon hospital admission. British Thoracic Society pneumonia study group. Respir Med. 2000;94(10):954–63.
5. Torres A, Peetermans WE, Viegi G, Blasi F. Risk factors for community-acquired pneumonia in adults in Europe: a literature review. Thorax. 2013;68(11):1057–65.
6. Baik I, Curhan GC, Rimm EB, Bendich A, Willett WC, Fawzi WWA. Prospective study of age and lifestyle factors in relation to community-acquired pneumonia in US men and women. Arch Intern Med. 2000;160(20):3082–8.
7. Almirall J, Bolibar I, Balanzo X, Gonzalez CA. Risk factors for community-acquired pneumonia in adults: a population-based case–control study. Eur Respir J. 1999;13(2):349–55.
8. Koivula I, Sten M, Makela PH. Risk factors for pneumonia in the elderly. Am J Med. 1994;96(4):313–20.
9. Farr BM, Woodhead MA, Macfarlane JT, Bartlett CL, McCraken JS, Wadsworth J, et al. Risk factors for community-acquired pneumonia diagnosed by general practitioners in the community. Respir Med. 2000;94(5):422–7.
10. Mannino DM, Davis KJ, Kiri VA. Chronic obstructive pulmonary disease and hospitalizations for pneumonia in a US cohort. Respir Med. 2009;103(2):224–9.
11. Rose RM, Pinkston P, O'Donnell C, Jensen WA. Viral infection of the lower respiratory tract. Clin Chest Med. 1987;8(3):405–18.
12. Bosch AA, Biesbroek G, Trzcinski K, Sanders EA, Bogaert D. Viral and bacterial interactions in the upper respiratory tract. PLoS Pathog. 2013;9(1):e1003057.
13. Weinberger DM, Klugman KP, Steiner CA, Simonsen L, Viboud C. Association between respiratory syncytial virus activity and pneumococcal disease in infants: a time series analysis of US hospitalization data. PLoS Med. 2015;12(1):e1001776.
14. Aston SJ, Rylance J. Community-acquired pneumonia in sub-Saharan Africa. Semin Respir Crit Care Med. 2016;37(6):855–67.
15. Penner J, Meier AS, Mwachari C, Ayuka F, Muchina B, Odhiambo J, et al. Risk factors for pneumonia in urban-dwelling HIV-infected women: a case–control study in Nairobi, Kenya. J Acquir Immune Defic Syndr. 2003;32(2):223–8.
16. Chen Y, Li W, Influence YS. Of passive smoking on admissions for respiratory illness in early childhood. Br Med J (Clin Res Ed). 1986;293(6542):303–6.
17. Fergusson DM, Horwood LJ, Shannon FT, Taylor B. Parental smoking and lower respiratory illness in the first three years of life. J Epidemiol Community Health. 1981;35(3):180–4.
18. Strachan DP, Cook DG. Health effects of passive smoking. 1. Parental smoking and lower respiratory illness in infancy and early childhood. Thorax. 1997;52(10):905–1.
19. Pershagen G. Smokeless tobacco. Br Med Bull. 1996;52(1):50–7.
20. Odenwald M, Neuner F, Schauer M, Elbert T, Catani C, Lingenfelder B, et al. Khat use as risk factor for psychotic disorders: a cross-sectional and case–control study in Somalia. BMC Med. 2005;3:5.
21. Patel NB. "Natural amphetamine" Khat: a cultural tradition or a drug of abuse. Int Rev Neurobiol. 2015;120:235–55.
22. Pantelis C, Hindler CG, Taylor JC. Use and abuse of khat (Catha Edulis): a review of the distribution, pharmacology, side effects and a description of psychosis attributed to khat chewing. Psychol Med. 1989;19(3):657–68.
23. Grijalva CG, Zhu Y, Williams DJ, Self WH, Ampofo K, Pavia AT, et al. Association between hospitalization with community-acquired laboratory-confirmed influenza pneumonia and prior receipt of influenza vaccination. JAMA. 2015;314(14):1488–97.
24. Ferdinands JM, Gargiullo P, Haber M, Moore M, Belongia EA, Shay DK. Inactivated influenza vaccines for prevention of community-acquired pneumonia: the limits of using nonspecific outcomes in vaccine effectiveness studies. Epidemiology. 2013;24(4):530–7.
25. Jackson ML, Nelson JC, Weiss NS, Neuzil KM, Barlow W, Jackson LA. Influenza vaccination and risk of community-acquired pneumonia in immunocompetent elderly people: a population-based, nested case–control study. Lancet. 2008;372(9636):398–405.
26. Talbot HK, Zhu Y, Chen Q, Williams JV, Thompson MG, Griffin MR. Effectiveness of influenza vaccine for preventing laboratory-confirmed influenza hospitalizations in adults, 2011–2012 influenza season. Clin Infect Dis. 2013;56(12):1774–7.
27. Johnston IDA, Strachan DP, Anderson HR. Effect of pneumonia and whooping cough in childhood on adult lung function. N Engl J Med. 1998;338(9):581–7.
28. Grimwood K, Chang AB. Long-term effects of pneumonia in young children. Pneumonia. 2015;6(1):101–14.
29. Munywoki PK, Ohuma EO, Ngama M, Bauni E, Scott JAG, Nokes DJ. Severe lower respiratory tract infection in early infancy and pneumonia hospitalizations among children, Kenya. Emerg Infect Dis. 2013;19(2):223–9.
30. Hedlund JU, Kalin ME, Ortqvist AB, Henrichsen J. Antibody response to pneumococcal vaccine in middle-aged and elderly patients recently treated for pneumonia. Arch Intern Med. 1994;154(17):1961–5.
31. Gordon SB, Bruce NG, Grigg J, Hibberd PL, Kurmi OP, Lam KB, et al. Respiratory risks from household air pollution in low and middle income countries. Lancet Respir Med. 2014;2(10):823–60.
32. Ezzati M, Kammen D. Indoor air pollution from biomass combustion and acute respiratory infections in Kenya: an exposure-response study. Lancet. 2001;358(9282):619–24.
33. Smith KR, Samet JM, Romieu I, Bruce N. Indoor air pollution in developing countries and acute lower respiratory infections in children. Thorax. 2000;55(6):518–32.
34. Dherani M, Pope D, Mascarenhas M, Smith KR, Weber M, Bruce N. Indoor air pollution from unprocessed solid fuel use and pneumonia risk in children aged under five years: a systematic review and meta-analysis. Bull World Health Organ. 2008;86(5):390–8c.
35. Jary H, Simpson H, Havens D, Manda G, Pope D, Bruce N, et al. Household air pollution and acute lower respiratory infections in adults: a systematic review. PLoS One. 2016;11(12):e0167656.
36. Jary H, Mallewa J, Nyirenda M, Faragher B, Heyderman R, Peterson I, et al. Study protocol: the effects of AIR pollution exposure and chronic respiratory disease on pneumonia risk in urban Malawian adults–the acute infection of the respiratory tract study (the AIR study). BMC Pulm Med. 2015;15:96.
37. Vinogradova Y, Coupland C, Hippisley-Cox J. Risk of pneumonia in patients taking statins: population-based nested case–control study. Br J Gen Pract. 2011;61(592):e742–8.
38. Vinogradova Y, Hippisley-Cox J, Coupland C. Identification of new risk factors for pneumonia: population-based case–control study. Br J Gen Pract. 2009;59(567):e329–38.
39. Okeyo TMBG, Stover J. Johnston a,. AIDS in Kenya: background, projections, impact, and interventions. Nairobi. Kenya: National AIDS and STDs Control Programme (NASCOP; 1998.
40. Flanagan KL, Plebanski M. Sex-differential heterologous (non-specific) effects of vaccines: an emerging public health issue that needs to be understood and exploited. Expert review Vaccine. 2017;16(1):5–13.
41. Aaby P, Kollmann TR, Benn CS. Nonspecific effects of neonatal and infant vaccination: public-health, immunological and conceptual challenges. Nature Immunology. 2014;15(1529–2916 (Electronic)).
42. Roth A, Sodemann M, Jensen H, Poulsen A, Gustafson P, Weise C, et al. Tuberculin reaction, BCG scar, and lower female mortality. Epidemiology. 2006;17(5):562–8.
43. Aaby P, Gustafson P, Roth A, Rodrigues A, Fernandes M, Sodemann M, et al. Vaccinia scars associated with better survival for adults. An observational

study from Guinea-Bissau. Vaccine. 2006;24(29–30):5718–25.
44. Meeting of the Strategic Advisory Group of Experts on immunization, April 2014 – conclusions and recommendations. Wkly Epidemiol Rec. 2014;89(21):221–36.
45. Grubb JR, Moorman AC, Baker RK, Masur H. The changing spectrum of pulmonary disease in patients with HIV infection on antiretroviral therapy. AIDS. 2006;20(8):1095–107.
46. Segal LN, Methé BA, Nolan A, Hoshino Y, Rom WN, Dawson R, et al. HIV-1 and bacterial pneumonia in the era of antiretroviral therapy. Proc Am Thorac Soc. 2011;8(3):282–7.

13

Impact of viral multiplex real-time PCR on management of respiratory tract infection

Lena M. Mayer[1,4], Christian Kahlert[2,4], Frank Rassouli[3], Pietro Vernazza[4] and Werner C. Albrich[4*]

Abstract

Background: Significance and clinical utility of multiple virus detection by multiplex real-time polymerase chain reaction (rtPCR) in respiratory tract infection remain unclear.

Methods: This retrospective cohort study analyzed how virus detection affected clinical management. During a 27-month period, clinical and laboratory information was collected from all children and adults in two Swiss tertiary centres whose respiratory samples were tested for respiratory viruses with a 16-plex rtPCR test.

Results: Pathogens were identified in 140 of 254 patients (55%); of those patients, there was ≥1 virus in 91 (65%), ≥ 1 bacterium in 53 (38%), and ≥1 virus and bacterium in 11 (8%). Of 80 patients with viral infection, 59 (74%) received antibiotics. Virus detection was associated with discontinuation of antibiotics in 2 of 20 adults (10%) and 6 of 14 children (43%). Overall 12 adults (34%) and 18 children (67%) were managed correctly without antibiotics after virus detection ($p = 0.01$). When taking biomarkers, radiologic presentations, and antibiotic pre-treatment into account, the impact of rtPCR and appropriateness of therapy for clinically viral infections increased to 100% in children and 62% in adults.

Conclusions: A substantial reduction of unnecessary antibiotic prescriptions seems possible. Appropriate application of rtPCR results in respiratory tract infections should be encouraged.

Keywords: Multiplex real-time PCR, Respiratory viruses, Antibiotic management

Background

Establishing the etiology of respiratory tract infections (RTI) is often difficult due to the lack of a diagnostic gold standard and the inability to detect the causative pathogen. A large proportion of RTI is believed to be caused by respiratory viruses [1–6]. With widespread availability of molecular methods such as multiplex real-time polymerase chain reaction (rtPCR), clinical work-flow has changed dramatically and the sensitivity of viral diagnostics has increased remarkably compared to conventional methods [3, 7–13]. However, the significance of virus detection remains unclear as the presence of a virus does not prove causality. Many respiratory viruses can be carried by asymptomatic children [4, 6, 14] and can be shed over prolonged periods, thus discrimination between carriage and infection is challenging [13–15]. Viral infection was reported previously to predispose to bacterial super-infection and concerns about possible bacterial co-infection remain [3, 7–13, 16–19]. Ruling out a bacterial infection with traditional microbiological techniques is frequently impossible [1, 5]. The predictive value of clinical signs to differentiate between viral and bacterial infection is also low [13, 17, 20–22]. On these grounds, clinical management of patients after respiratory virus diagnosis is controversial and surprisingly poorly studied. Overall, extensive yet often unnecessary use of antibiotics in RTI is common [1, 5, 6]. This adult and pediatric retrospective cohort study analyzed whether identification of a virus by multiplex rtPCR was associated with changes in the antibiotic treatment.

* Correspondence: Werner.Albrich@kssg.ch
[4]Division of Infectious Diseases & Hospital Epidemiology, Kantonsspital St. Gallen, Rorschacherstrasse 95, 9007 St. Gallen, Switzerland
Full list of author information is available at the end of the article

Methods

Study design and population

This was a retrospective cohort study of all pediatric and adult in- and outpatients in whom a 16-plex rtPCR assay for respiratory viruses was performed for upper and lower RTI, from either the Kantonsspital St. Gallen or Children's hospital of Eastern Switzerland. Both hospitals are tertiary-care Swiss teaching hospitals with active infectious diseases consult services and easily accessible web-based local guidelines (www.guidelines.ch) for the treatment of community-acquired or hospital-acquired pneumonia. The guidelines are strongly recommended for use but not strictly reinforced, and include use of rtPCR as optional diagnostic in hospitalized patients, particularly with immune suppression. The study period was from September 2012 (when this assay was introduced) to November 2014. The documented application dates of anti-infective medication were matched with the date of rtPCR analysis in order to determine whether treatment was changed in response to rtPCR results. The main outcome of interest was whether antibiotic therapy was modified according to results of multiplex rtPCR. Secondary outcomes were prevalence and distribution of positive results of rtPCR, complications, length of stay (LOS), and antibiotic therapy depending on identified pathogens.

Data collection

To identify patients, the database of the Centre for Laboratory Medicine was searched. Medical records were retrospectively analyzed to obtain basic demographic, clinical, laboratory and radiological parameters and data on clinical management. All chest radiographs (CXR) and computed tomographies (CT) for adults and children were reviewed by a pulmonologist and a pediatrician, respectively.

Clinical definitions

rtPCR results were available within 24 hours after testing. The application dates of anti-infective medication as documented in the medical records were correlated with the day of, or the day after, rtPCR analysis in order to define whether treatment initiation or discontinuation was associated with the results of viral testing.

The identified pathogens were retrospectively determined as relevant by an infectious disease specialist who integrated all available information. Etiologies were divided in four mutually exclusive groups: (i) bacterial (≥1 bacteria); (ii) viral (≥1 respiratory viruses); (iii) mixed (≥1 bacteria and ≥1 respiratory viruses); or (iv) no pathogen (including fungi, non-respiratory virus, bacterial contaminant including coagulase-negative staphylococci, propionibacterium, corynebacterium, colonizing oral and respiratory flora). For some children, rapid detection tests (Alere BinaxNOW Influenza A&B, Quidel QuickVue RSV Test) for respiratory syncytial virus (RSV) and influenza A/B virus were available. These results were additionally considered in forming the different groups.

For each patient, changes of antibiotic management, i.e. either starting or stopping antibiotics, were determined. All other situations were defined as no change.

Management was considered correct for viral infections if there was no antibiotic treatment before and after rtPCR *or* antibiotics were stopped after positive rtPCR results became available; for bacterial or mixed infections, if antibiotics were given before and after rtPCR *or* were started after a negative rtPCR result. Patients with an indication other than RTI for antibiotic therapy were excluded. For patients with febrile neutropenia without a specific focus, the antibiotic indication was defined as "other" because antibiotics would usually not be stopped despite a viral detection. If a patient underwent repeated testing for respiratory viruses within 3 weeks, only the first positive result was counted. If the time interval was longer or the detected viruses diverged, a different episode was presumed and analyzed separately [23].

To reflect clinical decision making in real-life situations, sub-analyses were performed. Cases without detection of bacteria (i.e. patients with viral etiology or with no pathogen) were evaluated as clinically bacterial if they fulfilled one of the following criteria: unilobar or multilobar pulmonary infiltrate on CT or CXR; C-reactive protein (CRP) >100 mg/l; procalcitonin (PCT) >0.25 μg/l; antibiotic therapy before rtPCR *and* with indeterminate biomarkers (CRP >100 mg/l *and* PCT ≤0.25 μg/l *or* CRP 51–100 mg/l *and* PCT not available). These criteria were adapted from earlier publications [17, 21] regarding the diagnosis of bacterial lower RTI.

The subgroup of patients with a viral etiology who had no clinically bacterial infection was considered to have a clinically viral infection. Children (<18 years) and adults (≥18 years) were analyzed separately. Sepsis was defined according to standard criteria at the time [24]. Systemic inflammatory response syndrome (SIRS) criteria for children were defined as age-specific [25].

For the imaging, if patients had interstitial infiltrates or ground glass opacities in the absence of unilobar or multilobar infiltrates, only therapy against "atypical" pathogens (macrolide, quinolone, tetracycline; but not antibiotics for coverage of "typical" bacterial pathogens) was considered appropriate. If both CXR and CT were available, only CT readings were used for further analyses. An infiltrate was required for the diagnosis of pneumonia but no radiography was needed to diagnose a RTI in general.

Laboratory procedures

The multiplex rtPCR was performed according to the manufacturer's instruction (Seegene, Korea). The Anyplex™ II RV16 detection kit (Seegene, Korea) detects the

Table 1 Baseline characteristics for adult patients

	Missing values	*Total (n = 182)*	*Viral[a] (n = 40)*	*Any virus[b] (n = 46)*	*Other[c] (n = 142)*	*p-value[d]*	
						Viral vs. any virus	*Viral vs. other*
Demographics							
Age, mean years ± SD (range)		55.9 ± 16.1 (18–88)	53.6 ± 16.1 (18–83)	53.9 ± 15.9 (18–83)	56.6 ± 16.1 (18–88)	0.93	0.30
Female sex, n (%)		76 (41.8)	14 (35.0)	19 (41.3)	62 (43.7)	0.55	0.33
Outpatients, n (%)		20 (11.0)	5 (12.5)	5 (10.9)	15 (10.6)	1.00	0.92
Comorbidities, n (%)							
Asthma		13 (7.1)	2 (5.0)	4 (8.7)	11 (7.7)	0.81	0.85
COPD		27 (10.6)	5 (12.5)	7 (15.2)	22 (15.5)	0.72	0.64
Other chronic lung disease[e]		26 (14.3)	2 (5.0)	2 (4.3)	24 (16.9)	1.00	0.06
Solid cancer[f]		25 (13.7)	3 (7.5)	3 (6.5)	22 (15.5)	1.00	0.20
Hematologic malignancy		38 (20.9)	13 (32.5)	15 (32.6)	25 (17.6)	0.99	0.04
Organ transplantation		13 (7.1)	3 (7.5)	3 (6.5)	10 (7.0)	1.00	1.00
Neutropenia		20 (11.0)	9 (22.5)	9 (19.6)	11 (7.7)	0.74	0.03
HIV infection		6 (3.3)	1 (2.5)	2 (4.3)	5 (3.5)	1.00	1.00
Diabetes mellitus		27 (14.8)	6 (15.0)	7 (15.2)	21 (14.8)	0.98	0.97
Collagen vascular disease/ Vasculitis		33 (18.1)	4 (10.0)	5 (10.9)	29 (20.4)	1.00	0.13
Systemic steroids		49 (26.9)	11 (27.5)	14 (30.4)	38 (26.8)	0.77	0.93
Other Immunosuppression[g]		21 (11.5)	5 (12.5)	6 (13.0)	16 (11.3)	0.94	1.00
Chronic renal failure		45 (24.7)	11 (27.5)	13 (28.3)	34 (23.9)	0.94	0.65
Clinical findings							
Systolic blood pressure, mmHg, mean ± SD (range)	9	125 ± 24 (63–207)	129 ± 27 (63–207)	128 ± 28 (63–207)	123 ± 22 (67–197)	0.87	0.17
Heart rate, beats/min, mean ± SD (range)	8	94 ± 20 (51–155)	91 ± 19 (51–150)	94 ± 19 (51–150)	94 ± 20 (56–155)	0.47	0.40
Respiratory rate, breaths/min, mean ± SD (range)	130	26 ± 9 (10–60)	23 ± 8 (12–36)	27 ± 13 (12–60)	27 ± 10 (10–60)	0.39	0.23
Body temperature, °C, mean ± SD (range)	20	37.6 ± 1.0 (35.4–42.0)	37.5 ± 0.9 (35.6–39.6)	37.5 ± 0.9 (35.6–39.6)	37.6 ± 1.0 (35.4–42.0)	1.00	0.59
Laboratory findings[h], mean ± SD (range)							
C-reactive protein (maximum), mg/l	13	151 ± 127 (1–500)	159 ± 148 (1–500)	166 ± 152 (1–500)	148 ± 121 (1–499)	0.83	0.64
White blood cells (maximum), G/l	11	11.5 ± 10.2 (0.0–97.0)	12.2 ± 16.8 (1.8–97.0)	12.6 ± 16.3 (1.8–97.0)	11.3 ± 7.3 (0.0–41.1)	0.91	0.75
Platelets (minimum), G/l	11	202 ± 128 (4–713)	159 ± 117 (5–513)	165 ± 117 (5–513)	215 ± 129 (4–713)	0.82	0.02
Discharge diagnosis, n (%)							
Bronchitis		22 (12.1)	7 (17.5)	7 (15.2)	15 (10.6)	0.78	0.36
Acute exacerbation of COPD		5 (2.7)	1 (2.5)	1 (2.2)	4 (2.8)	1.00	1.00
Upper respiratory tract infection		8 (4.4)	4 (10.0)	4 (8.7)	4 (2.8)	1.00	0.14
Respiratory tract infection, unspecified		7 (3.8)	2 (5.0)	4 (8.7)	5 (3.5)	0.81	0.96
Community-acquired pneumonia		65 (35.7)	21 (52.5)	25 (54.3)	44 (31.0)	0.86	0.01
Hospital-acquired pneumonia		12 (6.6)	0 (0.0)	0 (0.0)	12 (8.5)	n/a	0.09

Table 1 Baseline characteristics for adult patients *(Continued)*

Aspiration pneumonia	1 (0.5)	0 (0.0)	0 (0.0)	1 (0.7)	n/a	1.00
Tuberculosis	3 (1.6)	0 (0.0)	0 (0.0)	3 (2.1)	n/a	0.95
Other[i]	59 (32.4)	5 (12.5)	5 (10.9)	54 (38.0)	1.00	0.002

°C, degree Celsius, *COPD* chronic obstructive pulmonary disease, *HIV* human immunodeficiency virus, *n* number, *SD* standard deviation
[a]Cases in which only one or more respiratory viruses were detected
[b]Cases in which one or more respiratory viruses were detected (as single or mixed infection)
[c]Includes bacterial etiology, mixed etiology, no pathogen
[d]For continuous variables, 2-sample independent t-test was used. For categorical variables, Mantel-Haenszel chi square or Fisher exact test were used
[e]Other chronic lung diseases, e.g. cystic fibrosis, pulmonary sarcoidosis, pulmonary hypertension
[f]All solid tumors including bronchial carcinoma
[g]Patients with one of the following conditions: primary or secondary antibody deficiency, congenital immunodeficiency, immunosuppressive therapy other than steroids, severe malnutrition with cachexia
[h]Highest/lowest value within a time period of 3 days before and 3 days after date of rtPCR
[i]Other infections ($n = 10$); neoplastic diseases ($n = 6$); collagen vascular; other rheumatologic or autoimmune ($n = 14$); sarcoidosis ($n = 3$); non-infectious non-neoplastic pulmonary diseases ($n = 23$); cardiovascular diseases ($n = 3$)

following viruses: adenovirus, influenza A virus, influenza B virus, parainfluenza virus 1, parainfluenza virus 2, parainfluenza virus 3, parainfluenza virus 4, rhinovirus A/B/C, RSV A, RSV B, bocavirus 1/2/3/4, human metapneumovirus, coronavirus 229E, coronavirus NL63, coronavirus OC43, and enterovirus. Specimens that arrived before mid-morning from Monday to Friday were processed daily and results were provided by mid-afternoon. Specimens that arrived afterwards were processed on the following workday and reported by mid-afternoon. Dates of specimen collection and testing were available, but not date and time of reporting of results. For CRP, white blood cell count (WBC) and platelets, the most pathologic values within 3 days before and after rtPCR results were documented.

Statistical analyses

Quantitative variables are described as means ± standard deviations or median and interquartile range (IQR), as appropriate. Qualitative variables are presented as absolute counts and relative percentages. $\chi2$-test or Fisher's exact test were used to compare proportions, as appropriate. For continuous variables, the 2-sample independent t-test or the Mann-Whitney-U-test were used. *P*-values ≤0.05 (2-sided) were considered statistically significant. Multivariate logistic regression was used to examine whether different predictors were associated with virus detection. Variables with a *p*-value ≤0.05 in the univariate logistic regression were included. SPSS version 20.0 for Windows software, OpenEpi (www.openepi.com) and Microsoft Excel 2010 were used for statistical analyses.

Results

rtPCR for respiratory viruses was performed on 328 respiratory specimens, of which 74 samples were excluded due to insufficient clinical information or repeated testing of separate specimens for respiratory viruses in the same patient within 3 weeks. Data on 254 patients were analyzed, including 11 sputa, 47 nasopharyngeal swabs, 63 nasopharyngeal aspirates, 123 bronchoalveolar lavages, 9 tracheal aspirates and 1 pleural effusion.

Clinical characteristics

Baseline characteristics are presented in Tables 1, 2 and 3. One hundred and seven patients (42%) were female, and 72 were children (28%). Mean age in the group with viral infections was lower than in the remaining patients (29 vs. 47 years; $p < 0.001$) but the difference was not significant if children and adults were analyzed separately (children 4.3 vs. 5.7 years; $p = 0.28$; adults 53.6 vs. 56.6 years; $p = 0.31$). There were more patients with neutropenia, hematological malignancy or collagen vascular disease/vasculitis in the viral group ($p < 0.001$; $p = 0.04$; $p = 0.01$). Diagnosis of bronchitis and upper RTI were more common in the viral group ($p = 0.02$; $p = 0.004$).

Pathogen identification

Any pathogen was identified in 140 patients (55%), in 89 of 182 adults (49%) and in 51 of 72 children (71%). Among these patients, one or more respiratory virus was detected in 91 (65%), one or more bacteria in 53 (38%) and a mixed viral-bacterial infection in 11 (8%) patients. 45 of 72 children (63%) were infected with one or more respiratory viruses. Compared to children, viral detection in adults was less frequent (25%, $n = 46$; $p < 0.001$). A single pathogen was identified in 99 patients (39%); multiple pathogens were detected in 41 patients (16%). Distribution of detected pathogens and the differences between children and adults are shown in Table 4, and Figs. 1, 2a and b.

Antibiotic therapy

Of the 254 patients in the cohort, 61 (24%) received antibiotics before hospitalization, and 149 (59%) of all in- and outpatients received antibiotics at the time of rtPCR testing. Of 80 patients with a viral etiology, 59 (74%) received antibiotics at any time point, 28 of 40 children (70%) and

Table 2 Baseline characteristics for pediatric patients

	Missing values	*Total (n = 72)*	*Viral[a] (n = 40)*	*Any virus[b] (n = 45)*	*Other[c] (n = 32)*	*p-value[d]*	
						Viral vs. any virus	*Viral vs. other*
Demographics							
Age, mean years ± SD (range)		4.9 ± 5.7 (0–17)	4.3 ± 5.4 (0–16)	4.7 ± 5.5 (0–16)	5.7 ± 6.0 (0–17)	0.74	0.30
Female sex, n (%)		31 (43.1)	14 (35.0)	18 (40.0)	17 (53.1)	0.64	0.13
Outpatients, n (%)		3 (4.2)	2 (5.0)	2 (4.4)	1 (3.1)	1.00	1.00
Comorbidities, n (%)							
Asthma		1 (1.4)	1 (2.5)	1 (2.2)	0 (0.0)	1.00	1.00
Other chronic lung disease[e]		13 (18.1)	7 (17.5)	8 (17.8)	6 (18.8)	0.97	0.89
Solid cancer[f]		1 (1.4)	0 (0.0)	0 (0.0)	1 (3.1)	n/a	0.89
Haematologic malignancy		10 (13.9)	8 (20.0)	9 (20.0)	2 (6.3)	1.00	0.18
Organ transplantation		1 (1.4)	1 (2.5)	1 (2.2)	0 (0.0)	1.00	1.00
Neutropenia		9 (12.5)	8 (20.0)	8 (17.8)	1 (3.1)	0.79	0.06
Systemic steroids		8 (11.1)	5 (12.5)	6 (13.3)	3 (9.4)	0.91	0.98
Other Immunosuppression[g]		3 (4.2)	3 (7.5)	3 (6.7)	0 (0.0)	1.00	0.33
Clinical findings							
Systolic blood pressure, mmHg, mean ± SD (range)	29	100 ± 18 (59–140)	106 ± 15 (71–140)	105 ± 14 (71–140)	95 ± 18 (59–120)	0.82	0.04
Heart rate, beats/min, mean ± SD (range)	3	136 ± 33 (60–234)	138 ± 32 (60–186)	134 ± 32 (60–186)	135 ± 35 (72–234)	0.58	0.71
Respiratory rate, breaths/min, mean ± SD (range)	15	41 ± 20 (16–103)	41 ± 21 (18–103)	40 ± 21 (16–103)	40 ± 19 (16–88)	0.84	0.86
Body temperature, °C, mean ± SD (range)	3	37.6 ± 1.1 (35.0–40.1)	37.5 ± 1.1 (35.0–39.5)	37.5 ± 1.1 (35.0–39.5)	37.7 ± 1.1 (35.1–40.1)	1.00	0.46
Laboratory findings[h], mean ± SD (range)							
C-reactive protein (maximum), mg/l	2	85 ± 141 (5–999)	62 ± 77 (5–291)	67 ± 81 (5–293)	113 ± 191 (7–999)	0.78	0.16
White blood cells (maximum), G/l	2	16.0 ± 12.1 (0.2–63.1)	12.6 ± 10.0 (0.2–57.0)	13.6 ± 11.3 (0.2–57.0)	20.1 ± 13.3 (1.8–63.1)	0.68	0.01
Platelets (minimum), G/l	2	246 ± 144 (15–674)	257 ± 175 (15–674)	244 ± 169 (15–674)	234 ± 96 (16–488)	0.73	0.49
Discharge diagnosis, n (%)							
Bronchitis		10 (13.9)	9 (22.5)	9 (20.0)	1 (3.1)	0.78	0.04
Upper respiratory tract infection		14 (19.4)	9 (22.5)	10 (22.2)	5 (15.6)	0.98	0.47
Respiratory tract infection, unspecified		4 (5.6)	4 (10.0)	4 (8.9)	0 (0.0)	1.00	0.18
Community-acquired pneumonia		15 (20.8)	6 (15.0)	8 (17.8)	9 (28.1)	0.73	0.18
Hospital-acquired pneumonia		10 (13.9)	5 (12.5)	6 (13.3)	5 (15.6)	0.91	0.96
Aspiration pneumonia		2 (2.8)	1 (2.5)	2 (4.4)	1 (3.1)	1.00	1.00
Other[i]		17 (23.6)	6 (15.0)	6 (13.3)	11 (34.4)	0.83	0.06

°C, degree Celsius, *COPD* chronic obstructive pulmonary disease, *HIV* human immunodeficiency virus, *n* number, *SD* standard deviation

[a]Cases in which only one or more respiratory viruses were detected

[b]Cases in which one or more respiratory viruses were detected (as single or mixed infection)

[c]Includes bacterial etiology, mixed etiology, no pathogen

[d]For continuous variables, 2-sample independent t-test was used. For categorical variables, Mantel-Haenszel chi square or Fisher exact test were used

[e]Other chronic lung diseases, e.g. cystic fibrosis, pulmonary sarcoidosis, pulmonary hypertension

[f]All solid tumors including bronchial carcinoma

[g]Patients with one of the following conditions: primary or secondary antibody deficiency, congenital immunodeficiency, immunosuppressive therapy other than steroids, severe malnutrition with cachexia

[h]Highest/lowest value within a time period of 3 days before and 3 days after date of rtPCR

[i]Other infections ($n = 14$); neoplastic diseases ($n = 1$); collagen vascular; other rheumatologic or autoimmune ($n = 1$); gastroesophageal diseases ($n = 1$)

Table 3 Baseline characteristics for all patients

	Missing values	Total (n = 254)	Viral[a] (n = 80)	Any virus[b] (n = 91)	Other[c] (n = 174)	p-value[d]	
						Viral vs. any virus	Viral vs. other
Demographics							
Age, mean years ± SD (range)		41.5 ± 26.9 (0–88)	29.0 ± 27.5 (0–83)	29.6 ± 27.4 (0–83)	47.2 ± 24.7 (0–88)	0.89	<0.001
Female sex, n (%)		107 (42.1)	28 (35.0)	37 (40.7)	79 (45.4)	0.45	0.12
Children, n (%)		72 (28.3)	40 (50.0)	45 (49.5)	32 (18.4)	0.94	<0.001
Outpatients, n (%)		23 (9.1)	7 (8.8)	7 (7.7)	16 (9.2)	0.80	0.91
Comorbidities, n (%)							
Asthma		14 (5.5)	3 (3.8)	5 (5.5)	11 (6.3)	0.87	0.61
COPD		27 (10.6)	5 (6.3)	7 (7.7)	22 (12.6)	0.71	0.13
Other chronic lung disease[e]		39 (15.4)	9 (11.3)	10 (11.0)	30 (17.2)	0.96	0.22
Solid cancer[f]		26 (10.2)	3 (3.8)	3 (3.3)	23 (13.2)	1.00	0.02
Haematologic malignancy		48 (18.9)	21 (26.3)	24 (26.4)	27 (15.5)	0.99	0.04
Organ transplantation		14 (5.5)	4 (5.0)	4 (4.4)	10 (5.7)	1.00	1.00
Neutropenia		29 (11.4)	17 (21.3)	17 (18.7)	12 (6.9)	0.68	<0.001
HIV infection		6 (2.4)	1 (1.3)	2 (2.2)	5 (2.9)	1.00	0.77
Diabetes mellitus		27 (10.6)	6 (7.5)	7 (7.7)	21 (12.1)	0.96	0.28
Collagen vascular disease/Vasculitis		33 (13.0)	4 (5.0)	5 (5.5)	29 (16.7)	1.00	0.01
Systemic steroids		57 (22.4)	16 (20.0)	20 (22.0)	41 (23.6)	0.75	0.53
Other Immunosuppression[g]		24 (9.4)	8 (10.0)	9 (9.9)	16 (9.2)	0.98	0.84
Chronic renal failure		45 (17.7)	11 (13.8)	13 (14.3)	34 (19.5)	0.92	0.26
Clinical findings							
Systolic blood pressure, mmHg, mean ± SD (range)	38	120 ± 25 (59–207)	121 ± 26 (63–207)	119 ± 26 (63–207)	119 ± 24 (59–197)	0.67	0.60
Heart rate, beats/min, mean ± SD (range)	11	106 ± 31 (51–234)	114 ± 35 (51–186)	114 ± 33 (51–186)	102 ± 28 (56–234)	1.00	0.01
Respiratory rate, breaths/min, mean ± SD (range)	145	34 ± 18 (10–103)	37 ± 21 (12–103)	37 ± 20 (12–103)	32 ± 15 (10–88)	1.00	0.17
Body temperature, °C, mean ± SD (range)	23	37.6 ± 1.0 (35.0–42.0)	37.5 ± 1.0 (35.0–39.6)	37.5 ± 1.0 (35.0–39.6)	37.6 ± 1.0 (35.1–42.0)	1.00	0.48
Laboratory findings[h], mean ± SD (range)							
C-reactive protein (maximum), mg/l	15	132 ± 134 (1–999)	111 ± 127 (1–500)	117 ± 132 (1–500)	141 ± 137 (1–999)	0.77	0.11
White blood cells (maximum), G/l	13	12.8 ± 11.0 (0.0–97.0)	12.4 ± 13.8 (0.2–97.0)	13.1 ± 14.0 (0.2–97.0)	13.1 ± 9.4 (0.0–63.1)	0.75	0.69
Platelets (minimum), G/l	13	215 ± 134 (4–713)	208 ± 156 (5–674)	204 ± 149 (5–674)	218 ± 123 (4–713)	0.87	0.62
Discharge diagnosis, n (%)							
Bronchitis		32 (12.6)	16 (20.0)	16 (17.6)	16 (9.2)	0.69	0.02
Acute exacerbation of COPD		5 (2.0)	1 (1.3)	1 (1.1)	4 (2.3)	1.00	0.99
Upper respiratory tract infection		22 (8.7)	13 (16.3)	14 (15.4)	9 (5.2)	0.88	0.004
Respiratory tract infection, unspecified		11 (4.3)	6 (7.5)	8 (8.8)	5 (2.9)	0.76	0.18
Community-acquired pneumonia		80 (31.5)	27 (33.8)	33 (36.3)	53 (30.5)	0.73	0.60
Hospital-acquired pneumonia		22 (8.7)	5 (6.3)	6 (6.6)	17 (9.8)	0.93	0.36
Aspiration pneumonia		3 (1.2)	1 (1.3)	2 (2.2)	2 (1.1)	1.00	1.00

Table 3 Baseline characteristics for all patients *(Continued)*

Tuberculosis	3 (1.2)	0 (0.0)	0 (0.0)	3 (1.7)	n/a	0.64
Other[i]	76 (29.9)	11 (13.8)	11 (12.1)	65 (37.4)	0.75	<0.001

°C, degree Celsius, *COPD* chronic obstructive pulmonary disease, *HIV* human immunodeficiency virus, *n* number, *SD* standard deviation
[a]Cases in which only one or more respiratory viruses were detected
[b]Cases in which one or more respiratory viruses were detected (as single or mixed infection)
[c]Includes bacterial etiology, mixed etiology, no pathogen
[d]For continuous variables, 2-sample independent t-test was used. For categorical variables, Mantel-Haenszel chi square or Fisher exact test were used
[e]Other chronic lung diseases, e.g. cystic fibrosis, pulmonary sarcoidosis, pulmonary hypertension
[f]All solid tumors including bronchial carcinoma
[g]Patients with one of the following conditions: primary or secondary antibody deficiency, congenital immunodeficiency, immunosuppressive therapy other than steroids, severe malnutrition with cachexia
[h]Highest/lowest value within a time period of 3 days before and 3 days after date of rtPCR
[i]Other infections ($n = 24$); neoplastic diseases ($n = 7$); collagen vascular; other rheumatologic or autoimmune ($n = 15$); sarcoidosis ($n = 3$); non-infectious non-neoplastic pulmonary diseases ($n = 23$); cardiovascular diseases ($n = 3$); gastroesophageal diseases ($n = 1$)

Table 4 Relevant pathogens identified from respiratory specimens

	Total (n = 254)	*Adults (n = 182)*	*Children (n = 72)*
Bacteria, n (%)	66 (26.0)	54 (29.7)	12 (16.7)
Haemophilus influenzae	12 (4.7)	11 (6.0)	1 (1.4)
Klebsiella pneumoniae	8 (3.1)	6 (3.3)	2 (2.8)
Staphylococcus aureus	4 (1.6)	1 (0.5)	3 (4.2)
Escherichia coli	4 (1.6)	3 (1.6)	1 (1.4)
Pseudomonas aeruginosa	4 (1.6)	4 (2.2)	0 (0.0)
Streptococcus pneumoniae	3 (1.2)	2 (1.1)	1 (1.4)
Streptococcus pyogenes	3 (1.2)	2 (1.1)	1 (1.4)
Legionella pneumophila	3 (1.2)	3 (1.6)	0 (0.0)
Mycobacterium tuberculosis	3 (1.2)	3 (1.6)	0 (0.0)
Mycoplasma pneumoniae	1 (0.4)	0 (0.0)	1 (1.4)
Other bacteria	21 (8.3)	19 (10.4)	2 (2.8)
Viruses, n (%)	119 (46.9)	54 (29.7)	65 (90.3)
Rhinovirus A/B/C	33 (13.0)	16 (8.8)	17 (23.6)
Influenza A virus	17 (6.7)	11 (6.0)	6 (8.3)
Influenza B virus	4 (1.6)	0 (0.0)	4 (5.6)
Adenovirus	14 (5.5)	4 (2.2)	10 (13.9)
Bocavirus 1/2/3/4	9 (3.5)	0 (0.0)	9 (12.5)
Respiratory syncytial virus A	8 (3.1)	4 (2.2)	4 (5.6)
Respiratory syncytial virus B	6 (2.4)	5 (2.7)	1 (1.4)
Parainfluenza virus 1	1 (0.4)	1 (0.5)	0 (0.0)
Parainfluenza virus 2	1 (0.4)	0 (0.0)	1 (1.4)
Parainfluenza virus 3	6 (2.4)	3 (1.6)	3 (4.2)
Parainfluenza virus 4	5 (2.0)	2 (1.1)	3 (4.2)
Human Metapneumovirus	5 (2.0)	2 (1.1)	3 (4.2)
Enterovirus	3 (1.2)	0 (0.0)	3 (4.2)
Coronavirus 229E	1 (0.4)	1 (0.5)	0 (0.0)
Coronavirus NL63	2 (0.8)	1 (0.5)	1 (1.4)
Coronavirus OC43	1 (0.4)	1 (0.5)	0 (0.0)
Non respiratory viruses	3 (1.2)	3 (1.6)	0 (0.0)
Fungi, n (%)	10 (3.9)	9 (4.9)	1 (1.4)
Pneumocystis jirovecii	6 (2.4)	6 (3.3)	0 (0.0)
Other fungi	4 (1.6)	3 (1.6)	1 (1.4)

Pathogens associated with mixed infections were counted individually

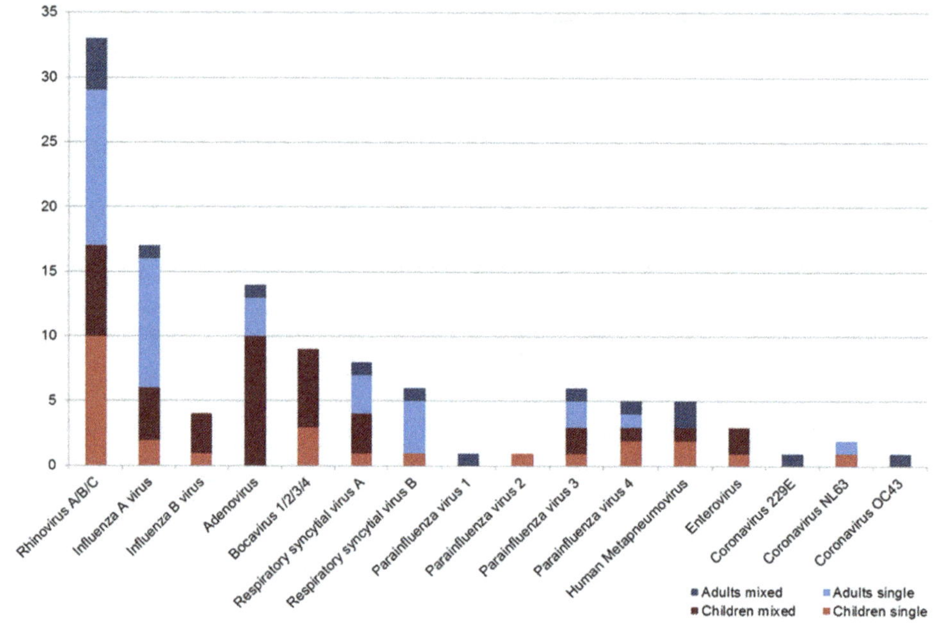

Fig. 1 Distribution of respiratory viruses detected as single or mixed pathogen

31 of 40 adults (78%). Inpatients with a bacterial etiology were treated with antibiotics in 92% ($p = 0.09$) and longer than those with a viral etiology or no pathogen ($p = 0.02$; $p = 0.01$). If children and adults were analyzed individually, similar but non-significant trends were observed (Tables 5, 6 and 7).

Influence of rtPCR testing on management

The effect of rtPCR analysis on antibiotic management is presented in Tables 8, 9 and 10. After exclusion of patients who received antibiotics for other indications virus detection was temporally associated with discontinuation of antibiotics in 2 of 20 adults (10%) and 6 of 14 children (43%). In patients with viral etiology, management was more frequently judged correct in children (18/27, 67%) than in adults (12/35, 34%; $p = 0.01$) after rtPCR results became available. In adults, management of viral etiology was less often judged correct compared to adults with bacterial etiology ($p = 0.002$). Among patients with clinically viral etiology, children were more frequently managed correctly (15/15, 100%) than adults (8/13, 62%; $p = 0.03$).

Eight adults and one child received oseltamivir. In four of five patients with proven influenza A virus infection, the antiviral medication was prescribed in response to the positive rtPCR analysis. In another child, oseltamivir was commenced after the third successive detection of influenza A virus within a month and stopped after 1 day. In two other patients, antiviral therapy was started or continued despite an rtPCR analysis negative for influenza and positive for other respiratory viruses. In another patient with identification of only bacterial

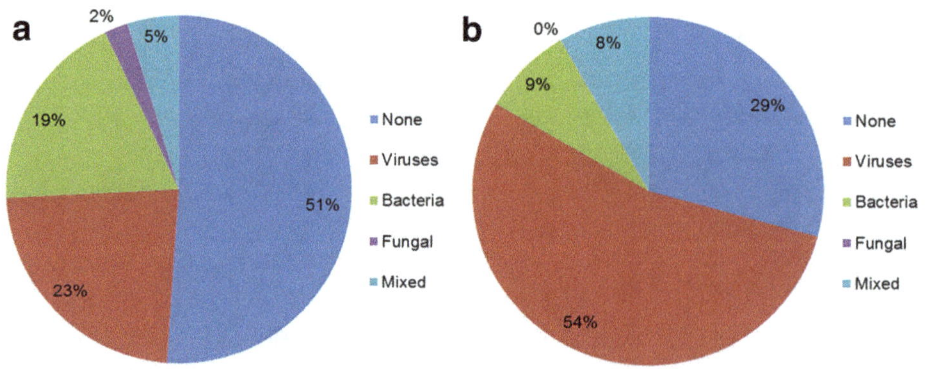

Fig. 2 a Distribution of identified pathogens for adults. **b** Distribution of identified pathogens for children

Table 5 Outcome depending on relevant detected pathogen for adult patients

	Viral	*Bacterial*	*Mixed*	*No pathogen*	*p-value*[a]		
	(n = 40)	*(n = 36)*	*(n = 6)*	*(n = 100)*	*Viral vs. bacterial*	*Viral vs. mixed*	*Viral vs. no pathogen*
LOS inpatients, median days (IQR)	8 (6–21)	21 (13–35)	11.5 (5–44.25)	15 (8–23.5)	<0.001	0.67	0.03
Complications, n (%)							
ICU admission	11 (27.5)	13 (36.1)	3 (50.0)	24 (24.0)	0.42	0.51	0.67
Mechanical ventilation	6 (15.0)	11 (30.6)	3 (50.0)	19 (19.0)	0.11	0.16	0.58
ARDS	3 (7.5)	5 (13.9)	2 (33.3)	6 (6.0)	0.60	0.24	1.00
Sepsis	24 (60.0)	24 (66.7)	5 (83.3)	6 (6.0)[b]	0.55	0.53	n/a
Mortality (all cause)	4 (10.0)	4 (11.1)	1 (16.7)	6 (6.0)	1.00	1.00	0.62
Antibiotic use (any indication)							
Any inpatient antibiotics, n (%)	30/35 (85.7)	29/32 (90.6)	4/6 (66.7)	72/89 (80.9)	0.81	0.54	0.53
Duration of inpatient use, mean days ± SD (range)	12.5 ± 14.3 (0–63)	18.1 ± 16.0 (0–72)	10.3 ± 12.1 (0–31)	10.8 ± 11.4 (0–63)	0.14	0.73	0.49
Discharged receiving oral antibiotics, n (%)	11 (30.6)[c]	17 (53.1)[d]	1 (20.0)[e]	23 (24.5)[f]	0.06	1.00	0.48

ARDS acute respiratory distress syndrome, *ICU* intensive care unit, *IQR* interquartile range, *LOS* length of stay, *n* number, *SD* standard deviation
[a]For continuous variables, 2-sample independent t-test or Mann-Whitney-U-test were used. For categorical variables, Mantel-Haenszel chi square or Fisher exact test were used
[b]Sepsis requires a pathogen per definition. In these six cases sepsis was exceptionally defined according to discharge papers
Missing values due to death or ongoing hospitalisation at time of analysis (number): c4; d4; e1; f6. For calculation of percentage and *p*-value missing values were excluded

pathogens, oseltamivir was stopped after negative rtPCR results were available. In an additional case with detection of bacteria only, antiviral medication was started 3 days after rtPCR analysis and it was stopped again on the next day.

Outcomes depending on etiology

Hospital length of stay (LOS) was longer in patients with bacterial etiology compared to patients with a viral etiology. For children, LOS did not significantly vary in the different groups between viral and bacterial etiologies

Table 6 Outcome depending on relevant detected pathogen for pediatric patients

	Viral	*Bacterial*	*Mixed*	*No pathogen*	*p-value*[a]		
	(n = 40)	*(n = 6)*	*(n = 5)*	*(n = 21)*	*Viral vs. bacterial*	*Viral vs. mixed*	*Viral vs. no pathogen*
LOS inpatients, median days (IQR)	18.5 (6–48.75)	47.5 (14–95.75)	34 (17.5–201.5)	37 (8–70)	0.19	0.10	0.45
Complications, n (%)							
ICU admission	18 (45.0)	4 (66.7)	5 (100.0)	12 (57.1)	0.58	0.06	0.37
Mechanical ventilation	8 (20.0)	4 (66.7)	4 (80.0)	11 (52.4)	0.07	0.03	0.01
ARDS	1 (2.5)	0 (0.0)	1 (20.0)	0 (0.0)	1.00	0.42	1.00
Sepsis	17 (42.5)	4 (66.7)	2 (40.0)	0 (0.0)	0.50	1.00	n/a
Mortality (all cause)	2 (5.0)	0 (0.0)	0 (0.0)	0 (0.0)	1.00	1.00	0.85
Antibiotic use (any indication)							
Any inpatient antibiotics, n (%)	28/38 (73.7)	6/6 (100.0)	5/5 (100.0)	18/20 (90.0)	0.38	0.49	0.26
Duration of inpatient use, mean days ± SD (range)	8.6 ± 13.4 (0–73)	14.2 ± 11.0 (0–34)	13.8 ± 7.8 (7–24)	6.2 ± 4.8 (0–18)	0.34	0.40	0.33
Discharged receiving oral antibiotics, n (%)	6 (15.8)[b]	0 (0.0)	1 (20.0)	3 (15.0)[c]	0.78	1.00	1.00

ARDS acute respiratory distress syndrome, *ICU* intensive care unit, *IQR* interquartile range, *LOS* length of stay, *n* number, *SD* standard deviation
[a]For continuous variables, 2-sample independent t-test or Mann-Whitney-U-test were used. For categorical variables, Mantel-Haenszel chi square or Fisher exact test were used
Missing values due to death or ongoing hospitalisation at time of analysis (number): b2; c1. For calculation of percentage and *p*-value missing values were excluded

Table 7 Outcome depending on relevant detected pathogen for all patients

	Viral	*Bacterial*	*Mixed*	*No pathogen*	*p-value*[a]		
	(n = 80)	*(n = 42)*	*(n = 11)*	*(n = 121)*	*Viral vs. bacterial*	*Viral vs. mixed*	*Viral vs. no pathogen*
LOS inpatients, median days (IQR)	12 (6–25.5)	22 (13–42.5)	27 (8–72)	16 (8–29.25)	0.004	0.20	0.20
Complications, n (%)							
ICU admission	29 (36.3)	17 (40.5)	8 (72.7)	36 (29.8)	0.65	0.05	0.34
Mechanical ventilation	14 (17.5)	15 (35.7)	7 (63.6)	30 (24.8)	0.03	0.01	0.22
ARDS	4 (5.0)	5 (11.9)	3 (27.3)	6 (5.0)	0.31	0.07	1.00
Sepsis	41 (51.3)	28 (66.7)	7 (63.6)	6 (5.0)[b]	0.10	0.44	n/a
Mortality (all cause)	6 (7.5)	4 (9.5)	1 (9.1)	6 (5.0)	0.94	1.00	0.65
Antibiotic use (any indication)							
Any inpatient antibiotics, n (%)	58/73 (79.5)	35/38 (92.1)	9/11 (81.8)	90/109 (82.6)	0.09	1.00	0.60
Duration of inpatient use, mean days ± SD (range)	10.5 ± 13.9 (0-73)	17.5 ± 15.3 (0–72)	11.9 ± 10.0 (0–31)	10.0 ± 10.6 (0–63)	0.02	0.75	0.80
Discharged receiving oral antibiotics, n (%)	17 (23.0)[c]	17 (44.7)[d]	2 (20.0)[e]	26 (22.8)[f]	0.02	1.00	0.98

ARDS acute respiratory distress syndrome, *ICU* intensive care unit, *IQR* interquartile range, *LOS* length of stay, *n* number, *SD* standard deviation
[a]For continuous variables, 2-sample independent t-test or Mann-Whitney-U-test were used. For categorical variables, Mantel-Haenszel chi square or Fisher exact test were used
[b]Sepsis requires a pathogen per definition. In these six cases sepsis was exceptionally defined according to discharge papers
Missing values due to death or ongoing hospitalisation at time of analysis (number): c6; d4; e1; f7. For calculation of percentage and *p*-value missing values were excluded

(Tables 5, 6 and 7). Patients with a mixed infection were more frequently admitted to the intensive care unit (ICU) and mechanically ventilated compared to patients with a viral etiology ($p = 0.05$; $p = 0.005$; respectively). If children and adults were analyzed separately, the differences within the adult population were not significant; in children, more patients with a mixed infection were mechanically ventilated ($p = 0.03$). All-cause and RTI-associated mortality was comparable between pathogen groups.

In patients with viral etiology there was no difference in mortality between those who discontinued antibiotics compared to those who did not (1/8 [13%] vs. 3/26 [12%]; $p = 1.00$). LOS was shorter in inpatients who discontinued antibiotics (median days 5 [IQR 3–11.75] vs. 10.5 [IQR 6–19.25]; $p = 0.05$). Patients in whom antibiotics were continued despite a viral detection were as frequently admitted to ICU (11/26 [42%] vs. 5/8 [63%]; $p = 0.55$) or mechanically ventilated (6/26 [23%] vs. 1/8 [13%]; $p = 0.93$) as patients in whom antibiotics were discontinued. The

Table 8 Change of antibiotic therapy after rtPCR, adult patients with another indication for antibiotics were excluded

	Viral	*Bacterial*	*Mixed*	*No pathogen*	*Clinically*	*Clinically*	*p-value*[c]		
	(n = 35)	*(n = 33)*	*(n = 6)*	*(n = 84)*	*bacterial*[a] *(n = 84)*	*viral*[b] *(n = 13)*	*Viral vs. bacterial*	*Viral vs. mixed*	*Viral vs. no pathogen*
No antibiotic treatment before and after rtPCR, n (%)	*10 (28.6)*	7 (21.2)	2 (33.3)	32 (38.1)	18 (21.4)	*8 (61.5)*	0.49	1.00	0.32
Antibiotic treatment stopped after rtPCR, n (%)	*2 (5.7)*	2 (6.1)	0 (0.0)	2 (2.4)	4 (4.8)	*0 (0.0)*	1.00	1.00	0.67
Antibiotic treatment started after rtPCR, n (%)	5 (14.3)	*4 (12.1)*	*2 (33.3)*	8 (9.5)	*7 (8.3)*	3 (23.1)	1.00	0.54	0.64
Antibiotic treatment before and after rtPCR, n (%)	18 (51.4)	*20 (60.6)*	*2 (33.3)*	42 (50.0)	*55 (65.5)*	2 (15.4)	0.45	0.71	0.89
Correct management, n (%)	*12 (34.3)*	*24 (72.7)*	*4 (66.7)*		*62 (73.8)*	*8 (61.5)*	*0.002*	0.30	n/a

n number; rtPCR, real-time polymerase chain reaction
[a]Cases without detection of bacteria were evaluated as clinically bacterial if they fulfilled one of the following criteria: unilobular or multilobular pulmonary infiltrate *or* CRP >100 mg/l *or* PCT >0.25 μg/l *or* antibiotic therapy before rtPCR and no bacterium detection and biomarkers indeterminate (CRP >100 mg/l and PCT ≤0.25 μg/l *or* CRP between 51 and 100 mg/l and PCT not available)
[b]Cases with a detected viral pathogen excluding those patients with a clinically bacterial co-infection (as described above)
[c]Mantel-Haenszel chi square test or Fisher exact test were used

Table 9 Change of antibiotic therapy after rtPCR, pediatric patients with another indication for antibiotics were excluded

	Viral (n = 27)	Bacterial (n = 4)	Mixed (n = 3)	No pathogen (n = 18)	Clinically bacterial[a] (n = 22)	Clinically viral[b] (n = 15)	p-value[c] Viral vs. bacterial		
							Viral vs. bacterial	Viral vs. mixed	Viral vs. no pathogen
No antibiotic treatment before and after rtPCR, n (%)	12 (44.4)	1 (25.0)	0 (0.0)	6 (33.3)	6 (27.3)	11 (73.3)	0.87	0.40	0.46
Antibiotic treatment stopped after rtPCR, n (%)	6 (22.2)	0 (0.0)	0 (0.0)	1 (5.6)	2 (9.1)	4 (26.7)	0.80	1.00	0.27
Antibiotic treatment started after rtPCR, n (%)	1 (3.7)	0 (0.0)	1 (33.3)	3 (16.7)	3 (13.6)	0 (0.0)	1.00	0.39	0.34
Antibiotic treatment before and after rtPCR, n (%)	8 (29.6)	3 (75.0)	2 (66.7)	8 (44.4)	11 (50.0)	0 (0.0)	0.23	0.50	0.32
Correct management, n (%)	18 (66.7)	3 (75.0)	3 (100.0)		14 (63.6)	15 (100.0)	1.00	0.66	n/a

n number; rtPCR, real-time polymerase chain reaction
[a]Cases without detection of bacteria were evaluated as clinically bacterial if they fulfilled one of the following criteria: unilobular or multilobular pulmonary infiltrate *or* CRP >100 mg/l *or* PCT >0.25 µg/l *or* antibiotic therapy before rtPCR and no bacterium detection and biomarkers indeterminate (CRP >100 mg/l and PCT ≤0.25 µg/l *or* CRP between 51 and 100 mg/l and PCT not available)
[b]Cases with a detected viral pathogen excluding those patients with a clinically bacterial co-infection (as described above)
[c]Mantel-Haenszel chi square test or Fisher exact test were used

proportion of patients with sepsis was comparable (16/26 [62%] vs. 6/8 [75%]; $p = 0.80$). These results were similar if adults and children were analyzed separately.

Radiological findings depending on etiology

Normal CXR findings were significantly more frequent in patients with viral infection compared to bacterial infections (30% vs. 9%; $p = 0.03$). Multilobar infiltrates and pleural effusion on CXR were observed less often among subjects with viral infection (Tables 11, 12 and 13).

Predictors of viral etiology

In multivariate logistic regression (Tables 14 and 15), the absence of pleural effusion in adults was associated with detection of respiratory viruses (odds ratio [OR] 0.31, 95% confidence interval [CI] 0.12–0.80). For children, the lack of multilobar infiltrates was a significant predictor of respiratory virus detection (OR 0.22, 95% CI 0.06–0.81).

Discussion

There are three main findings in this retrospective cohort study of the impact of viral multiplex rtPCR. First, the majority of patients with viral RTI received antibiotics and antibiotics were discontinued after viral detection in only a minority of patients. Second, when biomarkers, radiologic presentations and antibiotic pretreatment were taken into account and categories of clinically bacterial and clinically viral infections were created (which more closely reflect clinical decision making), the multiplex rtPCR showed a greater impact and considerably improved correct management of clinically viral infections, from 67 to 100% among children and from 34 to 62% among adults. Third, the impact of rtPCR testing seemed to be more accentuated in

Table 10 Change of antibiotic therapy after rtPCR, all patients with another indication for antibiotics were excluded

	Viral (n = 62)	Bacterial (n = 37)	Mixed (n = 9)	No pathogen (n = 102)	Clinically bacterial[a] (n = 106)	Clinically viral[b] (n = 28)	p-value[c]		
							Viral vs. bacterial	Viral vs. mixed	Viral vs. no pathogen
No antibiotic treatment before and after rtPCR, n (%)	22 (35.5)	8 (21.6)	2 (22.2)	38 (37.3)	24 (22.6)	19 (67.9)	0.15	0.71	0.82
Antibiotic treatment stopped after rtPCR, n (%)	8 (12.9)	2 (5.4)	0 (0.0)	3 (2.9)	6 (5.7)	4 (14.3)	0.40	0.64	0.03
Antibiotic treatment started after rtPCR, n (%)	6 (9.7)	4 (10.8)	3 (33.3)	11 (10.8)	10 (9.4)	3 (10.7)	1.00	0.16	0.82
Antibiotic treatment before and after rtPCR, n (%)	26 (41.9)	23 (62.2)	4 (44.4)	50 (49.0)	66 (62.3)	2 (7.1)	0.05	1.00	0.38
Correct management, n (%)	30 (48.4)	27 (73.0)	7 (77.7)		76 (71.7)	23 (82.1)	0.02	0.19	n/a

n number; rtPCR, real-time polymerase chain reaction
[a]Cases without detection of bacteria were evaluated as clinically bacterial if they fulfilled one of the following criteria: unilobular or multilobular pulmonary infiltrate *or* CRP >100 mg/l *or* PCT >0.25 µg/l *or* antibiotic therapy before rtPCR and no bacterium detection and biomarkers indeterminate (CRP >100 mg/l and PCT ≤0.25 µg/l *or* CRP between 51 and 100 mg/l and PCT not available)
[b]Cases with a detected viral pathogen excluding those patients with a clinically bacterial co-infection (as described above)
[c]Mantel-Haenszel chi square test or Fisher exact test were used

Table 11 Radiological findings for adult patients

	Viral (n = 40)	Bacterial (n = 36)	Mixed (n = 6)	No pathogen (n = 100)	p-value[a] Viral vs. bacterial	Viral vs. mixed	Viral vs. no pathogen
X-ray, (n)	33	26	5	81			
Unilobar infiltrate, n (%)	9 (27.3)	5 (19.2)	0 (0.0)	14 (17.3)	0.48	0.47	0.23
Multilobar infiltrates, n (%)	6 (18.2)	10 (38.5)	2 (40.0)	30 (37.0)	0.09	0.56	0.05
Interstitial infiltrates, n (%)	3 (9.1)	7 (26.9)	1 (20.0)	17 (21.0)	0.14	0.89	0.13
Pleural effusion, n (%)	5 (15.2)	11 (42.3)	0 (0.0)	24 (29.6)	0.02	0.95	0.11
Normal, n (%)	8 (24.2)	2 (7.7)	1 (20.0)	14 (17.3)	0.18	1.00	0.40
Computer tomography, (n)	23	29	5	71			
Unilobar infiltrate, n (%)	5 (21.7)	4 (13.8)	0 (0.0)	7 (9.9)	0.70	0.69	0.26
Multilobar infiltrates, n (%)	11 (47.8)	16 (55.2)	4 (80.0)	32 (45.1)	0.60	0.42	0.82
Ground glass opacity, n (%)	4 (17.4)	6 (20.7)	2 (40.0)	29 (40.8)	1.00	0.57	0.04
Pleural effusion, n (%)	5 (21.7)	13 (44.8)	1 (20.0)	25 (35.2)	0.09	1.00	0.23
Normal, n (%)	2 (8.7)	0 (0.0)	0 (0.0)	0 (0.0)	0.38	1.00	0.12

n number. Multiple findings were counted individually
[a]Mantel-Haenszel chi square test or Fisher exact test were used

children than in adults. More children than adults had an appropriate discontinuation of antibiotics, and the overall management of viral infections was superior in children compared to adults. Importantly, but with the caveat of small numbers, there was no evidence that outcome was worse in those with viral etiology who discontinued antibiotics compared to those who did not.

Several previous studies analyzed the impact of rapid availability of rtPCR results on antibiotic use. In a randomized controlled trial (RCT) of 107 adults with lower RTI, antibiotics were partially or totally discontinued in 6 (11%) of 55 patients for whom rtPCR results were available, albeit without overall reduction in antibiotic treatment duration [7]. In a controlled clinical trial enrolling 583 children with acute RTI, Wishaupt et al. [4] evaluated the diagnostic yield and effect of rapid communication of rtPCR results (within 12–36 h vs. 4 weeks after testing) and failed to show a significant influence on the duration of antibiotic treatment. In contrast, Brittain-Long et al. [20] demonstrated in a RCT with 406 adults that patients randomized to rapid rtPCR results received antibiotics less frequently for acute RTI in a primary care setting during their initial visit (4.5% vs. 12.3%; $p = 0.01$). However, at the 10-day follow-up the prescription rates were similar again (13.9% vs. 17.2%; $p = 0.36$) [20]. Contrary to these findings, a retrospective pre-post study of

Table 12 Radiological findings for pediatric patients

	Viral (n = 40)	Bacterial (n = 6)	Mixed (n = 5)	No pathogen (n = 21)	p-value[a] Viral vs. bacterial	Viral vs. mixed	Viral vs. no pathogen
X-ray, (n)	28	6	5	16			
Unilobar infiltrate, n (%)	6 (21.4)	0 (0.0)	1 (20.0)	2 (12.5)	0.56	1.00	0.76
Multilobar infiltrates, n (%)	6 (21.4)	2 (33.3)	4 (80.0)	6 (37.5)	0.88	0.04	0.42
Interstitial infiltrates, n (%)	2 (7.1)	1 (16.7)	1 (20.0)	2 (12.5)	0.91	0.80	0.93
Pleural effusion, n (%)	4 (14.3)	2 (33.3)	1 (20.0)	2 (12.5)	0.56	1.00	1.00
Normal, n (%)	10 (35.7)	1 (16.7)	0 (0.0)	3 (18.8)	0.70	0.28	0.40
Computer tomography, (n)	5	1	2	3			
Unilobar infiltrate, n (%)	2 (40.0)	0 (0.0)	0 (0.0)	0 (0.0)	1.00	0.95	0.71
Multilobar infiltrates, n (%)	2 (40.0)	1 (100.0)	2 (100.0)	3 (100.0)	1.00	0.57	0.36
Ground glass opacity, n (%)	0 (0.0)	0 (0.0)	1 (50.0)	0 (0.0)	n/a	0.57	n/a
Pleural effusion, n (%)	2 (40.0)	1 (100.0)	1 (50.0)	2 (66.7)	1.00	1.00	1.00
Normal, n (%)	1 (20.0)	0 (0.0)	0 (0.0)	0 (0.0)	1.00	1.00	1.00

n number. Multiple findings were counted individually
[a]Mantel-Haenszel chi square test or Fisher exact test were used

Table 13 Radiological findings for all patients

	Viral (n = 80)	Bacterial (n = 42)	Mixed (n = 11)	No pathogen (n = 121)	p-value[a] Viral vs. bacterial	Viral vs. mixed	Viral vs. no pathogen
X-ray, (n)	61	32	10	97			
Unilobar infiltrate, n (%)	15 (24.6)	5 (15.6)	1 (10.0)	16 (16.5)	0.32	0.57	0.21
Multilobar infiltrates, n (%)	12 (19.7)	12 (37.5)	6 (60.0)	36 (37.1)	0.06	0.03	0.02
Interstitial infiltrates, n (%)	5 (8.2)	8 (25.0)	2 (20.0)	19 (19.6)	0.06	0.51	0.05
Pleural effusion, n (%)	9 (14.8)	13 (40.6)	1 (10.0)	26 (26.8)	0.01	1.00	0.08
Normal, n (%)	18 (29.5)	3 (9.4)	1 (10.0)	17 (17.5)	0.03	0.37	0.08
Computer tomography, (n)	28	30	7	74			
Unilobar infiltrate, n (%)	7 (25.0)	4 (13.3)	0 (0.0)	7 (9.5)	0.26	0.35	0.10
Multilobar infiltrates, n (%)	13 (46.4)	17 (56.7)	6 (85.7)	35 (47.3)	0.44	0.14	0.94
Ground glass opacity, n (%)	4 (14.3)	6 (20.0)	3 (42.9)	29 (39.2)	0.82	0.25	0.02
Pleural effusion, n (%)	7 (25.0)	14 (46.7)	2 (28.6)	27 (36.5)	0.09	1.00	0.28

n number. Multiple findings were counted individually
[a]Mantel-Haenszel chi square test or Fisher exact test were used

1136 children showed that the introduction of an expanded multiplex rtPCR had a shorter turnaround time and decreased the duration of antibiotic use (2.8 vs. 3.2 days; $p = 0.003$) without reducing the proportion of antibiotic prescriptions [26].

As in most previous studies, typical respiratory bacteria were not included in the test panel. Due to this technical limitation, missing a treatable pathogen is of concern in light of potential bacterial-viral co-infections [3, 7–13, 16–19]. It was shown that clinical suspicion of a bacterial super-infection was one reason for physicians to not stop antibiotics in rtPCR-positive patients [3]. We tried to partially overcome this by creating categories of clinically bacterial and clinically viral infections. This definition, aided by providing a biomarker criterion, accounted for the possibility of a viral infection in the setting of bacterial carriage. One of the major differences and advantages of the current study compared to previous publications is that it not only assessed the impact of the rtPCR results, which themselves had a limited impact on appropriate therapy, but it also integrated other 'real-world' clinical and radiologic parameters into the decision process.

Advanced molecular diagnostic tests have to be interpreted in the context of available clinical and diagnostic information in order to improve clinical management. The results confirmed the important role of clinical judgement for appropriate antibiotic prescriptions, with rtPCR providing additional information rather than being solely responsible for treatment decisions.

Quantification of genomic viral load might improve specificity of virus detection, with higher organism burden being associated with higher risk of complications and severe disease in adults and children [27, 28]. Unfortunately, quantitative results were not available with the applied assay. Similarly, optimal timing of molecular testing in relation to symptom onset and inclusion of an ever-expanding number of respiratory viruses might be important to further increase sensitivity [27]. However, to the authors' knowledge, it has not yet been studied whether either of these two factors would improve clinical management.

A pathogen was identified in 140 (55%) patients in this study, in accordance with detection rates in other studies ranging from 38 to 82% [4, 12, 17, 19, 20, 22, 29–35]. A mixed bacterial-viral etiology was found in 11 (8%)

Table 14 Prediction of respiratory virus detection for adult patients

Predictor	Univariable analysis p-value	OR (95% CI)	Multivariable analysis p-value	OR (95% CI)
Neutropenia	0.01	3.46 (1.32–9.07)	0.27	2.11 (0.56–7.89)
Hematologic malignancy	0.04	2.25 (1.02–4.97)	0.59	1.35 (0.45–4.01)
Pleural effusion	0.02	0.36 (0.15–0.86)	0.02	0.31 (0.12–0.80)
Platelets (minimum), G/l	0.02	1.00 (0.99–1.00)	0.20	1.00 (0.99–1.00)

Table 15 Prediction of respiratory virus detection for pediatric patients

Predictor	Univariable analysis p-value	OR (95% CI)	Multivariable analysis p-value	OR (95% CI)
Neutropenia	0.06	7.75 (0.92–65.66)	0.10	7.44 (0.69–80.42)
Multilobular infiltrates	0.03	0.31 (0.11–0.91)	0.02	0.22 (0.06–0.81)
White blood cells (maximum), G/l	0.02	0.94 (0.89–0.99)	0.10	0.95 (0.90–1.01)

OR odds ratio, *CI* confidence interval

patients. Previously described rates varied between 2 and 23% [17, 19, 22, 29–35]. Some studies suggested that mixed bacterial-viral infections result in more severe clinical diseases (as measured by the CURB-65 score or the pneumonia severity index) [17, 34], a higher rate of mechanical ventilation, longer duration of ICU care [36, 37], longer hospital stays [22, 36], or higher mortality [37, 38], while other studies did not [29, 39, 40]. In this study, mixed bacterial-viral infections were associated with a higher rate of ICU admission and mechanical ventilation compared to pure viral ($p = 0.05$; $p = 0.005$) and pure bacterial ($p = 0.06$; $p = 0.19$) infections if all patients were considered. However, these results should not be viewed as representative of the etiology of lower RTI in East Switzerland as these hospitals presented a preselected group of patients.

In agreement with the findings of some studies [20, 22, 34] and in contrast to others [7, 29, 39], this study failed to identify specific predictors of viral detection in multivariate logistic regression. Advancing age was previously described as more common in viral infections [19, 22, 29, 35] but the evidence is inconclusive [31, 32]. In this study, younger age was a significant predictor of virus detection in univariable logistic regression if all patients were considered, but not in stratified analyses in children and adults. The mean age in the group with respiratory viral infections was lower than in the remaining patients (29 vs. 47 years; $p < 0.001$) but the differences were not significant if stratified for children and adults.

There are some limitations to the study. First, the change of anti-infective management was retrospectively matched with the date of the rtPCR analysis. Exact time specifications were not available, leaving room for potential inaccuracies. It is not known whether and to what extent these or other factors contributed to the clinical decisions in starting, stopping, or continuing antibiotic therapy. Due to the retrospective nature of the study, it was not possible to consider the clinical presentation in the analysis. Therefore, it was difficult to reproduce the decision-making process and the primary indication for antibiotic therapy. This is an important limitation because clinical judgement remains essential concerning the use of antibiotics [41]. Furthermore, data on the consequences of rtPCR results on antibiotic treatment are difficult to obtain in the ambulatory setting, which explains the relatively small number of enrolled outpatients. Prospective studies or ideally RCTs will be necessary to confirm the findings.

Second, creating categories of clinically bacterial and clinically viral etiology by means of biomarker, radiologic presentations and antibiotic pre-treatment was done arbitrarily to reflect real-life decision-making. These theoretical reflections were important to better understand the findings; however, and as noted above, retrospectively the actual decision-making process remained unclear.

Third, the study included patients with upper and lower respiratory tract infections and did not exclude patients with antibiotic pre-treatment or significant underlying pathologic conditions, which may have biased the results but reflects clinical routine. Not having algorithms in place when to perform rtPCR testing or how to apply the results likewise mirrors the real-world scenario.

Fourth, the study's multiplex rtPCR only included respiratory viruses. Newer generation assays additionally cover atypical and typical bacteria and increase the detection of potential respiratory pathogens, albeit with yet unresolved specificity issues as these typical bacterial pathogens might also represent carriage in the absence of disease [42].

Fifth, the prevalence of RSV was underestimated in this study. In the population of hospitalized children, rapid detection tests for RSV were performed initially and, if positive, no additional rtPCR was performed. Because the study included only patients in whom an rtPCR assay for respiratory viruses was performed, the number of RSV infections was lower than expected from epidemiological data.

Conclusion

This study reveals the real-life impact of viral multiplex rtPCR in both children and adults, which was more limited in adults but improved when results were seen in the context of biomarkers, radiology, and antibiotic pretreatment. As substantial reduction of unnecessary antibiotic prescriptions seems possible, it will be necessary to develop more structured management algorithms incorporating molecular diagnostics including bacterial pathogens, which need to be prospectively tested in their efficacy and safety in RTI.

Abbreviations

CRP: C-reactive protein; CT: Computer tomography; CXR: Chest radiograph; ICU: Intensive care unit; IQR: Interquartile range; LOS: Length of stay; PCT: Procalcitonin; RCT: Randomized controlled trial; RSV: Respiratory syncytial virus; RTI: Respiratory tract infection; rtPCR: Real-time polymerase chain reaction; SIRS: Systemic inflammatory response syndrome; WBC: White blood cells count

Acknowledgements

We are grateful to the laboratory team and the archive staff of Kantonsspital St. Gallen and Children's hospital of Eastern Switzerland for providing the necessary data. We thank Michael Mayer for input in statistics.

Funding

The study was funded by the Department of Infectious Diseases and Hospital Epidemiology, Kantonsspital St. Gallen and Children's Hospital of Eastern Switzerland.

Authors' contributions

All the authors met authorship criteria. LMM, WCA, CK conceived the study, generated and designed the research plan. Data collection was performed by LMM. Data analysis was conducted by LMM and supervised by WCA. CK,

FR and PV assisted with the clinical interpretation of the data. LMM and WCA wrote the first draft of the manuscript. All authors critically reviewed the manuscript for important intellectual content and agreed with the manuscript results and conclusions. All read and approved the final manuscript.

Competing interests

The authors declare that they have no competing interests.

Author details

[1]School of Medicine, University of Basel, Klingelbergstasse 61, 4056 Basel, Switzerland. [2]Children's Hospital of Eastern Switzerland, Claudiusstrasse 6, 9006 St. Gallen, Switzerland. [3]Clinic for Pulmonology & Sleep Medicine, Kantonsspital St. Gallen, Rorschacherstrasse 95, 9007 St. Gallen, Switzerland. [4]Division of Infectious Diseases & Hospital Epidemiology, Kantonsspital St. Gallen, Rorschacherstrasse 95, 9007 St. Gallen, Switzerland.

References

1. Musher DM, Roig IL, Cazares G, Stager CE, Logan N, Safar H. Can an etiologic agent be identified in adults who are hospitalized for community-acquired pneumonia: results of a 1-year study. J Infect. 2013;67:11–8. doi:10.1016/j.jinf. 2013.03.003.
2. Lieberman D, Korsonsky I, Ben-Yaakov M, Lazarovich Z, Friedman MG, Dvoskin B, et al. A comparative study of the etiology of adult upper and lower respiratory tract infections in the community. Diagn Microbiol Infect Dis. 2002;42:21–8.
3. van de Pol AC, Wolfs TF, Tacke CE, Uiterwaal CS, Forster J, Van Loon AM, et al. Impact of PCR for respiratory viruses on antibiotic use: theory and practice. Pediatr Pulmonol. 2011;46:428–34. doi:10.1002/ppul.21385.
4. Wishaupt JO, Russcher A, Smeets LC, Versteegh FG, Hartwig NG. Clinical impact of RT-PCR for pediatric acute respiratory infections: a controlled clinical trial. Pediatrics. 2011;128:e1113–20. doi:10.1542/peds.2010-2779.
5. Creer DD, Dilworth JW, Gillespie SH, Johnston AR, Ling C, Patel S, et al. Aetiological role of viral and bacterial infections in acute adult lower respiratory tract infection (LRTI) in primary care. Thorax. 2006;61:75–9.
6. Rhedin S, Lindstrand A, Rotzén-Östlund M, Tolfvenstam T, Ohrmalm L, Rinder MR, et al. Clinical utility of PCR for common viruses in acute respiratory illness. Pediatrics. 2014;133:e538–45. doi:10.1542/peds.2013-3042.
7. Oosterheert JJ, Van Loon AM, Schuurman R, Hoepelman AI, Hak E, Thijsen S, et al. Impact of rapid detection of viral and atypical bacterial pathogens by real-time polymerase chain reaction for patients with lower respiratory tract infection. Clin Infect Dis. 2005;41:1438–44.
8. van de Pol AC, Wolfs TF, Jansen NJ, Van Loon AM, Rossen JW. Diagnostic value of real-time polymerase chain reaction to detect viruses in young children admitted to the pediatric intensive care unit with lower respiratory tract infection. Crit Care. 2006;10:R61.
9. Nolte FS. Molecular diagnostics for detection of bacterial and viral pathogens in community-acquired pneumonia. Clin Infect Dis. 2008;47:S123–6. doi:10. 1086/591392.
10. Templeton KE, Scheltinga SA, van den Eeden WC, Graffelman AW, van den Broek PJ, Claas EC. Improved diagnosis of the etiology of community-acquired pneumonia with real-time polymerase chain reaction. Clin Infect Dis. 2005;41:345–51.
11. Sanghavi SK, Bullotta A, Husain S, Rinaldo CR. Clinical evaluation of multiplex real-time PCR panels for rapid detection of respiratory viral infections. J Med Virol. 2012;84:162–9. doi:10.1002/jmv.22186.
12. Johansson N, Kalin M, Tiveljung-Lindell A, Giske CG, Hedlund J. Etiology of community-acquired pneumonia: increased microbiological yield with new diagnostic methods. Clin Infect Dis. 2010;50:202–9. doi:10.1086/648678.
13. Ruuskanen O, Lahti E, Jennings LC, Murdoch DR. Viral pneumonia. Lancet. 2011;377:1264–75. doi:10.1016/S0140-6736(10)61459-6.
14. Martin ET, Fairchok MP, Stednick ZJ, Kuypers J, Englund JA. Epidemiology of multiple respiratory viruses in childcare attendees. J Infect Dis. 2013;207: 982–9. doi:10.1093/infdis/jis934.
15. Walsh EE, Peterson DR, Kalkanoglu AE, Lee FE, Falsey AR. Viral shedding and immune response to respiratory syncytial virus infection in older adults. J Infect Dis. 2013;207:1424–32. doi:10.1093/infdis/jit038.
16. Bakaletz LO. Viral potentiation of bacterial superinfection of the respiratory tract. Trends Microbiol. 1995;3:110–4.
17. Falsey AR, Becker KL, Swinburne AJ, Nylen ES, Formica MA, Hennessey PA, et al. Bacterial complications of respiratory tract viral illness: a comprehensive evaluation. J Infect Dis. 2013;208:432–41. doi:10.1093/infdis/jit190.
18. De Roux A, Ewig S, García E, Marcos MA, Mensa J, Lode H, et al. Mixed community-acquired pneumonia in hospitalised patients. Eur Respir J. 2006; 27:795–800.
19. Van Gageldonk-Lafeber AB, Wever PC, van der Lubben IM, De Jager CP, Meijer A, De Vries MC, et al. The etiology of community-acquired pneumonia and implications for patient management. Neth J Med. 2013;71:418–25.
20. Brittain-Long R, Westin J, Olofsson S, Lindh M, Andersson LM. Access to a polymerase chain reaction assay method targeting 13 respiratory viruses can reduce antibiotics: a randomised, controlled trial. BMC Med. 2011;9:44. doi:10.1186/1741-7015-9-44.
21. Stolz D, Christ-Crain M, Gencay MM, Bingisser R, Huber PR, Müller B, et al. Diagnostic value of signs, symptoms and laboratory values in lower respiratory tract infection. Swiss Med Wkly. 2006;136:434–40.
22. Huijskens EG, Koopmans M, Palmen FM, Van Erkel AJ, Mulder PG, Rossen JW. The value of signs and symptoms in differentiating between bacterial, viral and mixed etiology in patients with community-acquired pneumonia. J Med Microbiol. 2014;63:441–52. doi:10.1099/jmm.0.067108-0.
23. Ambrosioni J, Bridevaux PO, Wagner G, Mamin A, Kaiser L. Epidemiology of viral respiratory infections in a tertiary care centre in the era of molecular diagnosis, Geneva, Switzerland, 2011–2012. Clin Microbiol Infect. 2014;20: O578–84. doi:10.1111/1469-0691.12525.
24. Bone RC, Balk RA, Cerra FB, Dellinger RP, Fein AM, Knaus WA, et al. Definitions for sepsis and organ failure and guidelines for the use of innovative therapies in sepsis. The ACCP/SCCM Consensus Conference Committee. American College of Chest Physicians/Society of Critical Care Medicine. Chest. 1992;101:1644–55.
25. Goldstein B, Giroir B, Randolph A. International pediatric sepsis consensus conference: definitions for sepsis and organ dysfunction in pediatrics. Pediatr Crit Care Med. 2005;6:2–8.
26. Rogers BB, Shankar P, Jerris RC, Kotzbauer D, Anderson EJ, Watson JR, et al. Impact of a rapid respiratory panel test on patient outcomes. Arch Pathol Lab Med. 2015;139:636–41. doi:10.5858/arpa.2014-0257-OA.
27. Lee N, Chan MCW, Lui GCY, Li R, Wong RYK, Yung IMH, et al. High viral load and respiratory failure in adults hospitalized for respiratory syncytial virus infections. J Infect Dis. 2015;212(8):1237–40. doi:10.1093/infdis/jiv248.
28. Hasegawa K, Jartti T, Mansbach JM, Laham FR, Jewell AM, Espinola JA, et al. Respiratory syncytial virus genomic load and disease severity among children hospitalized with bronchiolitis: Multicenter cohort studies in the United States and Finland. J Infect Dis. 2015;211(10):1550–9. doi:10.1093/ infdis/jiu658.
29. Johnstone J, Majumdar SR, Fox JD, Marrie TJ. Viral infection in adults hospitalized with community-acquired pneumonia: prevalence, pathogens, and presentation. Chest. 2008;134:1141–8. doi:10.1378/chest.08-0888.
30. Cillóniz C, Ewig S, Polverino E, Marcos MA, Esquinas C, Gabarrús A, et al. Microbial etiology of community-acquired pneumonia and its relation to severity. Thorax 2011; 66: 340–346. Thorax. 2011;66:340–6. doi:10.1136/thx.2010.143982.
31. Viasus D, Marinescu C, Villoslada A, Cordero E, Gálvez-Acebal J, Fariñas MC, et al. Community-acquired pneumonia during the first post-pandemic influenza season: a prospective, multicentre cohort study. J Infect. 2013;67: 185–93. doi:10.1016/j.jinf.2013.05.006.
32. Michelow IC, Olsen K, Lozano J, Rollins NK, Duffy LB, Ziegler T, et al. Epidemiology and clinical characteristics of community-acquired pneumonia in hospitalized children. Pediatrics. 2004;113:701–7.
33. Choi SH, Hong SB, Ko GB, Lee Y, Park HJ, Park SY, et al. Viral infection in patients with severe pneumonia requiring intensive care unit admission. Am J Respir Crit Care Med. 2012;186:325–32. doi:10.1164/rccm.201112-2240OC.
34. Jennings LC, Anderson TP, Beynon KA, Chua A, Laing RT, Werno AM, et al. Incidence and characteristics of viral community-acquired pneumonia in adults. Thorax. 2008;63:42–8.
35. Jain S, Self WH, Wunderink RG, Fakhran S, Balk R, Bramley AM, et al. Community-Acquired Pneumonia Requiring Hospitalization among U.S. Adults. N Engl J Med. 2015;373:415–27. doi:10.1056/NEJMoa1500245.
36. Ghani AS, Morrow BM, Hardie DR, Argent AC. An investigation into the prevalence and outcome of patients admitted to a pediatric intensive care unit with viral respiratory tract infections in Cape Town, South Africa. Pediatr Crit Care Med. 2012;13:e275–81. doi:10.1097/PCC.0b013e3182417848.
37. Rice TW, Rubinson L, Uyeki TM, Vaughn FL, John BB, Miller 3rd RR, et al. Critical illness from 2009 pandemic influenza A virus and bacterial coinfection in the

United States. Crit Care Med. 2012;40:1487–98. doi:10.1097/CCM.0b013e3182416f23.

38. Diederen BM, Van Der Eerden MM, Vlaspolder F, Boersma WG, Kluytmans JA, Peeters MF. Detection of respiratory viruses and Legionella spp. by real-time polymerase chain reaction in patients with community acquired pneumonia. Scand J Infect Dis. 2009;41:45–50. doi:10.1080/00365540802448799.
39. Bello S, Mincholé E, Fandos S, Lasierra AB, Ruiz MA, Simon AL, et al. Inflammatory response in mixed viral-bacterial community-acquired pneumonia. BMC Pulm Med. 2014;14:123. doi:10.1186/1471-2466-14-123.
40. Marcos MA, Camps M, Pumarola T, Martinez JA, Martinez E, Mensa J, et al. The role of viruses in the etiology of community-acquired pneumonia in adults. Antivir Ther. 2006;11(3):351–9.
41. Filice GA, Drekonja DM, Thurn JR, Hamann GM, Masoud BT, Johnson JR. Diagnostic Errors that Lead to Inappropriate Antimicrobial Use. Infect Control Hosp Epidemiol. 2015;36:949–56. doi:10.1017/ice.2015.
42. Gadsby NJ, Russell CD, Mchugh MP, Mark H, Conway Morris A, Laurenson IF, et al. Comprehensive molecular testing for respiratory pathogens in community-acquired pneumonia. Clin Infect Dis. 2016;62(7):817–23. doi:10.1093/cid/civ1214.

14

Tuberculosis and pneumonia in HIV-infected children

Helena Rabie[1,2,3*] and Pierre Goussard[1]

Abstract

Pneumonia remains the most common cause of hospitalization and the most important cause of death in young children. In high human immunodeficiency virus (HIV)-burden settings, HIV-infected children carry a high burden of lower respiratory tract infection from common respiratory viruses, bacteria and *Mycobacterium tuberculosis*. In addition, *Pneumocystis jirovecii* and cytomegalovirus are important opportunistic pathogens. As the vertical transmission risk of HIV decreases and access to antiretroviral therapy increases, the epidemiology of these infections is changing, but HIV-infected infants and children still carry a disproportionate burden of these infections. There is also increasing recognition of the impact of *in utero* exposure to HIV on the general health of exposed but uninfected infants. The reasons for this increased risk are not limited to socioeconomic status or adverse environmental conditions—there is emerging evidence that these HIV-exposed but uninfected infants may have particular immune deficits that could increase their vulnerability to respiratory pathogens. We discuss the impact of tuberculosis and other lower respiratory tract infections on the health of HIV-infected infants and children.

Keywords: Human immunodeficiency virus, HIV, Children, Lower respiratory tract infection, Tuberculosis, Pneumonia

Background

To prevent vertical transmission of human immunodeficiency virus (HIV) from mother to child and to improve long-term outcomes for HIV-infected pregnant women, the current standard of care is to initiate lifelong suppressive antiretroviral therapy (ART) [1]. With this strategy, transmission should be less than 1% in women who either know their status, or are diagnosed early in pregnancy and are retained in care on an effective regimen [1, 2]. However, as vertical HIV transmission risk decreases there is increasing recognition of adverse health impacts suffered by HIV-exposed but uninfected (HEU) infants, including vulnerability to developing lower respiratory tract infections (LRTIs) and tuberculosis (TB) due to socioeconomic status and adverse environmental conditions such as maternal ill health and lack of breastfeeding [3]. In these infants there is also increasing recognition of immune dysfunction including immune activation, altered T-cell numbers and function, and possibly humoral immunity [3].

Despite major reductions in vertical HIV transmission among adequately treated mothers, large numbers of HIV-infected children continue to be born, especially in settings where HIV service delivery or maternal uptake of available services is sub-optimal. In 2013, it was estimated that globally there were 240,000 new pediatric HIV infections [4]. In the absence of antiretroviral therapy, perinatally infected infants and children have high morbidity and mortality, with 50% dying by the age of 2 years in low resource settings [5]. Despite the high early mortality without ART, many perinatally infected children have slowly progressive disease and some may only be diagnosed in late childhood or adolescence [6]. As established by clinical, epidemiological and postmortem studies, LRTIs are the major cause of morbidity and mortality in HIV-infected children. LRTIs in HIV-infected children are from common childhood respiratory pathogens (viral and bacterial), as well as opportunistic pathogens, such as *Pneumocystis jirovecii*, cytomegalovirus (CMV) and *Mycobacterium tuberculosis* [7–11].

* Correspondence: hrabie@sun.ac.za
[1]Department of Pediatrics and Child Health, University of Stellenbosch and Tygerberg Academic Hospital, Cape Town, South Africa
[2]Childrens Infectious Diseases Clinical Research Unit (KidCRU), University of Stellenbosch, Cape Town, South Africa
Full list of author information is available at the end of the article

Tuberculosis

Epidemiology

The overlap in the epidemiology of TB and HIV is well known, with its epicenter in sub-Saharan Africa. All of the countries with HIV prevalence of more than 10% in persons aged 15–49 years are in sub-Saharan Africa, and more than 90% of all HIV-infected children live in this region [3, 12, 13]. In addition, all of the countries with a TB incidence of more than 500 cases per 100,000 population are in sub-Saharan Africa, although large case numbers are also found in Asian countries with high population numbers [12]. In settings with a high burden of both TB and HIV, high rates of co-infection are reported and up to 56% of children treated for TB in sub-Saharan Africa are considered to be HIV-infected [8]. Studies of HIV cohorts confirm high rates of incident and prevalent TB. In Cape Town, South Africa, TB program data suggested a TB incidence of 1596 cases per 100,000 among HIV-infected infants prior to the implementation of universal ART [14], while clinical cohort data identified 53 cases per 100 patient-years in children not on ART [15]. A randomized-controlled trial to assess the effect of universal isoniazid preventive therapy (IPT) in HIV-infected children found a TB disease rate of 121 per 1000 patient-years in children who had early ART access [16].

Major differences in the number of children diagnosed in TB endemic settings with comparable adult TB incidence rates probably reflect varying ability to diagnose TB in young children [8]. Irrespective of the setting, it remains crucial to test all TB patients for HIV. This is highlighted by cohort reports from multiple settings; in the United Kingdom, 8 of 18 TB/HIV co-infected children presented with TB, which prompted their HIV diagnosis [17]. Studies of older children and adolescents in Zimbabwe found a high yield of new HIV diagnosis in adolescents presenting with TB [18]. Rates of TB are not only increased in HIV-infected infants, but evidence suggests that HEU infants are also at increased risk for TB. Data from South Africa suggest this risk may be 4-fold that of the general population [19], with rates of 41 cases per 1000 child-years reported in HEU infants [16].

Reasons for the high rates of TB in HIV-infected infants are multifactorial. HIV-infected and HEU infants and children are highly exposed to adult TB source cases. HIV-infected adults are 21–34 times more likely to develop TB in high burden settings, with TB accounting for up to a quarter of HIV-associated mortality [20]. Woman of child-bearing age are disproportionately affected [21], which implies a high risk of household TB exposure in vulnerable young HIV-infected and HEU children [22]. In a study of IPT in high TB burden settings, 10% of HIV-exposed infants had contact with potential source cases by the age of 14 weeks [23]. If TB in HIV-infected pregnant women is missed, the infants are not only at risk of TB, but have a 3-fold higher HIV acquisition rate [24]. Where there are no strategies to identify mothers with sputum smear-negative TB, there may be significant delays in diagnosis and extended exposure of young children to risk of infection [25, 26].

Alongside exposure and infection, young age is one of the most important risk factors for developing severe disease [27]. However, young age is poorly studied as a risk factor in HIV-infected children in resource-limited settings, but as many as 33% of infants starting ART at a median age of 8 months are already receiving anti-TB therapy [28]. Other risk factors are poor nutritional status (stunting, wasting and reduced mid-upper arm circumference), advanced immune suppression and anemia [8]. School attendance is also associated with disease in older children, reflecting poor ventilation in schools in low-resource, high-burden settings [22].

Prevention

The most important tools we have to mitigate the HIV-associated risk of developing TB infection and disease are (i) access to ART for adults and children with HIV; and (ii) use of IPT. In the Children with HIV Early Antiretroviral Therapy (CHER) trial, conducted in Cape Town and Johannesburg, South Africa, TB occurred in 8.3% of children receiving early ART (initiated before12 weeks of age) and in 20% of children receiving delayed ART (commenced only after specific clinical and immunologic criteria were met) [29]. When ART is initiated in older children, reductions in presumed and confirmed incident TB of 32–70% are documented [8]. Nevertheless, HIV-infected children have more TB than their uninfected peers, including in low-burden settings [8, 30]. A transient increase in risk can also be expected in the first 3 months of therapy as part of immune reconstitution inflammatory syndrome (IRIS) [31, 32].

Though there is a decline in the number of children commencing ART only when they are severely immunocompromised, this situation is still common. In 2010 in Asia, Africa and South America, 63% of HIV-infected children in low-income countries, 66% in low–middle-income and 58% in upper–middle-income countries were already severely immunocompromised when commencing ART, compared with 19% of HIV-infected children in the United States [33]. Access to ART with broad penetration into the community will impact the epidemiology of TB, because there will be a decrease in adult cases of pulmonary disease. This is already clear from the decline in adult and pediatric TB cases in South Africa as the adult ART uptake increased. In Soweto, South Africa, ART access in TB in HIV-uninfected children declined from 18.7 to 11.0 per 100,000 [34].

In 2014, The Joint United Nations Programme on HIV/AIDS (UNAIDS) defined its ambitious 90–90–90 targets. The three targets to be achieved by 2020 are: 90% of HIV-infected persons must be diagnosed, 90% of those diagnosed should be on sustained therapy, and 90% of those on therapy should have an undetectable viral load [35]. If ART coverage expands to 80% of infected persons and all infected persons are eligible for therapy, the incidence of TB should decline by 28–37%. However, even if these targets are achieved, finding and treating TB cases remains important as it will prevent mortality and reduce TB transmission [36].

IPT is a well known prevention strategy in HIV-uninfected children and adults with known exposure to TB. In HIV-infected children there are no studies assessing post-exposure prevention; however, in a cohort of 494 children beginning ART when younger than 24 months of age in Cape Town, 127 courses of post-exposure IPT were provided, with only two children developing confirmed TB. Both had fully drug-susceptible isolates [28]. In a prospective study of prevention in older HIV-infected children, many with a history of prior TB infection, both all-cause mortality (16% in the placebo arm vs. 8% in the IPT arm) and incident cases of TB (9.9% vs. 3.8%) declined [37]. A subsequent reanalysis assessing the role of IPT and ART in these children found that the greatest reduction was in children receiving both ART and IPT [38]. In contrast, a pre-exposure prevention study enrolling very young infants found high rates of TB in HIV-infected and HEU infants, but no differences between those receiving IPT and placebo [16]. In this study, drug resistance was found to play an important role in IPT failure [39]. When present, children typically have primary rather than secondarily acquired multidrug-resistant (MDR) TB. HIV infection was independently associated with prevalent TB disease among child household contacts of adult MDR-TB cases and with failure of MDR preventative therapy [40]. In South African children with MDR-TB, HIV infection was reported in 54, 77, and 22% of cases from Johannesburg, Kwa-Zulu Natal, and Cape Town, respectively [41–43]. Reviewing the susceptibility/resistance patterns of adult contacts with TB is an essential component of managing children with HIV, irrespective of whether or not they have TB at the time. In children with MDR-TB, HIV is associated with a poorer outcome [44, 45].

The temporal associations between TB, influenza, and pneumococcal disease in children suggest a complex interaction between these infections. There is an increase in TB diagnosis approximately 3 months after the annual influenza season and a reduction in culture-confirmed TB in HIV-infected children following receipt of pneumococcal conjugate vaccines [46, 47]. The Antiretroviral Research for Watoto (ARROW) study followed 1,206 HIV-infected children for 5 years after ART and it included a randomized intervention to stop or continue co-trimoxazole after 96 weeks on ART. In this study, reduction in TB was associated not only with the duration of ART, but also with continued co-trimoxazole preventative therapy [48].

Diagnosis

Pulmonary TB is the most common disease manifestation in HIV-infected children, with 85% diagnosed in an early series of hospitalized South African children [49]. However, both intra- and extra-thoracic disease may occur concurrently [49–52]. The principles of TB diagnosis include the following steps: 1) carefully assess TB contact history and/or seek proof of infection; 2) enquire about suggestive symptoms; and 3) seek evidence of active disease and bacteriologic confirmation. TB symptoms, though similar in HIV-infected and uninfected infants and children, overlap with symptoms of other infections and HIV itself. The chest radiograph may be very difficult to interpret, especially when there is underlying lung disease. TB may also be confused with acute pneumonia in HIV-infected children. It should also be remembered that HIV-infected children who have not yet been diagnosed with an underlying HIV infection may present to the health service with TB [6, 8, 15, 17, 18, 49, 50, 53].

Treatment

The potential drug interactions between the TB therapy and ART are well known and, in general, TB therapy should not change. A dual treatment plan should consider the following questions:

1) What is the suspected or confirmed susceptibility pattern of *M. tuberculosis* and which drugs should be used?
2) Are alternative rifamycins to rifampicin available?
3) Which ART regimen is preferred AND can a suppressive regimen be given safely?
4) What are the potential drug interactions AND can adjustments be made if rifampicin is the only rifamycin available?

In the absence of ART, high mortality in HIV-infected children with TB was reported [49, 54] and continued with delayed ART initiation, especially when TB was the presenting diagnosis. Most deaths occurred within the first 2 months of delayed ART initiation and were not always directly TB-related [28].

Pharmacokinetic studies illustrate that both efavirenz and lopinavir-ritonavir 1:1 in their usual doses provide appropriate drug levels when co-administered with rifampicin [55, 56]. There are, however, ongoing concerns over nevirapine dosing and recommendations on dose adjustments have been suggested [57]. Table 1 summarizes important considerations when treating TB/HIV

Table 1 Summary of the first and second line anti-tuberculosis medications with recommended doses and drug-drug interactions* [60–63]

Drug	Dose Recommended	Drug-drug interactions with antiretrovirals
Group 1		
Isoniazid	7–15 mg/kg once daily	None
Rifampicin	10–20 mg/kg once daily	Coadministration reduces concentrations of[a] NNRTIs, [b]PIs, integrase inhibitors
Pyrazinamide	30–40 mg/kg once daily	None
Ethambutol	15–25 mg/kg once daily	None
Rifabutin	10–20 mg/kg/day (Max Dose 300 mg/day)	Boosted PI: increase rifabutin levels and rifabutin dose reduction is needed NNRTI: Efavirence reduces the concentration of rifabutin, increasing the rifabutin dose is recommended in adults Nevirapine dose adjustment is not needed for rifabutin
Group 2		
Kanamycin	15–30 mg/kg once daily, max 1 g	
Amikacin	15–22.5 mg/kg once daily, max 1 g	
Capreomycin	15–30 mg/kg once daily, max 1 g	
Streptomycin	20–40 mg/kg once daily, max 1 g	
Group 3		
Ofloxacin	15–20 mg/kg once daily, max 800 mg	
Levofloxacin	(15–20 mg/kg once daily)†, 7.5–10 mg/kg once daily, max 750 mg	
Moxifloxacin	7.5–10 mg/kg once daily, max 400 mg	Moxifloxacin concentration could be reduced by ritonavir, though limited data; buffered didanosine may reduce oral absorption of all fluoroquinolones
Group 4		
Ethionamide/ Prothionamide	15–20 mg/kg once daily, max 1 g	Possible, unknown
Cycloserine/Terizidone	10–20 mg/kg once or twice daily, max 1 g	Unlikely, unknown
Para-aminosalicylic acid (PAS)	150 mg/kg granules daily in 2–3 divided doses, max 12 g	Co-administration with efavirenz may reduc PAS AUC by 50%
Group 5		
Linezolid	(10 mg/kg twice daily, once daily for >10 years of age)[c]	Unlikely
Clofazimine	(3–5 mg/kg once daily)[c]	Unknown; may be a weak CYP3A4 inhibitor
Amoxicillin-clavulanic acid, Meropenem-clavulanic acid, and Imipenem/cilastin	As for bacterial infections	Unlikely
Thiacetazone	5–8 mg/kg once daily	Contraindicated in HIV-infected individuals
High-dose isoniazid	15–20 mg/kg once daily	None
Clarithromycin	7.5–15 mg/kg twice daily	Clarithomycin levels increase with boosted atazanavir and lopinavir with increased risk of toxisity. Clarithomycin levels are decreased by efavirence, nevirapine and etravirine Azithromycinn is prefered
Azithromycin	10 mg/kg once daily	Prefered macrolide but limited activity and caution required

† Indicates bracketed recommended by some experts, but differs from formal WHO guideline
[a]*NNRTI* Non-nucleoside reverse transcriptase inhibitor, [b]*PI* Protease inhibitor
[c]No formal paediatric dose recommended in WHO guidelines, so presented dose based on experience and expert opinion

co-infection [58–61]. In co-treated children, efavirenz has not been associated with worse outcomes, but despite reassuring data on the pharmacokinetic outcomes of lopinavir-ritonavir 1:1 concurrent TB therapy may be a risk factor for failure in children on lopinavir-ritonavir treatment [62–64]. The World Health Organization (WHO) also recommends a non-suppressive regimen of zidovidine, lamivudine and abacavir in children needing rifampicin as a short-term measure to avoid drug interactions [65]. This is based on the ARROW study. In

ARROW, three nucleoside/nucleotide reverse transcriptase inhibitors (NRTIs) were studied as an intensive induction and maintenance strategy when combined with non-nucleoside reverse transcriptase inhibitors (NNRTIs). Fifty-nine of the 1143 children required a drug alteration for TB that included stopping or replacing the NNRTI nevirapine. In contrast, children taking efavirenz did not require a drug switch. Triple NRTI for HIV suppression was effective at 36 weeks, but not at 144 weeks. The advantage of this latter strategy is that, although viral suppression is inferior, the risk of progressive NNRTI and protease inhibitor (PI) ART resistance was avoided and drug–drug interactions and logistic complications were minimized [66]. There is no current guidance on using integrase inhibitors and other PIs such as darunavir in children, and no data on newer anti-TB agents such as bedaquiline and delamanid in HIV-infected children. Nevertheless, ART should be initiated 2–8 weeks after starting TB therapy so as to reduce the risk of IRIS occurring [61]. For example, in TB meningitis cases deterioration due to paradoxical IRIS can be devastating and ART should be delayed at least 4 weeks [67, 68]. In Table 2 we highlight key messages to consider in TB and HIV co-infected children. TB may be an important challenge and opportunity in achieving the UNAID 90–90–90 targets [69].

Table 2 Summary of key messages related to TB/HIV co-infection in children

HIV-infected and exposed uninfected (HEU) children are at high risk of developing TB	High likelihood of household TB exposure early in life; disproportionate TB/HIV burden in young mothers
	Advanced disease, low CD4 count and malnutrition are additional risk factors
	All children with HIV must be regularly screened for TB exposure and disease
	BCG vaccination is contra-indicated in children known to be HIV-infected
Strategies to prevent TB	High community penetration of adult ART will reduce TB transmission in communities
	Universal early ART initiation in all HIV-infected
	Appropriate use of INH preventative therapy
	Active TB Case finding
	Infection prevention and control strategies
	History of contact
Early diagnosis of TB	Symptoms can overlap with other opportunistic infections
	Pulmonary and extrapulmonary disease possible
	Pulmonary TB can present like acute pneumonia
	A positive TST (≥5 mm) or IGRA confirms TB infection but not disease
	CXR is important; HIV-infected children more likely to have alveolar opacification and lung cavities
	Collect specimens for culture and Xpert MTB/RIF® as appropriate
Treating TB/HIV co-infection	Use appropriate/standard TB treatment regimen
	Adapt the ART regimen and dosing
	Support adherence
	Monitor for efficacy and side effects

HIV human immunodeficiency virus, *TB* tuberculosis, *ART* antiretroviral treatment, *INH* isoniazid, *TST* tuberculin skin test, *IGRA* interferon gamma release assay, *CXR* chest radiograph

Pneumonia

Pneumonia remains the leading cause of pediatric mortality and morbidity. Globally, there are approximately 12–14 million hospitalizations and 0.68–0.92 million deaths annually from pneumonia in children [70–72]. HIV-infected children are at increased risk of pneumonia that requires hospital admission and death from this infection. In a meta-analysis and modelling study, Theodoratou and colleagues [7] calculated that in 2010 there were 0.6–3.3 million pneumonia episodes and 47,400–153,000 pneumonia deaths in HIV-infected children living in low-resource settings. Of these cases, 1.3 million (90%) pneumonia episodes and 93% of the deaths occurred in children younger than 5 years of age from the Africa region. HIV-infected children had a 6.5 (95% CI 5.9–7.2) increase in odds of pneumonia that required hospitalization and they had an increased risk of death (odds ratio 5.9, 95% CI 2.7–12.7) [7]. The authors showed that there is also a wide variation between countries; for example, in Zimbabwe 55% of all pneumonia deaths are attributed to HIV, compared to 1% in India [7].

Even with early access to ART, pneumonia remains common among HIV-infected infants and children. In the CHER study, pneumonia occurred at a rate of 12.2 infections/100 person-years in children accessing ART before 12 weeks of age and 26.5 infections/100 person-years in children accessing ART only after laboratory evidence of immune suppression and/or clinical features of HIV infection became apparent [29]. Poor general health and malnutrition, immune depletion, chronic lung disease, increasing household exposure and vaccine responsiveness may all contribute to the risk of LRTI. A wide range of pathogens causing LRTIs and pneumonia in children with HIV is reported [73]. The importance of polymicrobial infections—including combinations of bacterial, viral, *P. jirovecii* and mycobacterial infections—is well recognized. Mortality is increased significantly with increasing numbers of pathogens. Children with polymicrobial pneumonia have a 10-fold greater risk of dying than children in whom only a single organism is identified [74].

Acute bacterial pneumonia

HIV-infected children have a higher risk of developing bacterial pneumonia than uninfected children. This remains a significant problem, even after the introduction of ART. HIV-infected children with pneumonia are more likely to have severe disease (including bacteremia), more complications, higher rates of treatment failure and death, and possibly more antimicrobial resistance than HIV-uninfected children [74]. The most common cause of bacterial pneumonia remains *Streptococcus pneumoniae*, but *Staphylococcus aureus* is increasingly important. Amongst Gram-negative bacteria associated with pneumonia in HIV-infected children, *Klebsiella* species, *Haemophilus influenzae*, *Escherichia coli*, *Pseudomonas aeruginosa* and non-typhoidal *Salmonella* species are also important [73].

HIV does not affect the radiographic appearance of bacterial pneumonia. The two classic patterns of either diffuse patchy air-space disease of bronchopneumonia, or confluent air-space disease with air bronchograms of lobar or segmental pneumonia can be found [75]. Necrotizing pneumonia, a severe complication of community-acquired pneumonia in non-HIV infected children, is characterized by liquefaction and cavitation of lung tissue and is being seen increasingly [76, 77]. The most common cause is *S. pneumoniae*, and although in the authors' experience it also occurs in HIV-infected children, this has not been reported to date in the literature. The chest radiographs in necrotizing pneumonia frequently demonstrate both pleural and parenchymal involvement. The so-called 'atypical pneumonias' can present with a variable radiographic appearance, which includes reticulonodular infiltration, patchy or confluent air-space disease or a combination of all three patterns [78]. It is, therefore, very important to correlate the radiographic appearance with the clinical setting [78].

Without appropriate vaccination or ART, HIV-infected children experience a 40-fold increase in the risk of pneumococcal bacteremia, pneumonia and meningitis compared to vaccinated HIV-uninfected children, and they also often experience multiple episodes of invasive disease [79]. In South Africa, ART decreased the pneumonia burden by half with an even higher (65.2%) decline in mortality from invasive pneumococcal disease [80]. Vaccinating with the pneumococcal conjugate vaccine causes a significant reduction in vaccine-type serotype colonization and disease [79–81]. The reported increases in empyema with non-vaccine serotypes are mostly from areas with very low incidence of HIV and the real incidence of empyema in HIV-positive children is not known [82].

Viral pneumonia

Viral infections play a major role in LRTIs and viruses are commonly identified in HIV-infected children hospitalized with these infections. Viral LRTIs may also play an important role in the pathogenesis of bacterial pneumonia and in the epidemiology of TB. In a large study from South Africa at least one virus was identified in 68% of HIV-infected children younger than 5 years of age and in 58% of those aged 5–14 years presenting with symptoms of a LRTI. More than one respiratory virus was found in 28 and 19% of children within these age groups, respectively. In children younger than 5 years the most common viruses detected were human rhinovirus (36%), adenovirus (32%), respiratory syncytial virus (RSV) (13%), enterovirus (8%), parainfluenza (9%) and influenza viruses (7%) [83, 84]. In addition, human bocavirus, human polyomaviruses and human coronaviruses are increasingly found in children with LRTIs, including those with HIV [85]; however, it is difficult to attribute causality to these viruses [85].

RSV is a very important pathogen in infants and young children and a common cause of LRTIs that require healthcare visits and hospitalization. HIV is an important risk factor for severe RSV infections, especially in high-burden settings [86]. HIV-infected children are older and may develop RSV outside of the seasonal peaks. Compared with HEU children, there is an increased incidence of hospitalization (3–5-fold) in children with HIV, and they tend to stay in hospital longer and have a higher risk of death. In a South African study of RSV-associated LRTI infection, 49 of the 1157 children with confirmed RSV were HIV-infected. In this study, ART data was only available for 12 cases, 6 of whom received ART. Four of the 9 deaths in this study occurred in HIV-infected children; however, their ART data are unknown [87].

Influenza is an important cause of pneumonia hospitalization and death. ART naïve HIV-infected children are up to 8 times more likely to be hospitalized and have a higher case fatality rate (8% in HIV-infected vs. 2% in uninfected children) [88, 89]. In a prospective South African study, pandemic and seasonal H1N1 influenza had a similar clinical course in HIV-infected children [90]. Giannattasio et al. reported on 11 HIV-infected and 30 otherwise healthy children hospitalized for H1N1 influenza. Leukopenia was recorded in 64% of HIV-infected and in 20% of healthy children ($p = 0.01$). Interstitial pneumonia was more frequent in HIV-positive children and consolidation was more frequent in HIV-negative children. Overall, 91% of HIV-positive children received oseltamivir. The H1N1 influenza attack rate was very high (20%) in HIV-infected children, but it consistently ran a mild course [91]. Annual vaccination with the seasonal influenza vaccine is recommended, but efficacy may be influenced by decreased vaccine immunogenicity reported in some studies [92].

CMV is a common co-infection in HIV-infected children and is frequently isolated from urine and respiratory secretions [93, 94]. Congenital and post-partum acquisition of CMV is common in HIV-exposed and infected infants and CMV infection may be associated with breastfeeding acquisition of HIV [95, 96]. The role of co-infection with CMV in children, especially those suspected of having *P. jiroveci* pneumonia (PJP), is poorly understood, but CMV itself can cause fatal pneumonia [94, 97]. Postmortem studies from Africa reported that in the 0–5 months age group, CMV (42.1%) was the second most common cause of fatal pneumonia after *P. jirovecci* (51.3%) [9]. The isolation of CMV by culture or polymerase chain reaction (PCR) from various sites or specimens does not prove that the child has CMV pneumonia. The chest radiographic appearance of PJP and CMV pneumonia can be very similar (diffuse alveolar disease). In children being ventilated for PJP and not responding to treatment for PJP, CMV was histologically proven in 72% of cases and associated with a poor outcome [97, 98]. CMV viremia is common in all infants with pneumonia, and a viral logarithmic load (to the base 10) of 4.6 or more was predictive of pneumonia in a study of from Cape Town [99]. In HIV-infected infants with severe pneumonia from suspected PJP, we would suggest that empiric treatment for CMV infection with either ganciclovir or valgancyclovir be used wherever possible, until such time that CMV infection can be excluded.

Despite access to effective vaccination, measles remains an important pathogen in children [100]. In settings with a high HIV burden, a significant number of children hospitalized with measles are also infected with HIV—such as Zambia, where up to 17% of hospitalized children with measles had HIV infection [101]. HIV-infected children with measles are significantly younger than uninfected children and often have not yet received the first vaccination of their primary measles containing vaccine schedule, even if that is scheduled at 9 months of age [102, 103]. Consequently, the WHO recommends first dose of a measles containing vaccine be administered at the age of 6 months in HIV-infected children [104]. Measles is generally thought to be more severe in HIV-infected children—both the duration of illness prior to hospitalization and the duration of hospitalization is longer [102, 103]. In low-resource settings, the case fatality rate is 2–7-fold higher in children with HIV [103, 104]. The effect of ART in preventing measles or modifying its severity is not fully understood, but initiation of ART at the time of admission for measles did not prevent readmission during a recent large measles outbreak in Cape Town [102].

Pneumocystis jiroveci pneumonia

P. jirovecii is a common and important pathogen in HIV-infected children and causes a severe, rapidly progressive pneumonia with a high mortality rate despite access to antibiotic therapy [93, 94]. This pathogen is also increasingly reported in severe pneumonia in young HEU infants [105, 106]. The chest radiograph findings show increased lung volumes (78%) and diffuse parenchymal opacification (64%) that lead ultimately to diffuse alveolar opacification (92%). This usually happens within 72 h of presentation [107]. Clinically, lack of fever, high respiratory rate, low oxygen saturation and absence of co-trimoxazole preventative therapy is suggestive of PJP. Real-time PCR is better than immunofluorescence at making a microbiologic diagnosis [108]. When PJP is suspected, high-dose co-trimoxazole and steroids should be added to the management of severe LRTI.

The most important strategy to prevent PJP is by using co-trimoxazole prophylactic therapy from 6 weeks of age [109]. Stopping co-trimoxazole after CD4 recovery was studied in African children, and its continuation may have additional benefits beyond PJP prophylaxis, including TB prevention [48].

Conclusions

Acute respiratory compromise caused by *M. tuberculosis* and other lung pathogens is a major cause of disease and death in HIV-infected children. Furthermore, many also develop chronic lung disease with bronchiectasis due to recurrent lung infections [110, 111]. In children with delayed ART initiation, nearly a third (28%) develop chronic lung disease with significantly compromised lung function [112]. This highlights the need for early ART initiation and universal ART access for all HIV-infected children to reduce the high burden of lung disease. Finally, vaccination, appropriate use of preventive therapy and early effective treatment of lung infections, including TB, are also essential to ensure optimal lung health in HIV-infected children.

Abbreviations

ARROW: The Antiretroviral Research for Watoto; ART: Antiretroviral therapy; CHER: Children with HIV early antiretroviral; CMV: Cytomegalovirus; CXR: Chest radiograph; HEU: HIV-exposed but uninfected infants; HIV: Human immunodeficiency virus; IGRA: Interferon gamma release assay; IPT: Isoniazid preventive therapy; IRIS: Immune reconstitution inflammatory syndrome; LRTI: Lower respiratory tract infections; MDR: Multidrug-resistant; NNRTI: Non-nucleoside reverse transcriptase inhibitors; NRTI: Nucleoside/nucleotide reverse transcriptase inhibitors; PCR: Polymerase chain reaction; PI: Protease inhibitor; PJP: *P. jiroveci* pneumonia; RSV: Respiratory syncytial virus; TB: Tuberculosis; TST: Tuberculin skin test; UNAIDS: The Joint United Nations Programme on HIV/AIDS; WHO: World Health Organization

Acknowledgements

We would like to thank Prof BJ Marais for reviewing the manuscript and for suggestions.

Funding

Helena Rabie is supported by The National Research Foundation of South Africa.

Competing interests

The authors declare that they have no competing interests.

Authors' contributions

HR review literature on tuberculosis and pneumonia and prepared the manuscript. PG reviewed the data on pneumonia and reviewed the manuscript. All authors met ICMJE authorship criteria. All authors contributed equally to the writing of the first draft of the manuscript and writing of the manuscript. All authors critically reviewed the manuscript for important intellectual content. All authors agreed with the manuscript results and conclusions.

Author details

[1]Department of Pediatrics and Child Health, University of Stellenbosch and Tygerberg Academic Hospital, Cape Town, South Africa. [2]Childrens Infectious Diseases Clinical Research Unit (KidCRU), University of Stellenbosch, Cape Town, South Africa. [3]Division of Infectious Diseases, Department of Paediatrics and Child Health, Faculty of Medicine and Health Sciences, Stellenbosch University, PO Box 241, Cape Town 8000, South Africa.

References

1. Fowler MG, Qin M, Fiscus SA et al. PROMISE: Efficacy and safety of 2 strategies to prevent perinatal HIV transmission. CROI 2015. 2015 Conference on Retroviruses and Opportunistic Infections (CROI 2015), 23–26 February 2015, Seattle. Oral abstract 31LB.
2. World Health Organization. Consolidated guidelines on the use of antiretroviral drugs for treating and preventing HIV infection: recommendations for a public health approach. Geneva: World Health Organization; 2013.
3. Evans C, Jones CE, Prendergast AJ. HIV-exposed, uninfected infants: new global challenges in the era of paediatric HIV elimination. Lancet Infect Dis. 2016;16(6).
4. World Health Organization. Global update on the health sector response to HIV. 2014. http://www.who.int/hiv/pub/progressreports/update2014-executive-summary/en/.
5. Newell ML, Coovadia H, Cortina-Borja M, Rollins N, Gaillard P, Dabis F. Mortality of infected and uninfected infants born to HIV infected mothers in Africa: a pooled analysis. Lancet. 2004;364:1236–43.
6. Ferrand RA, Corbett EL, Wood R, et al. AIDS among older children and adolescents in Southern Africa: projecting the time course and magnitude of the epidemic. AIDS. 2009;23:2039–46.
7. Theodoratou E, McAllister DA, Reed C, et al. Global, regional, and national estimates of pneumonia burden in HIV infected children in 2010: a meta-analysis and modelling study. Lancet Infect Dis. 2014;14(12):1250–8.
8. Venturini E, Turkova A, Chiappini E, Galli L, de Martino M, Thorne C. Tuberculosis and HIV co-infection in children. BMC Infect Dis. 2014;14 Suppl 1:S5.
9. Bates M, Mudenda V, Mwaba P, Zumla A. Deaths due to respiratory tract infections in Africa: a review of autopsy studies. Curr Opin Pulm Med. 2013;19(3):229–37.
10. Chintu C, Mudenda V, Lucas S, et al. Lung diseases at necropsy in African children dying from respiratory illnesses: a descriptive necropsy study. Lancet. 2002;360:985.
11. Gupta RK, Lucas SB, Fielding KL, Lawn SD. Prevalence of tuberculosis in post-mortem studies of HIV infected adults and children in resource-limited settings: a systematic review and meta-analysis. AIDS. 2015;29(15):1987–2002.
12. World Health Organization. Global tuberculosis report. Contract No.: WHO/HTM/TB/2014.08. 2014. http://www.who.int/tb/publications/global_report/en/.
13. Dodd PJ, Gardiner E, Coghlan R, Seddon JA. Burden of childhood tuberculosis in 22 high-burden countries: a mathematical modeling study. Lancet Glob Health. 2014;2(8):e453_9.
14. Hesseling AC, Cotton MF, Jennings T, et al. High Incidence of Tuberculosis among HIV infected Infants: Evidence from a South African population-based study highlights the need for improved tuberculosis control strategies. Clin Infect Dis. 2009;48:10.
15. Walters E, Cotton MF, Rabie H, Schaaf HS, Walters LO, Marais BJ. Clinical presentation and outcome of tuberculosis in human immunodeficiency virus infected children on antiretroviral therapy. BMC Pediatr. 2008;8:1.
16. Madhi SA, Nachman S, Violari A, et al. Effect of primary isoniazid prophylaxis against tuberculosis in HIV-exposed children. N Eng J Med. 2011;365:21–31.
17. Cohen JM, Whittaker E, Walters S, Lyall H, Tudor-Williams G, Kampmann B. Presentation, diagnosis and management of tuberculosis in HIV infected children in the UK. HIV Med. 2008;9(5):277–84.
18. Ferrand RA, Bandason T, Musvaire P, et al. Causes of acute hospitalization in adolescence: burden and spectrum of HIV-related morbidity in a country with an early-onset and severe HIV epidemic: a prospective survey. PLoS Med. 2010;7(2):e1000178.
19. Cotton MF, Slogrove A, Rabie H. Infections in HIV-exposed Uninfected Children With Focus on Sub-Saharan Africa. Pediatr Infect Dis J. 2014;33(10):1085–6.
20. Lawn SD, Churchyard G. Epidemiology of HIV-associated tuberculosis. Curr Opin HIV AIDS. 2009;4:325–33.
21. Lawn SD, Bekker LG, Middelkoop K, Myer L, Wood R. Impact of HIV infection on the epidemiology of tuberculosis in a peri-urban community in South Africa: the need for age-specific interventions. Clin Infect Dis. 2006;42:1040–7.
22. Wood R, Johnstone-Robertson S, Uys P, et al. Tuberculosis transmission to young children in a South African community: modeling household and community infection risks. Clin Infect Dis. 2010;51:401–8.
23. Cotton MF, Schaaf HS, Lottering G, Weber HL, Coetzee J, Nachman S. Tuberculosis exposure in HIV-exposed infants in a high-prevalence setting. Int J Tuberc Lung Dis. 2008;12:225–7.
24. Gupta A, Bhosale R, Kinikar A, et al. Maternal tuberculosis: a risk factor for mother-to-child transmission of human immunodeficiency virus. J Infect Dis. 2011;203:358–63.
25. Tostmann A, Kik SV, Kalisvaart NA, et al. Tuberculosis transmission by patients with smear-negative pulmonary tuberculosis in a large cohort in the Netherlands. Clin Infect Dis. 2008;47:1135–42.
26. Lawn SD, Edwards D, Wood R. Tuberculosis transmission from patients with smear-negative pulmonary tuberculosis in sub-Saharan Africa. Clin Infect Dis. 2009;48:496–7.
27. Marais BJ, Gie RP, Schaaf HS, et al. The natural history of childhood intra-thoracic tuberculosis: a critical review of literature from the pre-chemotherapy era. Int J Tuberc Lung Dis. 2004;8(4):392–402.
28. Walters E, Duvenhage J, Draper HR, et al. Severe manifestations of extrapulmonary tuberculosis in HIV infected children initiating antiretroviral therapy before 2 years of age. Arch Dis Child. 2014;99(11):998–1003.
29. Violari A, Cotton MF, Gibb DM, et al. Early antiretroviral therapy and mortality among HIV infected infants. N Engl J Med. 2008;359:2233–44.
30. Turkova A, Chappell E, Judd A, et al. Prevalence, incidence, and associated risk factors of tuberculosis in children with HIV living in the UK and Ireland (CHIPS): a cohort study. Lancet HIV. 2015;2(12):e530–9. doi:10.1016/S2352-3018(15)00200-3. Epub 2015 Oct 29.
31. Orikiiriza J, Bakeera-Kitaka S, Musiime V, Mworozi EA, Mugyenyi P, Boulware DR. The clinical pattern, prevalence, and factors associated with immune reconstitution inflammatory syndrome in Ugandan children. AIDS. 2010;24:2009–17.
32. Bakeera-Kitaka S, Conesa-Botella A, Dhabangi A, et al. Tuberculosis in human immunodeficiency virus infected Ugandan children starting on antiretroviral therapy. Int J Tuberc Lung Dis. 2011;15:1082–6.
33. Koller M, Patel K, Chi BH, et al. Immunodeficiency in children starting antiretroviral therapy in low-, middle-, and high-income countries. J Acquir Immune Defic Syndr. 2015;68:62–72.
34. Dangor Z, Izu A, Hillier K, et al. Impact of the antiretroviral treatment program on the burden of hospitalization for culture-confirmed tuberculosis in South African Children: a time-series analysis. Pediatr Infect Dis J. 2013;32:972–7.
35. UNAIDS. 90–90–90 An ambitious treatment target to help end the AIDS epidemic. UNAIDS/JC2684. 2014. Available from: http://www.unaids.org/sites/default/files/media_asset/90-90-90_en_0.pdf. [cited 2015 Feb 13].
36. Pretorius C, Menzies NA, Chindelevitch L, et al. The potential effects of changing HIV treatment policy on tuberculosis outcomes in South Africa: results from three tuberculosis-HIV transmission models. AIDS. 2014;28 Suppl 1:S25–34. doi:10.1097/QAD.0000000000000085.
37. Zar HJ, Cotton MF, Strauss S, et al. Effect of isoniazid prophylaxis on mortality and incidence of tuberculosis in children with HIV: randomised controlled trial. BMJ. 2007;334:136.
38. Frigati LJ, Kranzer K, Cotton MF, Schaaf HS, Lombard CJ, Zar HJ. The impact of isoniazid preventive therapy and antiretroviral therapy on tuberculosis in children infected with HIV in a high tuberculosis incidence setting. Thorax. 2011;66:496–501.

39. Hesseling AC, Kim S, Madhi S, Nachman S, et al. High prevalence of drug resistance amongst HIV-exposed and -infected children in a tuberculosis prevention trial. Int J Tuberc Lung Dis. 2012;16:192–5.
40. Seddon JA, Hesseling AC, Finlayson H, et al. Preventive therapy for child contacts of multidrug-resistant tuberculosis: a prospective cohort study. Clin Infect Dis. 2013;57(12):1676–84.
41. Seddon JA, Hesseling AC, Willemse M, Donald PR, Schaaf HS. Culture-confirmed multidrug-resistant tuberculosis in children: clinical features, treatment, and outcome. Clin Infect Dis. 2012;54(2):157–66.
42. Hicks RM, Padayatchi N, Shah NS, et al. Malnutrition associated with unfavorable outcome and death among South African MDR-TB and HIV co-infected children. Int J Tuberc Lung Dis. 2014;18(9):1074–83.
43. Fairlie L, Beylis NC, Reubenson G, Moore DP, Madhi SA. High prevalence of childhood multi-drug resistant tuberculosis in Johannesburg, South Africa: a cross sectional study. BMC Infect Dis. 2011;11:28.
44. Seddon JA, Hesseling AC, Godfrey-Faussett P, Schaaf HS. High treatment success in children treated for multidrug-resistant tuberculosis: an observational cohort study. Thorax. 2014;69(5):458–64.
45. Isaakidis P, Casas EC, Das M, Tseretopoulou X, Ntzani EE, Ford N. Treatment outcomes for HIV and MDR-TB co-infected adults and children: systematic review and meta-analysis. Int J Tuberc Lung Dis. 2015;19(8):969–78.
46. Dangor Z, Izu A, Moore DP, et al. Temporal association in hospitalizations for tuberculosis, invasive pneumococcal disease and influenza virus illness in South African children. PLoS One. 2014;9(3):e91464.
47. Moore DP, Klugman KP, Madhi SA. Role of Streptococcus pneumoniae in hospitalization for acute community-acquired pneumonia associated with culture-confirmed Mycobacterium tuberculosis in children: a pneumococcal conjugate vaccine probe study. Pediatr Infect Dis J. 2010;1(2):1099–04.
48. Crook AM, Turkova A, Musiime V, et al. Tuberculosis incidence is high in HIV infected African children but is reduced by co-trimoxazole and time on antiretroviral therapy. BMC Med. 2016;14:50.
49. Madhi SA, Huebner RE, Doedens L, Aduc T, Wesley D, Cooper PA. HIV-1 co-infection in children hospitalised with tuberculosis in South Africa. Int J Tuberc Lung Dis. 2000;4:448–54.
50. Marais BJ, Schaaf HS. Tuberculosis in children. Cold Spring Harb Perspect Med. 2014;4(9):a017855. doi:10.1101/cshperspect.a017855.
51. Schaaf HS, Marais BJ, Whitelaw A, et al. Culture-confirmed childhood tuberculosis in Cape Town, South Africa: a review of 596 cases. BMC Infect Dis. 2007;7:140.
52. Hesseling AC, Schaaf SH, Westra AE, et al. Outcome of HIV infected children with culture-confirmed tuberculosis. Arch Dis Child. 2005;90:1171–4.
53. Maritz E, Liu L, Montepierda G, et al. Timing of tuberculosis sourse case contact information and tuberculosis in HIV infected and HIV-exposed non-infected children from southern Africa: IMPAACT 1041. 43rd Union World Conference on Lung Health 2012 Nov 13–17; Kuala Lumpur, Malaysia. Abstract PC 640 17.
54. Jeena PM, Pillay P, Pillay T, Coovadia HM. Impact of HIV-1 co-infection on presentation and hospital-related mortality in children with culture proven pulmonary tuberculosis in Durban, South Africa. Int J Tuberc Lung Dis. 2002;6:672–8.
55. Ren Y, Nuttall JJ, Eley BS, et al. Effect of rifampicin on efavirenz pharmacokinetics in HIV infected children with tuberculosis. J Acquir Immune Defic Syndr. 2009;50(5):439–43.
56. Ren Y, Nuttall JJ, Egbers C, et al. Effect of Rifampicin on Lopinavir Pharmacokinetics in HIV infected children with tuberculosis. J Acquir Immune Defic Syndr. 2008;47:566–9.
57. Oudijk JM, McIlleron H, Mulenga V, et al. Pharmacokinetics of nevirapine in HIV infected children under 3 years on rifampicin-based antituberculosis treatment. AIDS. 2012;26(12):1523–8.
58. Yapa HM, Boffito M, Pozniak A. Critical Review: What dose of rifabutin is recommended with antiretroviral therapy? J Acquir Immune Defic Syndr. 2016;72:138-52.
59. World Health Organization. Guidelines for the programmatic management of drug-resistant tuberculosis: Emergency Update 2008. 2008. http://whqlibdoc.who.int/publications/2008/9789241547581_eng.pdf.
60. Seddon JA, Hesseling AC, Marais BJ, et al. Paediatric use of second-line anti-tuberculosis agents: a review. Tuberculosis (Edinb). 2012;92(1):9–17. 3.
61. Coyne KM, Pozniak AL, Lamorde M, Boffito M. Pharmacology of second-line antituberculosis drugs and potential for interactions with antiretroviral agents. AIDS. 2009;23(4):437–46. 10.
62. Frohoff C, Moodley M, Fairlie L, et al. Antiretroviral therapy outcomes in HIV infected children after adjusting protease inhibitor dosing during tuberculosis treatment. PloS one. 2011;6:e17273. doi:10.1371/journal.pone.001727.
63. Meyers T, Sawry S, Wong JY, et al. Virologic failure among children taking lopinavir/ritonavir-containing first-line antiretroviral therapy in South Africa. Pediatr Infect Dis J. 2014:1.
64. Reitz C, Coovadia A, Ko S, et al. Initial response to protease-inhibitor-based antiretroviral therapy among children less than 2 years of age in South Africa: effect of cotreatment for tuberculosis. J Infect DIs. 2010;201:1121–31.
65. World Health Organization. Consolidated guidelines on the use of antiretroviral drugs for treating and preventing HIV infection: recommendations for a public health approach. 2013. Available from: http://www.who.int/publications/guidelines/en/. [cited 2015 Feb 13].
66. Arrow Trial Team. Routine versus clinically driven laboratory monitoring and first-line antiretroviral therapy strategies in African children with HIV (ARROW): a 5-year open-label randomised factorial trial. Lancet. 2013;381(9875):1391–403.
67. Bahr N, Boulware DR, Marais S, Scriven J, Wilkinson RJ, Meintjes G. Central nervous system immune reconstitution inflammatory syndrome. Curr Infect Dis Rep. 2013;15:583–93.
68. van Toorn R, Rabie H, Dramowski A, Schoeman JF. Neurological manifestations of TB-IRIS: a report of 4 children. Eur J Paediatr Neurol. 2012;16:676–82.
69. Rabie H, Frigati L, Hesseling AC, Garcia-Prats AJ. Tuberculosis: opportunities and challenges for the 90-90-90 targets in HIV infected children. J Int AIDS Soc. 2015;18 Suppl 6:20236.
70. Liu L, Oza S, Hogan D, et al. Global, regional, and national causes of child mortality in 2000–13, with projections to inform post-2015 priorities: an updated systematic analysis. Lancet. 2015;385(9966):430–40. published online Oct 1. http://dx.doi.org/10.1016/S0140-6736(14)61698-6.
71. Rudan I, O'Brien KL, Nair H, et al. Epidemiology and etiology of childhood pneumonia in 2010: estimates of incidence, severe morbidity, mortality, underlying risk factors and causative pathogens for 192 countries. J Glob Health. 2013;3:10401.
72. Nair H, Simoes EA, Rudan I, et al. Global and regional burden of hospital admissions for severe acute lower respiratory infections in young children in 2010: a systematic analysis. Lancet. 2013;381:1380–90.
73. Gray DM, Zar HJ. Community-acquired pneumonia in HIV infected children: a global perspective. Curr Opin Pulm Med. 2010;16(3):208–16.
74. McNally LM, Jeena PM, Gajee K, et al. Effect of age, polymicrobial disease, and maternal HIV status on treatment response and cause of severe pneumonia in South African children: a prospective descriptive study. Lancet. 2007;369:1440–51.
75. George R, Andronikou S, Theron S, et al. Pulmonary infections in HIV. Pediatr Radiol. 2009;39(6):545–54. doi:10.1007/s00247-009-1194-9.
76. Sawicki GS, Lu FL, Valim C, Cleveland RH, Colin AA. Necrotising pneumonia is an increasingly detected complication of pneumonia in children. Eur Respir J. 2008;31(6):1285–91.
77. Edinburgh KJ, Jasmer RM, Huang L, et al. Multiple pulmonary nodules in AIDS: usefulness of CT in distinguishing among potential causes. Radiology. 2000;214:427–32.
78. El-Atrouni W, Berbari E, Temesgen Z. HIV-associated opportunistic infections. Bacterial infections. J Med Liban. 2006;54:80–3.
79. Bliss SJ, O'Brein KL, Janoff EN. The evidence for using conjugate vaccines to protect HIV infected children against pneumococcal disease. Lancet Infect Dis. 2008;8:67–80.
80. Nunes MC, von Gottberg A, de Gouveia L, et al. The impact of antiretroviral treatment on the burden of invasive pneumococcal disease in South African children: a time series analysis. AIDS. 2011;25(4):453–62.
81. Madhi SA, Izu A, Nunes MC, et al. Longitudinal study on Streptococcus pneumoniae, Haemophilus influenzae and Staphylococcus aureus nasopharyngeal colonization in HIV infected and -uninfected infants vaccinated with pneumococcal conjugate vaccine. Vaccine. 2015;33(23):2662–9.
82. Fletcher MA, Schmitt HJ, Syrochkina M, Sylvester G. Pneumococcal empyema and complicated pneumonias: global trends in incidence, prevalence, and serotype epidemiology. Eur J Clin Microbiol Infect Dis. 2014;33:879–910.
83. Cohen C, Walaza S, Moyes J, et al. Epidemiology of viral-associated acute lower respiratory tract infection among children <5 years of age in a high HIV prevalence setting, South Africa, 2009–2012. Pediatr Infect Dis J. 2015;34(1):66–72.
84. Cohen C, Walaza S, Moyes J, et al. Epidemiology of severe acute respiratory illness (SARI) among adults and children aged ≥5 years in a high HIV-prevalence setting, 2009–2012. PLoS One. 2015;10(2):e0117716.
85. Nunes MC, Kuschner Z, Rabede Z, et al. Clinical epidemiology of bocavirus, rhinovirus, two polyomaviruses and four coronaviruses in HIV infected and HIV-uninfected South African children. PLoS One. 2014;9(2):e86448.

86. Shi T, Balsells E, Wastnedge E, et al. Risk factors for respiratory syncytial virus associated with acute lower respiratory infection in children under five years: systematic review and meta-analysis. J Glob Health. 2015;5(2):020416.
87. Moyes J, Cohen C, Pretorius M, et al. Epidemiology of respiratory syncytial virus-associated acute lower respiratory tract infection hospitalizations among HIV infected and HIV-uninfected South African children, 2010–2011. J Infect Dis. 2013;208 Suppl 3:S217–26.
88. Madhi SA, Schoub B, Simmank K, Blackburn N, Klugman KP. Increased burden of respiratory viral associated severe lower respiratory tract infections in children infected with human immunodeficiency virus type-1. J Pediatr. 2000;137(1):78–84.
89. Madhi SA, Ramasamy N, Bessellar TG, Saloojee H, Klugman KP. Lower respiratory tract infections associated with influenza A and B viruses in an area with a high prevalence of pediatric human immunodeficiency type 1 infection. Pediatr Infect Dis J. 2002;21:291–7.
90. Madhi SA, Kuwanda L, Venter M, Violari A. Prospective cohort study comparing seasonal and H1N1(2009) pandemic influenza virus illnesses in HIV infected children during 2009. Pediatr Infect Dis J. 2014;33(2):174–6.
91. Giannattasio A, Lo Vecchio A, Russo MT, et al. Pandemic flu: a comparative evaluation of clinical, laboratory, and radiographic findings in HIV-positive and negative children. AIDS. 2010;24(14):2292–4.
92. Cerevalolo A, Orsi A, Parodi V, Ansaldi F. Influenza vaccination in HIV-positive subjects: latest evidence and future perspective. J Prev Med Hyg. 2013;54(1):1–10.
93. Jeena PM, Coovadia HM, Chrystal V. Pneumocystis carinii and cytomegalovirus infections in severely ill, HIV infected African infants. Ann Trop Paediatr. 1997;76:124–8.
94. Williams AJ, Duong T, McNally LM, et al. Pneumocystis carinii pneumonia and cytomegalovirus infection in children with vertically acquired HIV infection. Aids. 2001;15:335–9.
95. Gumbo H, Chasekwa B, Church JA, et al. Congenital and postnatal CMV and EBV acquisition in HIV infected Zimbabwean infants. PLoS One. 2014;9(12):e114870.
96. Chang TS, Wiener J, Dollard SC, et al. Effect of cytomegalovirus infection on breastfeeding transmission of HIV and on the health of infants born to HIV infected mothers. AIDS. 2015;29(7):831–6.
97. Goussard P, Kling S, Gie RP, Nel ED, Heyns L, Rossouw GJ, Janson JT. CMV pneumonia in HIV infected ventilated infants. Pediatr Pulmonol. 2010;45:650–5.
98. Zampoli M, Morrow B, Hsiao NY, Whitelaw A, Zar HJ. Prevalence and outcome of cytomegalovirus-associated pneumonia in relation to human immunodeficiency virus infection. Pediatr Infect Dis J. 2011;30(5):413–7.
99. Hsiao NY, Zampoli M, Morrow B, Zar HJ, Hardie D. Cytomegalovirus viraemia in HIV exposed and infected infants: prevalence and clinical utility for diagnosing CMV pneumonia. J Clin Virol. 2013;58(1):74–8.
100. Moss WJ, Griffin DE. Measles. Lancet. 2012;379:153–64.
101. Moss WJ, Monze M, Ryon JJ, Quinn TC, Griffin DE, Cutts F. Prospective study of measles in hospitalized, human immunodeficiency virus (HIV)-infected and HIV-uninfected children in Zambia. Clin Infect Dis. 2002;35:189–96.
102. le Roux DM, le Roux SM, Nuttall JJ, Eley BS. South African measles outbreak 2009–2010 as experienced by a paediatric hospital. S Afr Med J. 2012;102:760–4.
103. Measles vaccines: WHO position paper. Wkly Epidemiol Rec 2009;84:349–60.
104. Moss WJ, Fisher C, Scott S, et al. HIV type 1 infection is a risk factor for mortality in hospitalized Zambian children with measles. Clin Infect Dis. 2008;46:523–7.
105. Mussi-Pinhata MM, Freimanis L, Yamamoto AY, et al. Infectious disease morbidity among young HIV-1-exposed but uninfected infants in Latin American and Caribbean countries: the National Institute of Child Health and Human Development International Site Development Initiative Perinatal Study. Pediatrics. 2007;119:e694–704.
106. Slogrove AL, Cotton MF, Esser MM. Severe infections in HIV-exposed uninfected infants: clinical evidence of immunodeficiency. J Trop Pediatr. 2010;56(2):75–81.
107. Pitcher RD, Daya R, Beningfield SJ, Zar HJ. Chest radiographic presenting features and radiographic progression of pneumocystis pneumonia in South African children. Pediatr Pulmonol. 2011;46(10):1015–22.
108. Morrow BM, Samuel CM, Zampoli M, Whitelaw A, Zar HJ. Pneumocystis pneumonia in South African children diagnosed by molecular methods. BMC Res Notes. 2014;7:26.
109. Chintu C, Bhat GJ, Walker AS, et al. Co-trimoxazole as prophylaxis against opportunistic infections in HIV infected Zambian children (CHAP): a double-blind randomised placebo-controlled trial. Lancet. 2004;364(9448):1865–71.
110. Berman DM, Mafut D, Djokic B, Scott G, Mitchell C. Risk factors for the development of bronchiectasis in HIV infected children. Pediatr Pulmonol. 2007;42(10):871 5.
111. Sheikh S, Madiraju K, Steiner P, Rao M. Bronchiectasis in pediatric AIDS. Chest. 1997;112(5):1202. 7.
112. McHugh G, Rylance J, Mujuru H, et al. Chronic morbidity among older children and adolescents at diagnosis of HIV infection. J Acquir Immune Defic Syndr. 2016. [Epub ahead of print].

15

Development of PCRSeqTyping—a novel molecular assay for typing of *Streptococcus pneumoniae*

Geetha Nagaraj, Feroze Ganaie, Vandana Govindan and Kadahalli Lingegowda Ravikumar*

Abstract

Background: Precise serotyping of pneumococci is essential for vaccine development, to better understand the pathogenicity and trends of drug resistance. Currently used conventional and molecular methods of serotyping are expensive and time-consuming, with limited coverage of serotypes. An accurate and rapid serotyping method with complete coverage of serotypes is an urgent necessity. This study describes the development and application of a novel technology that addresses this need.

Methods: Polymerase chain reaction (PCR) was performed, targeting 1061 bp cpsB region, and the amplicon was subjected to sequencing. The sequence data was analyzed using the National Centre for Biotechnology Information database. For homologous strains, a second round of PCR, sequencing, and data analysis was performed targeting 10 group-specific genes located in the capsular polysaccharide region. Ninety-one pneumococcal reference strains were analyzed with PCRSeqTyping and compared with Quellung reaction using Pneumotest Kit (SSI, Denmark).

Results: A 100% correlation of PCRSeqTyping results was observed with Pneumotest results. Fifty-nine reference strains were uniquely identified in the first step of PCRSeqTyping. The remaining 32 homologous strains out of 91 were also uniquely identified in the second step.

Conclusion: This study describes a PCRSeqTyping assay that is accurate and rapid, with high reproducibility. This assay is amenable for clinical testing and does not require culturing of the samples. It is a significant improvement over other methods because it covers all pneumococcal serotypes, and it has the potential for use in diagnostic laboratories and surveillance studies.

Keywords: Molecular serotyping, PCRSeqTyping, *Streptococcus pneumoniae*, cpsB sequencing

Background

Streptococcus pneumoniae, found in the upper respiratory tract of healthy children and adults, causes a range of infections including meningitis, septicemia, pneumonia, sinusitis, and otitis media. Children < 2 years of age and adults aged ≥65 years of age are particularly susceptible [1]. According to the Morbidity and Mortality Weekly Report, April 26 2013 [2], an estimated 14.5 million cases of serious pneumococcal disease (including pneumonia, meningitis, and sepsis) occur each year in children aged <5 years worldwide, which has resulted in approximately 500,000 deaths, mostly in low- and middle-income developing countries.

The high morbidity and mortality caused by pneumococci are not clearly understood. The pathogenicity of pneumococci has been linked to various virulence factors such as capsule, cell wall and its component polysaccharides, pneumolysin, PspA, complement factor H-binding component, autolysin, neuraminidase, peptide permeases, hydrogen peroxide, and IgA1 protease [3–5]. Capsular polysaccharide (CPS) is the primary virulence factor, and is also used to categorize, *S. pneumoniae*into more than 90 different serotypes [6–8]. Capsule is important for the survival of bacteria at infection site as it provides resistance to phagocytosis [9].

* Correspondence: klravikumar@gmail.com
Central Research Laboratory, KIMS Hospital and Research Centre, KR Road, VV Purum, Bangalore, Karnataka 560 004, India

Pneumococcal CPS is generally synthesized by the Wzx/Wzy-dependent pathway, except for types 3 and 37, which are produced by the synthase pathway [10, 11]. Most genes required for synthesis of capsule are within the capsule polysaccharide synthesis (*cps*) operon, which ranges from 10 kb (serotype 3) to 30 kb (serotype 38). *Cps* operon is flanked by *dexB* in 5′ end and *aliA* at 3′ end. Neither of these participates in capsule synthesis. The 5′-end of the CPS loci starts with regulatory and processing genes *wzg, wzh, wzd,* and *wze* (also known as *cpsABCD*), which are conserved with high sequence identity in all serotypes, followed by the central region consisting of serotype specific genes [12, 13].

Pneumococcal serotyping is necessary for epidemiological and vaccine impact studies. It also aids in understanding the pathogenicity of the organism and closely monitors for the emergence of non-vaccine strains, replacement serotypes, and new serovars [14, 15]. Widespread use of pneumococcal vaccines has led to replacement with serotypes that are not included in the vaccines. Continuous monitoring of serotypes is therefore essential for epidemiological surveillance and long-term vaccine impact studies [16–20].

Several phenotypic and genotypic methods are currently used to identify pneumococcal group and type. The phenotypic serotyping methods of capsular swelling reaction, latex agglutination and coagglutination tests are costly, require skilled personnel, and cannot detect all serotypes. Genotypic typing methods that assess genome variation include sequential multiplex polymerase chain reaction (PCR), sequential real-time PCR, restriction fragment length polymorphism (RFLP), microarray, sequetyping, and matrix-assisted lazer desorption ionization-time of flight (MALDI-TOF) analysis. In addition to general applicability and a high discriminatory power, these genotypic assays are economical, detect pneumococci directly from the clinical specimen, and detect emerging serovars, replacement strains, and vaccine escape recombinants [21]. However, many of these methods are multistep, intricate, and do not discriminate all serotypes [22–26].

It is crucial to develop a robust, simple method with complete serotype coverage for serotype detection and pneumococcal serogroup/serotype surveillance [27]. Herein, the authors describe an innovative serotyping approach that relies on sequencing of assembly genes located in the capsular operon to identify all pneumococcal serotypes.

Methods

Reference strains

There were 91 reference serotype strains of *S. pneumoniae* obtained from Staten Serum Institute, Copenhagen, Denmark (Table 1).

Clinical isolates

There were 28 clinical isolates of *S. pneumoniae* selected from isolates submitted to Central Research Laboratory, KIMS Hospital, Bangalore (Table 2). They were isolated from blood ($n = 23$), cerebrospinal fluid (CSF) ($n = 3$) and pleural fluid ($n = 2$).

Media and culture conditions

Strains were stored in skim milk, tryptone, glucose, and glycerol (STGG) media at −80 °C. They were cultured on 5% sheep blood agar (Chromogen, Hyderabad) for 18–24 hrs at37°C with 5% CO_2. The isolates were characterized as *S. pneumoniae* by colony morphology, alpha hemolysis, bile solubility, and optochin susceptibility.

Serotyping

Quellung reaction was performed using Pneumotest kit and type-specific antisera (SSI, Denmark), as recommended by the manufacturer.

PCRSeqTyping

PCRSeqTyping assay was performed in two steps. Step I involved PCR amplification and sequencing of the *cpsB* gene from genomic DNA. There were 91 serotypes that were divided into non-homologous group (Group I, 59 serotypes) and homologous group (Group II, 32 serotypes) based on the *cpsB* sequence data. The homologous group was further subdivided into 10 subgroups based on the sequence homology. The second step involved PCR and sequencing of each homology group by using specific primers in order to identify the unique serotypes.

Nucleic acid extraction

Genomic DNA was extracted from bacterial strains using QIAamp DNA mini kit (Qiagen, Germany), as per the manufacturer's protocol.

PCR amplification

PCR reaction was performed using the primers designed by Leung et al. [26] with modifications. Primers used in the study were *cps1-FP* (5′-GCAATGCCAGACAGT AACCTCTAT-3)′, *cps2-RP* (5′-CCTGCCTGCAAGTCT TGATT-3′) and cps-2538-RP (5′-CTTTACCAACCTT TGTAATCCAT-3′). The reaction mixture was modified to contain 50–100 ng of genomic DNA, 0.75 units XT-5 polymerase (3 U/µl, Merck, which is a mixture of thermo stable enzymes Taq DNA polymerase and proof-reading [PR] polymerase), 1X XT5A-Assay buffer, 1 µl deoxynucleoside triphosphates (dNTPs, 2.5 mM each [Fermentas, United States]), 1 µl forward primer (100 ng/µl), 1 µl of reverse primer mix (100 ng/µl). The final reaction volume was made up to 25 µl with DNase/RNase-free distilled water (Gibco, United States). Thermal

Table 1 PCRseqtyping results for 91 SSI strains

Sl. NO	Serogroup	Serotype	NCBI ACCESSION NO	PCRSeqTyping results	
				Step I	Step 2
1	1	1	CR931632	1	
2	2	2	CR931632	2/41A	2
3	3	3	CR931634	3	
4	4	4	CR931635	4	
5	5	5	CR931637	5	
6	6	6A	CR931638	6A	
7		6B	CR931639	6B	
8		6C	EF538714	6C	
9	7	7 F	CR931643	7 F	
10		7A	CR931640	7A	
11		7B	CR931641	7B/40	7B
12		7C	CR931642	7C	
13	8	8	CR931644	8	
14	9	9A	CR931645	9A/9 V	9A
15		9 L	CR931646	9 L	
16		9 N	CR931647	9 N	
17		9 V	CR931648	9A/9 V	9 V
18	10	10 F	CR931652	10 F/10C	10 F
19		10A	CR931649	10A	
20		10B	CR931650	10B	
21		10C	CR931651	10 F/10C	10C
22	11	11 F	CR931657	11 F	
23		11A	CR931653	11A/11D/18 F	11A
24		11B	CR931654	11B	
25		11C	CR931655	11C	
26		11D	CR931656	11A/11D/18 F	11D
27	12	12 F	CR931660	12 F/44	12 F
28		12A	CR931658	12A	
29		12B	CR931659	12B	
30	13	13	CR931661	13/20	13
31	14	14	CR931662	14	
32	15	15 F	CR931666	15 F	
33		15A	CR931663	15A	
34		15B	CR931664	15B	
35		15C	CR931665	15C	
36	16	16 F	CR931668	16 F	
37		16A	CR931667	16A	
38	17	17 F	CR931670	17 F	
39		17A	CR931669	17A/34	17A
40	18	18 F	CR931674	11A/11D/18 F	18 F
41		18A	CR931671	18A	
42		18B	CR931672	18B	

Table 1 PCRseqtyping results for 91 SSI strains *(Continued)*

43		18C	CR931673	18C	
44	19	19 F	CR931678	19 F	
45		19A	CR931675	19A	
46		19B	CR931676	19B	
47		19C	CR931677	19C	
48	20	20	CR931679	13/20	20
49	21	21	CR931680	21	
50	22	22 F	CR931682	22 F/22A	22 F
51		22A	CR931681	22 F/22A	22A
52	23	23 F	CR931685	23 F	
53		23A	CR931683	23A	
54		23B	CR931684	23B	
55	24	24 F	CR931688	24 F	
56		24A	CR931686	24A	
57		24B	CR931687	24B	
58	25	25 F	CR931690	25 F/25A	25 F
59		25A	CR931689	25 F/25A	25A
60	27	27	CR931691	27	
61	28	28 F	CR931693	28 F	
62		28A	CR931692	28A	
63	29	29	CR931694	29	
64	31	31	CR931695	31	
65	32	32 F	CR931697	32 F/32A	32 F
66		32A	CR931696	32 F/32A	32A
67	33	33 F	CR931702	33 F/33A/35A	33 F
68		33A	CR931698	33A	
69		33B	CR931699	33B	
70		33C	CR931700	33C	
71		33D	CR931701	33D	
72	34	34	CR931703	17A/34	34
73	35	35 F	CR931707	35 F/47 F	35 F
74		35A	CR931704	33 F/33A/35A	35A
75		35B	CR931705	35B/35C	35B
76		35C	CR931706	35B/35C	35C
77	36	36	CR931708	36	
78	37	37	CR931709	37	
79	38	38	CR931710	38	
80	39	39	CR931711	39	
81	40	40	CR931712	7B/40	40
82	41	41 F	CR931714	41 F	
83		41A	CR931713	2/41A	41A
84	42	42	CR931715	42	
85	43	43	CR931716	43	
86	44	44	CR931717	44	

Table 1 PCRseqtyping results for 91 SSI strains *(Continued)*

87	45	45	CR931718	45	
88	46	46	CR931719	46	
89	47	47 F	CR931721	35 F/47 F	47 F
90		47A	CR931720	47A	
91	48	48	CR931722	48	

cycling was performed in GeneAmp PCR system 9700 (Applied Biosystems, United States) under the following conditions: 94 °C for 5 min, followed by 35 amplification cycles of 94 °C for 30 s, 50 °C for 30 s, and 72 °C for 1 min and final extension at 72 °C for 5 min. The PCR products were separated by electrophoresis on 1.2% agarose gel for 45 min at 80 V in 1X Tris-acetate EDTA buffer. Ethidium bromide-stained DNA products were visualized under ultraviolet (UV) illumination and size of the DNA products was determined by using a 1–kb DNA molecular size marker (Fermentas).

Sequencing and data analysis

PCR products were purified using QIA quick PCR purification kit (Qiagen, Germany) following manufacturer's protocol. Purified PCR products were subjected

Table 2 Serotype distribution of the clinical isolates of *Streptococcus pneumoniae* from Central Research Laboratory, KIMS Hospital, Bangalore, India

Sl.No	Sample ID	SEX	AGE YRS	SOURCE	PCRSeq Typing data	Quellung data	Homologous(H) & Non-homologous (NH)
1	PIDOPS-01	M	5	Blood	6B	6B	NH
2	PIDOPS-02	F	2y5m	Blood	14	14	NH
3	PIDOPS-03	M	5	Pleural fluid	7 F	7 F	NH
4	PIDOPS-04	M	6 m	Blood	20	20	H- HG5
5	PIDOPS-05	M	5	Blood	14	14	NH
6	PIDOPS-07	M	1y6m	CSF	15B	15B	NH
7	PIDOPS-08	M	2	Blood	19 F	19 F	NH
8	PIDOPS-09	M	4y3 m	Blood	19 F	19 F	NH
9	PIDOPS-10	M	2y2 m	Blood	6B	6A	NH
10	PIDOPS-11	M	5	Blood	6B	6B	NH
11	PIDOPS-14	M	3	Blood	1	1	NH
12	PIDOPS-17	M	1y6m	Blood	19 F	19 F	NH
13	PIDOPS-18	M	4	Blood	1	1	NH
14	PIDOPS-19	M	1y6m	Blood	1	1	NH
15	PIDOPS-20	M	3	Blood	1	1	NH
16	PIDOPS-22	F	9 m	Blood	6A	6A	NH
17	PIDOPS-23	F	3y8m	Blood	11A	11A	H-HG1
18	PIDOPS-24	M	5	Blood	8	8	NH
19	PIDOPS-25	F	4y6m	CSF	5	5	NH
20	PIDOPS-28	M	9 m	Blood	1	1	NH
21	PIDOPS-30	F	3y3 m	Blood	15B	15B	NH
22	PIDOPS-31	M	3 m	Blood	19A	19A	NH
23	PIDOPS-32	M	2y6m	Pleural fluid	19A	19A	NH
24	PIDOPS-33	M	4y2 m	Blood	7B	7B	H-HG2
25	PIDOPS-42	M	2 m	CSF	6B	6B	NH
26	PIDOPS-45	F	6 m	Blood	7 F	7 F	NH
27	PIDOPS-46	F	10 m	Blood	19A	19A	NH
28	PIDOPS-50	M	5y	Blood	3	3	NH

to sequencing, employing the Big Dye Sequence Terminator kit V3.1 (Applied Biosystems) and analyzed on ABI 3730 XL Genetic Analyzer (Applied Biosystems). Sequencing was performed in one direction using forward primer (cps1), 5′-GCA ATG CCA GAC AGT AAC CTC TAT-3′ and Long Seq Module (ABI). DNA sequences that were obtained were analyzed for sequence similarity using GenBank database (http://www.ncbi.nlm.nih.gov/blast) and then assigned to serotype [26]. Serotype of the *cpsB* nucleotide sequence was determined from GenBank with the highest BLAST bit score of > 99% sequence identity with the query 'amplicon nucleotide sequence'.

Homology group assignment and PCRSeqTyping

Homology groups

Amplifiable serotypes that shared identical interceding sequences (e.g. sequences for serotypes 2 and 41A, 7B, and 40) were grouped into 10 different groups based on their homology by *in silico* analysis of *cpsB* region. Individual primer sets were designed for each subgroup. Sequetyping data obtained in Step I was used to assign the homologous strains into subgroups (Fig. 1). Serotypes were considered homologous when the highest bit score was shared between two or more serotypes (i.e. the same amount of nucleotide variation between query and database sequences), and then assigned to one of the 10 groups (Table 3).

For homologous strains, a second round of PCR was performed using group specific primers as specified in Table 3. PCR products were subjected to sequencing reaction. The nucleotide sequence data was used to assign the serotype.

Results

PCRSeqTyping results for reference strains

The 91 pneumococcal serotype reference strains (sourced from SSI) were tested with PCRSeqTyping protocol. All 91 strains were amplified using the modified method. In Step I of amplification and sequencing, 59 strains of the non-homologous group (Group I) were correctly assigned to their respective serotype. There were 32 strains (Group II) identified along with their homologous type. The homologous types were correctly assigned to their respective type in Step II by performing a second round of amplification using group specific primers and sequencing. Quellung reaction performed using Pneumotest kit (SSI), in parallel with PCRSeqTyping, showed 100% concordant results (Table 1).

The results were further evaluated by blinded testing of PCRSeqtyping. Samples were evaluated randomly by assigning codes. Quellung reaction data showed no discrepancies between serotypes assigned by Quellung and PCRSeqTyping for all reference strains.

PCRSeqTyping results for clinical isolates

Twenty eight pneumococcal isolates tested in the study were from children <5 years with invasive pneumococcal disease. The predominant serotypes were 1, 6B, 19A, 19 F, 14 and 7 F (Table 2). PCRSeqTyping results and serotyping results by Quellung reaction were in concordance, without any discrepancies. Among 28 isolates,

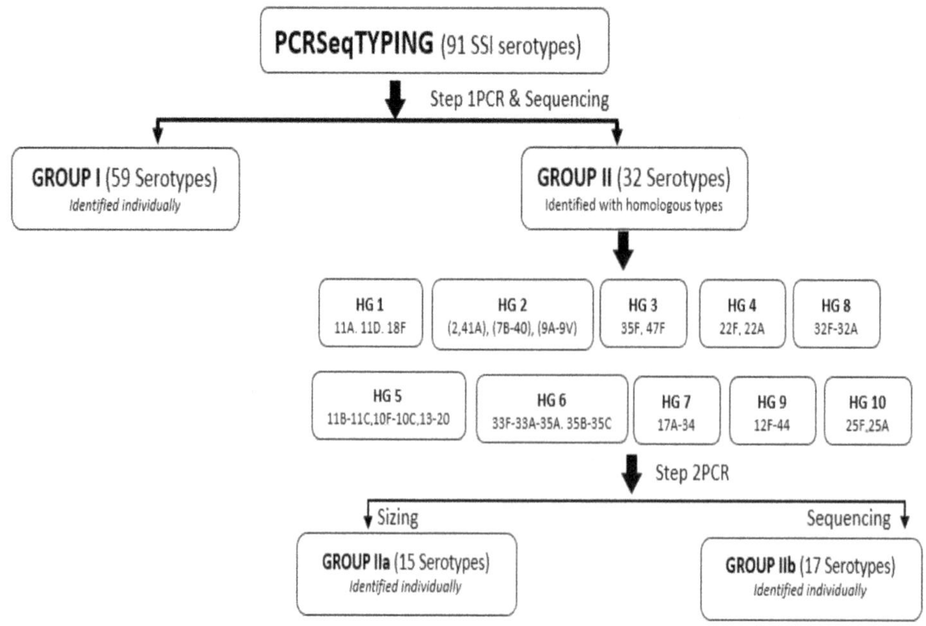

Fig. 1 Homology group assignment for 91 pneumococcal serotypes

Table 3 Primers used in PCRSeqTyping assay

	Primers		Sequence (5′-3′)	Product size (in bp)	Serotype
GROUP I	FP1	CPS-1FP	GCAATGCCAGACAGTAACCTCTAT	1061	
	RP1	CPS-2RP	CCTGCCTGCAAGTCTTGATT		
	RP2	2538-RP	CTTTACCAACCTTTGTAATCCAT	1109	
GROUP II					
HG1	HG1-FP	FP1	TGTCCAATGAAGAGCAAGACTTGAC	1109	11A
	HG1-RP	RP1	AAGTATATCCCTCCACAAACCCATC	435	11D
				316	18 F
HG2	HG2-FP	FP1	TGTCCAATGAAGAGCAAGACTTGAC	1628	2
	HG2-RP	RP5	ATATCACTTTTTTACGGTAATGTCTA	1820	41A
				1185	7B
				1820	40
				1819	9 V
				1502	9A
HG3	HG3-FP	FP1	TGTCCAATGAAGAGCAAGACTTGAC	1797	35 F
	HG3-RP	RP7	CACCTTTATTTTCACTATCTGCATC	1479	47 F
HG4	HG4-FP	FP8	ACTAGGAAGCTAGCCGTAGGTTGC	366	22 F
	HG4-RP	RP8	TCTCACCTTTAGTGCTTGAACCT	No Amplification	22A
HG5	HG5-FP	FP9	CCATGGGATGCTTTCTGTGTGGA	1061	10 F
	HG5-RP	RP9	TATATCACTTTTTTACGGTAATGTCTA	1004	10C
				1416	11B
				2958	11C
				1395	13
				1395	20
HG6	HG6-FP	FP1	TGTCCAATGAAGAGCAAGACTTGAC	929	33 F
	HG6-RP	RP4	AGCACCTAGCACCTGTTTAGAT	929	33A
				924	35A
				927	35B
				925	35C
HG7	HG7-FP	FP3	CAGAGTTCGTCTTACTTGGCAGCT	737	34
	HG7-RP	RP3	GAATCTTGCAAGCTATTAATGATCG	737	17A
HG8	HG8-FP	FP6	AGCAACTAGCCAAGTTAGCCAGAGT	643	32 F
	HG8-RP	RP6	ACTGTGCTTCCATCTGGGACATCATG	648	32A
HG9	HG9-FP	FP1	TGTCCAATGAAGAGCAAGACTTGAC	970	12 F
	HG9-RP	RP2	CAGAAAAAGTAGCCTTATTTCTTAAGA	996	44
HG10	HG10-FP	FP10	ATGAAGCTATTCAAAGTTTGTTAGC	656	25 F
	HG10-RP	RP10	TGAATCCTCTAATCCTTGCATGA	656	25A

25 isolates were assigned to their serotype with the first step of PCRSeqTyping. Three isolates belonging to the homologous group were subsequently identified with the second step of PCRSeqTyping.

Discussion

There is a renewed interest in pneumococcal capsular typing techniques, as a result of an increased complexity in the management of pneumococcal disease and the widespread use of pneumococcal vaccines [8]. The ability to differentiate pneumococcal strains efficiently is essential to track the emerging serovars, and for epidemiological investigations. The limitations of the Quellung serotyping method, many DNA-based typing protocols, PCR, restriction fragment length polymorphisms, hybridization assays, microarrays and sequencing for *S. pneumoniae* are well known. Different PCR strategies, namely multiplex PCR, sequential PCR, serotype-specific PCR, and real time multiplex PCR [25, 28–36] targeting serotype-specific regions of *cps* could detect only 22 serotypes uniquely, and 48 serotypes along with their homologous types [37, 38]. Despite the fact these methods cover imited serotypes, PCR is a widely used technique, which avoids the use of serological reagents and requires specific expertise to conduct.

Methods using multiple restriction enzymes and long *cps* fragments [39, 40] for PCR make the amplification difficult and inconsistent. Another protocol based on sequencing of regulatory region of *cps* [30, 31] shows poor resolution with cross reactivity of serotypes. An approach targeting serotype-specific glycosyl transferase genes [6] was only tested for serogroup 6 and serotype 19 F. The cross reactivity of serotypes, along with the requirement for a higher number of primers, and poor resolution limits their wide usage.

With the characterization of the *cps* locus of 92 serotypes [13], Leung et al. [26] developed sequetyping protocol using single primer pair, which binds in all pneumococcal serotypes. Recently, several research groups [27, 41–43] have published their results using sequetyping assay. Limitations of the sequetyping protocol were as follows: (i) only 84 serotypes out of 92 were predicted to be amplified by *in silico* analysis; (ii) cross-reacting serotypes (30/84) belonging to homologous groups could not be uniquely identified; and (iii) considering the central 732 bp region of the *cpsB* amplicon which could be sequenced, only 46 of 54 serotypes could be sequetyped.

In the first step of this study's modified approach, successful amplification of all 91 serotypes was achieved with the addition of a new reverse primer to amplify 25A, 25 F and 38 serotypes specifically. Additionally, XT-5 polymerase used in the PCR amplification reactions contains *Taq* DNA polymerase and *Pfu* enzyme. This enzyme blend utilizes the powerful 5′-3′ polymerase activity of Taq DNA polymerase and the 3′-5′ exonuclease-mediated proof-reading activity of PR polymerase, resulting in high fidelity PCR products [44]. PCR annealing temperature of 50 °C and extension time of 1 min were found to be optimal for amplification of *cpsB* gene of all 91 strains.

The serotypes were grouped into homologous (32) and non-homologous (59) based on *cpsB* sequence. Non-homologous types were identified uniquely. The 32 homologous strains were further subdivided into 10 groups (HG 1–10) based on their sequence similarity. Homology group-specific primers were designed and evaluated for their ability to differentiate between strains. HG primers were designed to be able to assign the serotype accurately with second step of PCR and sequencing.

The limitation of using 732 bp region of *cpsB* amplicon in sequetyping assay, resulting in prediction of 46 of 54 serotypes, was overcome with the use of Long Seq module. Approximately 1.0 kb quality reads in a single sequencing reaction were obtained with modification. This resulted in providing good quality reads up to the end of the PCR template, identifying cross-reacting serotypes (15B/15C, 7 F/7A, 18B/18C, 9 L/9 N, 15B/C, 17 F/33C, 18B/C, 7A/F, 12A/46, 6C/6D) which have a single SNP in the *cpsB* region.

A 100% concordance of serotype results of PCRSeq-Typing and Quellung testing was seen for the 28 clinical isolates. Moving forward, the study will be extended for serotyping a larger number of clinical isolates and clinical samples. The limitation of the protocol will be in quantification and serotype identification in multiple carriage; however, studies are underway to address these issues. For multiple carriage, the PCR amplicon obtained in the first step will be subcloned into T/A cloning vector and the individual clones will be sequenced for assigning the specific serotype. As the corresponding *cpsB* gene sequence of the recently discovered serotypes 6E, 6 F, 6G, 6H, 11E, 20A, 20B and 23B1 [45–47] were unavailable at the time of the study design, they will be included in future studies.

In the study's center, the typing cost with Pneumotest Kit (SSI, Denmark) was US$35/isolate, while PCRSeq-Typing cost was US$10 for Group I (non-homologous strains) and US$15 for Group II (homologous strains). With the easy availability of outsourced sequencing services, the accurate and reliable PCRSeqTyping test can be adopted in a regular microbiology laboratory, even without the sequencing facility.

This modified typing method has several advantages over other reported methods. It involves techniques with a workflow that many microbiology laboratories can easily implement. The high throughput PCRSeqTyping method features good discriminatory power, reproducibility, and portability, making it suitable for epidemiological studies. The assay has the flexibility of incorporating additional primers for the characterization of emerging serotypes. An added advantage of this method is that raw data from experiments can be reanalyzed upon the addition of new entries to the serotyping database.

Conclusion

PCRSeqTyping assay is a cost-effective alternative to currently available phenotypic and molecular typing methods. The method is simple to perform, robust, and economical. It can identify all 91 serotypes specifically and uniquely.

Abbreviations

Cps: Capsular polysaccharide; DNA: DeoxyRibo Nucleic Acid; EDTA: Ethylenediaminetetraacetic acid; MALDI-TOF: Matrix Assisted Laser Desorption Ionization - Time of Flight; PCR: Polymerase chain reaction; RFLP: Restriction fragment length polymorphism; SSI: Staten Serum Institute; STG: Serotype/group; STGG: Skim milk, tryptone, glucose, and glycerol

Acknowledgements
Not applicable.

Funding
No funding agencies involved.

Authors' contributions
GN - concept, designing the experiment, executing, data analysis and writing the manuscript. RKL - Guided the experimentation process and execution, reviewed the manuscript. FG and VG assisted during experimentation. All authors read and approved the final manuscript.

Competing interests
The authors declare that they have no competing interests.

References

1. Pneumococcal Disease. Atlanta: Centers for Disease control and prevention. Available from https://www.cdc.gov/pneumococcal/clinicians/streptococcus-pneumoniae.html. Accessed 23 Mar 2016.
2. Progress in Introduction of Pneumococcal Conjugate Vaccine — Worldwide, 2000–2012. Morb Mortal Wkly Rep. 2013: 62(16);308–311. Available from: https://www.cdc.gov/mmwr/preview/mmwrhtml/mm6216a4.htm
3. Velasco EL, Verheul AFM, Verhoef J, Snippe H. *Streptococcus pneumoniae*: Virulence Factors, Pathogenesis, and Vaccines. Microbiol Rev. 1995;59:591–603.
4. Shenoy AT, Orihuela CJ. Anatomical site-specific contributions of pneumococcal virulence determinants. Pneumonia. 2016;8:7.
5. Normark BH, Tuomanen EI. The Pneumococcus: Epidemiology, Microbiology, and Pathogenesis. Cold Spring HarbPerspect Med. 2013;3:a010215.
6. Tomita Y, Okamoto A, Yagi T, Hasegawa Y, Ohta M. Capsulartype prediction by phylogenetic tree of glycosyltransferase gene polymorphism in *Streptococcus pneumoniae*. Open Access Bioinforma. 2011;3:67–73.
7. Kim JO, Weiser JN. Association of intrastrain phase variation in quantity of capsular polysaccharide and teichoic acid with the virulence of *Streptococcus pneumonia*. J Infect Dis. 1998;177:368–77.
8. Ashu EE, Jarju S, Dione M, Mackenzie G, Ikumapayi UN, Manjang A, et al. Population structure, epidemiology and antibiotic resistance patterns of *Streptococcus pneumoniae* serotype 5: prior to PCV-13 vaccine introduction in Eastern Gambia. BMC Infect Dis. 2016;16:33.
9. Elberse KE, van de Pol I, Witteveen S, van der Heide HG, Schot CS, van Dijk A, et al. Population structure of Invasive *Streptococcus pneumoniae* in the Netherlands in the Pre-vaccination era assessed by MLVA and capsular sequence typing. PLoS ONE. 2011;6:e20390.
10. Llull D, Munoz R, Lopez R, Garcia E. A single gene (tts) located outside the cap locus directs the formation of *Streptococcus pneumoniae* type 37 capsular polysaccharide. Type 37 pneumococci are natural, genetically binary strains. J Exp Med. 1999;190:241–51.
11. Cartee RT, Forsee WT, Jensen JW, Yother J. Expression of the *Streptococcus pneumoniae* type 3 synthase in Escherichia coli. Assembly of type 3 polysaccharide on a lipid primer. J Biol Chem. 2001;276:48831–9.
12. Varvio SL, Auranen K, Arjas E, Makela PH. Evolution of the Capsular Regulatory Genesin*Streptococcus pneumonia*. J Infect Dis. 2009;200:1144–51.
13. Bentley SD, Aanensen DM, Mavroidi A, Saunders D, Rabbinowitsch E, Collins M, et al. Genetic analysis of the capsular biosynthetic locus from all 90 pneumococcal serotypes. PLoS Genet. 2006;2:e31.
14. Vernet G, Saha S, Satzke C, Burgess DH, Alderson M, Maisonneuve JF, et al. Laboratory-based diagnosis of pneumococcal pneumonia: state of the art and unmet needs. ClinMicrobiol Infect. 2011;17 (Suppl 3):1–13.
15. Jauneikaite E, Jefferies JMC, VereChurton NW, Pin Lin RT, Hibberd ML, Clarke SC. Genetic diversity of *Streptococcus pneumoniae* causing meningitis and sepsis in Singapore during the first year of PCV7 implementation. Emerging Microbes and Infect. 2014;3:e39.
16. Hausdorff WP, Bryant J, Paradiso PR, Siber GR. Which pneumococcal serogroups cause the most invasive disease: implications for conjugate vaccine formulation and use, part I. Clin Infect Dis. 2000;30:100–21.
17. Johnson HL, Deloria-Knoll M, Levine OS, Stoszek SK, FreimanisHance L, Reithinger R, et al. Systematic evaluation of serotypes causing invasive pneumococcal disease among children under five: the pneumococcal global serotype project. PLoS Med. 2010;7:e1000348. doi:10.1371/journal.pmed.1000348.
18. Weinberger DM, Malley R, Lipsitch M. Serotype replacement in disease after pneumococcal vaccination. Lancet. 2011;378:1962–73.
19. Obaro SK, Adegbola RA, Banya WA, Greenwood BM. Carriage of pneumococci after pneumococcal vaccination. Lancet. 1998;348:271–2.
20. Habib M, Porter BD, Satzke C. Capsular Serotyping of *Streptococcus pneumoniae*using the Quellung Reaction. J Vis Exp. 2014;84:e51208.
21. Bonofiglio L, Gardella N, Mollerach M. In: Magdeldin S, editor. Application of Molecular Typing Methods to the Study of Medically Relevant Gram-Positive Cocci, Gel Electrophoresis - Advanced Techniques. 2012. ISBN 978-953-51-0457-5.
22. Gonzalez TB, Rivera-Olivero IA, Sisco MC, Spadola E, Herman PW, de Waard JH. PCR deduction of invasive and colonizing pneumococcal serotypes from Venezuela: a critical appraisal. J Infect DevCtries. 2014;8:469–73. doi:10.3855/jidc.3274.
23. Slinger R, Hyde L, Moldovan I, Chan F, Pernica M. Direct *Streptococcus pneumoniae* real-time PCR serotyping from pediatric parapneumoniceffusions. BMC Pediatr. 2014;14:189.
24. Raymond F, Boucher N, Allary R, Robitaille L, Lefebvre B, et al. Serotyping of *Streptococcus pneumoniae*Based on Capsular Genes Polymorphisms. PLoS ONE. 2013;8:e76197. doi:10.1371/journal.pone.0076197.
25. Pai R, Gertz RE, Beall B. Sequential multiplex PCR approach for determining capsular serotypes of Streptococcus pneumoniae isolates. J Clin Microbiol. 2006;44:124–31.
26. Leung MH, Bryson K, Freystatter K, Pichon B, Edwards G, Charalambous BM, et al. Sequetyping: serotyping *Streptococcuspneumoniae* by a single PCR sequencing strategy. J Clin Microbiol. 2012;50:2419–27.
27. Jin P, Wu L, Oftadeh S, Kudinha T, Kong F, Zeng Q. Using a practical molecular capsular serotype prediction strategy to investigate *Streptococcus pneumoniae*serotypedistribution and antimicrobial resistance in Chinese local hospitalized children. BMC Pediatr. 2016;16:53.
28. Lawrence ER, Griffiths DB, Martin SA, George RC, Hall LM. Evaluation of semiautomated multiplex PCR assay for determination of *Streptococcus pneumoniae* serotypes and serogroups. J Clin Microbiol. 2003;41:601–7.
29. Jiang SM, Wang L, Reeves PR. Molecular characterization of *Streptococcus pneumoniae* type 4, 6B, 8, and 18C capsular polysaccharide gene clusters. Infect Immun. 2001;69:1244–55.
30. Kong F, Gilbert GL. Using cpsA-cpsB sequence polymorphisms and serotype-/group-specific PCR to predict 51 *Streptococcus pneumoniae* capsular serotypes. J Med Microbiol. 2003;52:1047–58.
31. Kong F, Wang W, Tao J, Wang L, Wang Q, Sabananthan A, et al. A molecular-capsular-type prediction system for 90 *Streptococcus pneumoniae* serotypes using partial cpsA-cpsB sequencing and wzy- or wzx-specific PCR. J Med Microbiol. 2005;54:351–6.
32. Rubin LG, Rizvi A. PCR-based assays for detection of *Streptococcus pneumoniae* serotypes 3, 14, 19 F and 23 F in respiratory specimens. J Med Microbiol. 2004;53:595–602.
33. O'Halloran DM, Cafferkey MT. Multiplex PCR for identification of seven *Streptococcus pneumoniae* serotypes targeted by a 7-valent conjugate vaccine. J Clin Microbiol. 2005;43:3487–90.
34. Billal DS, Hotomi M, Tasnim S, Fujihara K, Yamanaka N. Evaluation of serotypes of *Streptococcus pneumoniae* isolated from otitis media patients by multiplex polymerase chain reaction. ORLJ Otorhinolaryngol Relat Spec. 2006;68:135–8.
35. Park IH, Park S, Hollingshead SK, Nahm MH. Genetic basis for the new pneumococcal serotype, 6C. Infect Immun. 2007;75:4482–9.
36. Brito DA, Ramirez M, de Lencastre H. Serotyping *Streptococcus pneumoniae*by multiplex PCR. J Clin Microbiol. 2003;41:2378–84.
37. Singleton RJ, et al. Invasive pneumococcal disease caused by nonvaccine serotypes among Alaska native children with high levels of 7-valent pneumococcal conjugate vaccine coverage. JAMA. 2007;297:1784–92.
38. Brugger SD, Frey P, Aebi S, Hinds J, Muhlemann K. Multiple colonization with *S. pneumoniae*before and after introduction of the seven valent conjugated pneumococcal polysaccharide vaccine. PLoS One. 2010;5:e11638. doi:10.1371/journal.pone.0011638.

39. Lawrence ER, et al. Evaluation of serotype prediction by cpsA-cpsB gene polymorphism in *Streptococcus pneumoniae*. J Clin Microbiol. 2000;38:1319–23.
40. Batt SL, Charalambous BM, McHugh TD, Martin S, Gillespie SH. Novel PCR-restriction fragment length polymorphism method for determining serotypes or serogroups of *Streptococcus pneumoniae* isolates. J Clin Microbiol. 2005;43:2656–61.
41. Dube FS, van Mens SP, Robberts L, Wolter N, Nicol P, Mafofo J, et al. Comparison of a Real-Time Multiplex PCR and Sequetyping Assay for Pneumococcal Serotyping. PLoS ONE. 2015;10:e0137349.
42. Satzke C, Dunne EM, Porter BD, Klugman KP, Mulholland EK, et al. The PneuCarriage Project: A Multi-Centre Comparative Study to Identify the Best Serotyping Methods for Examining Pneumococcal Carriage in Vaccine Evaluation Studies. PLoS Med. 2015;12:e1001903.
43. Zhenzhen D, Erqing Z, Wei G, Kaihu Y, Sangjie Y, Yonghong Y. Analysis of serotype results of 94 *Streptococcus pneumoniae* isolates with partial cpsA-cpsB serotype prediction system. J Appl Clin Pediatr. 2015;12:934–7.
44. Cline J, Braman JC, Hogrefe HH. PCR fidelity of Pfu DNA polymerase and other thermostable DNA polymerases. Nucleic Acids Res. 1996;24:3546–51.
45. Calix JJ, Porambo RJ, Brady AM, Larson TR, Yother J, Abeygunwardana C, Nahm MH. Biochemical, Genetic, and Serological Characterization of Two Capsule Subtypes among *Streptococcus pneumoniae* Serotype 20 Strains. J Biol Chem. 2012;287(33):27885–94.
46. Geno KA, Gilbert GL, Song JY, Skovsted IC, Klugman KP, Jones C, et al. Pneumococcal Capsules and Their Types: Past, Present, and Future. Clin Microbiol Rev. 2015;28:871–99.
47. Oliver MB, van der Linden MP, Küntzel SA, Saad JS, Nahm MH. Discovery of *Streptococcus pneumoniae* Serotype 6 Variants with Glycosyltransferases Synthesizing Two Differing Repeating Units. J Biol Chem. 2013;288(36):25976–85.

16

Non-adherence to community oral-antibiotic treatment in children with fast-breathing pneumonia in Malawi– secondary analysis of a prospective cohort study

Rebecca Nightingale[1], Tim Colbourn[1], David Mukanga[2], Limangeni Mankhambo[3], Norman Lufesi[4], Eric D. McCollum[5] and Carina King[1*]

Abstract

Background: Despite significant progress, pneumonia is still the leading cause of infectious deaths in children under five years of age. Poor adherence to antibiotics has been associated with treatment failure in World Health Organisation (WHO) defined clinical pneumonia; therefore, improving adherence could improve outcomes in children with fast-breathing pneumonia. We examined clinical factors that may affect adherence to oral antibiotics in children in the community setting in Malawi.

Methods: We conducted a sub-analysis of a prospective cohort of children aged 2–59 months diagnosed by community health workers (CHW) in rural Malawi with WHO fast-breathing pneumonia. Clinical factors identified during CHW diagnosis were investigated using multivariate logistic regression for association with non-adherence, including concurrent diagnoses and treatments. Adherence was measured at both 80% and 100% completion of prescribed oral antibiotics.

Results: Eight hundred thirty-four children were included in our analysis, of which 9.5% and 20.0% were non-adherent at 80% and 100% of treatment completion, respectively. A concurrent infectious diagnosis (OR: 1.76, 95% CI: 0.84–2.96/OR: 1.81, 95% CI: 1.21–2.71) and an illness duration of >24 h prior to diagnosis (OR: 2.14, 95% CI: 1.27–3.60/OR: 1.88, 95% CI: 1.29–2.73) had higher odds of non-adherence when measured at both 80% and 100%. Older age was associated with lower odds of non-adherence when measured at 80% (OR: 0.41, 95% CI: 0.21–0.78).

Conclusion: Non-adherence to oral antibiotics was not uncommon in this rural sub-Saharan African setting. As multiple diagnoses by the CHW and longer illness were important factors, this provides an opportunity for further investigation into targeted interventions and refinement of referral guidelines at the community level. Further research into the behavioural drivers of non-adherence within this setting is needed.

Keywords: Pneumonia, Non-adherence, Oral antibiotics, iCCM, Child, Sub-Saharan Africa, Treatment failure

* Correspondence: c.king@ucl.ac.uk
[1]Institute for Global Health, University College London, London, UK
Full list of author information is available at the end of the article

Background

Pneumonia is the second leading cause of death among children under five years of age and the leading cause of death from an infectious disease, accounting for nearly 1 million deaths annually, with the greatest burden of disease falling in Africa [1, 2]. The World Health Organisation (WHO) recommends the use of integrated community case management (iCCM) at the community health worker (CHW) level [3]. These guidelines categorise pneumonia into non-severe pneumonia or 'fast-breathing pneumonia' (presence of a cough and/or difficult breathing with a fast respiratory rate for age) and advise treatment with oral antibiotics in the community, or severe pneumonia (presence of cough and/ or difficult breathing with chest in-drawing or danger signs, irrespective of an increased respiratory rate for age), which requires referral to a hospital [4]. Treatment failure in those who have sought healthcare within the community setting may contribute to the high mortality rate from pneumonia in developing countries [5]. A recent systematic review reported treatment failure rates in fast-breathing pneumonia ranging between 7.8–22.9% [5], with a range of possible causes including incorrect diagnosis, host comorbidities, concurrent diagnoses, antibiotic resistance, and non-adherence to oral antibiotics [6–8].

The development of tools to predict treatment failure have tended to focus on clinical presentation; however, with evidence demonstrating that non-adherence increases treatment failure only [6], it stands to reason that if adherence to oral antibiotics in community treated pneumonia were improved, treatment failure rates could be reduced. Therefore, approaches that aim to improve adherence to oral antibiotics should be considered.

There are few studies that relate to short-term medication use in children that report a vast range of non-adherence, from 3–60% [9–12]. To our knowledge, there are no published articles with a primary outcome of factors affecting adherence in children taking oral antibiotics in sub-Saharan Africa. Several publications have described different aspects of adherence related to chronic conditions in sub-Saharan Africa and acute conditions within the developed world. There is substantial evidence that prescribing 'patient friendly drugs'—for example, reducing the duration of a course or number of tablets per day—improved adherence [8, 13–17]. When treating children in sub-Saharan Africa diagnosed with pneumonia, a three-day course of amoxicillin has been shown to be as effective as a five-day course, and improved adherence rates from 85% to 94% [18]. Other factors that were shown to have some influence on adherence included therapy-related reasons (such as taste and texture) [11]; a patient's relationship with the health provider; access to healthcare; socioeconomic status; and condition-related factors (e.g. how unwell the patient is) [13, 19]. However, there is limited and conflicting evidence surrounding all these factors, particularly in acute conditions such as pneumonia, with a synthesis of systematic reviews finding over 770 separate factors in 51 systematic reviews of long-term treatments, yet found no publication focusing on short-term treatments [13].

In light of this evidence gap, we aimed to investigate clinical and diagnostic factors associated with non-adherence to oral antibiotic treatment of fast-breathing pneumonia in children at the community level, using data from a prospective cohort in rural Malawi.

Method

This study is a sub-analysis of data collected during a prospective cohort, between September 2013 and June 2014, of children treated with oral co-trimoxazole for community-treated iCCM pneumonia in Mchinji District, Malawi.

Data collection

The full methods of data collection have previously been published [6]. Briefly, the study population comprised all children aged 2–59 months diagnosed with fast-breathing pneumonia by 34 government-employed CHWs (called Health Surveillance Assistants) at their village clinics in rural Mchinji and Lilongwe districts, central region, Malawi. All children were dispensed oral co-trimoxazole to take in the community. All eligible participants who presented to CHWs and consented were recruited. Data were collected from 18 clinics in Mchinji and 16 in rural Lilongwe. Diagnoses and clinical assessments, including pulse oximetry, were recorded by CHWs on case report forms. These forms were barcoded, checked by supervisors, entered into a database, and regularly cleaned throughout the project. Lay village-level data collectors were recruited from the local area and received one week's training on the project protocol and clinical measurements. They conducted interviews at day 5 and day 14 in the home setting, with day 0 being the day of diagnosis. When subjects were not at home on day 5, re-visits were made up to day 7. At these follow-up visits the data collectors repeated a clinical examination for pneumonia, visually confirmed reported antibiotic adherence with pill counts, and asked about further care seeking and treatments.

Definitions

Community treated iCCM pneumonia was defined as as the observation or caregiver report of cough and/or difficult breathing and observed fast breathing (>50 breaths per minute for infants 2–11 months; >40 breaths per minute for children 12–59 months), in the absence of any danger signs or chest in-drawing [20]. Danger signs included vomiting everything, inability to feed, convulsions, sleepiness or unconsciousness, and signs of severe respiratory distress including grunting, oxygen saturation <90%, nasal flaring and head nodding. These were assessed based on the caregivers report and clinical assessment by the village data collectors or CHWs.

Non-adherence was measured using pill counts at the day 5 visit. For the purpose of comparison we defined non-adherence as both those who completed less than 80% (i.e. 7 or less of the 10 doses) and those who completed less than 100% (i.e. missed any dose) of the 5-day, twice-daily course of co-trimoxazole. This regime is the same as for amoxicillin and therefore the definition of non-adherence can be applied as countries transition from co-trimoxazole to amoxicillin. As per the standard Malawi guidelines one dose is ½ tablet for 2–11 months and 1 tablet 12–59 months.

Treatment failure was defined as the presence of any of the following on the day after the final dose of antibiotics: fast breathing for age, axillary temperature >37.5 °C, lower chest in-drawing, any danger sign, change of antibiotic, hospital admission or death.

Analysis

Data were analysed using Stata version 13.1 statistical software. We described non-adherence and conducted multivariate analysis using logistic regression with 80% and 100% adherence as the outcome variables in separate models. Based on the literature and prior knowledge, we included clinical presentation and concurrent diagnoses and treatments in the multivariate model. Clinical presentation was included using the following variables: temperature (normal: <=37.4 °C, fever: > 37.4 °C); oxygen saturation (normal = > 95%, abnormal <95%); age-adjusted respiratory rate as breaths per minute (fast: 40–59 [age 12–59 months] 50–69 [age 2–11 months], very fast: > = 60 [age 12–59 months] > =70 [age 2–11 months]); and heart rate as beats per minute (normal: <159 [age 2–11 months] <149 [age 12–23 months] <139 [age 24–59 months]). Concurrent diagnoses at presentation included: presumptive malaria (not laboratory or rapid diagnostic test confirmed), diarrhoea; ear infection, rash and other specified infection. Concurrent medications included: Paracetamol, Lumefantrine Artemether (LA) and others specified (including aspirin, topical creams, oral salbutamol). Duration of illness prior to seeking care (caregiver reported as over 24 h or under 24 h), child vomiting after antibiotics, age (2–12 months, 1–2 years and 2–5 years) and gender were also included.

To determine the inclusion of individual or composite formulations of medication and concurrent diagnosis variables, we looked at the correlation between these individual and composite variables; variables that had a correlation of above 0.7 were not included in the same model [21]. This resulted in the composite diagnosis/medication variables being analysed separately from the individual diagnosis and medication variables. The overall percentage of missing data was low, with all variables having less than 5% missing data, and overall 12% of records with any missing data. A complete case analysis approach was taken.

Results

A total of 974 cases were presented for analysis. Of these, 23 did not meet the criteria of fast-breathing pneumonia (had no cough or difficulty breathing), and 117 were not at home on day 5 when the pill count was completed. These patients were not included for analysis, which resulted in a total of 834 cases being analysed.

Table 1 summarises the baseline characteristics of the sample population and description of the clinical variables. Previously published baseline variables show those lost to follow up had lower rates of malnutrition but also lower rates of uptake of the PCV vaccination [6]. The percentage of children diagnosed with another condition concurrently to pneumonia was high (50.7%). Malaria was the most common concurrent diagnosis, occurring in 41.4% of children, and 61.8% of children received any medication in addition to oral co-trimoxazole. Caregiver histories revealed that 58% of children were brought to the clinic for assessment on the day they became unwell or within 24 h of illness onset. Just over 12% of children vomited after taking any dose of co-trimoxazole.

Non-adherence to oral co-trimoxazole was 9.5% when measured at 80%, and 20.0% at 100% completion. Treatment failure at day 5 was 14.9%, and 7.0% at day 14. While our aim was not to investigate treatment failure, the percentage of children failing treatment was slightly higher in those that were non-adherent (19.0%; 95% CI: 16.3–22.0) versus adherent (14.4%; 95% CI: 12.0–17.1); however, this study was not powered to look at this association. The results of the multivariate model are presented in Table 2 (bivariate analysis is available in the Appendix). For non-adherence measured at both 80% and 100%, children with any concurrent diagnosis had higher odds of being non-adherent to medication (OR: 1.76, 95% CI: 1.00–3.07/OR: 1.81 95% CI: 1.21–2.71, respectively). In the multivariate model, concurrent malaria diagnosis alone was not significantly associated with non-adherence (OR: 1.20; 95% CI: 0.67–2.15/OR: 1.41 95% CI: 0.93–2.17). Children who were unwell for more than 24 h before CHW diagnosis had significantly increased odds of non-adherence at 80% and 100% (OR: 2.14, 95% CI: 1.27–3.58/OR: 1.88, 95% CI: 1.29–2.73).

Table 1 Characteristics and description of the study population

N = 834			
		N (%)	
Age	2–11 months	268 (32.1%)	
	12–23 months	273 (32.7%)	
	24–59 months	293 (35.1%)	
Gender	Female	429 (51.4%)	
	Male	391 (46.9%)	
	Missing	14 (1.7%)	
District	Kabudula	479 (57.4%)	
	Mchinji	355 (42.6%)	
Clinical malaria diagnosis	Yes	345 (41.4%)	
	No	489 (58.6%)	
Diarrhoea diagnosis	Yes	28 (3.4%)	
	No	806 (96.6%)	
Any concurrent diagnosis[a]	Yes	423 (50.7%)	
	No	411 (49.3%)	
Prescribed LA[b]	Yes	430 (51.6%)	
	No	404 (48.4%)	
Prescribed paracetamol	Yes	430 (51.6%)	
	No	404 (48.4%)	
Prescribed multiple drugs	Yes	515 (38.2%)	
	No	319 (38.3%)	
Duration of illness before diagnosis	<24 h	482 (58.1%)	
	>24 h	347 (41.9%)	
Vomited after taking antibiotics	Yes	726 (12.7%)	
	No	106 (87.3%)	
		Number	Median[c] (range)
Respiratory rate (breaths/min)	Age 2–11 mths	253	55 (40–83)
	Age 12–59 mths	545	46 (40–100)
Temperature (°C)		803	42.0 (34.3–42)
Oxygen Saturation (%)		826	97 (90–100)
		Number	Mean[c] (SD)
Heart rate (beats/min)	Age 2–11 mths	260	136 (24.7)
	Age 12–23 mths	260	138 (24.9)
	Age 24–59 mths	279	129 (23.2)

LA lumefantrine artemether, *SD* standard deviation
[a]Diagnoses included: malaria, diarrhoea, ear infection, rash and other specified
[b]The child was presumptively prescribed the anti-malaria Lumefantrine Artemether (LA) by the community health worker
[c]Median used for skewed data, mean for normally distributed data

Being in the older age group was associated with lower odds of <80% adherence (OR: 0.41, 95% CI: 0.21–0.78), but this was not the case for <100% adherence. Children prescribed multiple medications showed increased odds of non-adherence in bivariate analysis, but not in the adjusted analysis. The clinical severity of the child's pneumonia at diagnosis did not show a significant relationship with non-adherence, nor did a child vomiting after their antibiotics.

Discussion

We sought to describe the effect of clinical presentation on adherence to oral antibiotics in children diagnosed with community-treated iCCM pneumonia in rural Malawi.

Table 2 Multivariable regression for clinical and diagnostic factors associated with non- adherence

	Adherence measured at 80%			Adherence measured at 100%		
Variable	Odds Ratio	P Value	CI	Odds ratio	P Value	CI
Any Concurrent Diagnosis[a]	1.75	0.050	1.00–3.07	1.81	0.004	1.21–2.71
Prescribed multiple drugs[b]	1.57	0.159	0.84–2.96	1.09	0.711	0.70–1.68
Duration of illness > 24 h	2.14	0.004	1.27–3.58	1.88	0.001	1.29–2.73
Abnormal oxygen saturation[c]	0.82	0.606	0.39–1.73	1.44	0.148	0.88–2.36
Very fast breathing[d]	0.82	0.754	0.22–2.92	0.66	0.355	0.27–1.60
Abnormal heart rate[e]	0.80	0.419	0.41–1.45	1.41	0.123	0.91–2.17
Fever[f]	1.50	0.150	0.86–2.60	1.06	0.777	0.70–1.61
Vomited antibiotics	0.82	0.605	0.38–1.77	0.85	0.574	0.48–1.50
Age (12–23months)	0.68	0.206	0.38–1.23	1.05	0.822	0.67–1.65
Age (24–56 month)	0.41	0.007	0.21–0.78	0.68	0.111	0.43–1.09
Sex (Male)	0.91	0.740	0.54–1.51	1.06	0.750	0.73–1.54
Pseudo R2 = 0.061				Pseudo R2 = 0.045		

[a]Diagnoses included: malaria, diarrhoea, ear infection, rash and other specified
[b]Drugs included: Paracetamol, Lumefantrine Artemether (LA) and others specified (including aspirin, topical creams, oral salbutamol)
[c]Normal: = > 95%; Abnormal: <= 94%
[d]Fast breathing (breaths per minute): 40–59 (age 12–59 months) 50–69 (age 2–11 months); Very fast breathing: > = 60 (age 12–59 months) > =70 (age 2–11 months)
[e]Normal (beat per minute): <159 (age 2-11months), <149 (age 12–23 months), <139 (age 24–59 months); Abnormal: > = 159 (age 2-11months), > = 149 (age 12–23 months), > = 139 (age 24–59 months)
[f]Normal: <=37.4 °C; Fever: > 37.4 °C

Our results highlighted that there is a level of non-adherence to oral antibiotics within these communities, with 20% of children not finishing their full course of antibiotics and nearly 10% not completing 80% of the course. There is limited data to compare this to, with available literature reporting a vast range of non-adherence from 3–60% [9–12]. Having a secondary diagnosis and presenting for treatment having been unwell for more than 24 h before diagnosis were associated with non-adherence amongst this population.

Clinical severity

The limited literature available suggests that the more seriously sick a child is, the more likely they are to be adherent to medication [22]; however, our results did not find severity to be a main driver of adherence in this group. It is plausible that the way this study has measured clinical presentation is not how a caregiver would assess it, since measures such as oxygen saturation are non-visible whereas a fever or faster respiratory rate may be visible to a caregiver. As these children were being treated in the community, caregivers may not have perceived them as seriously unwell. This is supported by the fact that they were seeking care in the community. However, with no studies reviewing children with pneumonia in an African setting, it is possible that the different cultural and local health beliefs mean severity and risk are viewed differently, giving alternative results. Evidence suggests that in Malawi, especially in areas with endemic tropical disease, health beliefs vary greatly from Western models, particularly when understanding the risk of disease [23]. There is also potential that parents did not see a benefit in continuing to give their child medication if the child (potentially with viral infections) improved or, alternatively, caregivers saw no to minimal improvement after completing 3 or 4 days of treatment. Research aiming to predict pneumonia treatment failure in Malawi showed limited success in using clinical severity as a possible predictor for failing treatment at the community level [6].

Concurrent diagnosis and medication

Children with a concurrent diagnosis were less likely to be adherent to oral antibiotics. In this study, a large proportion of children had malaria as a secondary diagnosis, yet concurrent malaria alone does not appear to be the reason for non-adherence. Due to a lack of evidence surrounding this topic, we speculate about possible reasons. It is possible that once the child recovered from the concurrent disease, their symptoms were much better and therefore the caregiver stopped giving the antibiotics. Alternatively, as the course of medication for malaria and many other diseases are shorter than 5 days, all medications may have been stopped together. Where a caregiver receives instructions for treatment of multiple conditions, confusion and lack of understanding could result in errors following the correct prescription. It would be expected that concurrent medications and concurrent diagnosis would have almost 100% correlation, yet this was not the case. Although moderate correlation existed, the relationship was not as strong as expected (correlation = 0.50). This could be attributed to an inaccurate caregiver reporting, as well as poor implementation of the iCCM guidelines by CHWs.

At the time of this study, CHWs in Malawi were not using rapid diagnostic testing for malaria. It is well documented that over-prescription of medication, particularly in non-confirmed malaria, is a common problem in sub-Saharan Africa [24]. It is also recognised that where rapid malaria tests are available, there is a reduction in prescription of malaria medication [25]. A limitation of this work is that human immunodeficiency virus (HIV) status of children was not collected due to practical and ethical considerations because pediatric HIV testing was not widely performed by government-sector CHWs in Malawi at the time of this study [6]. Co-trimoxazole is used as a prophylactic drug in children with HIV. HIV prevalence is approximately 8% amongst adults, and therefore a substantial percentage of these children could already be taking co-trimoxazole [26]. Beliefs about the drug itself, which parents could associate with a diagnosis of HIV, may affect adherence.

Duration of illness

Children whose caregivers reported that they had symptoms for more than 24 h were less likely to complete the course of antibiotics. We are not aware of any other comparable literature. Caregivers who took longer to present their unwell child to clinic may have experienced more problems with accessing the clinic, or may have a lower socioeconomic status with limited ability to ensure children took the medication. Similarly, a caregiver's health beliefs may influence the length of time taken to present to the clinic or result in a perception their child was not as sick. These reasons have been shown to increase non-adherence in other conditions and could be causes of non-adherence in those who have been unwell for longer [13].

Age

Older age was associated with improved adherence when measured at 80%, but not 100%. Co-trimoxazole prescribed in Malawi is a tablet that has to be split and crushed for young children. Evidence suggests that 'patient friendly' medication tends to improve adherence, particularly taste and texture with children [11]. Giving crushed tablets to a young baby is potentially not 'patient friendly' and difficult for the caregiver. Similar results have been seen in other studies, and suggest that alternative treatment types (e.g. syrups or dispersible tablets) should be investigated for improved adherence [13].

Treatment failure and non-adherence

This study was not powered to determine if non-adherence was statistically associated to treatment failure. The slight increase in treatment failure in those who were non-adherent needs further investigation with an appropriately powered study. Furthermore the limitation of WHO guidelines should be taken into account, since infections treated with antibiotics in this study may have been viral and thus reasonably be expected to have improved by day 5 or 14 without treatment. There is a potential tension when refining guidelines between encouraging non-specific antibiotic prescription for possible bacterial infections (where adherence will be beneficial and shorter-term mortality benefits will be maximized) and reducing unnecessary antibiotic use for self-resolving viral infections largely responsible for the development of increasing antimicrobial resistance rates, a longer term public health concern.

Limitations

This study was limited by the lack of socioeconomic data, with further research needed on the drivers of non-adherence from a socioeconomic and behavioural stand point. Records of a concurrent diagnosis and medication and duration of illness were from caregiver reports, where answers could be influenced by a range of socioeconomic and social desirability issues, which could lead to both over- and under-reporting. Measuring adherence by pill count assumes that the child swallowed the tablets that are not left, but it is possible they were thrown away, misplaced or lost, or sold. Over-reporting of adherence is therefore possible when using pill count as the measure [19]. Caution should also be given to the clinical measurement used in this study, there is consistent evidence that even with monthly supportive supervision and annual refresher trainings, that accurate assessment of clinical signs is poor in the community in Malawi [27, 28]. This is a significant limitation of establishing clinical severity effects on non-adherence within a community setting.

Conclusions

This analysis suggests that non-adherence to oral antibiotics is an issue in children diagnosed with community treated iCCM pneumonia in Malawi. Although different clinical severity (mild–moderate) at diagnosis is not associated with adherence, concurrent diagnoses, treatments and duration of illness could be important factors in driving treatment decisions and behaviour. Treatment failure was higher in non-adherent children, despite not demonstrating a statistically significant association, and therefore improving adherence is a potential area for improved community case management of pneumonia. As multiple diagnoses and treatments were highlighted as risks for poor adherence, refined diagnosis and treatment pathways in these potentially clinically complex children needs more investigation. Further research is required into the drivers of treatment decisions by caregivers and CHWs for acute infections in a sub-Saharan African community setting to inform this process, and to fill a considerable evidence gap.

Appendix

Table 3 Bivariate analysis of clinical and diagnostic factors associated with non-adherence at 80% and 100% completion

		80% adherence					100% adherence				
		Adherent	Non-adherent	OR	*p*-value	95% CI	Adherent	Non-adherent	OR	*p*-value	95% CI
Fever[a]	Normal	493	45				432	106			
	High	234	31	1.45	0.129	0.89, 2.36	208	57	1.12	0.549	0.78, 1.60
Oxygen Saturation[b]	Normal	643	66				566	134			
	Abnormal	113	13	1.11	0.754	0.59, 2.07	93	33	1.50	0.070	0.96, 2.33
Respiratory Rate[c]	High	680	75				599	156			
	V.High	40	3	0.68	0.526	0.21, 2.25	35	8	0.88	0.745	0.40, 1.93
Heart Rate[d]	Normal	541	60				477	112			
	High	182	16	0.79	0.429	0.45, 1.41	162	48	1.26	0.232	0.86, 1.85
Clinical Malaria	No	453	36				408	81			
	Yes	302	43	1.79	0.013	1.12, 2.86	259	86	1.67	0.003	1.19, 2.36
Diarrhoea	No	733	73				648	158			
	Yes	22	6	2.74	0.028	1.07, 6.99	19	9	1.94	0.103	0.86, 4.38
Any Concurrent Diagnosis	No	397	26				361	62			
	Yes	358	53	2.26	0.001	1.38, 9.71	306	105	2.00	0.001	1.40, 2.82
LA[e]	No	377	27				340	64			
	Yes	378	52	1.92	0.008	1.80, 3.13	327	103	1.67	0.004	1.18, 2.37
Paracetamol	No	381	23				342	62			
	Yes	374	56	2.48	0.001	1.49, 4.13	325	105	1.78	0.001	1.25, 2.53
Multiple Drugs	No	300	19				269	50			
	Yes	455	60	2.08	0.006	1.21, 3.57	398	117	1.58	0.013	1.10, 2.28
Duration of illness	<24h	450	32				408	74			
	>24h	301	46	2.15	0.001	1.33, 3.46	255	92	1.99	0.001	1.41, 2.82
Vomited after antibiotics	No	658	68				581	145			
	Yes	96	10	1.01	0.982	0.50, 2.03	85	21	0.99	0.969	0.59, 1.65
Age	2–11mths	233	35				213	55			
	12–23mths	247	26	0.70	0.195	0.41, 1.20	210	63	1.16	0.472	0.77, 1.75
	24–59mths	275	18	0.44	0.006	0.24, 0.79	244	49	0.79	0.248	0.52, 1.21
Sex	Male	355	36				311	80			
	Female	386	43	0.91	0.693	0.57, 1.45	342	87	1.01	0.949	0.72, 1.42

[a]Normal: <=37.4 °C, High: > 37.4 °C ; [b]Normal: = > 95% Abnormal: <= 94%; [c]High: 40–59 (age 12–59 months) 50–69 (age 2–11 months), Very High: > = 60 (age 12–59 months) > =70 (age 2–11 months); [d]Normal: <159 (age 2–11months), <149 (age 12–23 months), <139 (age 24–59 months). LA: Lumefantrine Artemether [e]Lumefantrine Artemether prescribed by the community health worker

Acknowledgements
We would like to thank all the respondents for taking the time to participate in this study. We would also like to thank all the data collectors, field supervisors and community health workers for their hard work. The other members of the study team included: Anthony Costello, James Beard and Bejoy Nambiar (Institute for Global Health, University College London), Gibson Masache and Tambosi Phiri (Parent and Child Health Initiative, Malawi), Rasa Izadnegahdar (Bill and Melinda Gates Foundation), Debbie C. Hay Burgess (Kimataifa Diagnostics & Devices Consulting LLC), Charles Mwansambo (Malawi Ministry of Health), Eric S. Johnson (Kaiser Permanente) and Robert W. Platt (McGill University).

Funding
This work was supported by the Bill & Melinda Gates Foundation [#23591].

Authors' contributions
The paper was conceived by RN and CK. The cohort study was designed by CK, DM, EDM and LM and data collection was supervised by CK and LM. Data cleaning was done by RN and CK and checked by James Beard and TC. Analysis was done by RN, with input from CK and TC. All authors read, commented and approved the final draft.

Competing interests
The author declare that they have no competing interests.

Author details
[1]Institute for Global Health, University College London, London, UK. [2]Science

and Health Impact Group (SHI), Kampala, Uganda. [3]Parent and Child Health Initiative, Lilongwe, Malawi. [4]Acute Respiratory Infection Unit, Ministry of Health, Lilongwe, Malawi. [5]Department of Pediatrics, Division of Pulmonology, Johns Hopkins School of Medicine, Baltimore, USA.

References

1. Liu L, Oza S, Hogan D, Perin J, Rudan I, Lawn JE, Cousens S, Mathers C, Black RE. Global, regional, and national causes of child mortality in 2000–13, with projections to inform post-2015 priorities: an updated systematic analysis. Lancet. 2015;385:430–40.
2. Walker CLF, Rudan I, Liu L, Nair H, Theodoratou E, Bhutta ZA, O'Brien KL, Campbell H, Black RE. Global burden of childhood pneumonia and diarrhoea. Lancet. 2013;381(9875):1405–16.
3. Integrated Community Case Management (iCCM) [http://www.unicef.org/health/files/iCCM_Joint_Statement_2012.pdf].
4. Caring for the Sick Child in the Community. Adpation for high HIV and TB Setting [http://www.who.int/maternal_child_adolescent/documents/9789241548045.pdf].
5. McCollum ED, King C, Hollowell R, Zhou J, Colbourn T, Nambiar B, Mukanga D, Burgess DC. Predictors of treatment failure for non-severe childhood pneumonia in developing countries–systematic literature review and expert survey–the first step towards a community focused mHealth risk-assessment tool? BMC Pediatr. 2015;15(1):74.
6. King C, McCollum E, Mankhambo L, Colborn T, Beard J, Hay Burgess D, Costello A, Izadnegahdar R, Lufesi N, Masache G, et al. Can we predict oral antibiotic treatment failure in children with fast-breathing pneumonia managed at a community level? A prospective cohort study in Malawi. PLoS One. 2015;10(8), e0136839.
7. Grant GB, Campbell H, Dowell SF, Graham SM, Klugman KP, Mulholland EK, Steinhoff M, Weber MW, Qazi S. Recommendations for treatment of childhood non-severe pneumonia. Lancet Infect Dis. 2009;9(3):185–96.
8. MASCOT. Clinical efficacy of 3 days versus 5 days of oral amoxicillin for treatment of childhood pneumonia: a multicentre double-blind trial. Lancet. 2002;360(9336):835–41.
9. Hazir T, Fox LM, Nisar YB, Fox MP, Ashraf YP, MacLeod WB, Ramzan A, Maqbool S, Masood T, Hussain W. Ambulatory short-course high-dose oral amoxicillin for treatment of severe pneumonia in children: a randomised equivalency trial. Lancet. 2008;371(9606):49–56.
10. Rajesh SM, Singhal V. Clinical Effectiveness of Co-trimoxazole vs. Amoxicillin in the Treatment of Non-Severe Pneumonia in Children in India: A Randomized Controlled Trial. Int J Prevent Med. 2013;4(10):1162.
11. Baguley D, Lim E, Bevan A, Pallet A, Faust SN. Prescribing for children–taste and palatability affect adherence to antibiotics: a review. Arch Dis Child. 2012;97(3):293–7.
12. Reyes H, Guiscafre H, Muñoz O, Perez-Cuevas R, Martinez H, Gutierrez G. Antibiotic noncompliance and waste in upper respiratory infections and acute diarrhea. J Clin Epidemiol. 1997;50(11):1297–304.
13. Kardas P, Lewek P, Matyjaszczyk M. Determinants of patient adherence: a review of systematic reviews. Front Pharmacol. 2013;4.
14. Falagas ME, Karagiannis AK, Nakouti T, Tansarli GS. Compliance with Once-Daily versus Twice or Thrice-Daily Administration of Antibiotic Regimens: A Meta-Analysis of Randomized Controlled Trials. PLoS One. 2015;10(1), e0116207.
15. Francis NA, Gillespie D, Nuttall J, Hood K, Little P, Verheij T, Coenen S, Cals JW, Goossens H, Butler CC. Antibiotics for acute cough: an international observational study of patient adherence in primary care. Br J Gen Pract. 2012;62(599):e429–37.
16. Pechère J-C, Hughes D, Kardas P, Cornaglia G. Non-compliance with antibiotic therapy for acute community infections: a global survey. Int J Antimicrob Agents. 2007;29(3):245–53.
17. Kardas P. Patient compliance with antibiotic treatment for respiratory tract infections. J Antimicrob Chemother. 2002;49(6):897–903.
18. ISCAP. Three day versus five day treatment with amoxicillin for non-severe pneumonia in young children: a multicentre randomised controlled trial. BMJ. 2004;328(7443):791.
19. Lehmann A, Aslani P, Ahmed R, Celio J, Gauchet A, Bedouch P, Bugnon O, Allenet B, Schneider MP. Assessing medication adherence: options to consider. Int J Clin Pharm. 2014;36(1):55–69.
20. Revised WHO classification and treatment of childhood pneumonia at health facilities [http://apps.who.int/iris/bitstream/10665/137319/1/9789241507813_eng.pdf].
21. Tabachnick BG, Fidell LS. Using multivariate statistics. In: Using multivariate statistics. 6th ed. Harlow: Peasrson Education Limited; 2014. p. 123–4.
22. DiMatteo MR, Haskard KB, Williams SL. Health beliefs, disease severity, and patient adherence: a meta-analysis. Med Care. 2007;45(6):521–8.
23. Morrison V, Ager A, Willock J. Perceived risk of tropical diseases in Malawi: evidence of unrealistic pessimism and the irrelevance of beliefs of personal control? Psychol Health Med. 1999;4(4):361–8.
24. Chandler CI, Jones C, Boniface G, Juma K, Reyburn H, Whitty CJ. Guidelines and mindlines: why do clinical staff over-diagnose malaria in Tanzania? A qualitative study. Malar J. 2008;7(1):53.
25. Cundill B, Mbakilwa H, Chandler CI, Mtove G, Mtei F, Willetts A, Foster E, Mwinyishehe R, Mandike R, Olomi R. Prescriber and patient-oriented behavioural interventions to improve use of malaria rapid diagnostic tests in Tanzania: facility-based cluster randomised trial. BMC Med. 2015;13(1):118.
26. Demographic and Health Survey: Malawi 2010 [https://dhsprogram.com/pubs/pdf/FR247/FR247.pdf].
27. Gilroy KE, Callaghan-Koru JA, Cardemil CV, Nsona H, Amouzou A, Mtimuni A, Daelmans B, Mgalula L, Bryce J. Quality of sick child care delivered by Health Surveillance Assistants in Malawi. Health Policy Plan. 2013;28(6):573–85.
28. Bjornstad E, Preidis GA, Lufesi N, Olson D, Kamthunzi P, Hosseinipour MC, McCollum ED. Determining the quality of IMCI pneumonia care in Malawian children. Paediatr Int Child Health. 2014;34(1):29–36.

17

Economic burden of community-acquired pneumonia among elderly patients: a Japanese perspective

Keiko Konomura[1], Hideaki Nagai[2] and Manabu Akazawa[1*]

Abstract

Background: This study aimed to estimate the economic burden of community-acquired pneumonia (CAP) among elderly patients in Japan. In addition, the study evaluated the relationship between total treatment cost and CAP risk factors.

Methods: An administrative database was searched for elderly patients (≥ 65 years old) who had pneumonia (ICD-10 code: J12–J18) and an antibiotic prescription between 1 June 2014 and 31 May 2015. The all-cause total healthcare costs of outpatient and inpatient CAP episodes were calculated.

Results: This study evaluated data from 29,619 patients with CAP who experienced 14,450 outpatient CAP episodes and/or 20,314 inpatient CAP episodes. The mean ages were 77.5 ± 8.0 years and 81.5 ± 8.2 years among the outpatient and inpatient groups, respectively. The median treatment costs were US$346 (interquartile range: $195–551) per outpatient episode and US$4851 (interquartile range: $3313–7669) per inpatient episode. More severe cases had increased treatment costs at the treating hospitals. Male sex, diabetes, chronic obstructive pulmonary disease, and liver dysfunction were associated with increased total treatment costs, while dementia, dialysis, and rheumatism were associated with high costs of treating a CAP episode.

Conclusions: The economic burden of CAP might be decreased by reducing the number of hospitalizations for mild CAP and the incidence of severe CAP. Therefore, preventative care (e.g. oral hygiene or pneumococcus vaccination) is recommended for patients with related risk factors, such as male sex, older age, diabetes, chronic obstructive pulmonary disease, liver dysfunction, rheumatism, dementia, or dialysis.

Keywords: Community-acquired pneumonia, Economic burden of disease, Cost analysis, A-DROP system, Invasive pneumococcal disease, Pneumonia

Background

Community-acquired pneumonia (CAP) is a common acute infectious disease among elderly people, and is associated with high rates of hospital admission and mortality. In Japan, there are approximately 1.9 million new CAP cases every year, with approximately 70% of cases involving patients who are >65 years old and approximately 70% of these elderly patients being hospitalized [1]. Thus, pneumonia is the third leading cause of death among elderly people in Japan. Age and male sex are known risk factors for CAP among adults [2–5], and many comorbidities are also risk factors for CAP, such as chronic obstructive pulmonary disease (COPD), diabetes, cancer, dementia, congestive heart failure, and liver function failure [2, 5–10]. Prescriptions for inhaled medication or oral corticosteroids are associated with an increased risk of CAP [6]. Several methods are used to classify the severity of CAP, and the most commonly used methods for selecting the CAP treatment location are the CURB-65 and pneumonia severity index (PSI) systems. Cases with higher PSI classification (most mild: class I, most severe: class V) have increased values for mortality rate, length of stay, rate of subsequent hospitalization, and rate of admission to the intensive care unit (ICU) [11].

* Correspondence: makazawa@my-pharm.ac.jp
[1]Public Health and Epidemiology, Meiji Pharmaceutical University, 2-522-1, Noshio, Kiyose, Tokyo 204-8588, Japan
Full list of author information is available at the end of the article

CAP is associated with both clinical and economic burdens, based on its high incidence, admission rate, and mortality rate [12, 13]. Many studies from various countries have estimated the economic burden of CAP among elderly individuals [14–20], and those studies have revealed that increased treatment costs are associated with older age and treatment setting [21]. For example, Dutch patients who were ≥50 years old had treatment costs of > US$5000 per CAP episode, and a Spanish population-based study revealed that direct costs for outpatient and inpatient CAP treatment were approximately US$200 and US$1700, respectively [22]. The total CAP treatment costs among inpatients increase for PSI classes I–III and reach a plateau for classes IV–V [23]. Sato et al. have also stratified the CAP-related risk based on the patient's immune status and chronic comorbidities [12], and reported that the all-cause total healthcare costs were higher for high-risk cases, compared to low-risk cases. Although Japan is the most aged country in the world, the economic burden of CAP according to risk factors and severity remains unclear. Furthermore, it is difficult to directly compare the treatment costs in various countries because of differences in the treatment approach and insurance systems. Nevertheless, it would be useful for healthcare providers and policy makers to understand the effects of risk factors and severity on treatment costs, which could help facilitate the appropriate distribution of medical resources.

There are several prophylactic treatments for CAP. Pneumococcal disease among adults can be prevented using the 13-valent pneumococcal conjugate vaccine or the 23-valent pneumococcal polysaccharide vaccine (PPV23). Many countries, including Japan, are also introducing age-based pneumococcal vaccination programs, and the PPV23 vaccine is thought to prevent 50–85% of invasive pneumococcal disease (IPD) cases [24], although the vaccination coverage rate remains low [25, 26]. Oral hygiene is also known to reduce pneumonia onset among elderly patients [27]. Thus, based on the aging global population, a strategy is needed to reduce the economic burden of CAP by identifying patients with high predicted healthcare costs and targeting individuals who should receive prophylactic treatment. However, the effects of CAP severity and risk factors on treatment costs remain unclear, and these factors are an important part of cost-effective or cost-utility analyses. The present study used a large administrative database to estimate the economic burden of CAP among elderly Japanese patients, as well as the per-episode and total treatment costs according to disease severity and risk factors.

Methods

Data source

The retrospective protocol of this study was approved by the ethical committee of Meiji Pharmaceutical University (Tokyo, Japan). Patient and treatment records from 1 April 2010 to 31 May 2015 were obtained from an administrative database that is maintained by Medical Data Vision Co. Ltd. (Tokyo, Japan). Pneumonia episodes were identified between 1 June 2014 and 31 May 2015, while patient characteristics were searched up until 1 June 2014. The database includes claims data from approximately 5 million patients who received treatment at 200 acute care hospitals, and were tracked using the Japanese Diagnosis Procedure Combination/Per-Diem Payment System (DPC/PDPS). These mainly consisted of small- and medium-sized hospitals that were distributed throughout Japan. Previous reports have provided detailed explanations of the DPC/PDPS [28–31], which is a case-mix system that tracks patients based on their diagnoses and procedures. Fixed medical payments are determined according to the case-mix system and additional fees for service. In addition to the medical costs that are calculated using the DPC/PDPS, the database also contains information regarding the total healthcare costs based on the provided medical services and their related fees. Anonymized data in the database include demographic characteristics, prescriptions, diagnosis (based on the International Classification of Diseases, 10th revision [ICD-10] code), medical treatments, treatment dates, hospital admission and discharging dates, discharge status, and pneumonia severity scores at the admission based on the A-DROP system, which is advocated by the Japanese Respiratory Society [32, 33]. The A-DROP system uses a modification of the CURB-65 score, which has been adjusted to reflect Japan's aging population. The system evaluates five factors: age of >69 years for male patients and >74 years for female patients, blood urea nitrogen of >20 mg/dL or dehydration, an SpO_2 value of ≤90% or a PaO_2 value of ≤60 Torr, presence of disorientation, and a systolic blood pressure of ≤90 mmHg. Cases are defined as mild, moderate, severe, or very severe, based on total scores of 0, 1–2, 3, and 4–5, respectively. The database also includes outpatient treatment records that are not covered by the DPC/PDPS.

Definition of CAP episodes

The present study included patients who were ≥65 years old with a confirmed diagnosis of pneumonia (ICD-10 code: J12–J18) and a prescription for antibiotic treatment between 1 June 2014 and 31 May 2015. The CAP episodes were classified as outpatient episodes or inpatient episodes. The outpatient index date was defined as the date of a pneumonia diagnosis with any antibiotic prescription. The treatment period extended from the index date until the end of the antibiotic prescription. If a second antibiotic prescription was provided within 7 days after the previous prescription's end date, the second treatment was considered part of the same outpatient episode. The inpatient index date was defined as the admission date for cases with a diagnosis of pneumonia, and the treatment period was defined as the length of stay (LOS). Inpatient CAP episodes were categorized based on treatment in the general ward or ICU (a minimum 1-night stay in the ICU). Death records (all-cause deaths based on discharge records) were only available for inpatient episodes. To ensure the study only considered cases of CAP, patients with a discharge date that was ≤14 days before the index date were excluded.

Treatment costs

CAP-related costs can be calculated as the CAP-related healthcare costs and/or the all-cause total healthcare costs. The CAP-related healthcare costs are calculated based on treatments that are directly related to the CAP, while the all-cause total healthcare costs are calculated based on the total costs during a CAP treatment period. The former method is difficult to use for elderly patients with CAP, as they typically have one or more comorbidities, which makes it difficult to differentiate between the treatments for the CAP and the exacerbation of comorbidities. Thus, the present study used the all-cause total healthcare costs in the analyses.

All-cause total healthcare costs were calculated by combining all recorded treatment costs during a single CAP episode. The treatment costs were classified as being related to inpatient stays, office visits, drug treatments, examinations, medical procedures, and other costs. The costs for inpatient stays and office visits included the facility's fixed costs and any service fees. The costs for drug treatments, examinations, and other costs were variable. The costs for medical procedures and other categories included service fees. A detailed breakdown of these categories is shown in Additional file 1: Table S1. Treatment costs were estimated based on medical fees and drug prices from April 2014. Because the fees and prices are revised every 2 years in Japan, the corresponding values for the period during which the treatment costs were calculated were selected.

CAP severity

The A-DROP system scores range from 0 to 5, with the most severe cases assigned a score of 5. CAP severity was also defined based on IPD episodes (severe CAP), as the related care is typically provided in a hospital. The IPD diagnoses were classified as bacteremia or meningitis. Bacteremia cases were identified based on a bacteremia diagnosis (ICD-10: A403, A409, A419, A491, A499), blood culture records, and antibiotic drug treatment during the CAP treatment period. Meningitis cases were identified based on a meningitis diagnosis (ICD-10: G001, G009), lumbar puncture, and antibiotic drug treatment during the CAP treatment period.

Other variables

Comorbidities were defined based on the patients' previous medications and/or diagnoses before the index date. The present study considered diabetes (ICD-10: E11–E14), COPD (ICD-10: J42–J44), dementia (ICD-10: F00), liver function failure (ICD-10: K70–K76), rheumatism (ICD-10: M059, M060, M068, M069), and cancer (ICD-10: C00–C99, D00–D09). Liver function failure does not have any specific medications, and was defined for the study as the presence of ≥2 diagnoses before the index date. Severe renal dysfunction was identified based on at least one dialysis treatment before the index date. The detailed definitions are shown in Additional file 1: Table S2. Medications that affected pneumonia were defined as oral steroids, inhaled steroids, angiotensin-converting enzyme inhibitors, and statins. To be considered as influencing the development of CAP, these drugs had to have been prescribed at least once during the 6 months before the index date. The definitions of medications are listed in Additional file 1: Table S3.

Analysis

All-cause total healthcare costs were calculated for outpatient and inpatient CAP episodes, as well as breakdowns of the total treatment costs. The costs of inpatient CAP episodes were also subdivided into cases that received treatment in the general ward or in the ICU. Treatment costs were also calculated according to mortality and CAP severity (based on the A-DROP score and episodes with or without IPD). The costs were stratified according to the presence of comorbidities and prescriptions, and all costs were expressed as median and interquartile range (IQR) values in US dollars (in May 2017, one US dollar equaled approximately 111.3 yen). All results were reported as mean, standard deviation, median, and IQR, as appropriate. All analyses were performed using SAS software (version 9.3; SAS Institute Inc., Cary, North Carolina, USA).

Results

Patient characteristics

There were 70,539 patients who were ≥65 years old and had a pneumonia diagnosis in the database. The study evaluated data from 29,619 patients with CAP, who experienced 14,450 outpatient CAP episodes and/or 20,314 inpatient CAP episodes. The study selection criteria is shown in Fig. 1. The mean ages were 77.5 ± 8.0 years and 81.5 ± 8.2 years among the outpatient and inpatient groups, respectively. Across both treatment settings, 61% of the patients were men (Table 1). The median CAP treatment periods were 7 days (IQR: 4–9 days) per outpatient episode and 14 days (IQR: 9–25 days) per inpatient episode. Liver function failure was the most prevalent comorbidity among both inpatient and outpatient cases, and was followed by COPD. Outpatient episodes were associated with a

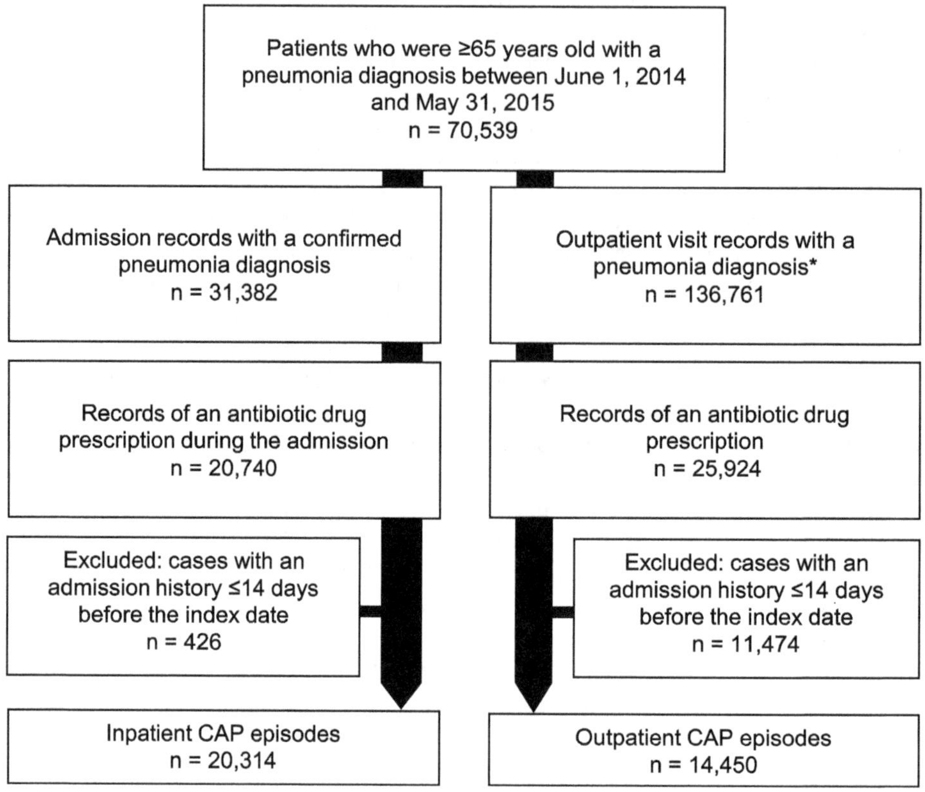

Fig. 1 The study selection criteria. *These records included both the first records of pneumonia diagnosis and subsequent follow-up visit records

higher rate of cancer, compared to inpatient episodes (16% vs. 7%).

All-cause CAP treatment costs

The median treatment costs were $346 (IQR: $195–551) per outpatient episode and $4851 (IQR: $3313–7669) per inpatient episode. Drug costs and laboratory test costs accounted for 82% of the outpatient CAP episode costs, while 61% of inpatient treatment costs were related to the inpatient stays (Fig. 2). Approximately 58% of the episodes (20,145/34,764) involved hospitalization in the general ward, and relatively few episodes involved ICU treatment (0.5%, 169/34,764). However, the treatment costs of ICU episodes were approximately 2.6× higher, compared to general ward episodes ($12,728 [IQR: $8059–21,512] vs. $4824 [IQR: $3301–7591], respectively). The combined total cost of CAP during the study period was $136,575,963, with outpatient episodes accounting for 6% of these costs, general ward episodes accounting for 92%, and ICU episodes accounting for 2%. The median treatment costs for cases of in-hospital mortality ($n = 2389$) were significantly higher than cases with survival until discharge ($6474 [IQR: $3372–10,639] vs. $4741 [IQR: $3308–7287], respectively).

CAP severity data were available for 83% of the inpatient episodes (16,931/20,314). The mean treatment costs of CAP episodes according to severity score are shown in Table 2. Higher severity was associated with increased treatment costs at the treating hospital, as well as with a higher mortality rate and prolonged treatment period. Approximately 1.3% of inpatient episodes involved IPD (263/20,314), and 4.6% (12/263) of the IPD episodes were treated in the ICU. The mean age of patients with IPD episodes was 80.7 ± 7.5 years, and 67% of the patients were men. The LOS for IPD episodes was longer than the LOS for non-IPD episodes (21 days vs. 14 days). The mortality rate for non-IPD episodes was 11%, compared to 35% for IPD episodes. Additional detailed data are shown in Additional file 1: Table S4. The median treatment cost per IPD episode was $7766 (IQR: $4411–12,762), and that cost was higher than the cost for non-IPD episodes ($4831 [IQR: $3304–7603]). Approximately 62% of the IPD episodes (162/263) had available CAP severity data. Cases with a severity score of 5 had the highest IPD rate (8%). Figure 3 shows the median treatment costs and mortality rates for IPD and non-IPD episodes. IPD episodes had higher median treatment costs and an increased mortality rate. Compared to non-IPD episodes, the mortality rate for IPD episodes was increased by 11–32%.

Table 1 Patient characteristics

	All patients		Outpatient CAP episodes		Inpatient CAP episodes	
	n = 29,619		*n* = 14,450		*n* = 20,314	
Age in years, mean (SD)	80.1	(8.4)	77.5	(8.0)	81.5	(8.2)
Age group, *n* (%)						
65–74 years	8403	(28%)	5787	(40%)	4499	(22%)
75–84 years	11,519	(39%)	5612	(39%)	7965	(39%)
≥ 85 years	9697	(33%)	3051	(21%)	7850	(39%)
Sex, *n* (%)						
Male	17,687	(60%)	8853	(61%)	12,314	(61%)
Median treatment period, days (IQR)	–	–	7	(4–9)	14	(9–25)
Death, *n* (%)	–	–	–	–	2389	(12%)
Comorbidities, *n* (%)						
Diabetes mellitus	3134	(11%)	1950	(13%)	2032	(10%)
Chronic obstructive pulmonary disease	3527	(12%)	2426	(17%)	2509	(12%)
Dementia	194	(1%)	103	(1%)	135	(1%)
Dialysis	525	(2%)	293	(2%)	382	(2%)
Liver function failure	4506	(15%)	3020	(21%)	2773	(14%)
Rheumatism	845	(3%)	620	(4%)	489	(2%)
Cancer	2718	(9%)	2284	(16%)	1322	(7%)
Prescriptions during previous 6 months, *n* (%)						
Oral antibiotics	2682	(9%)	2244	(16%)	1586	(8%)
Inhaled steroids	1691	(6%)	1279	(9%)	1155	(6%)
Angiotensin-converting enzyme inhibitors	882	(3%)	505	(3%)	586	(3%)
Statins	2634	(9%)	1678	(12%)	1583	(8%)

CAP community-acquired pneumonia, *SD* standard deviation, *IQR* interquartile range

All-cause CAP treatment costs according to risk factors

Total costs were associated with male sex, diabetes, COPD, and liver function failure (Table 3). Approximately 90% of the total costs were spent on general ward episodes for each risk factor. Increasing age was associated with higher hospitalization rates and total treatment costs. CAP episodes that involved dementia and dialysis were also associated with high admission rates. Table 4 shows the median treatment costs per CAP episode, the median treatment periods, and the mortality rates according to the risk factors. Inpatient CAP episodes that involved dementia, dialysis, and rheumatism were associated with high treatment costs (likely because of the prolonged LOS) and high mortality rates. Inpatient CAP episodes that involved cancer were associated with a high mortality rate, a short LOS, and low treatment costs.

Discussion

The present study evaluated the economic burden of CAP in Japan according to severity, as well as the relationship between treatment costs and risk factors. The study found that CAP episodes with hospitalization were 14× more

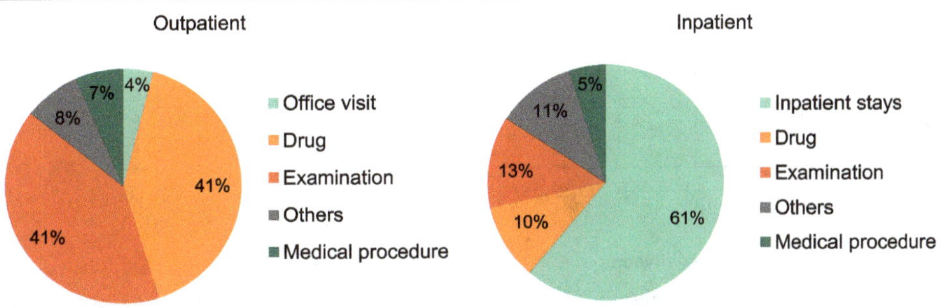

Fig. 2 The specific treatment costs as percentages of the total treatment cost

Table 2 All-cause total treatment costs according to severity and community-acquired pneumonia treatment setting

All cases (n = 16,931)	n	%	Median cost	Median treatment period (days)	Mortality rate (%)
Score 0	1006	6%	3508	10	2%
Score 1	5514	33%	4085	12	4%
Score 2	5644	33%	4706	14	8%
Score 3	3387	20%	5630	16	15%
Score 4	1126	7%	6175	17	35%
Score 5	254	2%	6578	19	52%
General ward (n = 16,809)	n	%	Median cost	Median treatment period (days)	Mortality rate (%)
Score 0	1005	6%	3507	10	2%
Score 1	5502	33%	4079	12	4%
Score 2	5602	33%	4679	13	8%
Score 3	3353	20%	5597	16	15%
Score 4	1104	7%	6099	17	35%
Score 5	243	1%	6410	18	52%
Intensive care unit (n = 122)	n	%	Median cost	Median treatment period (days)	Mortality rate (%)
Score 0	1	1%	4556	10	0%
Score 1	12	10%	13,264	34	0%
Score 2	42	34%	11,406	21	24%
Score 3	34	28%	11,763	26	18%
Score 4	22	18%	10,583	18	55%
Score 5	11	9%	14,117	22	55%

expensive, compared to outpatient episodes, and that stay-related costs accounted for 61% of inpatient treatment costs. It also found that CAP severity, male sex, diabetes, COPD, and liver function failure were associated with high total treatment costs. Furthermore, CAP episodes that involved dementia, dialysis, and rheumatism were associated with high treatment costs, which was likely because of the high admission rate. However, CAP episodes that involved cancer were associated with low inpatient treatment costs, which was likely related to the high mortality rate and short LOS.

Although it was observed that severe CAP, based on the A-DROP system, was associated with high treatment costs, no significant relationship was observed between cost and CURB-65 in a prospective non-interventional clinical study [34]. Another study revealed that total

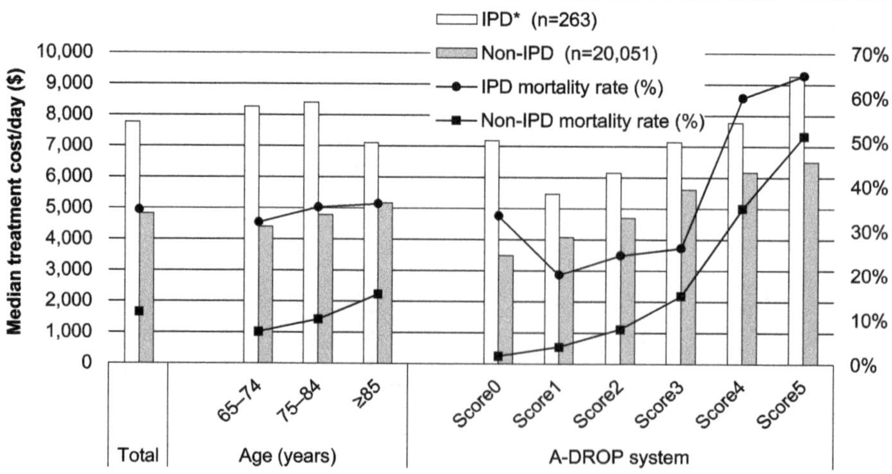

Fig. 3 The median all-cause treatment costs of community-acquired pneumonia episodes with or without invasive pneumococcal disease episodes. *IPD: invasive pneumococcal disease

Table 3 A breakdown of all-cause total treatment costs according to risk factors

	Total episodes	Proportion of CAP episodes (%)			Total costs		Proportion of total costs (%)		
Risk factors	*n*	Outpatient episodes	GW episodes	ICU episodes	$	%	Outpatient episodes	GW episodes	ICU episodes
Total	34,764	41.6%	57.9%	0.5%	136,575,963	100.0%	5.6%	92.2%	2.2%
Sex									
Male	21,167	41.8%	57.6%	0.6%	83,776,408	61.3%	5.8%	91.7%	2.5%
Female	13,597	41.2%	58.5%	0.4%	52,799,556	38.7%	5.4%	93.0%	1.6%
Age group									
65–74 years	10,286	56.3%	43.3%	0.5%	31,437,785	23.0%	10.8%	85.5%	3.7%
75–84 years	13,577	41.3%	58.1%	0.6%	54,022,674	39.6%	5.6%	92.4%	2.0%
≥ 85 years	10,901	28.0%	71.6%	0.4%	51,115,505	37.4%	2.5%	96.1%	1.3%
Comorbidities									
Diabetes mellitus	3982	49.0%	50.3%	0.8%	14,534,072	10.6%	8.9%	88.2%	3.0%
COPD	4935	49.2%	50.3%	0.6%	16,749,527	12.3%	8.2%	89.6%	2.3%
Liver function failure	5793	52.1%	47.4%	0.5%	19,154,382	14.0%	9.2%	88.5%	2.2%
Dementia	238	43.3%	55.9%	0.8%	936,780	0.7%	5.5%	90.0%	4.5%
Dialysis	675	43.4%	55.6%	1.0%	3,592,463	2.6%	9.1%	83.9%	7.0%
Rheumatism	1109	55.9%	43.7%	0.4%	3,533,324	2.6%	11.4%	84.9%	3.7%
Cancer	3606	63.3%	36.4%	0.3%	9,999,506	7.3%	18.6%	80.0%	1.4%
Prescriptions during previous 6 months									
Oral antibiotics	3830	58.6%	40.8%	0.6%	11,646,586	8.5%	13.7%	82.8%	3.5%
Inhaled steroids	2434	52.5%	46.6%	0.8%	7,329,868	5.4%	9.7%	86.9%	3.4%
ACE-I	1091	46.3%	53.0%	0.7%	4,087,905	3.0%	7.0%	90.8%	2.2%
Statins	3261	51.5%	47.7%	0.9%	10,744,840	7.9%	9.0%	87.2%	3.9%

CAP community-acquired pneumonia, *GW* general ward, *ICU* intensive care unit, *COPD* chronic obstructive pulmonary disease, *ACE-I* angiotensin-converting enzyme inhibitors

CAP treatment costs among inpatients increased for PSI classes I–III and reached a plateau at classes IV–V [23]. Thus, the relationship between CAP severity and treatment costs may differ depending on the severity score that is used.

The most important factor that influenced treatment cost was hospitalization, which accounted for 94% of total costs. Furthermore, treatment of episodes in the general ward was associated with high total treatment costs, while treatment of episodes in the ICU only accounted for 2% of total costs, despite these episodes clearly involving serious cases (i.e. high treatment costs, high mortality rate, and prolonged LOS). Interestingly, the costs of drug treatment and laboratory testing did not account for a large proportion of the total inpatient costs, and a prospective observational study in a Spanish public tertiary hospital also confirmed that the costs could be broken down into room costs (69%), drug costs (13%), laboratory costs (12%), and diagnostic procedures (6%) [15]. Therefore, the economic burden of CAP could be reduced by decreasing the number of admissions.

A previous study revealed that 61% of mild CAP cases were admitted to a hospital [34], although the rate was only 6% in the present study. This is likely related to differences in the definitions that are used for the CURB-65 and A-DROP systems, as the A-DROP system has one mild category (score 0) and the CURB-65 system has two mild categories (scores 0 and 1). When the CURB-65 system was applied, the results indicated that 34% of mild CAP cases were hospitalized, which suggests that the A-DROP system may underestimate the proportion of mild CAP cases. Thus, the present study's results highlight the importance of minimizing the hospitalization of mild CAP cases, and other previous studies have also provided similar findings [14, 35–37].

In the present study, the cost per inpatient episode tended to increase with age, although a Dutch administrative database study revealed that the median treatment cost per episode in the general ward remained relatively stable at approximately $5600 for patients who were ≥50 years old [21]. This difference is likely related to the fact that the LOS increased with age in the present study, but was stable in the Dutch study. For Dutch outpatient episodes, the cost was approximately $850 per episode for patients who were 50–84 years old, while the costs were approximately 50% lower for patients who were ≥85 years

Table 4 The median treatment costs, treatment periods, and mortality rates according to risk factors

Risk factors	Median treatment cost per episode ($)			Treatment period (days)			Mortality rate (%)	
	Outpatient episodes	GW episodes	ICU episodes	Outpatient episodes	GW episodes	ICU episodes	GW episodes	ICU episodes
Total	346	4824	12,728	7	14	24	12%	30%
Sex								
Male	356	4791	12,518	7	14	22	12%	30%
Female	330	4872	12,792	7	15	27	11%	31%
Age group								
65–74 years	353	4391	19,485	8	12	34	7%	20%
75–84 years	352	4778	11,098	7	14	17	10%	32%
≥ 85 years	323	5162	13,105	6	16	28	16%	39%
Comorbidities								
Diabetes mellitus	384	4878	10,035	8	15	21	10%	30%
COPD	355	4836	11,238	8	14	18	10%	39%
Liver function failure	338	4738	10,029	8	15	21	12%	37%
Dementia	320	5567	21,078	7	17	60	19%	0%
Dialysis	732	6389	23,136	6	15	37	15%	14%
Rheumatism	412	4910	20,673	8	15	34	10%	50%
Cancer	377	4528	8064	8	14	14	15%	50%
Prescriptions during previous 6 months								
Oral antibiotics	375	4821	11,218	8	14	20	13%	46%
Inhaled steroids	346	4622	11,388	7	13	22	8%	30%
ACE-I	298	5124	8778	7	15	19	11%	13%
Statins	352	4705	11,372	7	14	20	7%	21%

GW general ward, *ICU* intensive care unit, *COPD* chronic obstructive pulmonary disease, *ACE-I* angiotensin-converting enzyme inhibitors

old. However, in the present study, the treatment cost per CAP episode only decreased slightly for patients who were ≥85 years old. One possible explanation for this difference is that Dutch patients who were ≥85 years old had shorter outpatient treatments, as most patients in this age group were hospitalized.

Based on the findings of the present study, prophylactic treatment (e.g. oral hygiene or pneumococcal vaccination) is recommended to reduce treatment costs for patients who are male and/or have comorbidities (e.g. diabetes, COPD, and liver function failure). In addition, patients with dementia, dialysis, or rheumatism may be an important group to target, given their high treatment costs per CAP episode.

The present study determined the exact CAP treatment costs using a nationally representative data set, while previous studies were limited by only evaluating patients at a few hospitals. In addition, the present study's calculations were not influenced by changing costs based on the patient's income or insurance status, as Japanese medical service fees are determined based on a payment list that is approved by the government. Furthermore, healthcare claims data that are used for reimbursement can provide an accurate record of the provided medical services.

The study calculated the all-cause total healthcare costs according to CAP severity and risk factors. This is because the treatment of underlying disease could not be separated from the treatment of CAP exacerbation. By comparing patients with or without CAP, further study is planning to estimate the additional costs of CAP. The treatment costs of CAP episodes that were encountered by general practitioners were not estimated, as the study's database only included hospital records. However, the authors speculate that outpatient treatment costs of CAP episodes are comparable between hospitals and clinics. This is because almost all residents of Japan are covered by the national health insurance system, which provides equal reimbursement for hospital-based outpatient visits and clinic visits. The reimbursement rates are pre-determined by the Japanese government, and even patients who visit a large hospital without a referral would only make an extra out-of-pocket payment of < $72. However, the study's database mainly included small- or middle-sized hospitals, which suggests that patients would incur similar treatment costs at a hospital or clinic if they received the same treatment. Moreover, patients can select any hospital or clinic throughout Japan, regardless of the severity of their disease. Therefore, it is expected that there would be little difference in the outpatient treatment costs of CAP episodes at hospitals and clinics.

The present study also has several limitations. First, CAP cases that were caused by *Streptococcus pneumoniae* were not able to be identified, as culture results were not available in the database. Therefore, it was difficult to distinguish between specified or unspecified pneumonia. As there is very little evidence regarding IPD-related treatment costs, further studies are needed to more precisely estimate the IPD treatment costs using culture results. Second, compared to outpatients in the database, the hospitalized patients included fewer immunocompromised patients (e.g. patients with cancer and rheumatism). It is possible that many patients with cancer and a poor general status were included in the database. Another explanation is that all elderly people (> 65 years old) can receive the PPV23 vaccine in Japan, although the vaccination rate in 2014 was only 20% (based on vaccine shipment records), which could indicate that high-risk patients had been vaccinated and were less likely to develop CAP or other serious conditions. Third, a claims database was used for the present study, and this type of study is limited by various issues. For example, there can be differences between diagnostic and reimbursement records, and it would be useful to combine data regarding diagnoses and specific medications. However, there is no specific medication for treating liver function failure, and the present study arbitrarily defined these cases as patients who had ≥2 diagnoses before their index date. Therefore, these diagnoses may have been overestimated.

Conclusion

This study found that severe CAP cases had high rates of mortality and prolonged hospitalization, which were associated with high treatment costs. In addition, many hospitalizations that involved cases of mild CAP were detected. Therefore, to reduce the economic burden of CAP, clinicians should aim to decrease the number of hospitalized mild CAP cases and to prevent the development of severe CAP. For example, prophylactic treatment (e.g. oral hygiene or vaccination) may be effective for elderly patients who are male, ≥ 85 years old, or have comorbidities (e.g. diabetes, COPD, liver function failure, rheumatism, dementia, or dialysis). These findings can be used to identify population(s) that should be targeted by the vaccine program, based on their burden of diseases, and will help to estimate the value of the vaccine program. Furthermore, vaccination coverage remains low in Japan, and efforts should be made to increase pneumococcus vaccination coverage.

Abbreviations

CAP: Community-acquired pneumonia; COPD: Chronic obstructive pulmonary disease; DPC/PDPS: Diagnosis Procedure Combination/Per-Diem Payment System; ICD-10: International Classification of Diseases, 10th revision; ICU: Intensive care unit; IPD: Invasive pneumococcal disease; IQR: Interquartile range; LOS: Length of stay; PPV23: 23-Valent pneumococcal polysaccharide vaccine; PSI: Pneumonia severity index; SD: Standard deviation

Acknowledgements

None.

Funding

This research was supported by the Emerging/Re-emerging Infectious Diseases Project, which is administered by the Japanese Agency for Medical Research and Development (AMED).

Authors' contributions

MA and KK conceived and designed the research plan. KK analyzed and interpreted the patient data, under the supervision of MA, and was a major contributor in writing the manuscript. NH assisted with the clinical interpretation of the data. All authors read and approved the final manuscript.

Competing interests

The authors declare that they have no competing interests.

Author details

[1]Public Health and Epidemiology, Meiji Pharmaceutical University, 2-522-1, Noshio, Kiyose, Tokyo 204-8588, Japan. [2]Center for Pulmonary Diseases, National Hospital Organization Tokyo National Hospital, 3-1-1 Takeoka, Kiyose-shi, Tokyo 204-8585, Japan.

References

1. Morimoto K, Suzuki M, Ishifuji T, et al. The burden and etiology of community-onset pneumonia in the aging Japanese population: a multicenter prospective study. PLoS One. 2015;10:1–18.
2. Farr BM, Woodhead MA, MacFarlane JT, et al. Risk factors for community-acquired pneumonia diagnosed by general practitioners in the community. Respir Med. 2000;94:422–7.
3. Baik I, Curhan GC, Rimm EB, et al. A prospective study of age and lifestyle factors in relation to community-acquired pneumonia in US men and women. Arch Intern Med. 2000;160:3082–8.
4. Jackson ML, Neuzil KM, Thompson WW, et al. The burden of community-acquired pneumonia in seniors: results of a population-based study. Clin Infect Dis. 2004;39:1642–50.
5. Vila Corcoles A, Ochoa Gondar O, Rodriguez Blanco T, et al. Epidemiology of community-acquired pneumonia in older adults: a population-based study. Respir Med. 2009;103:309–16.
6. Millett ERC, De Stavola BL, Quint JK, et al. Risk factors for hospital admission in the 28 days following a community-acquired pneumonia diagnosis in older adults, and their contribution to increasing hospitalisation rates over time: a cohort study. BMJ Open. 2015;5:e008737.
7. Benjamin AL, Edward JB, Thomas SI, et al. Risk factors for acquiring pneumococcal infections. Arch Intern Med. 1986;146:2179–85.
8. Koivula I, Sten M, Makela PH. Risk factors for pneumonia in the elderly. Am J Med. 1994;96:313–20.
9. Almirall J, Bolíbar I, Balanzó X, et al. Risk factors for community-acquired pneumonia in adults: a population-based case-control study. Eur Respir J. 1999;13:349–55.
10. Sanz Herrero F, Blanquer OJ. Microbiology and risk factors for community-

acquired pneumonia. Semin Respir Crit Care Med. 2012;33:220–31.
11. Fine MJ, Auble TE, Yealy DM, et al. A prediction rule to identify low-risk patients with community acquired pneumonia. N Engl J Med. 1997;336:243–50.
12. Sato R, Gomez Rey G, Nelson S, et al. Community-acquired pneumonia episode costs by age and risk in commercially insured US adults aged >/=50 years. Appl Health Econ Health Policy. 2013;11:251–8.
13. File TM Jr, Marrie TJ. Burden of community-acquired pneumonia in north American adults. Postgrad Med. 2010;122:130–41.
14. Huang SS, Johnson KM, Ray GT, et al. Healthcare utilization and cost of pneumococcal disease in the United States. Vaccine. 2011;29:3398–412.
15. Reyes S, Martinez R, Vallés JM, et al. Determinants of hospital costs in community-acquired pneumonia. Eur Respir J. 2008;31:1061–7.
16. Cascini S, Agabiti N, Incalzi RA, et al. Pneumonia burden in elderly patients: a classification algorithm using administrative data. BMC Infect Dis. 2013;13:559.
17. Tichopad A, Roberts C, Gembula I, et al. Clinical and economic burden of community-acquired pneumonia among adults in the Czech Republic, Hungary, Poland and Slovakia. PLoS One. 2013;8:e71375.
18. Yoo KH, Yoo CG, Kim SK, et al. Economic burden and epidemiology of pneumonia in Korean adults aged over 50 years. J Korean Med Sci. 2013;28:888–95.
19. Thomas CP, Ryan M, Chapman JD, et al. Incidence and cost of pneumonia in medicare beneficiaries. Chest. 2012;142:973–81.
20. Kawakami K, Ohkusa Y, Kuroki R, et al. Effectiveness of pneumococcal polysaccharide vaccine against pneumonia and cost analysis for the elderly who receive seasonal influenza vaccine in Japan. Vaccine. 2010;28:7063–9.
21. Rozenbaum MH, Mangen MJ, Huijts SM, et al. Incidence, direct costs and duration of hospitalization of patients hospitalized with community acquired pneumonia: a nationwide retrospective claims database analysis. Vaccine. 2015;33:3193–9.
22. Bartolomé M, Almirrall J, Morera J, et al. A population-based study of the costs of care for community-acquired pneumonia. Eur Respir J. 2004;23:610–6.
23. Bauer TT, Welte T, Ernen C, et al. Cost analyses of community-acquired pneumonia from the hospital perspective. Chest. 2005;128:2238–46.
24. Butler JC, Breiman RF, Campbell JF, et al. Pneumococcal polysaccharide vaccine efficacy. An evaluation of current recommendations. JAMA. 1993; 270:1826–31.
25. Poethko Müller C, Schmitz R. Vaccination coverage in German adults: Results of the German Health Interview and Examination Survey for Adults (DEGS1). Vol. 56. Bundesgesundheitsblatt - Gesundheitsforschung - Gesundheitsschutz; 2013. p. 845–57.
26. Australian Institute of Health and Welfare. 2009 Adult vaccination survey: summary results. 2011. http://www.aihw.gov.au/publication-detail/?id=10737418409. Accessed 15 Apr 2017.
27. Yoneyama T, Yoshida M, Ohrui T, et al. Oral care reduces pneumonia in older patients in nursing homes. J Am Geriatr Soc. 2002;50:430–3.
28. Nakamura K. Diagnosis procedure combination database would develop Nationwide clinical research in Japan. Japanese Circ Soc. 2016;80:2289–90.
29. Milea D, Azmi S, Reginald P, et al. A review of accessibility of administrative healthcare databases in the Asia-Pacific region. J Mark Access Health Policy. 2015. doi.10.3402/jmahp.v3.28076.
30. Tanaka S, Seto K, Kawakami K. Pharmacoepidemiology in Japan: medical databases and research achievements. J Pharm Heal Care Sci. 2015. doi.10.1186/s40780-015-0016-5.
31. Uematsu H, Kunisawa S, Yamashita K, et al. The impact of patient profiles and procedures on hospitalization costs through length of stay in community-acquired pneumonia patients based on a Japanese administrative database. PLoS One. 2015;10:1–13.
32. Shindo Y, Sato S, Maruyama E, et al. Comparison of severity scoring systems A-DROP and CURB-65 for community-acquired pneumonia. Respirology. 2008;13:731–5.
33. Miyashita N, Matsushima T, Oka M, et al. The JRS guidelines for the management of community-acquired pneumonia in adults: an update and new recommendations. Intern Med. 2006;45:419–28.
34. Cupurdija V, Lazic Z, Petrovic M, et al. Community-acquired pneumonia: economics of inpatient medical care vis-à-vis clinical severity. J Bras Pneumol. 2015;41:48–57.
35. Choudhury G, Chalmers JD, Mandal P, et al. Physician judgement is a crucial adjunct to pneumonia severity scores in low-risk patients. Eur Respir J. 2011; 38:643–8.
36. Aliberti S, Ramirez J, Cosentini R, et al. Low CURB-65 is of limited value in deciding discharge of patients with community-acquired pneumonia. Respir Med. 2011;105:1732–8.
37. Spoorenberg SM, Bos WJ, Heijligenberg R, et al. Microbial aetiology, outcomes, and costs of hospitalisation for community-acquired pneumonia; an observational analysis. BMC Infect Dis. 2014;14:335.

18

Corynebacteria as a cause of pulmonary infection

Katharine Yang[1], Robert L. Kruse[1], Weijie V. Lin[1] and Daniel M. Musher[1,2*]

Abstract

Background: In most cases of community-acquired pneumonia (CAP), an etiologic agent is not determined; the most common report from the microbiological evaluation of sputum cites "normal respiratory flora." Non-diphtheria *Corynebacterium* spp., a component of this flora, is commonly viewed as a contaminant, but it may be the cause of pneumonia and the frequency with which it causes CAP may be underestimated.

Case presentations: This report present 3 cases of CAP in which *Corynebacterium* spp. was clearly the predominant isolate; identification was confirmed by matrix-assisted laser desorption ionization time of flight (MALDI-TOF) mass spectrometry. Two cases were caused by *C. propinquum* and one by *C. striatum*. Two patients had a tracheostomy and one was on hemodialysis. Patients who received an appropriate antibiotic responded well.

Conclusion: When identified as the predominant isolate in sputum from a patient with CAP, *Corynebacterium* spp. should be considered as a potential cause of the infection. In cases with patients who have compromised airway clearance or who are immunocompromised, microaspiration may be responsible. While some *Corynebacterium* spp. are suspectible to antibiotics usually prescribed for CAP, others are susceptible only to vancomycin or aminoglycosides. Vancomycin is thus the appropriate empiric antibiotic, pending speciation and susceptibility test results. The number of reported cases with result of antibiotic susceptibility testing, however, remains limited, and further investigation is needed. Non-diphtheria *Corynebacterium* spp. represent a noteworthy clinical cause of pneumonia. Identification by Gram stain and as a predominant organism on culture demands careful consideration for management.

Keywords: Pneumonia, Corynebacteria, Diphtheroids, Normal respiratory flora

Background

Pneumonia is an important cause of medical morbidity and mortality worldwide; pneumonia and influenza are listed as the 8th leading cause of death in the United States, with 57,062 deaths in 2015 [1]. Well-recognized and common causes of community-acquired pneumonia (CAP) in adults include bacteria such as *Streptococcus pneumoniae, Haemophilus influenzae*, and *Staphylococcus aureus*, and viruses such as influenza virus, respiratory syncytial virus, human metapneumovirus, and parainfluenza virus. Intensive recent investigations have failed to identify a causative organism in 50–62% of patients hospitalized for CAP [2, 3].

The most common laboratory report for sputum samples submitted for microbiological study is "mixed respiratory flora." Pneumonia caused by *S. pneumoniae* is thought to result from unrecognized microaspiration of pneumococci that have colonized the nasopharynx [4]. The authors of the present study have previously hypothesized that unrecognized aspiration of less virulent bacteria that normally inhabit the nasopharynx might also cause pneumonia, especially in persons whose upper airways are bypassed or whose ability to clear aspirated organisms is damaged [5]. The present study examined the possibilities that: (i) careful examination of Gram-stained sputum and culture plates may reveal a predominant bacterium such as *Corynebacterium* spp. that are not generally regarded as a pulmonary pathogen; (ii) quantitative cultures may document a high concentration of these bacteria in sputum; and (iii) these organisms are in fact the cause of some cases of pneumonia.

* Correspondence: Daniel.Musher@va.gov
[1]Baylor College of Medicine, Houston, TX 77030, USA
[2]Infectious Disease Section, Michael E. DeBakey Veterans Affairs Medical Center, 2002 Holcombe Boulevard, Houston, TX 77030, USA

Corynebacterium spp. Gram-positive bacilli that are often dismissed as contaminants have been reported to cause pneumonia (Table 1). New technologies, such as matrix-assisted laser desorption ionization time of flight (MALDI-TOF) mass spectrometry enable rapid and precise identification of bacterial species [6], and highly sensitive techniques such as polymerase chain reaction (PCR) can help exclude a role for viruses, mycoplasma, and chlamydia. With the advent of these new technologies, there has been greater interest in Corynebacteria, and these organisms have been cited as emerging pathogens [7].

The present study reports on 3 well-documented cases of CAP due to Corynebacteria (2 cases of *C. propinquum*, 1 case of *C. striatum*) that were diagnosed in a 6-month period at a large tertiary care hospital. The study reviews the medical literature on *Corynebacterium* spp. as etiologic agents of pneumonia, with the goal of increasing awareness of the possibility that so-called "normal respiratory flora" may actually be responsible for an as-yet undetermined proportion of cases of CAP.

Case presentations

Case 1

A 75-year-old man on hemodialysis for end-stage renal disease was hospitalized for cough, fever, and altered mental status. His temperature was 103 °F, pulse 68, blood pressure 124/69, respiratory rate 22, and O_2 saturation 96% on 2 L of O_2 by nasal cannula. He was lethargic, with bibasilar crackles and a normal cardiac examination. His white blood cell (WBC) count was 20,100 cells/mm^3 and his plasma procalcitonin was 1.1 ng/mL. Chest X-ray showed bibasilar infiltrates. Microscopic examination of Gram-stained sputum showed profuse polymorphonuclear leukocytes (PMNs) and Gram-positive rods, many of which appeared to be intracellular (Fig. 1). Sputum culture yielded overwhelmingly predominant Corynebacteria, with rare *P. aeruginosa*. The Corynebacteria was identified as *C. propinquum* by MALDI-TOF. Blood cultures and viral PCR were negative. The patient was initially treated with vancomycin, cefepime, and metronidazole. Based on the predominance of Corynebacteria with the absence of other bacteria on Gram stain and a negative PCR for respiratory viruses, his pneumonia was attributed to *C. propinquum*, and only vancomycin was continued. He responded and was discharged to complete a 10-day course of linezolid.

Case 2

A 61-year-old man was found unresponsive post laryngectomy and tracheostomy for laryngeal squamous cell carcinoma. His temperature was 97.8 °F, pulse 99, blood pressure 114/86, and respiratory rate 22. Breath sounds were decreased bilaterally. WBC count was 7200 cells/mm^3, lactate 1.2 mg/dL. Chest X-ray showed a new left-sided infiltrate. Sputum Gram stain revealed many Gram-positive rods, including those found within PMNs. Sputum yielded many Corynebacteria, identified by MALDI-TOF as *C. propinquum*, and few *S. aureus*. Sputum was liquefied with 2% N-acetyl cysteine and diluted serially; aliquots were cultured on blood agar and the number of colony forming units (CFU) was calculated [8]. The specimen contained 2×10^9 CFU of Corynebacteria and $< 10^5$ CFU of *S. aureus* per mL. Blood cultures and viral PCR were negative. The patient was initially given vancomycin, cefepime, and ampicillin; treatment was switched to ampicillin/sulbactam after the *Corynebacterium* was reported susceptible. His mental status rapidly improved, and he was subsequently discharged to complete a 10-day course of amoxicillin/clavulanate.

Case 3

A 59-year-old male with widely metastatic squamous cell carcinoma of the tongue was admitted for bleeding from his tracheostomy site. His temperature was 99 °F, blood pressure 108/84, pulse 119, respiratory rate 24, and oxygen saturation 82% on room air. He had blood at the tracheostomy site and bibasilar rhonchi. WBC count was 22,000 cells/mm^3, hemoglobin 11.1 g/dL, and lactate 1.8 mg/dL. Chest X-ray revealed a left upper-lobe infiltrate. Sputum sample showed profuse PMNs and Gram-positive rods. Culture yielded *C. striatum* (confirmed by MALDI-TOF) and few *Escherichia coli*. The patient was placed on comfort care and died 8 days later.

Discussion

Epidemiology

Non-diphtheria *Corynebacterium* spp.--commensal flora of the skin, respiratory tract, and mucous membranes [9, 10]-- have been characterized as emerging pathogens [7]. Among reported cases, infections of the respiratory tract are second in frequency only to those of the urinary tract [11]. The literature search revealed 67 reported cases of pulmonary infection due to non-diphtheria *Corynebacterium* spp., summarized in Table 1. Cases include pneumonia (community-acquired, hospital-acquired, or ventilator-associated), necrotizing pneumonia, and empyema, although pneumonia predominated. Implicated *Corynebacterium* spp. include *C. pseudodiphtheriticum* [12, 13], *C. propinquum* [14], *C. striatum* [14–18], *C. afermentans* [19], *C. xerosis* [20], *C. jeikeium* [10, 21–23], *C. pseudotuberculosis* [24, 25], *C. mucifaciens* [26], *C. ulcerans* [27], and *C. macginleyi* [28].

Table 1 Previously documented cases of *Corynebacterium* pulmonary infection

Organism isolated	No. of cases	Age/Sex	Co-morbid conditions	Diagnosis	Methods of Diagnosis	Mortality N (%)
C. accolens [46]	1	72F	DM, myocardial infarction, triple aortic bypass, heart failure	Pneumonia	Bronchoalveolar brush sample. Culture also yielded small numbers of *P. aeruginosa*	1 (100%)
C. afermentans [19]	1	27F	HIV	Empyema	Pleural fluid and blood culture positive. Sputum culture reported "normal respiratory flora"	0 (0%)
C. jeikeium [10, 22, 23, 47]	5	48F, 28F, 29F, 76M, 77F	2 Acute myelogenous leukemia, 1 Hodgkin's lymphoma and Acute myelomonocytic leukemia, 1 old pulmonary tuberculosis, and 1 COPD	Pneumonia, (necrosis and hemorrhage in 1 case)	Positive gram stain and culture from 1 post-mortem pneumonia; 4 positive respiratory cultures (including 1 TTA). In 1 case, sputum yielded 10^6 *C. jeikeium*, > 10^7 *S. aureus* and 10^3 *P. aeruginosa* per ml; TTA culture yielded > 10^8 *C. jeikeium*, 10^4 *P. aeruginosa*, and 10^3 *S. aureus*; FNA yielded pure growth of *C. jeikeium*	4 (80%)
C. macginleyi [28]	1	73F	Metastatic lung adenocarcinoma, chemotherapy, intubated post-bronchoscopy	Ventilator-associated pneumonia	Sputum culture had 10^5 CFU/mL *C. macginleyi*	0 (0%)
C. mucifaciens [26]	1	51M	DM	Cavitary pneumonia	Not described	0 (0%)
C. propinquum [14, 48]	4	72F, 79M, 83M, 7F	2 DM, 1 non-Hodgkin's MALT lymphoma, 2 Rheumatoid arthritis, 2 COPD, 1 ataxia telangiectasia on inhaled corticosteroids	Pneumonia	3 sputum culture; 1 case with bronchial aspirate and broncho-alveolar lavage yielding only *C. propinquum* and blood culture positive for *S. pneumoniae*	0 (0%)
C. pseudo-diphtheriticum [12–14, 33–38, 49–55]	40	91F, 40M, 79F, 70 M, 71M, 68M, 72M, 70F, 74M, 76F, 83M, 75M, 68M, 76M, 65M, 68F, 64M, 67M, 62M, 66M, 50F, 27F, 68F, 29M, 47M, 41M, 24M, 43M, 34M, 33M, 33M, 43M, 34M, 29M, 30M, 80F, 9F, 59M, 46M, 75M	2 CKD, 3 CHF, 10 COPD, 4 DM, 2 asthma, SLE, 1 Adult T-cell lymphotrophic virus Ab+, 1 tracheostomy, 2 lung cancers, 1 epidermoid carcinoma, 2 autoimmune disorder on steroid therapy, 2 intubations, 1 amyotrophic lateral sclerosis, 10 HIV/AIDS, 3 previous tuberculosis, 2 recent *Pneumocystis jiroveci* pneumonia, 1 cystic fibrosis	Pneumonia	15 sputum Gram stains, 2 bronchial secretions, 1 bronchial wash; Cultures also yielded fewer numbers of other bacteria: *S. aureus* (2), *H. influenzae* (1), *S. pneumoniae* (3), *S. maltophila* (1), *P. aeruginosa* (1), *E. cloacae* (1)	4 (10%); 9 status unknown, 27 resolved
C. pseudotuberculosis [24, 25]	2	23F, 28M	2 veterinary students (1 known exposure to sick horses)	Pneumonia	TTA or CT guided transthoracic biopsy	0 (0%)
C. striatum [14–17, 56–58]	7	68F, 47F, 28M, 27M, 69M, 58M, 69F	1 DM, 2 HIV/AIDS, 1 alcohol use, 1 COPD, 1 heart transplant, 1 RA on prednisone	6 pneumonia, 1 empyema	2 sputum, 2 BAL cultures (4×10^3 CFU/mL and > 10^5 CFU/mL), 1 bronchoscopy brush sample, 1 empyema, 1 pleural fluid +1 lung tissue culture	1 (14%)
C. ulcerans [27, 59]	2	78M, 80F	1 Metastatic squamous cell carcinoma of the lung, 1 HTN	Pneumonia	2 positive sputum cultures, 1 confirmed by BAL	2 (100%)
C. urealyticum [60]	1	72M	CHF, COPD	Pneumonia	Transtracheal aspirate	0 (0%)
C. xerosis [20]	1	63M	AML	Pneumonia	BAL culture yielded 10^5 *C. xerosis* /mL	1 (100%)
"Aerobic diphtheroids" [61]	1	68M	Heavy smoking history, dental extractions	Empyema	Pleural fluid culture grew only "diphtheroids"	0 (0%)

DM **Diabetes Mellitus, *HTN* Hypertension, *HLD* Hyperlipidemia, *HIV* Human Immunodeficiency Virus, *CFU* colony forming units, *COPD* Chronic Obstructive Pulmonary Disease, *RML* Right middle lobe of lung, *TTA* transtracheal aspiration, *FNA* Fine Needle Aspiration, *cx* culture, *MALT* Mucosa-associated lymphoid tissue, *CKD* Chronic kidney disease, *CHF* Congestive heart failure, *SLE* Systemic Lupus Erythematosis, *AIDS* Acquired Immunodeficiency Syndrome, *RA* Rheumatoid arthritis, *BAL* bronchoaveolar lavage**

Microbiology, pathogenesis, and immunity

"Coryneform bacteria" is the umbrella term for the class of bacteria comprised of facultative intracellular, non-spore-forming, catalase-positive, non-acid-fast, non-motile, and irregularly-shaped Gram-positive rods [29]. Based on 16S rRNA sequencing studies, *Corynebacterium* belongs to a subdivision of Gram-positive eubacteria with high guanine-to-cytosine content, which also contains *Arthrobacter, Mycobacterium, Nocardia,* and *Streptomyces* [30]. Coryneform bacteria are pleomorphic throughout their life cycle, and may have thickenings at either end, giving the "coryneform" name, meaning "club-shaped"; they may be clustered, forming shapes that resemble a "V," "palisades," or "Chinese letters" [29]. Because of their relation to *C. diphtheriae,* their common name is "diphtheroids."

Little is known about the virulence factors of the non-diphtheria *Corynebacterium* spp. that may contribute to CAP and other infections [31]. *C. pseudodiphtheriticum,* the species most commonly implicated as a cause of pneumonia, has an ability to invade human epithelial type 2 (HEp-2) cells and survive for 24 h after infection, suggesting a potential mechanism to escape killing by the innate immune system [31]. Invasive strains form biofilms and bind fibrinogen and fibronectin, which may be facilitated by fimbrial subunits [31, 32].

Predisposing conditions

With the exception of 2 cases of pneumonia due to *C. pseudotuberculosis* in veterinary workers [24, 25], all other reported cases of Corynebacterial pneumonia have occurred in persons whose upper airways are bypassed, whose ability to clear aspirated organisms is damaged, or who have immunocompromising conditions (Table 2). The great majority of patients have had conditions that affect pulmonary clearance, including chronic obstructive pulmonary disease (COPD), cystic fibrosis [33], and previous radiotherapy to the thorax [27]. Some have had procedures that bypass protective mechanisms of the upper airways such as recent endotracheal intubation [28, 34, 35] or laryngectomy [36], as seen in Cases 2 and 3 in the present study. Among patients who are immunocompromised, co-morbidities included HIV infection [17, 37, 38], chemotherapy [10, 28], hematologic malignancies or conditions that compromise PMN function such as diabetes mellitus, alcohol use disorder [16] or end-stage renal disease, as seen in Case 1 in the present study.

Clinical description

The presentation of pneumonia due to Corynebacteria does not differ from that due to bacterial pneumonia of any other cause: cough, fever, and altered mental status are usually present, as observed in the present study's 3 cases. Cases of community-acquired or ventilator-associated pneumonia, cavitary pneumonia, empyema, and bacteremia have been described (Table 1). Only 5 (7.5%) of the 67 reported patients with Corynebacterial pneumonia have been bacteremic with Corynebacteria. This suggests that blood cultures may be of minimal utility for confirming any sputum findings. Pneumonia caused by the quintessential pulmonary pathogen, *S. pneumoniae,* is bacteremic in no more than approximately 25% of cases [39], and the rate of bacteremia is far lower in pneumonia due to less pathogenic organisms, such as nontypable *H. influenzae* [40] or *Moraxella catarrhalis* [41].

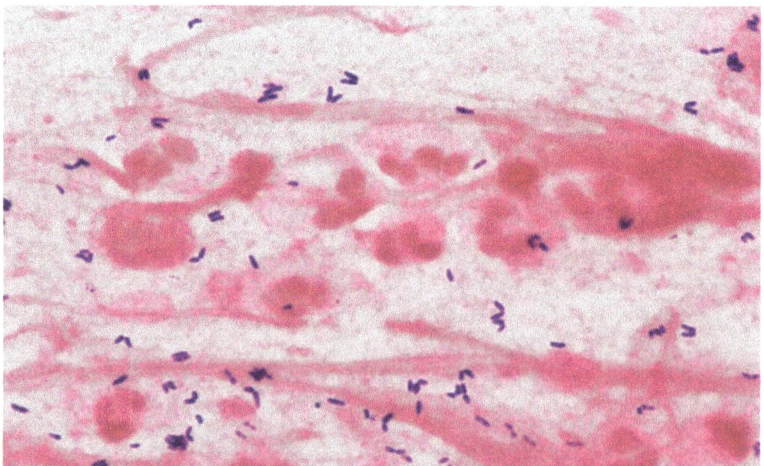

Fig. 1 Gram-stain observed in sputum from patient with Corynebacterial pneumonia. A sputum sample collected from the patient in Case 1 depicts Gram-positive bacilli (purple) within and surrounding polymorphonuclear cells (pink). The "club-shaped" appearance pathognomonic for the group "Coryneform" is appreciated

Table 2 Risk factors in reported cases of Corynebacterial pneumonia

Risk Category	Examples
Decreased clearance / Damaged lung structure	Chronic obstructive pulmonary disease Previous radiation to thorax Cystic fibrosis Heavy smoking history
Bypass of airway protection	Active or recent endotracheal intubation Laryngectomy
Immunodeficiency	Human immunodeficiency virus (HIV) infection Ongoing or recent cancer chemotherapy Conditions that compromise function of PMNs (e.g. poorly controlled diabetes mellitus, end-stage renal disease) Steroid use secondary to autoimmune disease Immunosuppressive drug use secondary to transplant
Miscellaneous factors	Alcohol use disorder
Environmental	Exposure to sick animals (*C. pseudotuberculosis* only)

Laboratory diagnosis

Given the limited utility of blood cultures in diagnosing Corynebacterial pneumonia, diagnosis requires a multifaceted approach. In most previous case reports, diagnosis has been based on microscopic examination of a Gram-stained sputum and careful examination of culture plates [42]. In the 3 cases discussed in this report, the sputum Gram stain showed profuse numbers of Corynebacteria. In 12 of the previously reported cases, quantitative studies were carried out on sputum, bronchoalveolar lavage samples, or protected bronchial brush samples (Table 1) with few or no colonies of other potentially pathogenic bacteria, as in Case 2 in which quantitative sputum culture revealed 1.2×10^9 CFU/mL. Pneumonia due to Corynebacteria may occur far more commonly than has been reported, because the finding of these organisms is usually dismissed as "normal mouth flora" or "normal respiratory flora."

MALDI-TOF is useful in providing precise speciation, as was employed in the 3 cases discussed in this report. An analysis of 83 Corynebacterial samples compared MALDI-TOF with API Coryne V2.0 (bioMérieux, Marcy l'Etoile, France), which is the method that has been most widely used to speciate Corynebacteria in the past few decades. Identification matched in 73 of 83 (88%) samples [43]. 16S rRNA sequencing was used to resolve the discrepancy in the remaining 10 samples. All 10 matched with MALDI-TOF's identification, which demonstrates the superiority of this methodology [43, 44].

Management

Corynebacterium spp. that have been identified as causes of pneumonia or empyema are delineated in Table 1. *C. pseudodiptheriticum,* the cause of about two-thirds of reported Corynebacterial pneumonia cases, is susceptible to penicillin, cephalosporins, and vancomycin, but resistant to macrolides, clindamycin, trimethoprim/sulfamethoxazole, quinolones, and/or rifampin (Table 3). Some species, including *C. jeikeium, C. macginleyi,* and *C. xerosis,* are resistant to all common antibiotics except glycopeptides such as vancomycin (Table 3). Intermediately resistant organisms such as *C. propinquum* and *C. striatum,* implicated in the present study's 3 cases, are also consistently susceptible to vancomycin and ampicillin, but variably susceptible to penicillin and cephalosporins, and commonly resistant to macrolides, clindamycin, trimethoprim-sulfamethoxazole, fluoroquinolines, and rifampin. The other reported *Corynebacterium* spp.—*C. accolens, C. afermentans, C. mucifaciens, C. pseudotuberculosis, C. urealyticum, and C. ulcerans*—had only 1–2 case reports each, and/or did not include comprehensive susceptibility reports. These cases are summarized in Table 3. Although only one pneumonia case report [17] included susceptibility to linezolid or tigecycline, a prospective study analyzing infections due to Corynebacteria from a variety of sites revealed that all isolates—the majority being *C. amycolatum, C. accolens, C. minutissimum,* and *C. glucuronolyticum* (strains that are not regularly implicated in pneumonia)—were susceptible to linezolid and tigecycline [45].

These results suggest that, when a Gram-stained sputum from a patient with pneumonia reveals Corynebacteria as the predominant isolate, vancomycin should be the initial antibiotic of choice. If MALDI-TOF identifies a species that is likely to be susceptible to other antibiotics, the empiric antibiotic of choice can be revised, or definitive antibiotic treatment can be given based on results of antibiotic susceptibility testing as determined by gradient diffusion strip testing. There is no accepted recommendation for length of treatment for Corynebacterial pneumonia. However, among case reports, treatment time has ranged from 10 days for a case of *C. macginleyi* pneumonia [28], to 8 weeks for a cavitating pneumonia due to *C. jeikeium* [22], to 14 months for pneumonia due to *C. pseudotuberculosis* [25]. It seems reasonable to select a duration of treatment based on the nature of the lung lesion. Infiltrates should respond

Table 3 Antibiotic susceptibilities of *Corynebacterium* spp. identified as causes of pulmonary infection

	Antibiotic													
Organism	**PCN**	**AMX**	**AMC**	**AMP**	**CEF**	**CFZ**	**CXM**	**CRO**	**CTX**	**SXT**	**ERY**	**AZM**	**CLI**	**CIP**
C. accolens (*n* = 1)	100		100						100	0	0		0	
C. afermentans (*n* = 1)										100				
C. jeikeium (*n* = 5)	0			0		0				0	0		0	
C. macginleyi (*n* = 1)	0				0	0	0	0	0					0
C. mucifaciens (*n* = 1)	100	100						100						
C. propinquum (*n* = 1)	100							100	100				0	
C. pseudodiphtheriticum (*n* = 24)	100	100	100	100	100	100	100	100	100	45	5		8	73
C. pseudotuberculosis (*n* = 2)	100							100		100	100		100	
C. striatum (*n* = 7)	60	100	100	100	67	0	0	0	75	0	50	0	0	0
C. ulcerans (*n* = 2)	50			100	100						100	100	50	100
C. urealyticum (*n* = 1)	100			100	100									
C. xerosis (*n* = 1)	0		0	0	0		0			0	0			0
Organism	**LCM**	**RIF**	**GEN**	**TOB**	**VAN**	**LZD**	**IPM**	**AMK**	**DOX**	**TET**	**TEC**	**CHL**	**FOF**	**DAP**
C. accolens (*n* = 1)		100	0	0	100			100		0			100	
C. afermentans (*n* = 1)					100		100							
C. jeikeium (*n* = 5)		100	50		100			100				50		
C. macginleyi (*n* = 1)					100									
C. mucifaciens (*n* = 1)					100			100						
C. propinquum (*n* = 1)					100		100							100
C. pseudodiphtheriticum (*n* = 24)	0	75	100	100	100		100	100	100	100	86	27		
C. pseudotuberculosis (*n* = 2)		100					100			100				
C. striatum (*n* = 7)	100	60	100	100	100	100	80	50		50	100			
C. ulcerans (*n* = 2)		100	100		100		100			100		100		
C. urealyticum (*n* = 1)										100				
C. xerosis (*n* = 1)			0		100			0						

Antibiotic susceptibility for each *Corynebacterium* spp. as reported in all previous cases of Corynebacterial pneumonia (see Table 1 for reference listing) was calculated from number of sensitive isolates as a percentage of the total number of isolates tested with that antibiotic. Blank boxes represent a lack of testing information. The total number of isolates of each species is provided (n). Not all isolates under each organism were tested for the same antibiotics.
PCN penicillin, *AMX* amoxicillin, *AMC* amoxicillin-clavulanic acid, *AMP* ampicillin, *CEF* cefalothin, *CFZ* cefazolin, *CXM* cefuroxime, *FOX* cefoxitin, *CRO* ceftriaxone, *CTX* cefotaxime, *OFX* ofloxacin, *SXT* trimethoprim-sulfamethoxazole, *ERY* erythromycin, *AZM* azithromycin, *CLI* clindamycin, *LCM* lincomycin, *RIF* rifampin, *GEN* gentamicin, *TOB* tobramycin, *VAN* vancomycin, *LZD* linezolid, *IPM* Imipenem, *AMK* amikacin, *DOX* doxycycline, *TET* tetracycline, *TEC* teicoplanin, *CHL* chloramphenicol, *FOF* Fosfomycin, *DAP* daptomycin

to the same 7 days of treatment that are used for other bacterial pneumonias, whereas cavitating pneumonia should be treated for longer periods, perhaps until the cavity is closed. In some cases, inadequate responses have been observed in cases of a lung abscess or cavitation, prompting surgical resection [16, 37].

Conclusions

Although traditionally regarded as part of normal respiratory flora, Corynebacteria has the capacity to cause pneumonia in immunocompromised patients, or in immunocompetent patients who have impaired airway clearance and/or structural damage to the airways. The presentation is similar to that of any other bacterial pneumonia. Such infections may be far more common than has been previously suggested, because the finding of Corynebacteria on Gram stain and culture is likely to lead to a report of "mixed" or "normal respiratory flora." A correct diagnosis can be made primarily by visualization of large numbers of diphtheroids in microscopic fields that contain > 20 WBC per epithelial cell, especially if the bacteria are located within PMNs, and supported by a culture in which the overwhelmingly predominant organism is Corynebacteria. Speciation by MALDI-TOF is increasingly available in clinical laboratories. Initial treatment should be with vancomycin. Speciation may guide antibiotic choice, but definitive therapy should be based on susceptibility testing using gradient diffusion strip testing methodology.

Abbreviations
CAP: Community-acquired pneumonia; CFU: Colony forming unit; COPD: Chronic obstructive pulmonary disease; HEp-2: Human epithelial type 2; MALDI-TOF: Matrix-assisted laser desorption ionization– time of flight; PMNs: Polymorphonuclear leukocytes; rRNA: Ribosomal RNA; spp.: Species; WBC: White blood cell

Authors' contributions
KY tabulated previous literature. KY and DMM drafted the manuscript. All authors contributed to the design of the study and the writing of the manuscript. All authors read and approved the final manuscript.

Competing interests
The authors declare that they have no competing interests.

References

1. National Center for Health Statistics. Health, United States, 2016: With Chartbook on Long-term Trends in Health. Hyattsville, MD. 2017.
2. Musher DM, Roig IL, Cazares G, et al. Can an etiologic agent be identified in adults who are hospitalized for community-acquired pneumonia: results of a one-year study. J Inf Secur. 2013;67:11–8.
3. Jain S, Self WH, Wunderink RG, Team CES. Community-acquired pneumonia requiring hospitalization. N Engl J Med. 2015;373:2382.
4. Janoff EN, Musher DM. Streptococcus pneumoniae. In: Bennett JEDR, Blaser MJ, editors. Mandell, Douglas, and Bennett's principles and practice of infectious diseases. Philadelphia: Saunders; 2015. p. 2310–27.
5. Musher DM, Abers MS, Bartlett JG. Evolving understanding of the causes of pneumonia in adults, with special attention to the role of pneumococcus. Clin Infect Dis. 2017;65:1736–44.
6. Sloan A, Wang G, Cheng K. Traditional approaches versus mass spectrometry in bacterial identification and typing. Clin Chim Acta. 2017;473:180–5.
7. Harrington AT, Clarridge Iii JE, Mahlen SD. Chapter 91 - Corynebacterium spp. as established and emerging respiratory pathogens A2 - Tang, Yi-Wei. In: Sussman M, Liu D, Poxton I, Schwartzman J, editors. Molecular Medical Microbiology. 2nd ed. Boston: Academic Press; 2015. p. 1627–33.
8. Thorsteinsson SB, Musher DM, Fagan T. The diagnostic value of sputum culture in acute pneumonia. JAMA. 1975;233:894–5.
9. von Graevenitz A, Punter-Streit V, Riegel P, Funke G. Coryneform bacteria in throat cultures of healthy individuals. J Clin Microbiol. 1998;36:2087–8.
10. Waters BL. Pathology of culture-proven JK Corynebacterium pneumonia. An autopsy case report. Am J Clin Pathol. 1989;91:616–9.
11. Camello TC, Souza MC, Martins CA, et al. Corynebacterium pseudodiphtheriticum isolated from relevant clinical sites of infection: a human pathogen overlooked in emerging countries. Lett Appl Microbiol. 2009;48:458–64.
12. Ahmed K, Kawakami K, Watanabe K, et al. Corynebacterium pseudodiphtheriticum: a respiratory tract pathogen. Clin Infect Dis. 1995;20:41–6.
13. Manzella JP, Kellogg JA, Parsey KS. Corynebacterium pseudodiphtheriticum: a respiratory tract pathogen in adults. Clin Infect Dis. 1995;20:37–40.
14. Diez-Aguilar M, Ruiz-Garbajosa P, Fernandez-Olmos A, et al. Non-diphtheriae Corynebacterium species: an emerging respiratory pathogen. Eur J Clin Microbiol Infect Dis. 2013;32:769–72.
15. Creagh R, Saavedra JM, Rodriguez FJ, et al. Pneumonia casued by Corynebacterium striatum in a patient with AIDS. Enferm Infecc Microbiol Clin. 2000;18:297–8.
16. Martinez-Martinez L, Suarez AI, Ortega MC, Rodriguez-Jimenez R. Fatal pulmonary infection caused by Corynebacterium striatum. Clin Infect Dis. 1994;19:806–7.
17. Roig-Rico P, Safont-Gaso P, Marin-Tordera D, Ortiz-De la Tabla V. Corynebacterium striatum pneumonia in an HIV patient. Enferm Infecc Microbiol Clin. 2011;29:402.
18. Renom F, Gomila M, Garau M, et al. Respiratory infection by Corynebacterium striatum: epidemiological and clinical determinants. New Microbes New Infect. 2014;2:106–14.
19. Minkin R, Shapiro JM. Corynebacterium afermentans lung abscess and empyema in a patient with human immunodeficiency virus infection. South Med J. 2004;97:395–7.
20. Wallet F, Marquette CH, Courcol RJ. Multiresistant Corynebacterium xerosis as a cause of pneumonia in a patient with acute leukemia. Clin Infect Dis. 1994;18:845–6.
21. Ifantidou AM, Diamantidis MD, Tseliki G, et al. Corynebacterium jeikeium bacteremia in a hemodialyzed patient. Int J Infect Dis. 2010;14(Suppl 3): e265–8.
22. McNaughton RD, Villanueva RR, Donnelly R, et al. Cavitating pneumonia caused by Corynebacterium group JK. J Clin Microbiol. 1988;26:2216–7.
23. Yoshitomi Y, Kohno S, Koga H, et al. Fatal pneumonia caused by Corynebacterium group JK after treatment of Staphylococcus aureus pneumonia. Intern Med. 1992;31:930–2.
24. Keslin MH, McCoy EL, McCusker JJ, Lutch JS. Corynebacterium pseudotuberculosis. A new cause of infectious and eosinophilic pneumonia. Am J Med. 1979;67:228–31.
25. Heggelund L, Gaustad P, Havelsrud OE, et al. Corynebacterium pseudotuberculosis pneumonia in a veterinary student infected during laboratory work. Open Forum Infect Dis. 2015;2:ofv053.
26. Djossou F, Bezian MC, Moynet D, et al. Corynebacterium mucifaciens in an immunocompetent patient with cavitary pneumonia. BMC Infect Dis. 2010;10:355.
27. Siegel SM, Haile CA. Corynebacterium ulcerans pneumonia. South Med J. 1985;78:1267.
28. Kebbe J, Mador MJ. Corynebacterium macginleyi: a cause of ventilator associated pneumonia in an immunocompromised patient. Respir Med Case Rep. 2015;16:154–6.
29. Funke G, von Graevenitz A, Clarridge JE 3rd, Bernard KA. Clinical microbiology of coryneform bacteria. Clin Microbiol Rev. 1997;10:125–59.
30. Woese CR. Bacterial evolution. Microbiol Rev. 1987;51:221–71.
31. Burkovski A. Corynebacterium pseudodiphtheriticum: putative probiotic, opportunistic infector, emerging pathogen. Virulence. 2015;6:673–4.
32. Souza MC, dos Santos LS, Sousa LP, et al. Biofilm formation and fibrinogen and fibronectin binding activities by Corynebacterium pseudodiphtheriticum invasive strains. Antonie Van Leeuwenhoek. 2015;107:1387–99.
33. Bittar F, Cassagne C, Bosdure E, et al. Outbreak of Corynebacterium pseudodiphtheriticum infection in cystic fibrosis patients, France. Emerg Infect Dis. 2010;16:1231–6.
34. Carranza Gonzalez R, Tena Gomez D, Prieto Gomez E, et al. Pneumonia by Corynebacterium pseudodiphteriticum: an infection to consider. An Med Interna. 2006;23:124–6.
35. Miller RA, Rompalo A, Coyle MB. Corynebacterium pseudodiphtheriticum pneumonia in an immunologically intact host. Diagn Microbiol Infect Dis. 1986;4:165–71.
36. Chiner E, Arriero JM, Signes-Costa J, et al. Corynebacterium pseudodiphtheriticum pneumonia in an immunocompetent patient. Monaldi Arch Chest Dis. 1999;54:325–7.
37. Gutierrez-Rodero F, Ortiz de la Tabla V, Martinez C, et al. Corynebacterium pseudodiphtheriticum: an easily missed respiratory pathogen in HIV-infected patients. Diagn Microbiol Infect Dis. 1999;33:209–16.
38. Roig P, Lopez MM, Arriero JM, et al. Corynebacterium pseudodiphtheriticum pneumonia in a patient diagnosed with HIV infection. An Med Interna. 1993;10:499–500.
39. Heffron R. Pneumonia with special reference to pneumococcus lobar pneumonia. New York: The Commonwealth Fund; 1939.
40. Musher DM, Kubitschek KR, Crennan J, Baughn RE. Pneumonia and acute febrile tracheobronchitis due to *Haemophilus influenzae*. Ann Intern Med. 1983;99:444–50.
41. Wallace RJ Jr, Musher DM. In honor of Dr. Sarah Branham, a star is born. The realization of Branhamella catarrhalis as a respiratory pathogen. Chest. 1986; 90:447–50.
42. Coyle MB, Lipsky BA. Coryneform bacteria in infectious diseases: clinical and laboratory aspects. Clin Microbiol Rev. 1990;3:227–46.
43. Vila J, Juiz P, Salas C, et al. Identification of clinically relevant Corynebacterium spp., Arcanobacterium haemolyticum, and Rhodococcus equi by matrix-assisted laser desorption ionization-time of flight mass spectrometry. J Clin Microbiol. 2012;50:1745–7.

44. Bao R, Gao X, Hu B, Zhou Z. Matrix-assisted laser desorption ionization time-of-flight mass spectrometry: a powerful tool for identification of Corynebacterium species. J Thorac Dis. 2017;9:3239–45.
45. Reddy BS, Chaudhury A, Kalawat U, et al. Isolation, speciation, and antibiogram of clinically relevant non-diphtherial Corynebacteria (Diphtheroids). Indian J Med Microbiol. 2012;30:52–7.
46. Losada I, Daza RM, Merino J, et al. Corynebacterium CDC G1: pathogen or colonizer? Enferm Infecc Microbiol Clin. 1996;14:510–1.
47. Riebel W, Frantz N, Adelstein D, Spagnuolo PJ. Corynebacterium JK: a cause of nosocomial device-related infection. Rev Infect Dis. 1986;8:42–9.
48. Malkocoglu G, Gencer H, Kaya A, et al. Corynebacterium propinquum bronchopneumonia in a child with ataxia telangiectasia. Turk J Pediatr. 2016;58:558–61.
49. Furiasse D, Gasparotto AM, Monterisi A, et al. Pneumonia caused byCorynebacterium pseudodiphtheriticum. Rev Argent Microbiol. 2016;48:290–2.
50. Chudnicka A, Szmygin-Milanowska K, Kieszko R, et al. The role of opportunistic species of Corynebacterium pseudodiphtheriticum in the pathogenesis of CAP (community acquired pneumonia). Ann Univ Mariae Curie Sklodowska Med. 2003;58:142–8.
51. Aspiroz Sancho C, Agustin Berne A, Navarro Pardos C, et al. Pneumonia caused by Corynebacterium pseudodiphteriticum, an entity worth knowing. An Med Interna. 2002;19:463–5.
52. Martaresche C, Fournier PE, Jacomo V, et al. A case of Corynebacterium pseudodiphtheriticum nosocomial pneumonia. Emerg Infect Dis. 1999;5:722–3.
53. Cohen Y, Force G, Gros I, et al. Corynebacterium pseudodiphtheriticum pulmonary infection in AIDS patients. Lancet. 1992;340:114–5.
54. Donaghy M, Cohen J. Pulmonary infection with Corynebacterium hofmannii complicating systemic lupus erythematosus. J Infect Dis. 1983;147:962.
55. Nishiyama A, Ishida T, Ito A, Arita M. Bronchopneumonia caused by Corynebacterium pseudodiphtheriticum. Intern Med. 2013;52:1847.
56. Cowling P, Hall L. Corynebacterium striatum: a clinically significant isolate from sputum in chronic obstructive airways disease. J Inf Secur. 1993;26:335–6.
57. Tarr PE, Stock F, Cooke RH, et al. Multidrug-resistant Corynebacterium striatum pneumonia in a heart transplant recipient. Transpl Infect Dis. 2003;5:53–8.
58. Verma R, Kravitz GR. Corynebacterium striatum empyema and osteomyelitis in a patient with advanced rheumatoid arthritis. BMJ Case Rep. 2016; https://doi.org/10.1136/bcr-2016-214691.
59. Mattos-Guaraldi AL, Sampaio JL, Santos CS, et al. First detection of Corynebacterium ulcerans producing a diphtheria-like toxin in a case of human with pulmonary infection in the Rio de Janeiro metropolitan area, Brazil. Mem Inst Oswaldo Cruz. 2008;103:396–400.
60. Jacobs NF Jr, Perlino CA. "Diphtheroid" pneumonia. South Med J. 1979;72:475–6.
61. Nazemi MM, Musher DM. Empyema due to aerobic diphtheroids following dental extraction. Am Rev Respir Dis. 1973;108:1221–3.

19

Cilostazol for the prevention of pneumonia

Hirotaka Nakashima[1,2*], Kazuhisa Watanabe[3], Hiroyuki Umegaki[3], Yusuke Suzuki[1,2] and Masafumi Kuzuya[3,4]

Abstract

Background: Pneumonia is a very common disease, especially among the elderly. Various drugs' preventive effects against pneumonia have been reported. The antiplatelet drug cilostazol is used to prevent pneumonia, but the robustness of its efficacy is unclear. This review estimates the effectiveness of cilostazol for preventing pneumonia in elderly individuals.

Methods: The following databases were searched from the earliest record to January 2016, without language restriction (the secondary search was conducted on February 2017): MEDLINE, Cochrane Library, CINAHL, and Ichushi-Web. Studies were included if they were published randomized controlled trials investigating the preventive effect of cilostazol on pneumonia in the elderly. The outcome was the incidence of pneumonia.

Results: Two trials were identified that met the search criteria (1423 participants). Both trials compared cilostazol with no antiplatelet in patients with a history of cerebral infarction. A meta-analysis was not performed because of the small number of trials and the heterogeneity of the data. Both trials suggested that cilostazol reduced the incidence of pneumonia (risk ratio [RR] 0.40; 95% confidence interval [CI] 0.22–0.73 in one trial, RR 0.20; 95% CI 0.06–0.69 in the other) and the recurrence of cerebral infarction (0.43; 0.21–0.90, 0.53; 0.34–0.81, respectively). The quality of evidence provided by the trials was very low, mainly because of the high risk of bias.

Conclusions: It is difficult to draw conclusions on the basis of two trials. Moreover, in the two trials, cilostazol could have reduced the incidence of pneumonia via a reduction of the recurrence of cerebral infarction, which suggests that other antiplatelets could also have the same effects. Stronger evidence is required from large trials assessing the effectiveness of cilostazol for the prevention of pneumonia.

Trial registration: PROSPERO (CRD42016036724).

Keywords: Antiplatelet, Cilostazol, Elderly, Pneumonia, Swallowing function

Background

Pneumonia is a very common disease, especially in the elderly. The mortality rate of pneumonia has not decreased despite advances in antimicrobial therapy [1]. In Japan, the country with the most aged population in the world, pneumonia has risen from the fourth most common cause of death to the third most common [2]. A preventive effect of various drugs against pneumonia has been reported [3, 4] and cilostazol is one of these drugs.

Cilostazol is an antiplatelet agent that has been commercially available for more than two decades. It has antiplatelet and vasodilatory effects via the inhibition of phosphodiesterase-3 (PDE3), and it presents a relatively small risk of bleeding compared to other antiplatelet agents [5]. Many studies have demonstrated the effectiveness of cilostazol in the management of intermittent claudication due to peripheral arterial disease, cerebrovascular disease, and coronary artery disease [5]. Despite the benefit of cilostazol, some patients discontinue the drug due to adverse effects such as headache and increased heart rate [5], and cilostazol is contraindicated in patients with heart failure because of the risk for exacerbation.

Pneumonia in the elderly is often caused by silent aspiration resulting from reduced swallowing and coughing reflexes [6]. Substance P, a neurotransmitter in the

* Correspondence: naka621@med.nagoya-u.ac.jp
[1]Centre for Community Liaison and Patient Consultations, Nagoya University Hospital, 65 Tsurumai-cho, Showa-ku, Nagoya, Aichi 466-8560, Japan
[2]Department of Geriatrics, Nagoya University Hospital, Nagoya, Japan
Full list of author information is available at the end of the article

nucleus of the solitary tract in the brainstem, plays important roles in these reflexes [7]. Cilostazol increases the level of substance P in the brain by inhibiting PDE3 [8] and thus could prevent pneumonia [9].

There are two systematic reviews that investigated the preventive effect of cilostazol on pneumonia, and the authors of those reviews concluded that although cilostazol seemed to help prevent pneumonia, the use of cilostazol was not recommended because of the risk of bleeding [3, 4]. However, those reviews did not focus on cilostazol; rather, the comprehensive prevention of pneumonia was the focus. Moreover, since those reviews were published, one randomized controlled trial (RCT) in this field has also been published [10].

In 2015, cilostazol was rated to have the best risk–benefit profile for secondary prevention after stroke among long-term antiplatelet mono- and dual therapies [11]. The frequency of cilostazol prescription is expected to increase in the future, and it would therefore be useful to elucidate its characteristics. This study represents an updated and specialized systematic review of RCTs to estimate the effectiveness of cilostazol in preventing pneumonia.

Methods

The protocol of the present review is registered at PROSPERO (the International Prospective Register of Systematic Reviews, of the UK's National Institute for Health Research) (#CRD42016036724) [12]. The methods used were based on the Cochrane Collaboration Handbook [13]. The recommendations of the Preferred Reporting Items for Systematic Reviews and Meta-Analyses (PRISMA) were followed [14].

Search strategy

This review searched the following databases from the earliest record to 5 January 2016 without language restriction: MEDLINE (EBSCOhost), Cochrane Library, CINAHL (the Cumulative Index to Nursing and Allied Health Literature), and Ichushi-Web (Japan Medical Abstracts Society, http://www.jamas.or.jp). Keywords and MeSH terms relevant to the intervention of interest were used, including "cilostazol" and "antiplatelet," and terms relevant to the medical condition of interest, including "pneumonia," "aspiration," and "dysphagia." An additional file shows the full search strategies [see Additional file 1]. A manual search of relevant journals and reference lists of eligible studies was also carried out. The secondary search was conducted on 26 February 2017.

Inclusion criteria

Studies were regarded as eligible for inclusion if they were published RCTs investigating the preventive effect of cilostazol on pneumonia in the elderly (i.e. patients ≥65 years old). Studies were included if they investigated the incidence of pneumonia, but other studies (such as studies on the swallowing function) were excluded. Studies of patients from community settings, long-term care settings, and hospitals were included. Studies of critically ill or ventilated patients were excluded. No restrictions were set on past medical history, concurrent medication (including antiplatelet medications), or the dosage of cilostazol. Eligible studies' diagnostic criteria for pneumonia had to include symptoms or clinical signs. Studies were included if they followed up their subjects for > 1 month.

Study selection

Two reviewers independently evaluated the studies for eligibility. Disagreements between the reviewers concerning the decision to include or exclude a study were resolved by consensus, and if necessary, by consultation with a third reviewer. After the titles and abstracts retrieved from the searches were assessed, the full texts of the studies were assessed for eligibility. Those studies fulfilling the eligibility criteria were included.

Data extraction and quality assessment

Data were extracted by two independent reviewers, and disagreements were resolved by consensus. Extracted data included details on the study design, setting, participants, intervention, control therapy, diagnostic criteria, and incidence of pneumonia. Missing data were not imputed. The two reviewers also independently assessed the risk of bias for each study included by using the Cochrane Collaboration risk of bias tool [13]. It was planned that reporting bias would be assessed using the visual asymmetry of a funnel plot if there were at least 10 trials.

Statistical analysis

The primary outcome was the incidence of pneumonia. A random-effects meta-analysis with risk ratios (RR) for binary outcomes was performed, and 95% confidence intervals (CI) and two-sided p-values using the software Review Manager 5.3 (RevMan, [Computer program] Version 5.3. Copenhagen: The Nordic Cochrane Centre, The Cochrane Collaboration 2014) were calculated. The review assessed heterogeneity between the studies in terms of their effect measured by the visual inspection of forest plots and the I^2 statistic. A subgroup analysis regarding the dosage of cilostazol was performed, and the subsequent sensitivity analyses included only (1) trials with a low risk of bias, and (2) trials comparing cilostazol with other antiplatelet medications. The Grades of Recommendation, Assessment, Development and Evaluation (GRADE) approach was used to assess the overall certainty of evidence [15].

Results

The search results

As illustrated in Fig. 1, search strategies identified 517 reports without duplicates. The screening of the titles and abstracts of these reports identified 15 reports as potentially eligible for this review. The full-text screening of these 15 reports excluded 13 reports. The remaining two RCTs met the inclusion criteria [10, 16].

Included studies

The two trials, which are described in detail in Table 1, examined 1423 randomized patients: the Yamaya et al. trial included 328 patients and was published in 2001 [16], and the Shinohara et al. trial investigated 1095 patients and was published in 2006 [10]. Both trials compared cilostazol with the absence of antiplatelet medication in patients with a history of cerebral infarction in Japan. The control groups of these trials did not take aspirin, because the use of aspirin to prevent the recurrence of cerebral infarction was not approved by the Japanese Ministry of Health, Labor and Welfare at that time.

The study by Yamaya et al. was designed to establish whether cilostazol lowers the incidence of pneumonia and reduces the recurrence of cerebral infarction in patients with a history of stroke [16]. The trial compared cilostazol with no active treatment without placebo. Because the trial was only reported as a 'Letter to the Editor', relatively few data from the trial appeared in the published article.

The study by Shinohara et al. [10] was a post-hoc analysis of the Cilostazol Stroke Prevention Study (CSPS) [17]. The CSPS was a multicenter, randomized, placebo-controlled double-blind study, and the CSPS group reported the efficacy and safety of cilostazol for the secondary prevention of cerebral infarction.

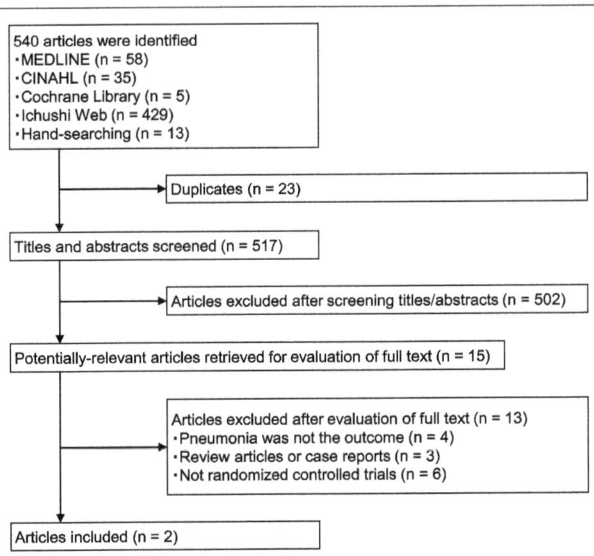

Fig. 1 Flow of studies through the review

Risk of bias in the two trials

Both the Yamaya et al. and Shinohara et al. trials had varying risks of bias, as follows.

Allocation

Both trials reported using random sequence generation processes and had low risks of bias. Regarding allocation concealment, the study by Yamaya et al. had an unclear risk of bias because the study's authors reported only that the allocation list was held independently of the investigators.

Blinding

In the Yamaya et al. study, blinding of the participants was impossible, and the diagnosis of pneumonia required symptoms that had to be assessed subjectively. This trial therefore had a high risk of bias. On the other hand, the trial had a low risk bias in terms of the blinding of the outcome assessment because radiologists who were not involved in the study diagnosed the participants' pneumonia. The Shinohara et al. study was a post-hoc analysis of a double-blind trial. The study had an unclear risk of bias for outcome assessment because the outcome assessors might have had information on the interventions used.

Incomplete outcome data

Yamaya et al. performed an as-treated analysis, so the trial had a high risk of bias. The study by Shinohara et al. had an unclear risk of bias because the reasons for post-randomization dropouts were unclear.

Selective reporting

The study protocol of Yamaya et al. study was not able to be obtained. Those authors did not report adverse events in the control group (no active treatment), and the trial had a high risk of bias. The study by Shinohara et al. had a high risk of bias because the study was a post-hoc analysis of the CSPS [17] and it did not set pneumonia as an outcome.

Other potential sources of bias

Both studies did not report any funding, but the CSPS [17] was supported by Otsuka Pharmaceutical Co., Ltd.

The effects of intervention

A meta-analysis was not performed because of the small number of trials and the heterogeneity of data (the heterogeneity will be described later in detail). Hence, the outcomes were addressed using a narrative description of the available evidence. Both the Yamaya et al. and

Table 1 Summary of the two included studies

Study and country	Yamaya et al. 2001 [16], Japan	Shinohara et al. 2006 [10], Japan
Population	History of cerebral infarction but not bedridden	History of cerebral infarction, age < 80 years
Mean age	Mean age: 76.5 ± 2.1 years	Mean age: 65.0 ± 8.7 years
Gender	No statement about gender	Female 34.4%
Risk factors	No statement about risk factors for pneumonia	No statement about risk factors for pneumonia
Criteria for diagnosis of pneumonia	New pulmonary infiltrate seen on chest radiographs (assessed by two radiologists not involved in the study) and one of the following: cough, body temperature > 37.8 °C, subjective dyspnea	Description by attending physician in the medical chart, chest radiographs and blood test
Intervention and control (n, allocated)	I: cilostazol 100 mg per day (n: not stated)	I: cilostazol 200 mg per day (n: 547)
	C: no active treatment (n: not stated)	C: placebo (n: 548)
	328 patients were allocated in total but the number of patients in each group at allocation was not reported	
Intervention period	3 years	3.3 years on average
Number of patients analyzed	*I* = 125, C = 145, see comments	*I* = 531, C = 533, see comments
Outcomes	Pneumonia	Pneumonia
	I: 12 (9.6%), C: 35 (24.1%)	I: 3 (0.56%), C: 15 (2.8%)
	RR = 0.40 (95% CI 0.22–0.73)**	RR = 0.20 (95% CI 0.06–0.69)**
	Cerebral infarction	Cerebral infarction [17]
	I: 9 (7.2%), C: 24 (16.6%)	I: 30 (5.6%), C: 57 (10.7%)
	RR = 0.43 (95% CI 0.21–0.90)*	RR = 0.53 (95% CI 0.34–0.81)*
	Bleeding	Bleeding [17]
	I: 12 (9.6%), severity of the bleeding events was not reported	Fatal intracranial hemorrhage
	C: No statement about adverse events	I: 0, C: 1
		Nonfatal intracranial hemorrhage
		I: 4 (0.75%), C: 6 (1.1%)
		Other bleeding
		I: 15[a] (2.8%), C: 11 (2.1%)
Risk of bias		
Random sequence generation	Low	Low
Allocation concealment	Unclear: Inadequate description	Low
Blinding of participants and personnel	High: Open-label trial	Low
Blinding of outcome assessment	Low	Unclear: Post-hoc analysis of a RCT [17]
Incomplete outcome data	High: As-treated analysis	Unclear: Reasons for dropouts were unclear
Selective reporting	High: No protocol available, No statement about adverse events in the control group	High: Post-hoc analysis of a RCT [17]
Other bias	Unclear: No statement about funding	Unclear: No statement about funding but original RCT [17] was supported by Otsuka Pharmaceutical
Comments	Reported in a Letter to the Editor	1095 patients were randomized but 31 patients were excluded from analysis because of "serious protocol violations"
	328 patients were randomized but 58 patients were excluded from analysis; 31 patients died from causes other than pneumonia; additionally, 27 patients in cilostazol group dropped out because of adverse events	Of 1064 patients, about half of the patients discontinued the treatment (I: 54%, C: 49%)

C control, *CI* confidence interval, *I* intervention, *RR* risk ratio
**P* < 0.05, ***P* < 0.01
[a] Including one gastrointestinal bleeding

Shinohara et al. studies described that the cilostazol groups had significantly lower incidences of pneumonia compared to the groups that did not use antiplatelets (RR 0.40; 95% CI 0.22–0.73 in Yamaya et al., RR 0.20; 95% CI 0.06–0.69 in Shinohara et al.) (Fig. 2). The cilostazol groups also had lower risks for the recurrence of cerebral infarction (RR 0.43; 95% CI 0.21–0.90, RR 0.53; 95% CI 0.34–0.81, respectively).

The incidence of pneumonia was considerably higher in the Yamaya et al. study (17.4%) compared to the Shinohara et al. study (1.7%). This was largely because the patients in the Yamaya study were older than those in the Shinohara study. The age difference could also affect the recurrence of cerebral infarction (12.2% in the Yamaya study; 8.2% in the Shinohara study), as advanced age is one of the major risk factors of pneumonia.

Adverse events

Yamaya et al. reported that 27 of the 152 (18%) patients who received cilostazol suffered adverse events: bleeding (12 patients), palpitation and/or tachycardia (11 patients), diarrhea (one patient), and headache (two patients). The severity of the bleeding was not reported. These 27 patients dropped out of the study. There was no statement about adverse events in the control group (no active treatment), suggesting that the trial did not collect or report the data on adverse events in the control group.

The details of the adverse events in the Shinohara et al. study were provided in the CSPS report [17] (Fig. 3). The incidence of bleeding events was not significantly different between the cilostazol and placebo groups (2.8% and 2.1%, respectively). The bleeding events included one gastrointestinal bleeding event in the cilostazol group. Apart from those bleeding events, 11 patients developed intracranial hemorrhages; one patient in the placebo group developed a fatal intracranial hemorrhage; 4 patients in the cilostazol group and 6 in the placebo group developed nonfatal intracranial hemorrhages. Headache (12.8% in the cilostazol group and 3.2% in the placebo group), palpitations (5.3% and 0.4%, respectively), and an increase in pulse rate (19% and 7.9%, respectively) occurred with greater frequency in the cilostazol group, and these adverse events resulted in a higher discontinuation rate in the cilostazol group.

Heterogeneity

Because only two trials were included in the present review, a formal testing of heterogeneity was not performed. However, the two trials were heterogeneous with respect to the following: the subjects' ages, the dosage of cilostazol, the interventions in the control groups (no active treatment or placebo), the incidence of pneumonia, the discontinuation rate, and the methods of analysis (as-treated analysis or intention-to-treat analysis).

Subgroup analyses, sensitivity analyses

A subgroup analysis or sensitivity analysis of the two trials was not performed.

Reporting bias

Reporting bias using a funnel plot was not explored because of the small number of trials in this review.

Excluded studies

Osawa et al. retrospectively compared cilostazol with the absence of cilostazol (most patients took some antiplatelets other than cilostazol) with regard to the preventive effect on pneumonia in patients with a history of cerebral infarction [18]. This study was excluded because it was not a RCT.

Teramoto et al. reported their double-blinded, placebo-controlled, three-period crossover study that compared the effects on the swallowing function of cilostazol, aspirin, and placebo in patients with a history of cerebral infarction [9]. This study was also excluded, because it did not examine the incidence of pneumonia.

Study or Subgroup	Cilostazol Events	Cilostazol Total	No Antiplatelet Events	No Antiplatelet Total	Risk Ratio M-H, Random, 95% CI	Year
1.1.1 Pneumonia						
Yamaya2001	12	125	35	145	0.40 [0.22, 0.73]	2001
Shinohara2006	3	531	15	533	0.20 [0.06, 0.69]	2006
1.1.2 Cerebral Infarction						
Yamaya2001	9	125	24	145	0.43 [0.21, 0.90]	2001
Shinohara2006	30	531	57	533	0.53 [0.35, 0.81]	2006

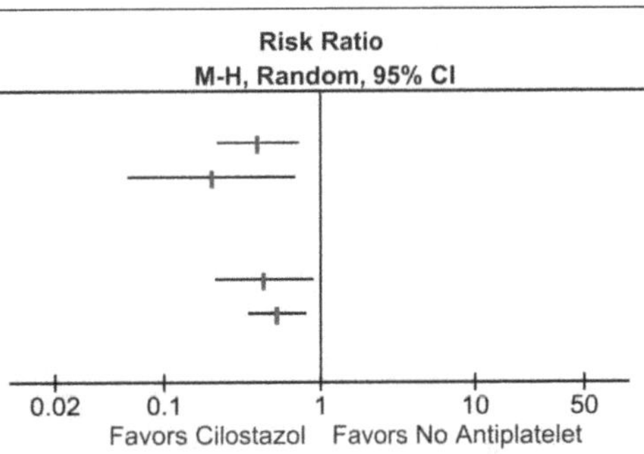

Fig. 2 Risk of pneumonia and cerebral infarction with cilostazol treatment compared with no antiplatelet. A meta-analysis was not performed because of the small number of trials. Yamaya et al. (2001) [16] compared cilostazol with no active treatment without placebo. Shinohara et al. (2006) [10] compared cilostazol with placebo

Study or Subgroup	Cilostazol Events	Cilostazol Total	Placebo Events	Placebo Total	Risk Ratio M-H, Random, 95% CI	Year
2.1.1 Fatal intracranial hemorrhage						
Shinohara2006	0	531	1	533	0.33 [0.01, 8.19]	2006
2.1.2 Nonfatal intracranial hemorrhage						
Shinohara2006	4	531	6	533	0.67 [0.19, 2.36]	2006
2.1.3 Other bleeding						
Shinohara2006	15	531	11	533	1.37 [0.63, 2.95]	2006
2.1.4 Headache						
Shinohara2006	68	531	17	533	4.02 [2.39, 6.74]	2006
2.1.5 Palpitations						
Shinohara2006	28	531	2	533	14.05 [3.36, 58.69]	2006
2.1.6 Increase in pulse rate						
Shinohara2006	77	531	34	533	2.27 [1.55, 3.34]	2006

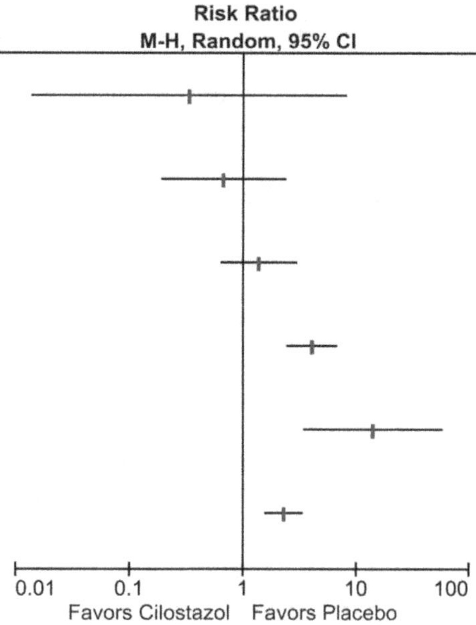

Fig. 3 Risk of adverse events with cilostazol treatment compared with placebo. Only one trial (Shinohara et al. 2006) was included in this figure because the other (Yamaya et al. 2001) did not describe adverse events in the control group

Discussion

Only two trials met the inclusion criteria for this study. Both trials compared cilostazol with the absence of any antiplatelet medication in patients with a history of cerebral infarction in Japan. Both trials showed that cilostazol significantly reduced the incidence of pneumonia and the recurrence of cerebral infarction.

According to the GRADE system [15] that we used to assess the quality of evidence, the two trials provide very low-quality evidence. The evidence was downgraded from high to very low quality because of a very high risk of bias (downgraded two levels) and imprecision due to the small sample size (one level).

Two systematic reviews investigated the preventive effect of cilostazol on pneumonia [3, 4], and both were published before the study by Shinohara et al. and therefore included only the Yamaya et al. study. The Shinohara et al. study, which was a larger placebo-controlled trial, was added to our systematic review.

The present review has a major limitation. Both of the trials examined herein compared cilostazol with the absence of antiplatelets, which resulted not only in a decrease in the incidence of pneumonia but also a low risk of the recurrence of cerebral infarction in the cilostazol group. Cerebral infarction is one of the major risk factors of pneumonia, and thus cilostazol could reduce the incidence of pneumonia by reducing the recurrence of cerebral infarction. This means that other antiplatelets could also have the same effect in terms of preventing pneumonia.

As described above, there is no conclusive evidence to recommend cilostazol to prevent pneumonia. However, Teramoto et al. reported that cilostazol but not aspirin improved the swallowing function of patients with a history of cerebral infarction [9]. In addition, Osawa et al. reported that in their retrospective study of patients with a history of cerebral infarction, the incidence of pneumonia was lower in the cilostazol group compared to the group in which most patients (95%) took an antiplatelet other than cilostazol [18]. These studies suggest that cilostazol but not other antiplatelet medications has a preventive effect on pneumonia by improving the swallowing function.

Further trials are needed to assess the preventive effects of cilostazol against pneumonia compared to other antiplatelets. Other trial designs would also be useful; for example, the co-administration of cilostazol and other antiplatelets. In the current clinical setting, cilostazol is used as an additional treatment to aspirin or clopidogrel, and thus such trial designs would provide more clinically meaningful outcomes. Trials comparing cilostazol with the absence of antiplatelets in patients who do not need to take antiplatelets would also be beneficial. Such trials could clarify the use of cilostazol as a preventive agent for pneumonia, rather than an antiplatelet. Cilostazol's potential risk of bleeding complications is an issue, but dosage adjustment might resolve the problem.

Conclusions

There is insufficient clinical trial evidence regarding the efficacy of cilostazol for preventing pneumonia. The result of two trials (Yamaya et al. and Shinohara et al.) suggested that cilostazol, compared to the absence of any antiplatelet medication, significantly reduced the incidence of pneumonia. However, these trials provided very low-quality evidence, mainly because of the high risk of bias. Moreover, in the two trials, cilostazol treatment may have reduced the incidence of pneumonia by reducing the recurrence of cerebral infarction, which suggests that other antiplatelets can also have the same effect. Stronger evidence is required from large trials assessing the effectiveness of cilostazol for the prevention of pneumonia.

Abbreviations
CI: Confidence interval; CSPS: Cilostazol Stroke Prevention Study; GRADE: Grades of Recommendation, Assessment, Development and Evaluation; RCT: Randomized controlled trial; RR: Risk ratio

Acknowledgements
Not applicable.

Funding
The authors have no support or funding to report.

Authors' contributions
Literature search: HN. Study selection: HN, KW, HU. Data extraction and quality assessment: HN, KW. Statistical analysis: HN. Drafting of the manuscript: HN. All authors performed a critical review of the manuscript. All authors read and approved the final manuscript.

Competing interests
The authors declare that they have no competing interests.

Author details
[1]Centre for Community Liaison and Patient Consultations, Nagoya University Hospital, 65 Tsurumai-cho, Showa-ku, Nagoya, Aichi 466-8560, Japan. [2]Department of Geriatrics, Nagoya University Hospital, Nagoya, Japan. [3]Department of Community Healthcare and Geriatrics, Nagoya University Graduate School of Medicine, Nagoya, Japan. [4]Institute of Innovation for Future Society, Nagoya University, Nagoya, Japan.

References
1. Plouffe JF Jr, Martin DR. Re-evaluation of the therapy of severe pneumonia caused by Streptococcus pneumoniae. Infect Dis Clin N Am. 2004;18:963–74.
2. Ministry of Health, Labour and Welfare, Japan. Cause of death. In: Vital Statistics of Japan Yearly Survey 2015. http://www.mhlw.go.jp/toukei/saikin/hw/jinkou/kakutei15/index.html (in Japanese). Accessed 15 Aug 2017.
3. Loeb MB, Becker M, Eady A, Walker-Dilks C. Interventions to prevent aspiration pneumonia in older adults: a systematic review. J Am Geriatr Soc. 2003;51:1018–22.
4. El Solh AA, Saliba R. Pharmacologic prevention of aspiration pneumonia: a systematic review. Am J Geriatr Pharmacother. 2007;5:352–62.
5. Rogers KC, Oliphant CS, Finks SW. Clinical efficacy and safety of cilostazol: a critical review of the literature. Drugs. 2015;75:377–95.
6. Sekizawa K, Ujiie Y, Itabashi S, Sasaki H, Takishima T. Lack of cough reflex in aspiration pneumonia. Lancet. 1990;335:1228–9.
7. Ujiie Y, Sekizawa K, Aikawa T, Sasaki H. Evidence for substance P as an endogenous substance causing cough in Guinea pigs. Am Rev Respir Dis. 1993;148:1628–32.
8. Zhang N, Miyamoto N, Tanaka R, Mochizuki H, Hattori N, Urabe T. Activation of tyrosine hydroxylase prevents pneumonia in a rat chronic cerebral hypoperfusion model. Neuroscience. 2009;158:665–72.
9. Teramoto S, Yamamoto H, Yamaguchi Y, Ishii M, Hibi S, Kume H, et al. Antiplatelet cilostazol, an inhibitor of type III phosphodiesterase, improves swallowing function in patients with a history of stroke. J Am Geriatr Soc. 2008;56:1153–4.
10. Shinohara Y. Antiplatelet cilostazol is effective in the prevention of pneumonia in ischemic stroke patients in the chronic stage. Cerebrovasc Dis. 2006;22:57–60.
11. Xie W, Zheng F, Zhong B, Song X. Long-term antiplatelet mono- and dual therapies after ischemic stroke or transient ischemic attack: network meta-analysis. J Am Heart Assoc. 2015;4:e002259.
12. Nakashima H, Watanabe K, Suzuki Y, Umegaki H, Kuzuya M. Cilostazol for prevention of pneumonia: systematic review and meta-analysis. 2016. https://www.crd.york.ac.uk/PROSPERO/display_record.asp?ID=CRD42016036724. Accessed 15 Aug 2017.
13. Higgins JP, Green S, eds. Cochrane handbook for systematic reviews of interventions, version 5.1.0. The Cochrane collaboration. 2011. http://training.cochrane.org/handbook. Accessed 28 Jan 2017.
14. Moher D, Liberati A, Tetzlaff J, Altman DG. Preferred reporting items for systematic reviews and meta-analyses: the PRISMA statement. Ann Intern Med. 2009;151:264–9.
15. Guyatt GH, Oxman AD, Vist GE, Kunz R, Falck-Ytter Y, Alonso-Coello P, et al. GRADE: an emerging consensus on rating quality of evidence and strength of recommendations. BMJ. 2008;336:924–6.
16. Yamaya M, Yanai M, Ohrui T, Arai H, Sekizawa K, Sasaki H. Antithrombotic therapy for prevention of pneumonia. J Am Geriatr Soc. 2001;49:687–8.
17. Gotoh F, Tohgi H, Hirai S, Terashi A, Fukuuchi Y, Otomo E, et al. Cilostazol stroke prevention study: a placebo-controlled double-blind trial for secondary prevention of cerebral infarction. J Stroke Cerebrovasc Dis. 2000;9:147–57.
18. Osawa A, Maeshima S, Tanahashi N. Efficacy of cilostazol in preventing aspiration pneumonia in acute cerebral infarction. J Stroke Cerebrovasc Dis. 2013;22:857–61.

The association between pre-hospital antibiotic therapy and subsequent in-hospital mortality in adults presenting with community-acquired pneumonia: an observational study

Biswajit Chakrabarti[1*], Dan Wootton[2,3], Steven Lane[4], Elizabeth Kanwar[5], Joseph Somers[1], Jacyln Proctor[6], Nancy Prospero[5] and Mark Woodhead[7,8]

Abstract

Background: The majority of patients with community acquired-pneumonia (CAP) are treated in primary care and the mortality in this group is very low. However, a small but significant proportion of patients who begin treatment in the community subsequently require admission due to symptomatic deterioration. This study compared patients who received community antibiotics prior to admission to those who had not, and looked for associations with clinical outcomes.

Methods: This study analysed the Advancing Quality (AQ) Pneumonia database of patients admitted with CAP to 9 acute hospitals in the northwest of England over a 12-month period.

Results: There were 6348 subjects (mean age 72 [SD 16] years; gender ratio 1:1) admitted with CAP, of whom 17% had been pre-treated with antibiotics. The in-hospital mortality was 18.6% for the pre-treatment group compared to 13.2% in the "antibiotic naïve" group ($p < 0.001$). On multivariate analysis, age, male gender and antibiotic pre-treatment were predictors of in-hospital mortality along with a history of cerebrovascular accident, congestive cardiac failure, dementia, renal disease and cancer. After adjustment for CURB-65 score, age, co-morbidities and pre-treatment with antibiotics remained as independent risk factors for in-hospital mortality (OR 1.43, 95% CI 1.19–1.71).

Conclusion: CAP patients admitted to hospital were more likely to die during admission if they had received antibiotics for the same illness pre-admission. Future studies should endeavor to determine the mechanisms underlying this association, such as microbiological factors and the role of comorbidities. Patients hospitalized with CAP despite prior antibiotic treatment in the community require close monitoring.

Keywords: Pneumonia, Antibiotics, Community, Mortality, Comorbidity, Severity

* Correspondence: biz@doctors.org.uk
[1]Aintree University Hospital NHS Foundation Trust, Liverpool, UK
Full list of author information is available at the end of the article

Background

Community-acquired pneumonia (CAP) constitutes a considerable worldwide burden in terms of morbidity, mortality and emergency medical admissions [1]. At the time of presentation to hospital up to 20% of patients diagnosed with CAP have been pre-treated with antibiotics in primary care for symptoms of a lower respiratory tract infection (LRTI) [2, 3]. A paucity of high quality data exists as to whether prior antibiotic therapy in the community is associated with an adverse outcome following hospitalization. However, prior antibiotic therapy is usually a specific criterion excluding entry into antibiotic clinical trials in CAP. CAP is observed with increasing prevalence in the elderly, the immunosuppressed and in those with significant co-morbidity, which are risk factors in themselves for mortality in pneumonia [2, 4]. In any study examining this issue, adequate separation of such variables from prior antibiotic therapy is essential to truly define the contribution of the latter as a potential risk factor in CAP. Advancing Quality (AQ) is a National Health Service (NHS)-recognized initiative set in the northwest of England, which aims to improve standards of healthcare delivery in alignment with national guidelines and encompasses a variety of conditions, including CAP [5]. This UK-based study involves analysis of the AQ Pneumonia database to determine whether in-hospital mortality in adults hospitalized with CAP is associated with prior antibiotic treatment.

Methods

The AQ Pneumonia program requires participating hospitals to submit data for all cases admitted with a diagnosis of CAP on a rolling monthly basis. The processes underpinning case identification and data entry for the AQ Pneumonia program are outlined in the supplement. For submission to the AQ program, it is necessary for the diagnosis of CAP to be made by a consultant physician following formal medical review within 24 h of hospital admission, along with compatible chest radiograph findings. For each case, key measures integral to the optimal management of CAP are captured; e.g. whether assessment of oxygenation status and CAP severity index were documented, the time to chest radiograph being performed and time to "1st dose inpatient antibiotic administration", and whether antibiotic selection was appropriate according to local guidelines. The AQ Pneumonia database specifically excludes subjects who do not have an abnormal chest radiograph reported on admission, those referred to palliative care following senior medical review or those on a "palliative care code" on hospital admission, those entered into a clinical trial, those diagnosed with hospital-acquired pneumonia (HAP), and subjects where there is no documentation of a diagnosis of pneumonia following senior consultant medical review after admission.

For each case being submitted to the AQ Pneumonia program, the official admission chest X-ray report (made by a consultant radiologist) is examined by an independent administrator at the time of data entry into the AQ program to ensure that it is compatible with a diagnosis of CAP prior to acceptance. Each hospital participating in the AQ Pneumonia program complies with regular independent NHS audits in order to ensure accuracy of data entry. For each case of CAP submitted to the AQ Pneumonia database, it is also mandatory to record (from analysis of the medical and prescribing records) whether antibiotics were administered in primary care in the 24 h prior to the admission episode, so called "prior-treatment".

For the analysis, in-patient mortality was defined as and restricted to patients who were recorded as having died at the end of their hospital stay. Patients who were discharged alive and died later are not included in the calculation. In-patient mortality was defined as patients who have a coded discharge method as defined by the NHS Data Dictionary (http://www.datadictionary.nhs.uk). A 30-day readmission was defined as any emergency or unplanned admission to hospital for the same patient within 30 days of the discharge date of the original index admission, while a 30-day readmission due to pneumonia was defined as any readmission based on whether the primary diagnosis code of the readmission is pneumonia, using the same ICD10 list used to identify the initial cohort. Patient comorbidities were identified using the Charlson Comorbidity Index (CCI) as defined in the Standardized Hospital Mortality Guide [6]. This uses ICD10 diagnosis codes in the patient spell to identify if the patient has any of the 17 different comorbidities listed, in which each comorbidity is allocated a different weight according to the burden of disease. The total comorbidity score is the sum weight of the patient's comorbidities. For this study, analysis of all the CAP cases submitted by the 9 participating hospitals in the AQ Pneumonia program for a 12-month period (April 2016–2017) was undertaken. The 9 hospitals studied were required to submit all cases of CAP to the AQ Pneumonia program during the study period. The analysis was performed by a group comprising respiratory physicians, a senior business intelligence analyst, a medical statistician, two healthcare managers and a respiratory specialist nurse.

Statistical analysis

Demographic information was summarized using mean and standard deviations for continuous data, unless the data was not normally distributed. In this case, the median and interquartile range was used to describe the average and variability in the data. Categorical data was presented using counts and percentages. The data was stratified depending on whether the patients had been on antibiotic treatment prior to admittance. Following this, formal hypothesis tests (using Pearson's chi-squared test) were undertaken to investigate possible differences between comorbidities and home antibiotic prescribing, and then between comorbidities and death. Logistic regression was used to construct a multivariate model, which combined demographic variables and comorbidities, along with antibiotic prescribing, to determine the major predictors of death. A further series of logistic regression models were constructed to determine the risk of death for individual comorbidities and antibiotic prescribing. Participant age and, where available, severity of condition (CURB-65) were also included as significant covariates in these models. To complete the analysis, antibiotic home prescribing and the risk of re-admittance with pneumonia was investigated using the chi-squared test. In all analysis, results were considered significant if $p < 0.05$. All analysis was undertaken using SPSS version 22.

Results

A total of 6348 adults admitted with CAP were submitted to the AQ Pneumonia database during the study period. The study population demographics are outlined in Table 1. The in-hospital mortality for the entire cohort was 14.4% (916/6348). There were 1059 subjects (17%) "pre-treated" with antibiotics prior to admission and 4973 (78%) who were not "pre-treated". It was not possible to determine whether antibiotics had been administered pre-admission in 316 (5%) subjects.

The incidence of specific comorbidities in the study population, along with the ICD-10 codes ascribed to each condition, is listed in the Additional file 1: Table S1. There were no subjects with a coded diagnosis of human immunodeficiency virus (HIV) or acquired immune deficiency syndrome (AIDS) in the cohort. Table 2 outlines the variables associated with in-hospital mortality in the entire CAP cohort. In-hospital mortality was associated with advanced age, higher CCI, "pre-treatment" with antibiotics in primary care and a higher CURB-65 score. The in-hospital mortality was 18.6% (197/1059) in the antibiotic "pre-treated" subjects, compared to 13.2% (658/4973) in those not "pre-treated" (chi square 26.80, df = 2; $p < 0.001$). In terms of specific co-morbidity, a history of congestive cardiac failure (CCF), cerebrovascular accident (CVA), myocardial infarction (MI), renal disease, dementia, cancer (including metastatic) and paraplegia were all associated with in-hospital mortality.

Table 1 Demographics of the study population

Age (mean/SD)	72 (16) years
Gender	3201 (50.4%) female
	3147 (49.6%) male
Length of stay (median/IQR)	5 (3–11) days
Charlson Comorbidity Index (median/IQR)	6 (3–17)
Admission "CURB 65" score	*N* (%)
CURB 65 score 0	547 (9%)
CURB 65 score 1	906 (14%)
CURB 65 score 2	1269 (20%)
CURB 65 score 3	992 (16%)
CURB 65 score 4	244 (3.8%)
CURB 65 score 5	35 (0.6%)
CURB 65 score not documented	2355 (37%)

When comparing the antibiotic "pre-treated" cohort to those not "pre-treated" with antibiotics, an elevated CCI score was observed in the "pre-treated cohort" with a non-significant trend observed for female gender. In terms of specific co-morbidity, the incidence of congestive cardiac failure (CCF) and renal disease was significantly higher in the "pre-treated" cohort. No differences were observed in terms of severity of pneumonia (distribution of CURB-65 scores), age, gender or 30 day readmission rate (see Table 3).

After applying multivariate analysis (Table 4), the following variables emerged as significant predictors of in-hospital mortality: age, male gender, antibiotic pretreatment, along with the following co-morbidities: CVA, CCF, dementia, renal disease and cancer. When controlling for age, pre-treatment with antibiotics and severity, gender was not a significant variable in these models. The comorbidities MI (adjusted odds ratio [aOR]1.40 [95% CI 1.09–1.79]), CVA (aOR 1.66 [95% CI 1.21–2.17]), CCF (aOR 2.06 [95% CI 1.69–2.51]), dementia (aOR 1.36 [95% CI 1.09–1.70]), renal (aOR 1.35 [95% CI 1.09–1.66]), metastatic cancer (aOR 2.55 [95% CI 1.66–4.07]) and cancer (aOR 1.57 [95% CI 1.21–2.05]) were all significant predictors of death. In each of these models antibiotic prescribing was also a significant predictor of death (aOR 1.43 [95% CI 1.19–1.71]).

When the analysis was restricted to only those patients with a CURB-65 score (3993 subjects), the CURB-65 score became a significant predictor of mortality (Table 5). Although it should be noted that as the CURB-65 variable only contained 6 categories, the variable was included in the model as 5 dummy indicator variables with the CURB-65 "Zero" score (547 observations) taken as reference. For this variable, the aOR ranged from 1.5 to 16.9, although the 95% confidence interval for the CURB-65 score of 5 was wide (6.2–45.8) due to there being only 35 observations in this category. Of the demographic variables age (aOR 1.03 [95% CI 1.02–1.04]), CCI (aOR 1.02 [95% CI 1.00–1.03]) and pre-treatment with antibiotics (aOR 1.54 [95% CI 1.20–1.99]) were significant predictors of mortality along with three co-morbidity indicators: CCF (aOR 1.62, [95% CI

Table 2 Comparison of subjects who died in-hospital against those surviving to discharge

	Discharged from hospital $n = 5432$	Died in-hospital $n = 916$	
Charlson Co-morbidity Index	4 (1–14)	14 (4–23)	$P < 0.001$
Gender			
Female	2761 (50.8%)	440 (48%)	$P = 0.12$
Male	2671 (49.2%)	476 (52%)	
Age (mean/SD years)	71 (16)	80 (11)	$P < 0.001$
History of MI *n* (%)	499 (9.2%)	137 (15.0%)	$P < 0.001$
History of CVA *n* (%)	248 (4.6%)	81 (8.8%)	$P < 0.001$
History of Congestive Cardiac Failure *n* (%)	733 (13.5%)	290 (31.7%)	$P < 0.001$
History of Dementia *n* (%)	581 (10.7%)	178 (19.4%)	$P = < 0.001$
History of Diabetes n(%)	1004 (18.5%)	161 (17.6%)	$P = 0.51$
History of Liver Disease *n* (%)	45 (0.8%)	9 (1.0%)	$P = 0.64$
History of Pulmonary Disease *n* (%)	2564 (47.2%)	405 (44.2%)	$P = 0.09$
History of Cancer *n* (%)	642 (11.8%)	166 (18.1%)	$P < 0.001$
History of Diabetes Mellitus with complications *n* (%)	58 (1.1%)	8 (0.9%)	$P = 0.59$
History of Paraplegia *n* (%)	95 (1.7%)	27 (2.9%)	$P = 0.02$
History of Renal Disease *n* (%)	740 (13.6%)	219 (23.1%)	$P < 0.001$
History of Metastatic Cancer *n* (%)	208 (3.8%)	75 (8.2%)	$P < 0.001$
History of Severe Liver Disease *n* (%)	18 (0.3%)	6 (0.7%)	$P = 0.14$
Admission CURB 65 score ($n = 3993$; 2355 cases not documented)	CURB 0: 538 (15.3%)	CURB 0: 9 (1.9%)	$P < 0.001$
	CURB 1: 863 (24.6%)	CURB 1: 43 (8.9%)	
	CURB 2: 1127 (32.1%)	CURB 2: 142 (29.4%)	
	CURB 3: 799 (22.8%)	CURB 3: 193 (40%)	
	CURB 4: 163 (4.6%)	CURB 4: 81 (16.8%)	
	CURB 5: 20 (0.6%)	CURB 5: 15 (3.1%)	

1.22–2.17]), cancer (aOR 1.40 [95% CI 1.01–1.95]) and metastatic cancer (aOR 1.88 [95% CI 1.03–3.47]).

Of the 5432 subjects who survived the index admission, 1095 (21%) were readmitted within 30 days. Of these, 362 (33.1%) were specifically coded for pneumonia as a primary diagnosis. The administration of pre-hospital antibiotics was not associated with a significantly increased risk of 30-day readmission either due to any cause or specifically due to pneumonia (Table 6).

Discussion

This study has shown that in adults admitted to hospital with a diagnosis of CAP, the in-hospital mortality was higher in those who had received antibiotic treatment immediately prior to admission. This finding remained even when controlling for variables that have traditionally been shown to be of prognostic value in CAP, such as co-morbidity, age, and the CURB-65 score. The clinical relevance of this lies in the fact that currently, national guidance for the management of CAP does not recommend a change in management strategy when clinicians in the emergency department encounter a patient with pneumonia "pre-treated" with antibiotics in the community. The evidence associating the outcome from CAP specifically with antibiotic pre-treatment has been conflicting to date [7–14]. A single-centre study of 2179 subjects hospitalized with CAP reported that 17% had been treated with antibiotics prior to admission, a proportion similar to the current study's findings, yet no significant differences were noted in 30-day mortality, length of stay, or incidence of intensive care unit (ICU) admission, although the frequency of bacteremia was less in the "pre-treatment" group [7]. However, in contrast to the current study, the "prior antibiotic" group had less in terms of co-morbidity in the form of diabetes and cardiac disease as well as a significantly lower proportion of "severe" pneumonia according to CURB-65 criteria, which may explain the authors' findings. In contrast to the current study's cohort, this group had less severe pneumonia as evidenced by lower CURB65 scores.

Table 3 Comparison of subjects "pre-treated" with antibiotics prior to admission against those not "pre-treated"

	Not pre-treated with antibiotics pre-admission ($n = 4973$)	Pre-treated with antibiotics pre-admission ($n = 1059$)	P value
Age	72.41 (16.71)	72.13 (15.88)	0.61
Gender			
Female	2484 (49.9%)	564 (53.3%)	0.051
Male	2498 (50.1%)	495 (46.7%)	
In-hospital Mortality	658 (13)	197 (19)	< 0.001
Length Of Stay (LOS)	5 (2–11)	5 (3–11)	0.15
Admission CURB-65 score ($n = 3993$; 2355 cases not documented)	CURB 0:463 (14%)	CURB 0: 84 (14%)	0.72
	CURB 1: 780 (23%)	CURB 1: 126 (21%)	
	CURB 2: 1073(32%)	CURB 2: 196 (32%)	
	CURB 3: 830 (25%)	CURB 3: 162 (27%)	
	CURB 4: 211(6%)	CURB 4: 33 (5%)	
	CURB 5: 29 (1%)	CURB 5: 6 (1%)	
Charlson Co-morbidity Index	4 (3–16)	7 (3–17)	0.001
History of MI	489 (9.8)	109 (10.3)	0.65
History of CVA	248 (5)	63 (5.9)	0.20
History of CCF	792 (15.1)	197 (18.6)	0.005
History of Pulmonary Disease	2314 (46.5)	498 (47)	0.78
History of Renal Disease	709 (14.3)	190 (17.9)	0.002
History of Diabetes Mellitus	922 (18.5)	183 (17.3)	0.34
History of Diabetes Mellitus with complications	54 (1.1)	11 (1)	0.89
History of Dementia	578 (11.6)	144 (13.6)	0.07
History of Paraplegia	93 (1.9)	25 (2.4)	0.30
History of Liver Disease	49 (1)	4 (0.4)	0.054
History of Severe Liver Disease	20 (0.4)	3 (0.3)	0.57
History of Cancer	633 (12.7)	133 (12.6)	0.88
History of Metastatic Cancer	224 (4.5)	48 (4.5)	0.97

Their patients also had less diabetic and cardiovascular comorbidity. The issue of prior outpatient therapy was addressed by Van de Garde who reported that of 1096 subjects hospitalized for CAP over a 5 year period in the Netherlands, 27% had been "pre-treated" with antibiotics with no significant difference reported in mortality [8]. However, the diagnosis of CAP was based on ICD coding which has been shown to carry limitations in diagnostic accuracy [9]. In contrast, the current study's AQ cohort had a more stringent process to ensure an accurate diagnosis of CAP; i.e. confirmed radiological diagnosis of CAP verified by an independent reviewer at the time of data

Table 4 Multivariate analysis of variables associated with in-hospital mortality

Variable	Adjusted odds ratio	95% confidence interval	Significance
Age	1.04	(1.03, 1.04)	$P < 0.001$
Male Gender	1.17	(1.01, 1.37)	$P = 0.04$
Pre-treatment with antibiotics	1.43	(1.19, 1.71)	$P = 0.001$
History of Cerebrovascular Accident (CVA)	1.55	(1.17, 2.05)	$P = 0.002$
History of Congestive Cardiac Failure (CCF)	2.28	(1.91, 2.71)	$P < 0.001$
History of Dementia	1.42	(1.15, 1.74)	$P = 0.001$
History of Renal Disease	1.27	(1.06, 1.54)	$P = 0.01$
History of Cancer	1.73	(1.41–1.72)	$P < 0.001$

Table 5 Analysis of subjects with a documented CURB-65 score

Variable	Regression coefficient	Adjusted odds ratio	95% confidence interval	Significance
Age	0.03	1.03	(1.02, 1.04)	$P < 0.001$
CCI	0.02	1.02	(1.00, 1.03)	$P = 0.008$
Pre-treatment with antibiotics	0.43	1.54	(1.20, 1.99)	$P = 0.001$
History of CCF	0.49	1.62	(1.22, 2.17)	$P = 0.001$
History of Cancer	0.34	1.40	(1.01, 1.95)	$P = 0.046$
History of metastatic cancer	0.64	1.88	(1.03, 3.47)	$P = 0.04$
CURB65 0		Reference		
CURB65 1	0.42	1.53	(0.72, 3.26)	$P = 0.27$
CURB65 2	1.05	2.85	(1.37, 5.92)	$P = 0.005$
CURB65 3	1.56	4.77	(2.38, 9.97)	$P < 0.001$
CURB65 4	2.25	9.48	(4.37, 20.56)	$P < 0.001$
CURB65 5	2.83	16.88	(6.22, 45.77)	$P < 0.001$

entry, coupled with the requirement that a documented diagnosis of CAP had to have been made by a senior physician within the first 24 h following admission to hospital. Similarly, a smaller retrospective North American study of 733 subjects admitted with CAP to 2 centres did not report a significant difference in mortality in the 17% of subjects who had received antibiotics prior to admission [13]. However, the definition of "prior antibiotic therapy" in this study included subjects who had received antibiotics within 30 days of the admission, as opposed to the current study where only those who were being treated with antibiotics within 24 h of admission were captured. Furthermore, the North American study excluded those who were nursing home residents and 32% of the pre-treated cohort was administered fluoroquinolones prior to admission, which would not be normal practice in the UK where the prescription of antibiotics in the primary care setting is more tightly regulated. A prospective single-centre study of 3364 subjects reported that similar to the findings of this study, 18% of subjects had been administered antibiotics in the 24 h prior to admission [10]. In contrast to the data from the current study, the authors reported improved outcomes in the "pre-treated" cohort, namely a reduced need for mechanical ventilation and a decrease in the incidence of septic shock, but no difference in overall mortality. However, such a difference may be explained due to this cohort having a higher incidence of "low severity" pneumonia (defined as a CURB score of 0–1) standing at 50% and 56% in the non-pretreated and pretreated groups, respectively, in comparison to 14% observed in both groups of the current cohort. Furthermore, as with earlier studies, the range of antibiotics administered in primary care settings was more diverse when compared to the UK (including cefotaxime and quinolones) and in addition, this study specifically excluded nursing home residents. Similarly, in the earlier described study of 733 pneumonia cases admitted to 2 US hospitals, the 30-day mortality in the entire cohort was reported to be 8.1% and 55% of the study population had pneumonia classified as "low risk", which suggests there may be differences in the study population from that represented in the current study's cohort [13]. Another retrospective study of more than 18,000 patients aged over 65 years hospitalized with pneumonia reported that 24.4% had received pre-hospital antibiotic therapy [14]. This study reported that pre-hospital antibiotics were likely to have been administered if subjects were female gender and from a "skilled nursing facility" and were more likely to have had decreased pneumonia severity when compared with those not receiving antibiotics pre-hospital, whilst the current study reported a non-significant trend to female gender and pre-hospital antibiotic therapy but not with pneumonia severity when using CURB-65 as opposed to the pneumonia severity index (PSI). Unsurprisingly, the authors reported that the subjects administered pre-hospital antibiotics were less likely to be admitted to intensive care although this may be explained by this group presenting with less severe CAP according to PSI score. Interestingly, the "pre-treated" group had higher 30-day mortality if antibiotics were administered within 8 h of hospital admission compared to administration beyond 8 h from admission.

Table 6 The relationship between 30-day readmission and "pre-treatment" with antibiotics

	Readmission due to any cause		
	No	Yes	
Not "pre-treated"	4118 (82.4%)	878 (82.5%)	$P = 0.94$
"Pre-treated"	855 (17.6%)	181 (17.5%)	
	Readmission with Pneumonia		
	No	Yes	
Not "pre-treated"	3877 (83.4%)	438 (83.1%)	$P = 0.88$
"Pre-treated"	273 (16.6%)	89 (16.9%)	

As in previous studies, the in-hospital mortality was considerably lower than reported in the current study's cohort, standing at 7%, which again suggests that the study population may have been less "sick" at presentation than the cohort from this current study.

There are a number of potential mechanisms to explain these observations and whether these differences in observed outcome can be explained solely by treatment failure at a microbiological level or reflect a complex interplay between co-morbidities and the host microbiome require further study. The subjects admitted following antibiotic treatment in primary care could have represented a "sicker" cohort with a greater burden of co-morbidity, as evidenced by the fact that there was a higher incidence of cardiac failure and renal disease in this group. However, interestingly, the CURB-65 score, a widely used measure to risk stratify CAP at admission in UK hospitals, was not found to differ significantly between the 2 groups nor did age itself when taken separately. Despite there being no observed difference in CAP severity, as measured by CURB65 score, between the pre-treated and non-pre-treated groups it is possible there are unmeasured markers of severity. The study observed a statistically significant increase in the frequency of renal and cardiac disease in pre-treated patients. These conditions cause fluid overload with associated changes in antibiotic absorption via the gut and across "wet" lungs. These conditions cause increased susceptibility to CAP and possible reduced efficacy of therapy and as a consequence primary care physicians are more likely to prescribe prompt antibiotics. Whilst the UK has a low level of pneumococcal resistance to beta-lactam antibiotics, a proportion of this cohort were also diagnosed with underlying chronic lung disease which may suggest the presence of an expanded range of pathogens causing CAP such as *Haemophilus influenzae*, and *Pseudomonas aeruginosa* [15]. An intriguing mechanism to explain these findings may lie in the fact that the traditional concept of a "sterile" lung has been challenged of late, and the pathogenesis of pneumonia in an individual has been linked to alterations in the lung microbiome [16]. Further studies are required to better understand the effect prior antibiotic therapy has in terms of causing imbalances in the lung biome in the specific setting of inpatients hospitalized with CAP. Irrespective of any potential mechanism, the authors propose that clinicians adopt a degree of vigilance when managing this cohort of patients following hospital admission and that such patients warrant close monitoring with early input from senior physicians and clinical microbiology. However, whether antibiotic prescribing should differ from established guidance when managing such a cohort of CAP patients from those who have not received antibiotics prior to admission requires more detailed prospective study [17].

A particular strength of this study is that the Advancing Quality database is a nationally recognized initiative adopted by multiple NHS hospitals in the northwest of England and data quality is subject to strict audit and regulation. The diagnosis of CAP was more robust in the study as it was not based solely on ICD coding as in previous studies, but from analysis of medical records documenting a diagnosis of CAP made by a consultant physician, exclusion of those with a normal chest radiograph from the AQ database, and an independent review at the time of data entry ensuring the official chest X-ray report was compatible with a diagnosis of CAP. Furthermore, subjects with a "Palliative" code were also excluded from the AQ analysis, as were cases of HAP and "Aspiration" pneumonia; hence, for the cases entered, CAP was more likely to play a more significant role in terms of contributing to in-hospital mortality. The fact that this multi-centre study involved 9 hospitals and more than 6000 subjects adds to the strength of this data. Furthermore, all the 9 hospitals studied were required to submit all cases of CAP to the AQ program during the study period, thus reducing the possibility of selection bias. The age, pattern of comorbidities and inpatient mortality was similar to that reported in the BTS audit cohort although lung disease was more frequent in this current group [1].

Limitations to this study include that antibiotic pretreatment was ascertained by inspection of medical and hospital pharmacy records, which may have missed certain cases where documentation did not take place. The analysis did not take into account differences in duration of antibiotic pre-treatment as a predictor of outcome; i.e. the study did not distinguish between the scenario of a patient admitted with CAP having been administered simply one dose of antibiotic prior to admission (therefore not necessarily deemed to have "failed" an antibiotic course in the community), compared to a different situation where a patient receives several courses of antibiotics in the weeks prior to admission yet still requires admission due to inadequate resolution of symptoms. Furthermore, the dose and type of antibiotic prescribed in primary care was not studied and this could have influenced outcome. However, in the UK, prescribing options in primary care are highly regulated according to national guidelines as opposed to "physician discretion" where the vast majority of patients will have received amoxicillin either as monotherapy or with clarithromycin or monotherapy with doxycycline or clarithromycin [18]. This study's dataset did not contain any specific information regarding microbiology testing from the cohort during the hospital admission, hence specific associations between microbiology results and the impact of antibiotic pre-treatment on outcomes were not examined. This requires detailed prospective study. A further limitation is that in this study's cohort, the "CURB-65 score" was not documented in 37% of cases. However, when taking only those cases where the "CURB-65" score had been documented, antibiotic pre-treatment still emerged as significant following multivariate analysis. This limitation should also be balanced with the large sample size of the study population coupled with the fact that the statistical analysis controlled for comorbidity.

Furthermore, whilst, the CURB-65 score itself represents a standard of care in terms of CAP severity assessment, the relationship between antibiotic pre-treatment and other markers of adverse outcome (such as ICU admission, incidence of multi-organ failure and oxygenation) was not examined. In addition, whilst this study did control for key conditions known to result in immunosuppression, such as hematological malignancy, it did not directly study the effect of immunosuppressive and other medications associated with an increased incidence CAP [19, 20]. Another limitation is that this dataset did not record detailed surrogate markers reflecting the severity of co-morbidity which may have influenced outcome, such as nursing home residence, frequency of hospital admissions in the preceding 12 months, or number of outpatient attendances; e.g. for dialysis. However, the 30-day readmission rate due to any cause was not found to differ between the antibiotic pre-treatment group and those subjects not pre-treated with antibiotics prior to admission.

Conclusion

In summary, this study reports a higher mortality for subjects hospitalized with CAP who had received antibiotic therapy in the community immediately prior to hospital admission, a relationship maintained independent of comorbidity and disease severity. Such patients require close clinical monitoring in hospital with early specialist input. Future prospective studies should endeavor to determine the underlying mechanisms responsible for this observation focusing on factors such as disease etiology, microbiological variables, alterations to the lung microbiome, and adherence to therapy.

Abbreviations

AIDS: Acquired Immune Deficiency Syndrome; aOR: Adjusted Odds Ratio; AQ: Advancing Quality; CAP: Community Acquired Pneumonia; CCF: Congestive Cardiac Failure; CCI: Charlson Comorbidity Index; CVA: Cerebrovascular Accident; HAP: Hospital Acquired Pneumonia; HIV: Human Immunodeficiency Virus; ICD: International Classification Of Diseases; ICU: Intensive Care Unit; LOS: Length Of Stay; LRTI: Lower Respiratory Tract Infection; MI: Myocardial Infarction; NHS: National Health Service; PSI: Pneumonia Severity Index; SuS PbR: Secondary Uses Service Payment by Results

Acknowledgements

Not applicable.

Funding

No other external sources of funding.

Authors' contributions

The analysis was performed by BC, DW, MW, NP, SL, JS, LK and JP. BC, DW, SL, NP and MW designed and wrote the manuscript. All authors read and approved the final manuscript.

Competing interests

The National Health Service employers of Dr Chakrabarti and Professor Woodhead were reimbursed for the time spent performing Clinical Advisor roles for the Advancing Quality Pneumonia Program.

Author details

[1]Aintree University Hospital NHS Foundation Trust, Liverpool, UK. [2]Institute of Infection and Global Health, University of Liverpool, Liverpool, UK. [3]Department of Respiratory Research, Aintree University Hospital NHS Foundation Trust, Liverpool, UK. [4]Institute of Translational Medicine, University of Liverpool, Liverpool, UK. [5]Advancing Quality Alliance, Manchester, UK. [6]Warrington and Halton Hospitals NHS Foundation Trust, Warrington, UK. [7]Department of Respiratory Medicine, Central Manchester University Hospitals NHS Foundation Trust, Manchester, UK. [8]Manchester Academic Health Science Centre and Faculty of Medical and Human Sciences, University of Manchester, Manchester, UK.

References

1. Lim WS, Smith DL, Wise MP, Welham SA. British Thoracic Society community acquired pneumonia guideline and the NICE pneumonia guideline: how they fit together. Thorax. 2015;70(7):698–700.
2. Fine MJ, Auble TE, Yealy DM, Hanusa BH, Weissfeld LA, Singer DE, et al. A prediction rule to identify low-risk patients with community-acquired pneumonia. N Engl J Med. 1997;336(4):243–50.
3. Minogue MF, Coley CM, Fine MJ, Marrie TJ, Kapoor WN, Singer DE. Patients hospitalized after initial outpatient treatment for community-acquired pneumonia. Ann Emerg Med. 1998;31(3):376–80.
4. Lim WS. Defining community acquired pneumonia severity on presentation to hospital: an international derivation and validation study. Thorax. 2003; 58(5):377–82. Available from: http://thorax.bmj.com/cgi/doi/10.1136/thorax.58.5.377
5. Sutton M, Nikolova S, Boaden R, Lester H, McDonald R, Roland M. Reduced mortality with hospital pay for performance in England. N Engl J Med. 2012;367(19):1821–8. Available from: http://www.nejm.org/doi/abs/10.1056/NEJMsa1114951
6. Charlson ME, Pompei P, Ales KL, MacKenzie CR. A new method of classifying prognostic comorbidity in longitudinal studies: development and validation. J Chronic Dis. 1987;40(5):373–83.
7. Simonetti AF, Viasus D, Garcia-Vidal C, Grillo S, Molero L, Dorca J, Carratala J. Impact of pre-hospital antibiotic use on community-acquired pneumonia. Clin Microbiol Infect. 2014;20(9):O531–7.
8. Van de Garde EMW, Souverein PC, van den Bosch JMM, Deneer VHM, Goettsch WG, Leufkens HGM. Prior outpatient antibacterial therapy as prognostic factor for mortality in hospitalized pneumonia patients. Respir Med. 2006;100(8):1342–8.
9. Van de Garde EMW, Oosterheert JJ, Bonten M, Kaplan RC, Leufkens HGM. International classification of diseases codes showed modest sensitivity for detecting community-acquired pneumonia. J Clin Epidemiol. 2007;60(8):834–8.
10. Amaro R, Sellares J, Polverino E, Cilloniz C, Ferrer M, Fernandez-Barat L, .Mensa J, Niederman M, Torres A. Antibiotic therapy prior to hospital admission is associated with reduced septic shock and need for mechanical ventilation in patients with community-acquired pneumonia. J Inf Secur 2017;74(5):442–449.
11. Johnson D, Carriere KC, Jin Y, Marrie T. Appropriate antibiotic utilization in seniors prior to hospitalization for community-acquired pneumonia is

associated with decreased in-hospital mortality. J Clin Pharm Ther. 2004;29(3):231–9.
12. Meehan TP, Fine MJ, Krumholz HM, Scinto JD, Galusha DH, Mockalis JT, et al. Quality of care, process, and outcomes in elderly patients with pneumonia. JAMA. 1997;278(23):2080–4.
13. Mortensen EM, Restrepo MI, Pugh JA, Anzueto A. Impact of prior outpatient antibiotic use on mortality for community acquired pneumonia: a retrospective cohort study. BMC Res Notes. 2008;1:120.
14. Houck PM, Bratzler DW, Nsa W, Ma A, Bartlett JG. Timing of antibiotic administration and outcomes for Medicare patients hospitalized with community-acquired pneumonia. Arch Intern Med. 2004;164(6):637–44.
15. Health Protection Report Vol 10 no 40; 18th November 2016.
16. Dickson RP, Erb-Downward JR, Huffnagle GB. The role of the bacterial microbiome in lung disease. Expert Rev Respir Med [Internet]. 2013;7(3):245–57.
17. Van de Garde EMW, Natsch S, Prins JM, van der Linden PD. Antibiotic prescribing on admission to patients with pneumonia and prior outpatient antibiotic treatment: a cohort study on clinical outcome. Br Med J. 2015;5(2):1–7.
18. NHS, Centre for Clinical Practice at NICE. Respiratory tract infections – antibiotic prescribing [Internet]. NICE Clinical Guidelines. 2008; Available from: http://www.ncbi.nlm.nih.gov/pubmed/21698847
19. Suissa S, Ernst P. Precision medicine urgency: the case of inhaled corticosteroids in COPD. Chest. 2017;152(2):227–31.
20. Ramsay EN, Pratt NL, Ryan P, Roughead EE. Proton pump inhibitors and the risk of pneumonia: a comparison of cohort and self-controlled case series designs. BMC Med Res Methodol [Internet]. 2013;13(1):82.

Decreased relative risk of pneumococcal pneumonia during the last decade

Carlos M. Luna[1*], Laura Pulido[1], Michael S. Niederman[4], Alberto Casey[1], Diego Burgos[1], Sebastián D. Leiva Agüero[1], Alejandra Grosso[1,2,3], Evangelina Membriani[1,2,3], Andrea C. Entrocassi[1,2,3], Marcelo Rodríquez Fermepin[2], Carlos A. Vay[3], Susana Garcia[3] and Angela Famiglietti[3]

Abstract

Background: *Streptococcus pneumoniae* (SP) is one of the most common pathogens of Community-Acquired Pneumonia (CAP), but recent reports suggest that its incidence may be declining in relation to the use of the conjugate 13-valent pneumococcal vaccine in children. We compared the result of the immunochromatographic SP urinary antigen test (SPUAT) and clinical outcomes in patients with CAP admitted in two periods of time: 2001–2002(CAP1) and 2015–2016(CAP2).

Methods: This was a matched nested case-control study of two prospectively recorded cohorts of patients admitted with CAP, with SPUAT and blood culture performed in all patients. CAP2 cases and CAP1 controls were matched for age ± 4 years, sex, and Pneumonia Severity Index (PSI) score ± 10 points. Odds ratios (OR) for having SPUAT positive was estimated by conditional logistic regression. A multivariate model assessed the contribution of individual variables.

Results: Four hundred ninety-eight patients were recruited; 307 during the CAP1 and 191 during the CAP2 periods. Comparing both periods we observed differences, in age, PSI score, and the percentage of smokers, outpatients, previously immunized with pneumococcal vaccine, and positive SPUAT. On the other hand, mortality, admission from nursing homes, pneumococcal bacteremia and hospital admission were not different. After matching, pneumonia due to SP per the SPUAT was observed in 34(23.4%) of CAP1 and in 12(8.3%) of CAP2 patients ($p < 0.001$), and 6/145 CAP1 vs 33/145 CAP2 patients had received pneumococcal immunization before their admission ($p < 0.001$). A multivariate analysis confirmed that, independent of falling into PSI class 5, having not received the pneumococcal vaccine and having not survived the episode of pneumonia, there were two factors that increased the probability of having SPUAT positive: developing pneumonia during the CAP1 period (OR = 1.23) and having pneumococcal bacteremia (OR = 2.66).

Conclusion: We observed a reduction of the role of SP as pathogen, along with an increase in the number of patients who received pneumococcal immunization before admission, in 2015-2016 compared to 2001-2002. In addition, the use of conjugate 13-valent vaccine, starting in 2012 for childhood immunization, could be an additional factor contributing to these changes, as a result of early herd immunity in adults pneumonia.

Keywords: Community acquired pneumonia, *Streptococcus pneumoniae*, Urinary antigen test, Prevalence, Pneumococcal conjugate vaccine

* Correspondence: dr.cm.luna@gmail.com
[1]Department of Medicine, Pulmonary Diseases Division; Hospital de Clínicas, Universidad de Buenos Aires, Ayacucho, 1850, piso 5 dto B, 1112 Buenos Aires, Argentina
Full list of author information is available at the end of the article

Background

Community acquired pneumonia (CAP) is one of the most common causes of morbidity and mortality worldwide [1] and *Streptococcus pneumoniae* (SP) has been found to be its most common pathogen [2]. The frecuency of pneumococcal pneumonia might be decreasing following widespread use of the 13-valent pneumococcal vaccine in children, and in people 65 years of age or older [3].

Disease caused by SP is a major public health problem worldwide, leading to invasive CAP, meningitis, and bacteremia. Non-invasive illnesses, such as non-bacteremic pneumonia, otitis media, bronchitis and upper airway infections are common but less severe [4]. Besides its role as a pathogen, SP is asymptomatically carried in the nasopharynx by up to 50% of infants and up to 5% of adults [5]. Colonization occurs before disease, and transmission is from child to child and from children to adults can occur [6]. In addition to the traditional microbiological diagnosis of pneumonia based on respiratory specimens and blood culture, the use of immunochromatographic SP urinary antigen test (SPUAT) in patients with CAP is also recommended for diagnosis by international guidelines [7]. Sensitivity and specificity of SPUAT in adults for the etiologic diagnosis of pneumococcal CAP have been found to be 57.9–75% and 96.6–99.7%, respectively [8–11]. Antibodies to capsular polysaccharide antigen provide serotype-specific protection against serious infection, and the pneumococcal vaccines are designed to cover the serotypes most commonly associated with severe pneumococcal disease [12]. Vaccination has greatly reduced the burden of pneumococcal disease.Two types of pneumococcal vaccines are available in Argentina (country where this study was performed): the 23-valent pneumococcal polysaccharide (non-conjugate), (PPV23) and the 13-valent polysaccharide conjugate vaccine (PCV13).

By 2016, the national committee on immunizations in Argentina (CoNain) recommended the PPV23 for all individuals ≥65 years of age and for those younger, with comorbidities. Universal PCV13 vaccination for children was initiated in Argentina in 2012 [at 2, 4 and 6 months and 1 year of age (3 + 1 schedule)], with a coverage higher than 90% [13]. Results of the Community-Acquired Pneumonia immunization Trial in Adults (CAPiTA), a randomized controlled trial in elderly adults in the Netherlands, demonstrated the efficacy of PCV13 to prevent IPD and pneumonia caused by homologous serotypes [14]. A decline in the incidence of pneumococcal pneumonia in adults has been observed after PCV13 introduction in children, indicating an early indirect protection (so called herd effect) on adult disease, as a consequence of childhood vaccination [15]. These effects may accrue over the coming years with implications for national pneumococcal vaccination policies in adults.

Objectives

To compare the SPUAT result (a sensitive and highly specific test to detect pneumococcal infection), the clinical findings and outcomes, in patients with CAP admitted during two different periods of time: 2001–2002 (CAP1) and 2015–2016 (CAP2), trying to define if there were any differences in the frequency and clinical features of pneumococcal CAP during these two periods.

Methods

Patients

The cases eligible for the study were adults over 17 years-old, with CAP (which met the inclusion criteria described below), consulting the Emergency Department or admitted to the wards of the Department of Medicine and the critical care areas of the Hospital de Clínicas, University of Buenos Aires, from January 1st 2015 to December 31st, 2016. The controls were patients admitted to the same institution from January 1st 2001 to December 31st, 2002. Cases and controls were evaluated in an identical fashion during the two periods of time. The criteria published in a National Clinical Practice Guideline were applied in decision making about the site of care to the patients who were admitted (Table 1) [16]. Inclusion criteria were: having a presumptive diagnosis of pneumonia within the first 24 h of admission to the study; presence of a new infiltrate on chest radiograph, and clinical findings confirmatory of at least one "major criterion" such as cough, sputum, or fever > 37.8C; or at least two "minor criteria", including pleuritic chest pain, dyspnea, altered mental status, findings consistent with consolidationon physical exam, and leukocyte count > 12,000/ mm^3 [17]; having had testing for the detection of SPUAT and blood cultures during their initial microbiological evaluation at admission. SPUAT was carried out from freshly obtained urine samples according to the manufacturer's instructions (results read visually at 15 min and recorded as positive, with no interpretation of color intensity, or negative). All samples were stored

Table 1 Criteria for hospital admission, Luna CM, et al. [16]

1) Presence of two or more of the following: age > 65 years; chronic pulmonary disease; congestive heart failure; chronic kidney failure; chronic liver disease; malignant neoplasm; diabetes mellitus; hospitalization for pneumonia during the past year.
2) Respiratory rate ≥ 30 / minute.
3) Low blood pressure: systolic < 90 and/or diastolic: < 60 mmHg).
4) Poor respiratory mechanics. (paradoxical respiration. Circulation. etc.).
5) Any of the following: PaO_2 < 60 mmHg; SaO_2 < 89%; PaCO2 > 50 mmHg with acidosis; white blood cell count < 4000 or > 30.000/ mm^3; BUN > 25 mg/dl; hematocrit < 30%.
6) Alteration of consciousness.
7) Serious swallowing disorder suggesting likely aspiration.
8) Suppurative complications (pericarditis. Arthritis. empyema. Etc.)
9) Severe chest radiograph involvement (multilobar, bilateral, cavitation, progression > 50% over a previous RX)
10) Reasons suggesting inaccurate treatment compliance.

at ≤ – 70 °C and assayed later, directly after thawing, Exclusion criteria included: having been hospitalized for any reason within the previous 14 days; no chest radiographic confirmation of a new infiltrate or attributing the abnormality only to a noninfectious etiology; a confirmed diagnosis of lung cancer before admission to the study; patients with a known diagnosis of HIV at the time of enrollment, or high doses of immunosuppressants (> 20 mg of prednisone or other corticosteroid dose equivalent) in chronic treatment (over 20 days).

Mortality: was defined as death that occurred within 30 days of the diagnosis of CAP.

Evaluation

Clinical evaluation included: risk factors such as smoking and comorbidities (chronic lung disease, diabetes; chronic heart, renal or liver disease and history of malignancy). Findings on the clinical exam were recorded for each patient. Pneumonia severity index (PSI) [18] was calculated .

Radiological assessment: the radiological patterns considered to support the diagnosis of pneumonia included the presence of: focal or multi-focal infiltrates, airspace infiltrates or an interstitial or miliary pattern. Pleural effusion without any parenchymal radiological findings was not included.

Microbiologic evaluation: urine samples collected in the emergency department or on the ward in the first 24 h to test for SPUAT (BinaxNOW ®, Portland, ME, and Alere Inc., Waltham, MA, USA) in accordance with the manufacturer's instructions. Blood cultures were drawn in all patients at admission. Culture of respiratory specimens for common aerobic bacteria were performed in a number of cases, but not systematically in all patients.

Blood analyses: all the hospitalized and some ambulatory patients entered into the study had blood drawn for white blood cell count and routine biologic analyses.

Demographic data (age and sex), the PSI score, site of care (ambulatory or admitted to the general ward or the ICU), presence of criteria for receiving pneumococcal vaccine, results of the blood culture, admission from a nursing home, past medical history including presence of comorbidities, smoking history and vaccination against SP were recorded.

Therapy and follow-up

Patients admitted to the study were treated per the criteria adopted by the attending physician and followed for up to 30 days. In brief, all patients received empiric antimicrobial therapy as early as possible and concordant with the National Guidelines, and fluid resuscitation with intravenous crystalloids for patients with hypotension.

Data analysis

We carried out a nested case-control, cohort study; cases (the CAP2 patients) and controls (the CAP1 patients) were prospectively enrolled during the two periods of study. Cases were matched to controls for age ± 4 years, sex, and PSI score ± 10 points, allowing for the possibility of finding different etiologies and frequencies of pathogens. Results are expressed as mean and standard deviation for age, or as number and percentages for categorical variables. Age was assessed by the *t- test* and categorical variables were assessed by the chi square or Fisher exact test. The relative risk (RR) and 95% confidence interval (95%CI) of the cathegorical variables and their change over the time periods studied, were analyzed. A multivariate analysis, using a conditional logistic regression model, suggested for matched case-control studies [19], with the dependent variable being the positivity of the SPUAT, was performed. Confounding factors including PSI class 5, having not received the pneumococcal vaccine and having not survived the episode of pneumonia, were used for adjustment to calculate the odds ratio (OR) and 95%CI. All data management and statistical analyses were performed using the SPSS 21 processor (SPSS Inc., Chicago, IL).

This study was approved by the ethics committee of the hospital, but patient-informed consent was considered unnecessary because of the observational nature of the study, but the study team explained the potential risks related to drawing blood, including the nature of potential risk of blood drawing.

Results

Clinical characteristics of the cohort

A total of 498 patients with a clinical diagnosis of CAP made on either an outpatient basis or during the first 24 h of hospitalization were consecutively recruited. In all patients, at least one specimen for SPUAT and two sets of blood cultures were collected during their initial microbiological evaluation. Among these patients, 307 were recruited during the CAP1 period and 191 during the CAP2 period, respectively (Fig. 1).

Some significant differences were observed comparing the characteristics of the patients (unmatched) recruited during the two different periods, CAP1 and CAP2, including: age, 64.6 ± 21.2 vs. 70.3 ± 19.1 years old (p = 0.002); PSI score, 110.7 ± 39.8 vs 93.8 ± 41.1 (p < 0.001); and percentages of smokers, 9.1% vs.17.3% (p = 0.007). The rates of hospitalization for each age group were 75.5% and 61.7%, for CAP1 and for CAP2, respectively (p = 0.001) (Table 2, panel A). Also, we found significant

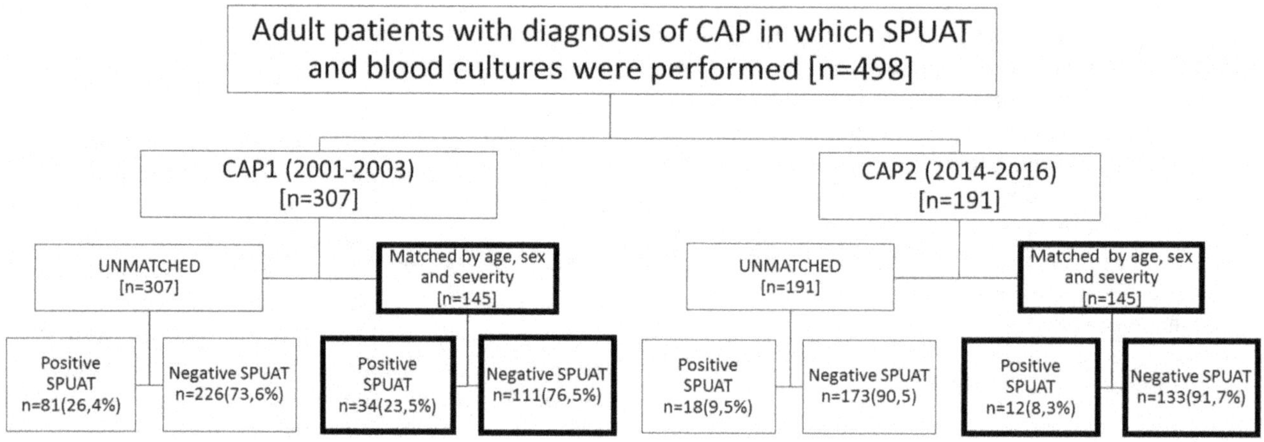

Fig. 1 Distribution of the patients in the cohorts CAP1 and CAP2 in general and considering the approaches analyzing both cohorts, unmatched and matched. The unmatched patients, both from CAP1 and CAP2 cohorts, were excluded because they had no pair with comparable age, sex and PSI score. The number of patients excluded from the case-control analysis were 162 from the CAP1 and 46 from the CAP2 cohorts

differences among the percentage of patients who had received pneumococcal immunization, 4.2% vs 18.8% (p = 0.001) and the positivity of the SPUAT, 25.0% vs 9.5% (p = 0.001) respectively, comparing CAP1 and CAP2.

Considering the indications for pneumococcal vaccination according to the national recommendations in Argentina (including age > 65 years, comorbidities, splenectomy, and cerebrospinal fluid leakage); 247 (80.4%) patients had an indication for pneumococcal vaccination in the CAP1 and 142 (74.2%) patients, in the CAP2 time period.

Nested case-control study

It was possible to successfully pair 145 CAP2 patients, age- (± 4 years), sex- and severity- (PSI score ± 5 points) matched, with 145 CAP1 control subjects. Forty-six cases were excluded because it was not possible to find a control among the CAP1 patients for them. The result of the comparison of CAP1 with CAP2 matched patients' findings in this nested case-control study is displayed in Table 2, panel B.

Comparing CAP2 with CAP1 matched patients, most of the variables were not different. The exceptions were the increasing rate of pneumococcal immunization, 4.1% versus 22.7%, (RR = 0.2549, 95% confidence interval [CI] {0.1205 to 0.5390} 0.), p < 0.001 and the declining rate of positive SPUAT, 23.4% vs. 8.3%, (RR = 1.6248, 95% CI [1.3041 to 2.0243]), p < 0.001, comparing the two periods (Table 2). This last finding represents a reduction in the RR of pneumococcal pneumonia that happened in the CAP2 period, compared with the CAP1 period.

Pneumococcal vaccination had been performed using the PPV23 vaccine in all cases during the CAP1 period. The same happened with the majority of those included in the CAP2 period, as PCV13 vaccine was approved for use in adults in 2012, and only indicated in adults older than 65 years-old by the CoNain in 2016, after the CAPiTA study was published. The CAPITA study demonstrated among this population that PCV13 was effective in preventing vaccine-type pneumococcal, bacteremic, and non-bacteremic CAP and vaccine type invasive pneumococcal disease, but not in preventing community-acquired pneumonia from any cause [14, 20].

Interestingly, although the positivity of the SPUAT was significantly different, showing a reduction in the RR of SP as a pathogen of pneumonia, the rate of bacteremia due to SP did not change during this time. All SP isolated in blood cultures were susceptible to penicillin (Clinical and Laboratory Standards Institute MIC breakpoints for patients without meningitis treated with intravenous penicillin were < 2 μg/mL).

Mortality was also not different comparing CAP1 with CAP2 periods, in the matched population.

The result of the univariate and multivariate analyses using the positivity of the SPUAT as the dependent variable, the variables evaluated and their OR, the 95% CI, and the p values are displayed in Tables 3 and 4. These results confirm that, independent of the presence of a PSI risk class 5, of having a history of receving pneumococcal vaccine and of not surviving the episode of pneumonia, there were two factors that increased the chance of having the SPUAT positive: developing pneumonia during the CAP1 period in 2001–2002 (with an OR of 1.23) and having pneumococcal bacteremia (with an OR of 2.66).

Discussion

The most important findings of our study are: (1) the relative risk of pneumococcal pneumonia, as per SPUAT

Table 2 Comparison of demographic and clinical characteristics among patients with CAP during the CAP1 and the CAP2 periods unmatched and matched (case control). Figures are means (±SD) and n (%). The *p* value and risk ratio (RR)

	PANEL A (UNMATCHED)			PANEL B (MATCHED)			
Variable	CAP1 ($n = 307$)	CAP2 ($n = 191$)	p value	CAP1 ($n = 145$)	CAP2 ($n = 145$)	p value	RR
Age, year (±SD)	64.6 ± 21.2	70.3 ± 19.1	0.002	67.8 ± 20.4	67.7 ± 20.4	0.484	
Male Sex	160 (58.6%)	93 (48.7%)	0.749	74 (51.0)	74 (51.0)	1.000	1.000
PSI class 5	106 (34.5%)	43 (22.5%)	< 0.001	37 (25.5%)	33 (22.8%)	0.575	1.077
Admitted from nursing home	43 (14.0%)	27 (14.1%)	0.972	12 (8.3%)	23 (15.9%)	0.082	0.657
Managed as outpatients	75 (24.4%)	73 (38.2%)	0.003	51 (35.12%	54 (37.2%)	0.706	0.956
Admitted to the hospital	232 (75.5%)	118 (61.7%)	< 0.001	94 (64.8%)	91 (62.8%)	0.716	0.968
Admitted (general ward)	176 (57.3%)	100 (52.3%)	0.402	83 (57.2%	77 (53.1%)	0.481	1.088
Admitted (ICU)	56 (18.2%)	18 (9.4%)	0.007	11 (7.6%)	14 (9.7%)	0.552	0.870
Positive blood culture	12 (3.9%)	7 (3.7%)	0.954	7 (4.8%)	6 (4.1%)	0.784	0.911
Requiring mechanical ventilation	16 (5.2%)	6 (3.1%)	0.012	4 (2.8%)	5 (3.4%)	0.748	0.886
Pneumococcal immunization	13 (4.2%)	36 (18.8%)	< 0.001	6 (4.1%)	33 (22.7%)	< 0.001	0.255
Pneumococcal. vaccine Indication	247 (80.4%)	142 (74.3%)	0.108	109 (75.2%)	103 (71.0%)	0.438	1.114
Positive SPUAT	81 (26.4%)	18 (9.5%)	< 0.001	34 (23.4%)	12 (8.3%)	< 0.001	2819
Current smoker	28 (9.1%)	33 (17.3%)	0.007	15 (10.3%)	20 (13.8%)	0.396	0.841
Chronic lung disease	91 (29.6%)	41 (21.5%)	0.041	37 (25.3%)	28 (19.3%)	0.184	1.186
Cardiac disease	68 (22.2%)	38 (19.9%)	0.558	21 (14.5%)	29 (20.1%)	0.243	0.813
Diabetes	29 (9.5%)	22 (11.5%)	0.464	10 (6.9%	13 (8.9%)	0.706	0.538
Hepatic disease	6 (1.9%)	6 (3.1%)	0.412	2 (1.4%)	3 (2.1%)	0.681	0.797
Renal failure	30 (10.8%)	19 (9.9%)	0.951	10 (6.9%)	5 (3.4%)	0.112	1.358
Descesed	64 (20.8%)	30 (15.5%)	0.143	23 (15.9%)	22 (15.2%)	0.870	1.026

Table 3 Conditional Logistic Regression model for matched cases and controls, Univariate Analysis, The odds ratio (OR), the 95% confidence index (CI 95%) and the *p* value are displayed

Variable	OR	CI 95%	*p* value
CAP1 versus CAP2 Period	1.23	0.30 to 1.80	0.006
Sex	0.62	−0.22 to 1.47	0.148
Nursing Home	−1.93	−4.00 to 0.14	0.067
PSI = 5	0.88	−0.01 to 1.77	0.053
CURB 65	0.26	− 0.11 to 0.64	0.168
Positive blood cultures	2.80	1.26 to 4.35	< 0.001
Positive sputum	2.44	0.20 to 4.67	0.033
Admitted to general ward	1.63	0.60 to 2.66	0.002
Outpatients	−1.85	−3.03 to −0.68	0.002
Admitted to the ICU	−0.19	−1.60 to 1.23	0.800
Decesed	0.89	−0.20 to 1.99	0.110
Pneumococcal vaccination	−0.25	−1.46 to 0.95	0.680

positivity in a cohort of patients treated for CAP in a University Hospital (Hospital de Clínicas, University of Buenos Aires), during a 2 year (CAP2), was reduced overall to a ratio of 0.34 ($p < 0.001$), compared with a control cohort, treated 14 years earlier (CAP1), matched by age, sex and severity of illness; (2) the f history of pneumococcal vaccination (mainly PPV23) among the CAP2 group of patients increased overall to a ratio of 0.55 ($p < 0.001$), even though the percentage of patients indicated to receive the vaccination did not change. In addition, rates of pneumococcal bacteremia and overall mortality did not change over the two time periods. Reported mortality was comparable to the rates observed in the UK (Chalmers JD, et al...) and US (Morril HJ, et al) [21, 22]. Out matched, nested case-control methods run the risk of over-matching, and thus we also analyzed the positivity of the SPUAT observed in this study using a multivariate method. This analysis was based on the linear logistic model (conditional logistic model), recomended for the analysis of case-control studies with pairwise matching. This technique enabled us to investigate the effect of several variables simultaneously in the analysis, while allowing for the matched design. This multivariate analysis demonstrated that only two factors increased the chance of having a positive positive SPUAT: developing pneumonia in the CAP 1 period (OR = 1.23) and having pneumococcal bacteremia (OR = 2.66). The latter was expected, but confirms the robustness of our analysis.

Table 4 Conditional Logistic Regression model for matched cases and controls, Multivariate Analysis, showing that regardless of PSI class = 5, having received pneumococcal vaccine, and age (in addition to all the variables by which the individuals were matched), the only two factors that increased the chance of having positive SPUAT were belonging to the CAP1 (OR 2.66) cohort and having positive blood cultures (OR 2.66)

Variable	OR	CI 95%	*p* value
CAP1 versus CAP2 Period	1.23	0.30 to 2.17	0.01
Positive blood cultures	2.66	0.80 to 4.52	0.005
PSI = 5	0.005	−0.013 to 0.023	0.590
Decesed	−0.19	−1.57 to 1.20	0.790
Pneumococcal vaccination	0.27	−1.2 to 1.73	0.720

The SPUAT test, provides results in 15 min, detecting the C-polysaccharide cell wall antigen common to all SP strains [23]. The sensitivity and specificity of the SPUAT have been evaluated and most studies demonstrated high specificity near 100% and moderate to high sensitivity. Horita et al., found in a meta-analysis, a pooled specificity of 0.75 and a pooled sensitivity was 0.95. This high sensitivity and specificity make SPUAT a useful tool in clinical practice to predict negatively or positively the role of SP in the etiology of CAP. Ortega et al. found evidence that links the degree of the SPUAT positivity to the severity of the pneumonia [24]. Some studies published between 2001 and 2007 in patients with a clinical diagnosis of CAP showed that SPUAT was positive in a range between 16 and 33% of patients [25–28].

The introduction of PCV7 into the infant immunization programs in developed countries beginning in 2006, was highly effective in reducing the incidence of invasive and non-invasive pneumococcal disease. Rodrigo et al., beginning in 2008, conducted a 5-year prospective cohort study of adults admitted to hospital with CAP in Nottingham, UK [15]; they observed a reduction in the incidence of the number of adult patients hospitalized for pneumococcal CAP [incidence rate ratio (IRR) per year 0.84, 95% CI 0.80–0.89; $p < 0.001$] over the 5-year period of the study. The incidence of CAP due to serotypes included in the PCV7 declined by 88% (IRR 0.12, 95% CI 0.08–0.20; $p < 0.001$), and CAP due to the additional 6 serotypes in PCV13 declined by 30% (IRR 0.70, 95% CI 0.51–0.96; $p = 0.024$). This study and other previous studies described the finding of so-called herd immunity, reducing the incidence of pneumococcal pneumonia in children and adults, after the introduction of PCV7 and PCV13 into the infant immunization programs [29, 30]. Other authors found that although PCV13 protects against key serotypes that increased after routine immunization with the PCV7, its potential for herd immunity and serotype replacement is uncertain [31–37]. In Argentina, the percentages of coverages for the 1st and 3rd doses of PCV13 have been appropriate and comparable with the coverage observed in developed countries such as the United States, after its introduction in 2012. Our study suggested a potential benefit to adults, of the immunization with pneumococcal vaccine in children, leading to a dramatic decline in non-invasive pneumooccal CAP, diagnosed by SPUAT, but no change in bacteremic pneumococcal CAP.

This study has several limitations, including: the diagnosis of pneumococcal pneumonia was based on the positivity of the SPAUT, a methodology that highly specific, but can produce between a 25% and 42.1% rate of false negatives [8–11]. Blood cultures were performed to all patients, but respiratory cultures and/or serotyping were not available for all patients. Also, we could not analyze the effect of concordant therapy, because this was not recorded in all patients in the CAP1 cohort.

Among the strengths of our study, is our comparison of two cohorts, one treated after the implementation of PCV vaccination in children in the calendar in 2012, with another comparable cohort treated before the implementation of this pneumococcal vaccine, allowing us to compare the frequency of pneumococcal pneumonia, including by multivariate analysis.

Conclusions

The result of this comparison demonstrated that the RR of pneumococcal pneumonia, diagnosed as per SPUAT positivity, was reduced in more recent years, leading us to speculate about possible explanations. The frequency of SP as the causative microorganism of CAP was reduced to a ratio of 0.34, compared with the control cohort, 23.4% vs 8.3% ($p < 0.001$), although there was no change in the frequency of bacteremic pneumococcal pneumonia. The introduction of pneumococcal vaccine might account for a decline in pneumococcal pneumonia by either inducing immunity in immunized at risk patients or by its herd immunity impact of childhood vaccination on the community, but this could be confirmed only in studies demonstrating a reduction of the serotypes represented by the vaccine.

Abbreviations

CAP: community-acquired pneumonia.; CAP1: 2001–2002 period of time; CAP2: 2015–2016 period of time; CAPiTA: Community-Acquired Pneumonia immunization Trial in Adults; CoNain: the national committee on immunizations in Argentina.; OR: odds ratio; PCV13: the 13-valent pneumococcal conjugate vaccine.; PPV23: the 23-valent pneumococcal polysaccharide (non-conjugate) vaccne.; PSI: Pneumonia severity index; RR: relative risk; SP: *Sterptococcus pneumoniae*; SPUAT: immunochromatographic *Streptococcus pneumoniae* urinary antigen test

Acknowledgements

The authors want to recognize to Sebastián García Zamora who performed the multivariate analysis of this study.

Funding

Study funding was provided by both an Independent Research Fund administered by the Cooperadora del Hospital de Clínicas (Pulmonary Division Account "Pneumonia Study") and a subsidy from the Secretaría de Ciencia y Técnica, University of Buenos Aires.

Authors' contributions

CML conceived of the study, and participated in its design, coordination and data interpretation, and helped to draft the manuscript; LP participated in the study design and coordination and helped to draft the manuscript; MSN participated in the study design, coordination and data interpretation, and helped to draft the manuscript; AC participate in the data acquisition and helped to draft the manuscript; DB, SLA, AG and EM participate in the data acquisitionand in the manuscript revision; MRF conceived of the study, and participated in its design, coordination and data interpretation and drafted the manuscript; ACE participate in the data acquisition, carried out the molecular studies and drafted the manuscript; CAV participate in the data acquisition and microbiological data analysis and drafted the manuscript; SG participate in the data acquisition and microbiological data analysis; AF participated in its design, coordination and microbilological data interpretation, and helped to draft the manuscript. All authors approved the final manuscript.

Competing interests

Dr. Luna reports personal fees from Pfizer and personal fees from Merk Sharp Dohne, outside the submitted work. Dr. Pulido, Dr. Niederman, Dr. Casey, Dr. Burgos1, Dr. Leiva Agüero, Dr. Grosso1, Dr. Membriani, Dr. Entrocassi, Dr. Rodríquez Fermepin, Dr. Vay1, Dr. Garcia, and Dr. Famiglietti, have no competing interests to disclose.

Author details

[1]Department of Medicine, Pulmonary Diseases Division; Hospital de Clínicas, Universidad de Buenos Aires, Ayacucho, 1850, piso 5 dto B, 1112 Buenos Aires, Argentina. [2]Department of Chemical Biochemistry, Immuno-Serology Section, Faculty of Pharmacy and Biochemistry; Hospital de Clínicas, Universidad de Buenos Aires, Buenos Aires, Argentina. [3]Department of Chemical Biochemistry, Section Microbiology, Faculty of Pharmacy and Biochemistry; Hospital de Clínicas, Universidad de Buenos Aires, Buenos Aires, Argentina. [4]Pulmonary and Critical Care, New York Presbyterian/ Weill Cornell Medical Center, New York, USA.

References

1. The top 10 causes of death, 2016. World Health Organization. Available from http://www.who.int/news-room/fact-sheets/detail/the-top-10-causes-of-death. Accessed 22 Aug 2018.
2. Bartlett JG. Diagnostic tests for agents of community-acquired pneumonia [abstract]. Clin Infect Dis. 2011;52(suppl 4):296–304S.
3. Jain S, Self WH, Wunderink RG, et al. Community-acquired pneumonia requiring hospitalization among U. S Adults N Engl J Med. 2015;373:415–27.
4. World Health Organization. Global Health Observatory data, update 2015. Available from: http://www.who.int/gho/mortality_burden_disease/en/. Accessed 22 Aug 2018.
5. Le Polain de Warroux O, Flasche S, Prieto-Merino D, Edmund WJ. Age-dependent prevalence of nasopharyngeal carriage of Streptococcus pneumoniae before conjugate vaccine introduction: a prediction model based on a meta-analysis. PLoS One. 2014;9:e86136.
6. Almeida ST, Nunes S, Santos Paulo AC, et al. Low prevalence of pneumococcal carriage and high serotype and genotype diversity among adults over 60 years of age living in Portugal. PLoS One. 2014;9(3):e90974. https://doi.org/10.1371/journal.pone.0090974.
7. Mandell LA, Wunderink RG, Anzueto A, et al. Infectious Diseases Society of America/American Thoracic Society consensus guidelines on the management of community-acquired pneumonia in adults. Clin Infect Dis. 2007;44(suppl 2):27–72.
8. Zhou F, Gu L, Qu JX, Liu YM, Cao B. Evaluating the utility of Binax NOW Streptococcus pneumoniae urinary antigen test in adults with community acquired pneumonia in China. Clin Respir J. 2018;12:425–32.
9. Zalacain R, Capelastegui A, Ruiz LA, et al. Streptococcus pneumoniae antigen in urine: diagnostic usefulness and impact on outcome of bacteraemic pneumococcal pneumonia in a large series of adult patients. Respirology. 2014;19:936–43.
10. Molinos L, Zalacain R, Menéndez R, et al. Sensitivity, specificity and positivity predictors of the pneumococcal urinary antigen test in community-acquired pneumonia. Ann Am Thorac Soc. 2015;12:1482–9.

11. Horita N, Miyazawa N, Kojima R, et al. Sensitivity and specificity of the Streptococcus pneumoniae urinary antigen test for unconcentrated urine from adult patients with pneumonia: a meta-analysis. Respirology. 2013;18: 1177–83.
12. Grabenstein JD, Manoff SB. Pneumococcal vaccines in adults: assessing the evolving evidence. Vaccine. 2011;29:4435–44.
13. Ministerio de Salud, Argentina. Calendario Nacional de Vacunación 2017. Available from: http://www.msal.gob.ar/index.php/component/content/article/46-ministerio/184-calendario-nacional-de-vacunacion-2017. Accessed 22 Aug 2018.
14. Bonten MJ, Huijts SM, Bolkenbaas M, et al. Polysaccharide conjugate vaccine against pneumococcal pneumonia in adults. N Engl J Med. 2015;372:1114–25.
15. Rodrigo C, Bewick T, Sheppard C, et al. Impact of infant 13-valent pneumococcal conjugate vaccine on serotypes in adult pneumonia. Eur Respir J. 2015;45:1632–41.
16. Luna CM, Efron ED, Schiavi E, et al. Community-acquired pneumonia in adults. Clinical practice guideline for Argentina. Study group on community acquired pneumonia. Medicina (B Aires). 1997;57:343–55.
17. Fine MJ, Auble TE, Yealy DM, et al. A prediction rule to identify low-risk patients with community-acquired pneumonia. N Engl J Med. 1997;336: 243–50.
18. Fang GD, Fine M, Orloff J, et al. New and emerging etiologies for community-acquired pneumonia with implications for therapy. A prospective multicenter study of 359 cases. Medicine (Baltimore). 1990;69:307–16.
19. Kuo C-L, Duan Y, Grady J. Unconditional or conditional logistic regression model for age-matched case–control data? Front Public Health. 2018;6:1–14.
20. van Werkhoven CH, Hollingsworth RC, Huijts SM, et al. Pneumococcal conjugate vaccine herd effects on non-invasive pneumococcal pneumonia in elderly. Vaccine. 2016;34:3275–82.
21. Chalmers JD, Campling J, Dicker A, Woodhead M, Madhava H. A systematic review of the burden of vaccine preventable pneumococcal disease in UK adults. BMC Pulmonary Medicine. 2016;16:77.
22. Morrill HJ, Caffrey AR, Noh E, LaPlante KL. Epidemiology of pneumococcal disease in a National Cohort of older adults. Infectious Diseases and Therapy. 2014;3:19–33.
23. Murdoch DR, Laings RT, Mills GD, et al. Evaluation of a rapid immunochromatographic test for detection os Streptococcus pneumoniae antigen in urine, utility and clinical impact on the reported etiology. J Infect Chemother. 2004;10:359–63.
24. Ortega L, Sierra M, Dominguez J, et al. Utility of a pneumonia severity index in the optimization of the diagnostic and therapeutic effort for community-acquired pneumonia. Scand J Infect Dis. 2005;37:657–63.
25. Andreo F, Domínguez J, Ruiz J, et al. Impact of rapid urine antigen tests to determine the etiology of community-acquired pneumonia in adults. Respir Med. 2006;100:884–91.
26. Gutiérrez F, Masiá M, Rodríguez JC, et al. Evaluation of the immunochromatographic Binax NOW assay for detection of Streptococcus pneumoniae urinary antigen in a prospective study of community-acquired pneumonia in Spain. Clin Infect Dis. 2003;36:286–92.
27. Ishida T, Hashimoto T, Arita M, et al. A 3-year prospective study of a urinary antigen-detection test for *Streptococcus pneumoniae* in community-acquired pneumonia: utility and clinical impact on the reported etiology. J Infect Chemother. 2004;10:359–63.
28. Marcos MA, Jiménez de Anta MT, de la Bellacasa JP, et al. Rapid urinary antigen test for rapid diagnosis of pneumococcal community-acquired pneumonia in adults. Eur Resp J. 2002;21:209–14.
29. Rodgers GL, Klugman KP. Surveillance of the impact of pneumococcal conjugate vaccines in developing countries. Hum Vaccin Immunother. 2016; 12:417–20.
30. Tsaban G, Ben-Shimol S. Indirect (herd) protection, following pneumococcal conjugated vaccines introduction: a systematic review of the literature. Vaccine. 2017;35:2882–91.
31. Grau I, Ardanuy C, Cubero M, Benitez MA, et al. declining mortality from adult pneumococcal infections linked to children's vaccination. J Inf Secur. 2016;72:439–49.
32. Hays C, Vermee Q, Agathine A, et al. Demonstration of the herd effect in adults after the implementation of pneumococcal vaccination with PCV13 in children. Eur J Clin Microbiol Infect Dis. 2017;36:831–8.
33. Nieddu F, Moriondo M, De Vitis E, et al. PCV13 serotype decrease in Italian adolescents and adults in the post-PCV13 era: herd protection from children or secular trend? Vaccine. 2017;35:1544–50.
34. Regev-Yochay G, Paran Y, Bishara J, et al. Early impact of PCV7/PCV13 sequential introduction to the national pediatric immunization plan, on adult invasive pneumococcal disease: a nationwide surveillance study. Vaccine. 2015;33:1135–42.
35. Regev-Yochay G, Katzir M, Strahilevitz J, et al. The herd effects of infant PCV7/PCV13 sequential implementation on adult invasive pneumococcal disease, six years post implementation; a nationwide study in Israel. Vaccine. 2017;35:2449–56.
36. Simonsen L, Taylor RJ, Schuck-Paim C, et al. Effect of 13-valent pneumococcal conjugate vaccine on admissions to hospital 2 years after its introduction in the USA: a time series analysis. Lancet Respir Med. 2014;2:387–94.
37. Waight PA, Andrews NJ, Ladhani SN, et al. Effect of the 13-valent pneumococcal conjugate vaccine on invasive pneumococcal disease in England and Wales 4 years after its introduction: an observational cohort study. Lancet Infect Dis. 2015;15:535–43.

22

Rationale and methods of a randomized controlled trial of immunogenicity, safety and impact on carriage of pneumococcal conjugate and polysaccharide vaccines in infants in Papua New Guinea

Deborah Lehmann[1*], Wendy Kirarock[2], Anita H. J. van den Biggelaar[1*], Megan Passey[3], Peter Jacoby[1], Gerard Saleu[2], Geraldine Masiria[2], Birunu Nivio[2], Andrew Greenhill[1,2,4], Tilda Orami[2], Jacinta Francis[2], Rebecca Ford[2], Lea-Ann Kirkham[1,5], Vela Solomon[2], Peter C. Richmond[1,5], William S. Pomat[1,2] and for the 10v13v PCV trial team

Abstract

Background: Children in third-world settings including Papua New Guinea (PNG) experience early onset of carriage with a broad range of pneumococcal serotypes, resulting in a high incidence of severe pneumococcal disease and deaths in the first 2 years of life. Vaccination trials in high endemicity settings are needed to provide evidence and guidance on optimal strategies to protect children in these settings against pneumococcal infections.

Methods: This report describes the rationale, objectives, methods, study population, follow-up and specimen collection for a vaccination trial conducted in an endemic and logistically challenging setting in PNG. The trial aimed to determine whether currently available pneumococcal conjugate vaccines (PCV) are suitable for use under PNG's accelerated immunization schedule, and that a schedule including pneumococcal polysaccharide vaccine (PPV) in later infancy is safe and immunogenic in this high-risk population.

Results: This open randomized-controlled trial was conducted between November 2011 and March 2016, enrolling 262 children aged 1 month between November 2011 and April 2014. The participants were randomly allocated (1:1) to receive 10-valent PCV (10vPCV) or 13-valent PCV (13vPCV) in a 1-2-3-month schedule, with further randomization to receive PPV or no PPV at age 9 months, followed by a 1/5th PPV challenge at age 23 months. A total of 1229 blood samples were collected to measure humoral and cellular immune responses and 1238 nasopharyngeal swabs to assess upper respiratory tract colonization and carriage load. Serious adverse events were monitored throughout the study. Of the 262 children enrolled, 87% received 3 doses of PCV, 79% were randomized to receive PPV or no PPV at age 9 months, and 67% completed the study at 24 months of age with appropriate immunization and challenge.

(Continued on next page)

* Correspondence: Deborah.Lehmann@telethonkids.org.au; Anita.vandenbiggelaar@telethonkids.org.au
[1]Telethon Kids Institute, University of Western Australia, 100 Roberts Road, Subiaco, WA 6008, Australia
Full list of author information is available at the end of the article

(Continued from previous page)

Conclusion: Laboratory testing of the many samples collected during this trial will determine the impact of the different vaccine schedules and formulations on nasopharyngeal carriage, antibody production and function, and immune memory. The final data will inform policy on pneumococcal vaccine schedules in countries with children at high risk of pneumococcal disease by providing direct comparison of an accelerated schedule of 10vPCV and 13vPCV and the potential advantages of PPV following PCV immunization.

Trial registration: ClinicalTrials.gov CTN NCT01619462, retrospectively registered on May 28, 2012

Keywords: Pneumococcal, Vaccine, PCV, PPV, Pneumococcal conjugate vaccine, Pneumococcal polysaccharide vaccine, Papua New Guinea, Randomized controlled trial, RCT

Background

An estimated 921,000 children die annually from pneumonia, with the majority of deaths occurring in third-world countries [1]. *Streptococcus pneumoniae* (pneumococcus) is the leading cause of pneumonia deaths in children under 5 years, being responsible for approximately 400,000 of these deaths annually [2]. The pneumococcus is also a leading cause of meningitis, septicemia and otitis media. Infants are at greatest risk of dying from pneumococcal disease [1].

In Papua New Guinea (PNG), acute lower respiratory infection (ALRI) is the most common reason for hospitalization and cause of death in children [3, 4] and the burden of invasive pneumococcal disease (IPD) remains high. In a 7-valent pneumococcal conjugate vaccine (7vPCV) trial that we conducted between 2005–2009 in the Asaro Valley, Eastern Highlands Province (the site of this study), the overall incidence rate of ALRI before age 18 months in 109 controls was 1175/1000 person-years; there were 62 episodes of moderate or severe ALRI (incidence rate 439/1000 person-years), 27% of which occurred between 10 and 18 months of age [5]. In the same trial, the estimated incidence rate of IPD in the first year of life was 4762/100,000 per annum (95% CI 1936–9665), approximately 100 times the rates reported in European infants [6]. Upper respiratory tract (URT) pneumococcal carriage starts within weeks of birth in PNG (median age of acquisition is 19 days) [7] and is persistent throughout early childhood, with average pneumococcal carriage rates of 70–80% from age 3 months to 5 years [8, 9]. Moreover, the distribution of pneumococcal serotypes in PNG is broad: in our 7vPCV trial more than 60 different pneumococcal serotypes were identified in the URT of infants followed from birth until 18 months of age, of which 53 were identified in the first month of life [8, 9]. Only 43% of pneumococcal carriage isolates among controls who had not received PCV would have been covered by 13vPCV [8].

Vaccines for pneumococcal disease

Protection against IPD is by circulating opsonophagocytic IgG antibodies binding to capsular polysaccharides, which determine serotype. More than 90 different pneumococcal serotypes have been identified to date. The recognition that immunity correlated with anti-capsular antibodies led to the development of multivalent polysaccharide vaccines [10, 11]. However, polysaccharides are T-cell independent antigens and therefore the pneumococcal polysaccharide vaccine (PPV) is poorly immunogenic in infants and does not induce immune memory [12, 13]. Pneumococcal conjugate vaccines (PCV) containing polysaccharide antigens of individual serotypes covalently bound to protein carriers, hence transforming polysaccharides into T-cell dependent antigens, became available in 2000. In contrast to PPV, PCVs induce immunological memory and serum antibodies with a strong opsonophagocytic capacity in infants [14, 15] and they are effective in preventing vaccine serotype-associated IPD, pneumonia and mortality in high-risk infants [16–19]. Furthermore, PCVs reduce URT carriage of vaccine serotypes in vaccinated children, thus interrupting circulation of vaccine serotypes in the community, which in turn reduces IPD incidence in unvaccinated individuals through herd immunity [20].

The Global Alliance for Vaccines and Immunization (Gavi) and the World Health Organization (WHO) committed to the introduction of PCVs for infants in Gavi-eligible countries (including PNG). Two PCVs are currently available: i) 10-valent PCV (10vPCV, Synflorix®, GlaxoSmith Kline [GSK], Belgium) containing serotypes 1, 4, 5, 6B, 7F, 9 V, 14, 18C, 19F & 23F; and ii) 13-valent PCV (13vPCV, Prevenar 13®, Pfizer, United States of America [USA]) containing serotypes 3, 6A and 19A in addition to the 10 serotypes in 10vPCV. Both vaccines have been shown to prevent vaccine serotype-associated IPD in high-risk populations [18, 19].

10vPCV also contains non-typeable *Haemophilus influenzae* (NTHi) Protein D as a carrier, which may offer protection against NTHi disease [21]. NTHi was frequently isolated in lung aspirates from children with pneumonia in PNG [22], is a predominant cause of otitis media worldwide [23], and has also been reported as a cause of invasive disease [24–27].

Policy on choice of PCV in low- and middle-income countries has been hampered by the lack of data comparing the two vaccines in high-risk infants. While the three additional serotypes included in 13vPCV improve coverage for prevention of pneumococcal disease, the potential benefits of protection against NTHi-related pneumonia and otitis media by 10vPCV need to be considered [19, 21, 28–30].

The broad range of serotypes causing IPD in PNG and other high-risk populations means that even 13vPCV provides limited coverage (50–70%) against IPD [31–34]. There are also concerns that serotype replacement is more likely to occur in high-risk populations, similar to what was reported for native Alaskan infants after 7vPCV introduction [35].

Despite limited immunogenicity in infants, PPV given to PNG children aged 6 months to 5 years of age has been shown to reduce mortality and severe morbidity due to ALRI [36, 37], with an age-related maturation of IgG responses correlating with efficacy data [38]. Therefore, in high-risk infants, priming with PCV followed by a single dose of PPV in later infancy could potentially increase protection against IPD, particularly for serotypes such as type 2 that is an important cause of meningitis but is not covered by either PCV [31, 39]. This strategy also has the potential to improve duration of protection and reduce the risk of serotype replacement disease compared to PCV alone.

A study in Fiji raised concerns on PPV immunization in young children by reporting that children primed with 7vPCV in infancy followed by a dose of PPV at 12 months of age failed to further boost the already high antibody titres following challenge with 1/5th of a normal PPV dose 5 months later. However, serotype-specific IgG responses in these children did not decline and were robust with high avidity and opsonic functional activity suggesting protective responses [40, 41]. Follow-up of the Fijian study participants at pre-school age showed that serotype-specific antibody levels were similar in those who had and those who had not received PPV at age 12 months, implying that there was no evidence of long-term hyporesponsiveness at pre-school age [42].

In the 7vPCV trial PPV was found to be immunogenic when given at age 9 months to PNG infants previously primed with 3 doses of PCV [5], and antibody titres to PCV and non-PCV serotypes rose in response to a 1/5th PPV challenge dose at age 3–4 years. These data further contribute to the evidence that long-lasting deleterious effects of PPV immunization in infancy are unlikely [43]. Limitations of the 7vPCV trial were the relatively long time interval between receipt of PPV at 9 months and assessment of response to challenge at 3–4 years of age, and that the study did not include a group of children who had received PCV with no PPV. To determine whether priming of high-risk infants with PCV followed by a single dose of PPV in later infancy could be a preferred strategy to increase serotype coverage for IPD, without compromising both short- and long-term protective immune responses, a randomized controlled trial including a control group not receiving PPV is required.

Rationale for the present study

This head-to-head randomized trial aims to demonstrate that 10vPCV and 13vPCV are suitable vaccines for use under PNG's accelerated immunization schedule by comparing the safety and immunogenicity of 10vPCV with that of 13vPCV in a 1-2-3-month schedule with and without a PPV booster at 9 months of age. This is important for the following reasons:

- With support from Gavi, an increasing number of low-resource countries are introducing PCV into routine immunization schedules, with a comparable number of 10vPCV and 13vPCV doses being used.
- At the time of the primary schedule of this trial, PCV had not been introduced into PNG and no data were available directly comparing the safety and immunogenicity of these two vaccines in a high-risk population such as PNG. While PNG infants have been receiving 13vPCV since 2014 (after completion of the primary schedule for this trial), it remains important to determine the safety and immunogenicity of 10vPCV should there be a shortage in the supply of 13vPCV or if future research shows that 10vPCV protects against NTHi disease.
- There are limited data on the immunogenicity of PCVs in children with very early onset of dense URT pneumococcal and NTHi carriage.
- The Expanded Program on Immunization (EPI) schedule is accelerated in PNG (ages 1, 2 and 3 months); neither 10vPCV nor 13vPCV13 have been evaluated under this schedule.
- Given the broad range of serotypes causing disease in PNG and in other high-risk populations, it is important to investigate the safety and immunogenicity of a booster dose of PPV at age 9 months following priming with PCV.
- Data are lacking on PCV-induced functional antibody responses and 10vPCV-induced NTHi Protein D antibody responses in populations with high URT carriage rates from a young age.
- While there is evidence that PCV impacts on vaccine serotype-specific URT pneumococcal carriage in high-risk settings [44, 45], there are limited data on the potential impact on carriage density in these settings.

Study objectives

The overarching aim of the study is to ensure that the PCVs under investigation are suitable for use under PNG's accelerated immunization schedule, and that a schedule including PPV in later infancy is safe and immunogenic in this high-risk population.

The primary objectives of this study are to:

1. Determine the safety and reactogenicity up to 24 months of age of 10vPCV and 13vPCV given in the accelerated 1-2-3-month PNG schedule;
2. Evaluate serotype-specific serum IgG and functional antibody responses at 4 and 9 months of age following completion of 3 doses of 10vPCV or 13vPCV, and antibody persistence and IgG avidity maturation at 23 months of age;
3. Compare serotype-specific serum IgG titres, functional antibody responses and circulating memory B-cells at 10 months of age and the persistence of these responses at 23 months of age in children primed with 10vPCV or 13vPCV who did or did not receive PPV at 9 months of age;
4. Assess the persistence of B-cell memory by measuring circulating vaccine serotype-specific memory B-cells, IgG and opsonophagocytic antibody responses and IgG avidity maturation 1 month after challenge at 23 months with 1/5th of a normal PPV dose in children who did or did not receive PPV at 9 months of age; and
5. Compare the relative impact of 10vPCV and 13vPCV on pneumococcal (total and vaccine type) and NTHi carriage rates and bacterial load up to 2 years of age and the effect of a PPV booster.

Secondary objectives of this study are to:

1. Compare development of IgG responses to NTHi Protein D between infants receiving 10vPCV and those receiving 13vPCV; and
2. Describe the frequency of pneumonia and otitis media with perforation associated with pneumococcal vaccine serotypes and/or NTHi isolated from the nasopharynx and/or middle ear discharge.

Methods

The following paragraphs describe the methods used for enrolment, clinical follow-up and specimen collection and storage.

Study design and location

Between November 2011 and March 2016, we conducted an open randomized controlled trial of safety and immunogenicity of 13vPCV and 10vPCV given in an accelerated 1-2-3-month schedule, with further randomization of children in each PCV group to receive PPV or no PPV at age 9 months, followed by a 1/5th challenge dose of PPV to all children at age 23 months. The study was conducted in Goroka Town and villages located within an hour's drive from Goroka in the Eastern Highlands Province of PNG. Goroka is the provincial capital (population ~25,000; altitude 1600 m) and the PNG Institute of Medical Research (PNGIMR) laboratories and clinic are adjacent to Eastern Highlands Provincial Hospital (EHPH), the only tertiary hospital in the area. Outside the urban area, people live in villages often accessible only by 4WD vehicles. Living standards vary widely between urban, peri-urban and rural settings.

Ethical considerations

Ethical approval was obtained from the PNG Medical Research Advisory Committee (#11.03) and PNGIMR Institutional Review Board (#1028). The study was conducted according to Declaration of Helsinki International Conference on Harmonisation Good Clinical Practice (ICH-GCP) and local ethical guidelines. The study is registered with ClinicalTrials.gov (CTN NCT01619462).

Recruitment, assent and consent process

Prior to starting the study, field staff visited communities around Goroka Town and surrounding villages to explain the study to community members and seek their willingness to participate in the trial. Pregnant women were invited by research nurses and health extension officers (HEOs) to take part in the study during these field visits or when women attended the PNGIMR clinic. Local drivers who were familiar to and respected by the local communities played an important role in introducing the study team to the communities. Assent was sought from pregnant women and their husbands, contact details were recorded and information sheets were provided. Women who had assented were seen again close to their expected delivery date or when they presented of their own accord at the PNGIMR clinic after delivery. Informed consent was sought at time of enrolment of the child.

Inclusion criteria for infants to be enrolled in the study were:

- Aged 28–35 days;
- Resident within 1 h drive from Goroka town; and
- Intending to remain in the study area for at least 2 years.

Exclusion criteria were:

- Birth weight < 2000 g;
- Severe congenital abnormality;
- Mother or child known to be positive for Human Immunodeficiency Virus (HIV); or
- Unable to or did not provide consent.

Study vaccines

A single dose (0.5 mL) of 10vPCV (Synflorix®, GSK, Belgium, batches ASPNA0099AB, ASPNA267DD) contains 1 μg of each pneumococcal polysaccharide for serotypes 1, 5, 6B, 7F, 9 V, 14 and 23F and 3 μg of serotype 4, each conjugated to Protein D of NTHi and 3 μg of serotypes 18C and 19F conjugated to tetanus and diphtheria toxoids, respectively. One dose (0.5 ml) of 13vPCV (Prevenar 13®, Pfizer, USA, batch numbers F36226, G71540) contains 2.2 μg of pneumococcal purified capsular polysaccharides for serotypes 1, 3, 4, 5, 6A, 7F, 9 V, 14, 18C, 19A, 19F and 23F, and 4.4 μg of pneumococcal purified capsular polysaccharides for serotype 6B and 0.125 mg aluminium adjuvant. Each serotype is individually conjugated to non-toxic diphtheria CRM_{197} protein.

Each 0.5 mL dose of PPV (Pneumovax®23 Merck & Co, USA, batch numbers T0861, V1200, K006913) contains 25 μg of purified capsular polysaccharides of each of serotypes 1, 2, 3, 4, 5, 6B, 7F, 8, 9 N, 9 V, 10A, 11A, 12F, 14, 15B, 17F, 18C, 19F, 19A, 20, 22F, 23F and 33F and 0.25% phenol preservative.

Enrolment, randomization, vaccination and follow-up

Children who met the eligibility criteria were randomized at 1 month of age to receive 10vPCV or 13vPCV using a computer-generated random number list. This assignment was specified inside a sealed envelope with the next sequential number and kept in the participant's personal folder. Throughout the study laboratory staff was blinded to the group allocation. The vaccine and specimen collection schedules are shown in Table 1. Prior to any vaccination (and PPV challenge at age 23 months), study nurses/HEOs obtained a medical history and examined children to exclude contraindications for vaccination (including temperature ≥ 38 °C, anaphylaxis to previous vaccination, serious neurological illness within 48 h of previous pentavalent vaccine) and specimens were collected. Routine childhood vaccines (including pentavalent whole-cell pertussis, diphtheria, tetanus, Hepatitis B and *Haemophilus influenzae* type B

Table 1 Vaccination and specimen collection schedule

Age	Birth	1 m	2 m	3 m	4 m	6 m	9 m	10 m	23 m	24 m
Vaccinations										
BCG[a]	✓									
HepB[a]	✓									
Pentavalent		✓	✓	✓						
PCV[b]		✓	✓	✓						
OPV		✓	✓	✓						
Measles						✓	✓			
PPV[b]							✓			
1/5th challenge dose PPV									✓	
Specimen collection										
NPS		✓			✓		✓	✓	✓	✓
Blood - Serum		✓			✓		✓	✓	✓	✓
Blood - PBMC					✓		✓	✓	✓	✓
Morbidity surveillance[c]		—	—	—	—	—	—	—	—	→

BCG Bacillus Calmette-Guérin vaccine; *HepB* Hepatitis B vaccine; Pentavalent is a diphtheria, tetanus, whole cell pertussis, *Haemophilus influenzae* type B, Hepatitis B combination vaccine; *PCV* 10-valent or 13-valent pneumococcal conjugate vaccine; *OPV* oral polio vaccine; *PPV* 23-valent pneumococcal polysaccharide vaccine; *NPS* nasopharyngeal swab; *PBMC* peripheral blood mononuclear cells

[a]Birth doses of BCG and Hepatitis B were given by hospital nurses before enrolment of infants into the study

[b]PCV and PPV are study vaccines while the other vaccines were routine EPI vaccines in PNG at the time of the trial

[c]Morbidity surveillance was conducted throughout the duration of the trial. Vitamin A was given at 6 and 9 months of age

(Hib) vaccine and oral polio vaccine; see Table 1) were administered by the study HEOs/nurses at 1, 2, and 3 months of age, together with the 10vPCV or 13vPCV study vaccines. Information on birth doses of Bacillus Calmette-Guérin (BCG) vaccine and Hepatitis B vaccines administered by hospital staff was collected from hospital records, as were birth weights. At the initial visit mothers were given a follow-up card on which dates for future visits were recorded. Children living in rural areas were generally transported to and from the clinic while urban residents were either brought in or came of their own accord to the clinic following a reminder by mobile phone. At age 4 months children attended the clinic for specimen collection only. At age 6 months, children received their first dose of measles vaccine and a dose of Vitamin A either at the PNGIMR clinic or at other child health clinics. At age 9 months children received a second dose of measles vaccine and Vitamin A, and were randomized within each PCV group to receive or not receive PPV. The PPV group allocation was assigned at enrolment, at the same time as PCV randomization, but kept in an unopened envelope until the 9-month visit. Specimens were collected before vaccination and again 4 weeks later.

All participants were given a 1/5th challenge dose of PPV at age 23 months with specimens collected immediately before the challenge and 4 weeks later. All vaccinations were documented in the child's health book held by the mother/guardian and also written on the child's follow-up card, which was stored electronically. Photocopies of records in the parent-held books (which include information on any illness episode) were stored in the child's personal folder.

Every effort was made to locate participants for follow-up in a timely manner. Between 10 and 23 months, nurses and field staff attempted to contact participants' caregivers at least twice to find out about any intervening illness and changes in address. Children were withdrawn from the study if the child could not be located on 3 home visits or information had been obtained from relatives that the family had moved out of the study area permanently, or if parents withdrew their consent for continuation in the study. Children were also withdrawn by the investigators following a protocol violation.

Monitoring for adverse reactions

Following each vaccination, children were observed at the clinic for 1 h for immediate local and systemic reactions and generally taken home by the study team. This helped locate participants for subsequent visits. Study nurses/HEOs visited children at home 24–48 h post-vaccination to assess local or systemic side effects and they provided treatment as required.

Specimen collection

A nasopharyngeal swab (NPS) to assess pneumococcal and NTHi carriage and bacterial load was collected at ages 1, 4, 9, 10, 23 and 24 months (Table 1) as previously described [8] except that a flocked swab (Copan Diagnostics, USA) was used. NPS samples were placed in skim-milk-tryptone-glucose-glycerol broth (STGGB) and stored at −80 °C within 2 h of collection. Culture and pneumococcal serotyping were conducted at PNGIMR as previously described [8]. Aliquots from the stored NPS were sent in liquid nitrogen to the University of Western Australia to measure bacterial load. If middle ear discharge was seen, a flocked swab was used to collect and store the purulent discharge in STGGB for culture, identification and characterisation of bacterial pathogens [8].

Venous blood samples (up to 3 mL) for *serum* collection were collected at ages 1, 4, 9, 10, 23 and 24 months (Table 1) to measure pneumococcal serotype-specific IgG antibody titres [5], IgG avidity [46], opsonophagocytic antibody titres [47], and NTHi Protein D-specific IgG antibody levels [48]. No more than 3 attempts to collect blood were undertaken at a single time point. On occasions when parents agreed, a further attempt at blood collection was undertaken a few days later. Serum samples were aliquoted and stored at −80 °C. Serotype-specific IgG antibody responses were measured at PNGIMR using a WHO standardized pneumococcal enzyme-linked immunosorbent assay (ELISA) [49]. Serum aliquots were sent in liquid nitrogen to the University of Western Australia (UWA) to conduct functional pneumococcal antibody assays and NTHi protein D antibody assays.

From age 4 months onwards, at each routine follow-up visit, we aimed to collect 2–7 mL of heparinized venous blood samples to isolate peripheral blood mononuclear cells (PBMCs) to measure pneumococcal serotype-specific B-cell responses and pneumococcal protein-specific T-cell responses as shown in Table 1 [50]. After immediate processing at PNGIMR, PBMCs were cryopreserved and sent in batches in liquid nitrogen vapour phase to UWA.

Detailed laboratory methods will be reported elsewhere with laboratory results.

Morbidity surveillance

Passive morbidity surveillance was conducted. Parents were encouraged to attend the PNGIMR clinic if their child was unwell. Generally parents liked to bring their children directly to the PNGIMR clinic as they were seen faster than at routine outpatient clinics, they knew the staff, and were assisted with transport if required. In addition, family members other than the study child could be seen at the PNGIMR clinic for the duration of the study. Children were referred to pediatricians at EHPH as required.

The EHPH pediatric ward was also monitored for any hospitalizations of study participants. Information on any intervening illnesses was documented on a morbidity report form and in the parent-held child's health book. Children were treated according to standard management protocols in PNG [51].

ALRI was defined as mild (cough and raised respiratory rate, namely >60/min in infants less than 2 months of age, or >40/min in infants aged 2 months and older), moderate (as for mild with chest wall in-drawing), or severe (as for moderate with cyanosis or inability to feed or restlessness or heart failure). This is a slight modification from that used generally in PNG. Standard treatment protocols in PNG recommend hospitalization for all moderate or severe ALRIs.

A serious adverse event (SAE) was defined as any event requiring hospitalization or resulting in death. In 2015 there were disruptions of EHPH services. During this period an SAE was also documented for illnesses (mainly moderate ALRI cases) deemed serious enough to require hospitalization, but the children had to be treated as outpatients and were monitored closely. Blood cultures and NPS were collected when children were seen with a temperature > 38 °C or a provisional diagnosis of moderate or severe ALRI, or meningitis.

Outcomes

PCV outcome measures are:

(1) Safety and reactogenicity of 10vPCV and 13vPCV in PNG infants;
(2) Serum PCV serotype-specific IgG and opsonizing antibody geometric mean titres (GMTs), and proportions of children with serum serotype-specific IgG antibody concentrations ≥0.35 μg/mL and opsonizing titres ≥8 for PCV serotypes at 4 and 9 months of age;
(3) Serum *H. influenzae* Protein D IgG GMTs at 4 and 9 months of age;
(4) Number of circulating memory B-cells specific for PCV serotypes and PCV carrier proteins (NTHi Protein D, Tetanus Toxoid and CRM_{197}) and PCV serotype-specific IgG avidity maturation at 4 and 9 months of age;
(5) T-cell responses to PCV carrier proteins (NTHi Protein D, Tetanus Toxoid and CRM_{197}) at 4 and 9 months of age;
(6) Nasopharyngeal carriage rates of *S. pneumoniae* (vaccine and non-vaccine serotypes) and serotypeable and non-serotypeable *H. influenzae* at 1, 4 and 9 months of age;
(7) Pneumococcal and *H. influenzae* nasopharyngeal density at 1, 4 and 9 months of age; and
(8) Rates for hospitalization with ALRI or record of otitis media with perforation between 4 and 9 months of age.

PPV outcome measures are:

(1) Serum PCV and PPV serotype-specific IgG and opsonizing antibody GMTs, and proportions of children with PCV and PPV serotype-specific IgG concentrations ≥0.35 μg/mL and opsonizing titres ≥8 at 10 and 23 months of age;
(2) Number of circulating memory B-cells and IgG avidity maturation for PCV and non-PCV serotypes included in PPV at 10, 23 and 24 months of age;
(3) Nasopharyngeal carriage rates and density of serotype-specific *S. pneumoniae*, and serotypeable and non-serotypeable *H. influenzae* at 10, 23 and 24 months of age; and
(4) Rates for hospitalization with ALRI or record of otitis media with perforation between 10 and 24 months of age.

Study and data management

To ensure any problems or queries were addressed as soon as possible, investigators in PNG and Australia attended monthly teleconferences.All data collection forms were checked manually before entry into a password-protected computer file using FileMaker Pro version 11 (Santa Clara, CA, USA).

Data safety monitoring board

A data safety monitoring board (DSMB) was established, which included independent clinicians in PNG and Australia. All SAEs were reported within 24 h to an appointed Papua New Guinean Safety Monitor and the Chair of the DSMB for review, followed by a final report with outcome. The Chair of the DSMB was informed immediately when a death occurred. A quarterly report was prepared by the investigators and sent to the Chair of the DSMB and distributed to other DSMB members. This included a summary of all serious adverse events, all morbidities, protocol violations, and status of enrolment and follow-up. A teleconference with DSMB members and the study investigators was held annually.

Sample size calculations

Sample size calculations were based on an anticipated 80% follow-up rate with evaluable samples to the final visit based on results from our 7vPCV trial (87% at age 18 months) [5]. Based on the study's primary outcome, it was postulated that 90% of children would achieve serotype-specific antibody concentrations ≥0.35 μg/ml at 4 months of age for serotypes included in the PCV children were given. Based on this assumption, a sample size of 100 children (receiving 10vPCV or 13vPCV) would give us 95% confidence that the true proportion is within 6% of this level of 90%. For bacterial load analysis, previous data for *H. influenzae* bacterial loads [52] indicate that a within-group standard deviation in $\log_{10}$ bacterial load (copies/ml) of 2.0 can be expected. With a sample size of 50 in each group (after randomization into PCV and PPV group), this would give 80% power to detect a between-group difference in mean $\log_{10}$ bacterial load of 0.9. In view of the higher loss to follow-up than anticipated during the first year of the study, the total number of children to be enrolled was increased from 200 to 260.

Statistical methods

Statistical analysis is by intention to treat. All serum antibody concentrations and opsonophagocytic titres were log-transformed and geometric mean concentrations (GMC) and geometric mean titres (GMT) calculated respectively with 95% confidence intervals. To compare continuous and categorical variables between groups, Mann-Whitney tests and Pearson chi-square tests were used respectively. Spearman rank correlation analysis was used to investigate correlations between serotype-specific opsonophagocytic and IgG antibody concentrations. Linear and logistic regression models were used for further analyses examining associations between specific outcomes and different factors incorporating generalised estimating equations to take into account multiple samples from individual children. For all analyses, test outcomes were considered to be significant if the p-value is smaller or equal to 0.05.

Results

Assent and enrolment

A total of 431 women assented to having their child participate in the study, of which 265 (61%) gave their informed consent. Three children did not meet inclusion criteria (2 were overage and 1 child's mother was HIV-positive). Hence 262 children were formally enrolled into the study between 14 November 2011 and 16 April 2014, including 131 children randomized to receive 10vPCV and 131 randomized to receive 13vPCV. A flow chart (Fig. 1) shows the number of women who assented, number of infants randomized to receive one or other PCV at 1 month of age, number of children seen at subsequent visits, number of withdrawals and reasons for withdrawal according to randomization schedule.

Withdrawals

A total of 86 (33%) children were withdrawn from the study (including deaths and protocol violations), the majority before age 9 months (41% before age 3-month visit, 63% before 9-month visits) (Fig. 1). Parents withdrew their consent for 20 children (8%) (8 in 10vPCV group and 12 in 13vPCV group); 25 children (9.5%) migrated with their parents to another location (12 in 10vPCV group and 13 in 13vPCV group); and 25 children (9.5%) were recorded as lost to follow-up after at least 3 unsuccessful home visits by field staff (13 in 10vPCV group and 12 in 13vPCV group). Of the children lost to follow up, two-thirds could not be located within 2 months of enrolment, while approximately one-third of those who migrated out of the study area did so before age 4 months. Approximately two-thirds of parents who withdrew consent did so before the 4-month visit. None of the withdrawals were related to an adverse event.

There were 7 deaths, none of which were related to any vaccination (4 in the 10vPCV group and 3 in the 13vPCV group). Documented causes of death, age at death and PCV/PPV status were as follows:

- Severe pneumonia and presumed pulmonary tuberculosis; 9 months; 13vPCV
- Blood dyscrasia, anaemia; 9 months; 10vPCV
- Moderate pneumonia, malnutrition, gastroenteritis; 15 months; 10vPCV, no PPV
- Malnutrition, anaemia, presumed pulmonary tuberculosis; 17 months; 10vPCV, no PPV
- Gastroenteritis with dehydration; 17 month; 13vPCV, PPV
- Gastroenteritis with severe dehydration; 18 months; 10vPCV, PPV
- Severe malnutrition, dysentery, anaemia; 19 months; 13vPCV, no PPV

One other child received the first dose of 13vPCV but soon after was diagnosed with a retroperitoneal tumour, at which time this child was withdrawn from the study and died at age 2 months.

There were 8 protocol violations: 3 were related to the PCV schedule (2 in the 10vPCV group, 1 in the 13vPCV group), 1 was related to PPV immunization (within the 13vPCV group) and 4 were related to the low-dose challenge at 23 months of age (1 in the 10vPCV/no PPV group, 2 in the 13vPCV/no PPV group and 1 in the 13vPCV/PPV group).

Follow-up of study participants

Of the 262 children enrolled in the study who received PCV at age 1 month, 93% received 2 doses of PCV and 87% received 3 doses of PCV. At age 9 months 79% of enrolled children were randomized to receive PPV or no PPV; 77% of the 262 children were seen at the 10 month visit; 69% at 23 months; and 67% completed the study at 24 months of age with appropriate immunization and challenge. Follow-up was similar for the different PCV/PPV groups.

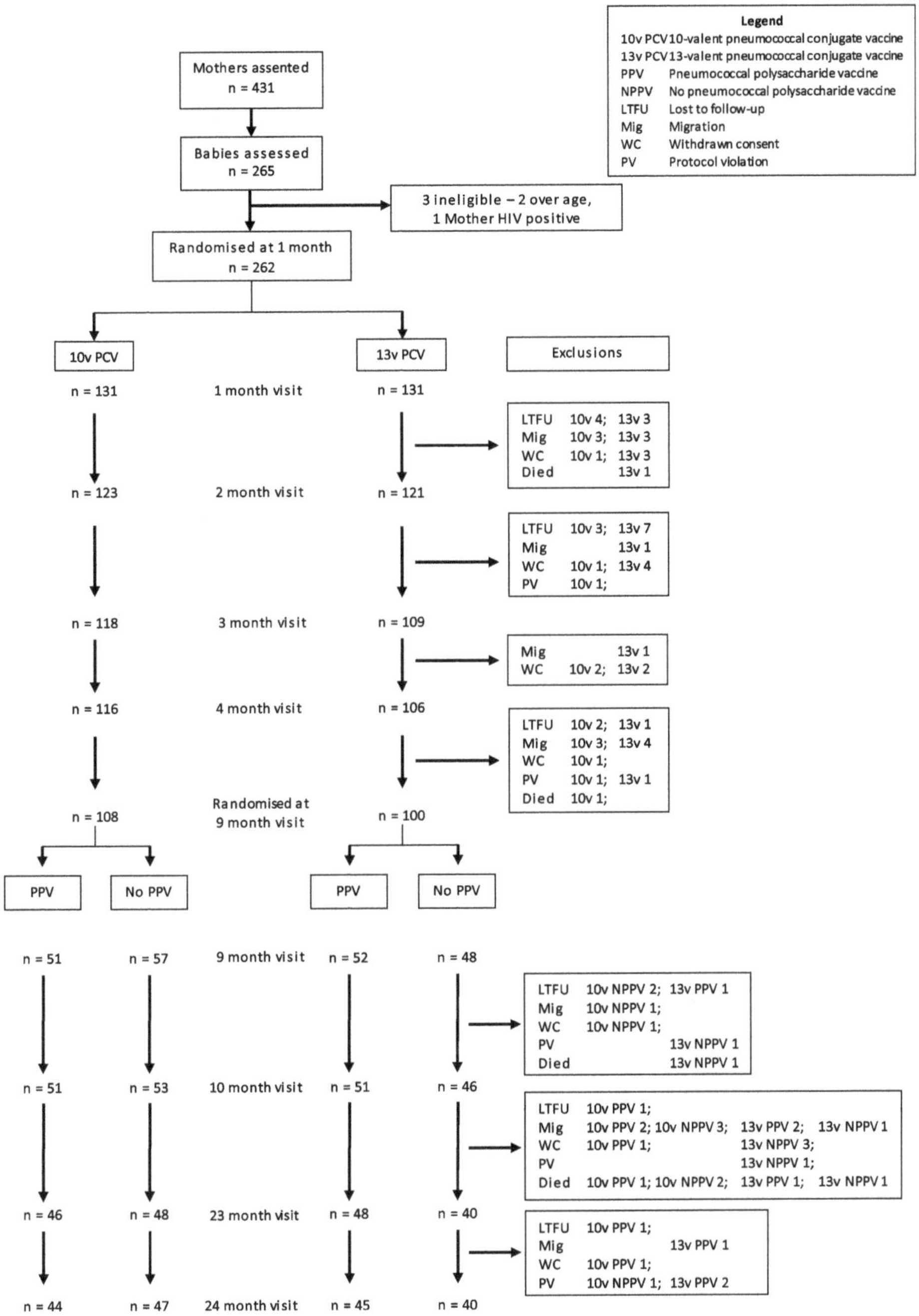

Fig. 1 flow chart

Table 2 shows that children received PCV and PPV in a timely manner with no difference in age at vaccination and follow-up between groups. The table also shows the gender distribution and average body weight according to PCV/PPV group at different time points. There were no differences between the groups.

Specimen collection

NPS and venous blood samples for serum collection were successfully obtained from more than 96% of attendees at different ages, while PBMCs were successfully isolated from 64 to 69% of blood samples (Table 3). On 4 occasions parents declined blood collection from their children.

Discussion

To our knowledge, our study is the only trial directly comparing safety and immunogenicity of two different PCVs followed by a PPV booster dose. A trial in The

Table 2 Description of study population according to randomization groups

	10vPCV		13vPCV	
Number enrolled	131		131	
Male, number (%) at enrolment	66 (50%)		72 (55%)	
Age (days) at study visits				
Visit 1 m/PCV1, mean ± sd	30.9 ± 2.5 (*n* = 131)		31.0 ± 2.2 (*n* = 131)	
(Min-Max)	(25–39)		(27–40)	
Visit 2 m/PCV2, mean ± sd	61.6 ± 3.4 (*n* = 122)		61.9 ± 4.0 (*n* = 121)	
(Min-Max)	(55–77)		(56–84)	
Visit 3 m/PCV3, mean ± sd	94.0 ± 7.8 (*n* = 119)		92.5 ± 4.4 (*n* = 109)	
(Min-Max)	(84–134)		(84–112)	
Weight (kg)				
Birth weight, mean ± sd	3.4 ± (*n* = 97)		3.3 ± (*n* = 105)	
(Min-Max)	(2.2–4.5)		(2.3–4.5)	
Visit 1 m, mean ± sd	4.4 ± 0.7 (*n* = 127)		4.3 ± 0.5 (*n* = 126)	
(Min-Max)	(2.5–6.1)		(2.7–5.7)	
Visit 2 m, mean ± sd	5.3 ± 0.7 (*n* = 122)		5.3 ± 0.7 (*n* = 120)	
(Min-Max)	(3.4–6.8)		(2.9–7.2)	
Visit 3 m, mean ± sd	6.1 ± 0.9 (*n* = 114)		6.0 ± 0.8 (*n* = 108)	
(Min-Max)	(4.0–8.5)		(4.1–8.1)	
	10vPCV		13vPCV	
	No PPV	PPV	No PPV	PPV
Number followed-up at 9 months	57	51	48	52
Male, number (%) at 9 months	29 (51%)	24 (43%)	26 (54%)	29 (54%)
Age (months)				
Visit 9 m, mean ± sd	9.2 ± 0.7 (*n* = 57)	9.5 ± 1.2 (*n* = 51)	9.06 ± 0.2 (*n* = 48)	9.2 ± 0.5 (*n* = 52)
(Min-Max)	(8.2–13.1)	(8.9–14.4)	(8.6–9.9)	(8.9–11.9)
Visit 23 m, mean ± sd	23.4 ± 0.8 (*n* = 47)	23.3 ± 0.6 (*n* = 46)	23.3 ± 0.8 (*n* = 40)	23.3 ± 0.7 (*n* = 46)
(Min-Max)	(22.1–27.1)	(22.9–26.3)	(22.9–26.5)	(22.6–26.0)
Visit 24 m, mean ± sd	24.5 ± 1.0 (*n* = 47)	24.6 ± 0.9 (*n* = 44)	24.4 ± 0.8 (*n* = 40)	24.5 ± 1.1 (*n* = 45)
(Min-Max)	(23.2–28.1)	(23.9–27.9)	(23.9–30.1)	(23.7–30.1)
Weight (kg)				
Visit 9 m, mean ± sd	8.4 ± 1.1 (*n* = 53)	8.1 ± 1.3 (*n* = 51)	8.1 ± 0.8 (*n* = 45)	8.0 ± 0.9 (*n* = 52)
(Min-Max)	(6.5–11.2)	(6.3–14.0)	(6.5–10.4)	(6.6–10.5)
Visit 23 m, mean ± sd	11.3 ± 1.2 (*n* = 44)	10.7 ± 1.4 (*n* = 42)	10.9 ± 1.3 (*n* = 38)	11.0 ± 1.5 (*n* = 37)
(Min-Max)	(9.7–14.0)	(7.7–14.0)	(8.8–14.0)	(8.9–15.0)
Visit 24 m, mean ± sd	11.7 ± 1.5 (*n* = 44)	11.3 ± 1.4 (*n* = 40)	11.3 ± 1.2 (*n* = 35)	11.17 ± 1.4 (*n* = 42)
(Min-Max)	(8.9–15.0)	(8.1–14.0)	(9.0–14.0)	(9.0–15.0)

Gambia directly compared safety and immunogenicity of 10vPCV and 13vPCV as part of a larger trial of new experimental pneumococcal protein-based vaccines, but did not include a PPV booster [53]. Two other trials comparing different schedules of the two PCVs are underway, one in Vietnam (NCT01953510) and another in Australian Aboriginal children (ACTRN12610000544077 and NCT01174849).

Study strengths and limitations

Despite logistical difficulties in conducting the study in urban and rural areas of the Eastern Highlands Province of PNG, a large enough number of samples were successfully collected to address study outcomes. Two-thirds of those enrolled in this study were fully followed up to 2 years of age, with sera and NPS collected at >1200 routine visits and high numbers of PBMCs (Table 3) isolated

Table 3 Number of collected specimens (% of participants seen at specified age), blood volumes and PBMCs[a] isolated at study visits

Age	1 month	4 months	9 months	10 months	23 months	24 months
Study participants[b]	262	222	208	201	182	176
Nasopharyngeal swabs	262 (100%)	215 (97%)	205 (99%)	199 (99%)	182 (100%)	175 (99%)
Blood (serum)	262 (100%)	213 (96%)	201 (97%)	196 (98%)	182 (100%)	175 (99%)
Mean volume (mL)	1.8	2.3	2.3	2.2	2.4	2.3
(Min-Max)	(0.1–5.0)	(0.2–5.0)	(0.2–5.0)	(0.1–4.0)	(0.5–4.0)	(0.3–4.0)
Blood (PBMCs[a])	–	142 (64%)	143 (69%)	128 (64%)	126 (69%)	119 (68%)
Mean volume (mL)	–	1.9	2.0	1.9	1.9	1.8
(Min-Max)		(0.1–4.5)	(0.5–4.0)	(0.4–4)	(0.3–4.0)	(0.3–3.0)
Mean number of cells $\times 10^6$ *(95% CI)*		8.5 (7.3–9.6)	10.1 (8.8–11.4)	9.4 (8.3–10.4)	8.7 (7.5–9.8)	8.8 (7.7–10.0)

[a]Peripheral blood mononuclear cells [b]Numbers exclude those who did not meet inclusion criteria and those who were lost to follow-up or withdrawn

from 658 blood samples from age 4 months onwards. This is a reflection of the long-established relationship and trust between the community and PNGIMR staff, in addition to the perseverance of field staff in locating participants.

The two-stage process of assent followed by formal consent was important, allowing parents to discuss their participation with family members. Providing medical treatment to participants and their families and close follow-up in the event of illness was appreciated and a motivation to take part in the study. In addition, all study children received hand-knitted sweaters donated by Australian volunteers, and at the end of the study parents received a certificate of participation with a photograph of their child.

Every vaccination entailed at least three trips to communities (pick-up and drop-off, and 24–48 h follow-up visit), with additional visits needed if not located the first time. Roads were at times impassable and locals repairing roads sometimes charged a 'toll'. In 2012 there were national elections and some families returned to their home villages outside the study area to vote and did not return. Furthermore, disputes between supporters of rival candidates at times restricted movement in the study area.

Despite every effort, approximately one-third of participants did not complete the study. This is in part the result of increasing mobility of the population: 10% of participants migrated out of the area during this study compared with 5% during the earlier 7vPCV study conducted between 2005 and 2009 [54]. Loss to follow-up and withdrawal of consent tended to occur at a young age, similar to the 7vPCV study [54]. In some cases, husbands had not been part of the assent and consent processes and subsequently indicated they did not want their children to participate in the study. While every effort was made to provide full information about what the study entailed, mothers may on further reflection have had doubts about taking part in the study. Some parents were concerned about the volume of blood that was being collected from their child. Collecting blood samples from young children was sometimes difficult, though the nurses/HEOs did not persevere if the child or parent was distressed.

Having a Papua New Guinean doctor to oversee the clinical activities and train nurses and HEOs was a great advantage and much appreciated by parents. When the study doctor left a year and a half into the study to pursue pediatric training, a succession of three competent HEOs oversaw the field and clinical activities. However, these staff changes reduced continuity over the course of the study.

In contrast to laboratory staff who were blinded to the vaccine randomization, study nurses were not blinded due to the limited number of nurses/HEOs available to administer vaccines and conduct follow-ups. However, whenever possible, different nurse/HEOs administered vaccines to those assessing reactogenicity. It is acknowledged that this could potentially impact on the interpretation of clinical outcomes, but cannot affect the primary immunogenicity outcomes.

Despite the launch of the 13vPCV program in PNG in 2014, vaccine was not available in the EHP until 2015 and has been introduced slowly since: coverage with one dose of 13vPCV was only around 25% and with three doses around 5% in late 2015 in the study area [55]. Herd protection following launch of the PNG 13vPCV program in PNG in late 2014 is therefore unlikely to have impacted on the results of the present study.

Notably, there were no deaths among study participants due to uncomplicated pneumonia in a country where pneumonia remains the most common cause of childhood death [3]. This is attributed to all study children receiving both pneumococcal and Hib vaccines and close monitoring of study participants when they were sick. While morbidity among study participants will be reported fully elsewhere, 2 of the 3 cases of culture-proven pneumococcal bacteraemia were due to non-PCV serotypes and the third child with a PCV serotype-related bacteraemia had only received one dose of PCV at the time of death [56]. The mean age at death was older than previously recorded [57], with 5 of the 8 deaths occurring in the second year of life. While a diagnosis of pulmonary tuberculosis was assigned for two children who died, these were not laboratory-confirmed. The emergence of malnutrition as an important cause of death in PNG has been highlighted elsewhere [58]. This may be related to undiagnosed tuberculosis, which was previously rare in the highlands of PNG, overall poverty, or a reflection of societal challenges including unwanted pregnancies [59, 60] and associated neglect of children [61]. Finally, infants with a birth weight of less than 2000 g were excluded as low birth weight was used as a surrogate marker for prematurity, which may affect immune responses to vaccines including PCVs [62], as well as that prematurity is hard to assess in this setting. As is true for randomized clinical trials in general, field studies conducted post-implementation may find different results in individuals due to the influence of various external factors. However, the authors believe that the results for 10vPCV and 13vPCV immunogenicity and safety are largely generalizable to newborns in PNG and other settings where pneumococcal infections are highly endemic.

Conclusions

The introduction of PCV in high-risk settings facilitated by Gavi is likely to have a significant impact on the burden of IPD, although the high proportion of pneumococcal disease due to non-vaccine serotypes raises concerns with regard to serotype replacement. The lack of data comparing PCVs has made it difficult for countries to choose the PCV likely to provide the most benefit. This study provides direct comparison of safety, immunogenicity (including functional antibody responses) and impact on carriage rates and bacterial load in a randomized controlled trial of an accelerated 3-dose schedule of 10vPCV and 13vPCV in a low-income setting. Following completion of the primary schedule in this trial without immediate concerns regarding reactogenicity and safety of either PCV, 13vPCV was introduced into the PNG EPI Program in 2014. In addition to comparison of currently available PCVs, this study will provide evidence on the potential advantages of PPV following PCV immunization in infancy in high-risk settings, including immune protection against important IPD-causing non-PCV serotypes [31, 34], boosting of immune responses against PCV serotypes to enhance long-term immunity, and will directly investigate any effects on B-cell memory. Samples collected in this cohort are currently undergoing laboratory testing to determine the impact of the different vaccine schedules and formulations on nasopharyngeal carriage, antibody production and function, and immune memory response. Assessment of antibody and T-cell responses to pneumococcal and NTHi proteins will aid an understanding of the development of natural immunity to these antigens relevant to development of protein-based vaccines. These studies will provide data to inform policy on pneumococcal vaccine schedules in countries with children at high risk of invasive pneumococcal disease.

Abbreviations

10vPCV: 10-valent pneumococcal conjugate vaccine; 13vPCV: 13-valent pneumococcal conjugate vaccine; AE: Adverse event; ALRI: Acute lower respiratory infection; BCG: Bacillus Calmette-Guérin; CSL: Commonwealth Serum Laboratories Ltd.; DSMB: Data safety monitoring board; EHPH: Eastern Highlands Provincial Hospital; ELISA: Enzyme-linked immunosorbent assay; EPI: Expanded Program on Immunization; Gavi: Global Alliance for Vaccines and Immunization; GMC: Geometric mean concentration; GMT: Geometric mean titre; HEO: Health extension officer; Hib: *Haemophilus influenzae* type B; HIV: Human Immunodeficiency Virus; ICH-GCP: International Conference on Harmonisation Good Clinical Practice; IPD: Invasive pneumococcal disease; NHMRC: National Health and Medical Research Council; NPS: Nasopharyngeal swab; NTHi: Non-typeable *Haemophilus influenzae*; PBMC: Peripheral blood mononuclear cells; PCV: Pneumococcal conjugate vaccine; PNG: Papua New Guinea; PNGIMR: PNG Institute of Medical Research; PPV: Pneumococcal polysaccharide vaccine; SAE: Serious adverse event; STGGB: Skim milk tryptone-glucose-glycerol broth; URT: Upper respiratory tract; UWA: University of Western Australia; WHO: Word Health Organization

Acknowledgements

We thank Professor John Vince (Chair) and Dr. Christopher Blyth for their support as members of the Data Safety Monitoring Board, and the Safety Monitors Drs Harry Poka and Paul Wari. We also would like to acknowledge Seqirus (formerly bioCSL) for donating Pneumovax for the study. Institutions and investigators in alphabetical order comprising the 10v13v PCV Trial team: *Papua New Guinea Institute of Medical Research:* L Bele, M Dreyam, A Elizah, R Ford, J Francis, A Gihigupa, A Greenhill, S Javati, J Kave, W Kirarock, M Lai, B Martin, G Masiria, A Michael (deceased), L Moliki, B Nagepu, M Nenikuro, B Nivio, C Opa, T Orami, WS Pomat, G Saleu, P Siba, V Solomon, S Wana, L Wawae, M Yoannes. *Eastern Highlands Provincial Hospital:* I Hwaihwanje, T Korowi, C Mond, P Wari. *Telethon Kids Institute:* P Jacoby, D Lehmann, A van den Biggelaar. *School of Paediatrics and Child Health, University of Western Australia:* K Corscadden, C de Gier, L Kirkham, T Rahman, P Richmond, R Thornton. *The University of Sydney, University Centre for Rural Health, School of Public Health Lismore:* M Passey.

Funding

This study was funded through the Papua New Guinea Institute of Medical Research Internal Competitive Research Award Scheme (ICRAS); Papua New Guinea Liquefied Natural Gas Project (a joint venture of Exxon Mobil Corporation, Oil Search, Santos, Nippon Oil, Mineral Resource Development Company and Eda Oil) and the Australian National Health and Medical Research Council (NHMRC) (APP 1087200); the Telethon Kids Institute's Wesfarmers Centre of Vaccines and Infectious Diseases provided salary support to DL and AVDB; LAK is supported by a NHMRC Career Development Fellowship (APP 1061428); MP was supported by fellowships from the NHMRC (GNT1072213) and the Cancer Institute NSW (13/ECF/1-11); Seqirus (formerly bioCSL) donated Pneumovax for the study. None of the funding bodies were involved in the design of the study and collection, analysis, and interpretation of data and in writing the manuscript.

Authors' contributions

DL, PR, and WP conceived and designed the study, acquired funding, and were responsible for overall oversight of the study; VS provided clinical supervision and was responsible for recruitment and follow up of study participants; WK provided program management support and was involved in participant recruitment and follow-up; GS, GM and BN conducted the recruitment and follow-up of the study participants; WP, AVDB and PR were responsible for design, oversight and interpretation of immunological experiments; JF was responsible for the processing of immunological samples and assay conduct in PNG; AG and RF were responsible for all aspects of bacterial analysis in PNG; LAK is responsible for design, oversight and interpretation of microbiological experiments in Australia; TO was responsible for processing microbiological samples and conducting analysis in PNG; PJ is responsible for statistical methods and analysis; MP contributed to design and implementation of the study. WK wrote the first draft of the manuscript and DL and AVDB wrote the final version; PR, LAK, and MP critically reviewed and edited the final version. All authors read and approved the final manuscript.

Competing interests

DL has received support from Pfizer Australia to attend conferences, an honorarium from Merck Vaccines to give a seminar at their offices in Pennsylvania and support from Merck Vaccines to attend a conference; and is an investigator on an investigator-initiated research grant that was funded by Pfizer Australia. PR has received non-financial support from Pfizer, grants from GlaxoSmithKline, grants from Pfizer, and non-financial support from GlaxoSmithKline for work outside the submitted work. WP has received funding from Pfizer Australia to attend a conference. AVDB was previously an employee of Janssen Pharmaceuticals, Johnson and Johnson. LAK has received educational grants and travel support from Pfizer and GSK to attend conferences, is an investigator on an investigator-initiated research grant funded by Pfizer Australia, and is an inventor on patents for a pneumococcal protein vaccine antigen. All other authors declare no competing interests.

Author details

[1]Telethon Kids Institute, University of Western Australia, 100 Roberts Road, Subiaco, WA 6008, Australia. [2]Papua New Guinea Institute of Medical Research, Homate Street, Goroka, Eastern Highlands Province 441, Papua New Guinea. [3]The University of Sydney, University Centre for Rural Health, School of Public Health, 61 Uralba Street, Lismore, NSW 2480, Australia. [4]School of Applied and Biomedical Sciences, Federation University, Northways Road, Churchill, VIC 3842, Australia. [5]School of Paediatrics and Child Health, University of Western Australia, Roberts Road, Subiaco, WA 6008, Australia.

References

1. Liu L, Oza S, Hogan D, Chu Y, Perin J, Zhu J, et al. Global, regional, and national causes of under-5 mortality in 2000-15: an updated systematic analysis with implications for the sustainable development goals. Lancet. 2016;388:3027–35.
2. Mortality GBD. Causes of death collaborators. Global, regional, and national life expectancy, all-cause mortality, and cause-specific mortality for 249 causes of death, 1980-2015: a systematic analysis for the global burden of disease study 2015. Lancet. 2016;388:1459–544.
3. Committee CHA. PNG Department of Health, PNG Paediatric society. Child morbidity and mortality, annual report 2015. Port Moresby: PNG National Department of Health and the PNG Paediatric Society; 2015.
4. Papua New Guinea Department of Health. Papua New Guinea child health plan 2008–2015. Port Moresby: Department of Health; 2008.
5. Pomat WS, Van den Biggelaar AHJ, Phuanukoonnon S, Francis J, Jacoby P, Siba PM, et al. Safety and immunogenicity of neonatal pneumococcal conjugate vaccination in Papua new Guinean children: a randomised controlled trial. PLoS One. 2013;8:e56698.
6. Isaacman DJ, McIntosh ED, Reinert RR. Burden of invasive pneumococcal disease and serotype distribution among Streptococcus Pneumoniae isolates in young children in Europe: impact of the 7-valent pneumococcal conjugate vaccine and considerations for future conjugate vaccines. Int J Infect Dis. 2010;14:e197–209.
7. Francis JP, Richmond PC, Pomat WS, Michael A, Keno H, Phuanukoonnon S, et al. Maternal antibodies to pneumolysin but not to pneumococcal surface protein a delay early pneumococcal carriage in high-risk Papua new Guinean infants. Clin Vaccine Immunol. 2009; 16:1633–8.
8. Aho C, Michael A, Yoannes M, Greenhill A, Jacoby P, Reeder J, et al. Limited impact of neonatal or early infant schedules of 7-valent pneumococcal conjugate vaccination on nasopharyngeal carriage of *Streptococcus pneumoniae* in Papua new Guinean children: a randomized controlled trial. Vaccine Rep. 2016;6:36–43.
9. Yoannes M, Michael A, Saleu G, Opa C, Greenhill A, Siba P, et al. High pneumococcal carriage in 3–5 year old Papua New Guinean children following 9-month Pneumovax23 dose with or without prior 7- valent conjugate vaccine. In: Program and Abstracts: Eight International Symposium on Pneumococci and Pneumococcal Diseases (ISPPD8). Iguacu; 2012. p. 360. Abstract no. 49. [Available online: http://io.teiion.gr/bitstream/handle/123456789/656/FinalAbstractbook.pdf].
10. Poolman JT. Pneumococcal vaccine development. Expert Rev Vaccines. 2004;3:597–604.
11. Feldman C, Anderson R. Review: current and new generation pneumococcal vaccines. J Inf Secur. 2014;69:309–25.
12. Zandvoort A, Timens W. The dual function of the splenic marginal zone: essential for initiation of anti-TI-2 responses but also vital in the general first-line defense against blood-borne antigens. Clin Exp Immunol. 2002;130:4–11.
13. Laferriere C. The immunogenicity of pneumococcal polysaccharides in infants and children: a meta-regression. Vaccine. 2011;29:6838–47.
14. Lee LH, Frasch CE, Falk LA, Klein DL, Deal CD. Correlates of immunity for pneumococcal conjugate vaccines. Vaccine. 2003;21:2190–6.
15. Selman S, Hayes D, Perin LA, Hayes WS. Pneumococcal conjugate vaccine for young children. Manag Care. 2000;9(9):49–52. 4, 6-7 passim
16. Klugman KP, Madhi SA, Huebner RE, Kohberger R, Mbelle N, Pierce N. A trial of a 9-valent pneumococcal conjugate vaccine in children with and those without HIV infection. N Engl J Med. 2003;349:1341–8.
17. Cutts FT, Zaman SM, Enwere G, Jaffar S, Levine OS, Okoko JB, et al. Efficacy of nine-valent pneumococcal conjugate vaccine against pneumonia and invasive pneumococcal disease in the Gambia: randomised, double-blind, placebo-controlled trial. Lancet. 2005;365:1139–46.
18. Mackenzie GA, Hill PC, Jeffries DJ, Hossain I, Uchendu U, Ameh D, et al. Effect of the introduction of pneumococcal conjugate vaccination on invasive pneumococcal disease in the Gambia: a population-based surveillance study. Lancet Infect Dis. 2016;16:703–11.
19. Plosker GL. 10-Valent pneumococcal non-typeable *Haemophilus influenzae* protein D-conjugate vaccine: a review in infants and children. Paediatr Drugs. 2014;16:425–44.
20. Whitney CG, Farley MM, Hadler J, Harrison LH, Bennett NM, Lynfield R, et al. Decline in invasive pneumococcal disease after the introduction of protein-polysaccharide conjugate vaccine. N Engl J Med. 2003;348:1737–46.
21. Prymula R, Peeters P, Chrobok V, Kriz P, Novakova E, Kaliskova E, et al. Pneumococcal capsular polysaccharides conjugated to protein D for prevention of acute otitis media caused by both *Streptococcus pneumoniae* and non-typable *Haemophilus influenzae*: a randomised double-blind efficacy study. Lancet. 2006;367:740–8.
22. Shann F, Gratten M, Germer S, Linnemann V, Hazlett D, Payne R. Aetiology of pneumonia in children in Goroka hospital, Papua New Guinea. Lancet. 1984;2:537–41.
23. Ngo CC, Massa HM, Thornton RB, Cripps AW. Predominant bacteria detected from the middle ear fluid of children experiencing otitis media: a systematic review. PLoS One. 2016;11:e0150949.
24. Desai S, Jamieson FB, Patel SN, Seo CY, Dang V, Fediurek J, et al. The epidemiology of invasive *Haemophilus influenzae* non-serotype B disease in Ontario, Canada from 2004 to 2013. PLoS One. 2015;10:e0142179.
25. Laupland KB, Schonheyder HC, Ostergaard C, Knudsen JD, Valiquette L, Galbraith J, et al. Epidemiology of *Haemophilus influenzae* bacteremia: a multi-national population-based assessment. J Inf Secur. 2011;62:142–8.
26. Mudhune S, Wamae M. Report on invasive disease and meningitis due to *Haemophilus influenzae* and *Streptococcus pneumoniae* from the network for surveillance of pneumococcal diseases in the east African region (netSPEAR). Clin Infect Dis. 2009;48(Suppl 2):S147–S52.
27. Van Eldere J, Slack MP, Ladhani S, Cripps AW. Non-typeable *Haemophilus influenzae*, an under-recognised pathogen. Lancet Infect

Dis. 2014;14:1281–92.

28. Leach AJ, Wigger C, Hare K, Hampton V, Beissbarth J, Andrews R, et al. Reduced middle ear infection with non-typeable Haemophilus influenzae, but not Streptococcus Pneumoniae, after transition to 10-valent pneumococcal non-typeable *H. influenzae* protein D conjugate vaccine. BMC Pediatr. 2015;15:162.
29. Prymula R, Hanovcova I, Splino M, Kriz P, Motlova J, Lebedova V, et al. Impact of the 10-valent pneumococcal non-typeable *Haemophilus influenzae* protein D conjugate vaccine (PHiD-CV) on bacterial nasopharyngeal carriage. Vaccine. 2011;29:1959–67.
30. Tregnaghi MW, Saez-Llorens X, Lopez P, Abate H, Smith E, Posleman A, et al. Efficacy of pneumococcal nontypable *Haemophilus influenzae* protein D conjugate vaccine (PHiD-CV) in young Latin American children: a double-blind randomized controlled trial. PLoS Med. 2014;11: e1001657.
31. Greenhill AR, Phuanukoonnon S, Michael A, Yoannes M, Orami T, Smith H, et al. *Streptococcus pneumoniae* and *Haemophilus influenzae* in paediatric meningitis patients at Goroka general hospital, Papua New Guinea: serotype distribution and antimicrobial susceptibility in the pre-vaccine era. BMC Infect Dis. 2015;15:485.
32. Lehmann D, Gratten M, Montgomery J. Susceptibility of pneumococcal carriage isolates to penicillin provides a conservative estimate of susceptibility of invasive pneumococci. Pediatr Infect Dis J. 1997;16:297–305.
33. Lehmann D, Willis J, Moore HC, Giele C, Murphy D, Keil AD, et al. The changing epidemiology of invasive pneumococcal disease in aboriginal and non-aboriginal western Australians from 1997 through 2007 and emergence of nonvaccine serotypes. Clin Infect Dis. 2010;50:1477–86.
34. Saha SK, Hossain B, Islam M, Hasanuzzaman M, Saha S, Hasan M, et al. Epidemiology of invasive pneumococcal disease in Bangladeshi children before introduction of pneumococcal conjugate vaccine. Pediatr Infect Dis. 2016;35:655–61.
35. Singleton RJ, Hennessy TW, Bulkow LR, Hammitt LL, Zulz T, Hurlburt DA, et al. Invasive pneumococcal disease caused by nonvaccine serotypes among Alaska native children with high levels of 7-valent pneumococcal conjugate vaccine coverage. JAMA. 2007;297:1784–92.
36. Lehmann D, Marshall TF, Riley ID, Alpers MP. Effect of pneumococcal vaccine on morbidity from acute lower respiratory tract infections in Papua new Guinean children. Ann Trop Paediatr. 1991;11:247–57.
37. Riley ID, Lehmann D, Alpers MP, Marshall TF, Gratten H, Smith D. Pneumococcal vaccine prevents death from acute lower-respiratory-tract infections in Papua new Guinean children. Lancet. 1986;2:877–81.
38. Pomat WS, Lehmann D, Sanders RC, Lewis DJ, Wilson J, Rogers S, et al. Immunoglobulin G antibody responses to polyvalent pneumococcal vaccine in children in the highlands of Papua New Guinea. Infect Immun. 1994;62:1848–53.
39. Saha SK, Al Emran HM, Hossain B, Darmstadt GL, Saha S, Islam M, et al. *Streptococcus pneumoniae* serotype-2 childhood meningitis in Bangladesh: a newly recognized pneumococcal infection threat. PLoS One. 2012;7:e32134.
40. Russell FM, Balloch A, Licciardi PV, Carapetis JR, Tikoduadua L, Waqatakirewa L, et al. Serotype-specific avidity is achieved following a single dose of the 7-valent pneumococcal conjugate vaccine, and is enhanced by 23-valent pneumococcal polysaccharide booster at 12 months. Vaccine. 2011;29: 4499–506.
41. Russell FM, Carapetis JR, Burton RL, Lin J, Licciardi PV, Balloch A, et al. Opsonophagocytic activity following a reduced dose 7-valent pneumococcal conjugate vaccine infant primary series and 23-valent pneumococcal polysaccharide vaccine at 12 months of age. Vaccine. 2011;29:535–44.
42. Licciardi PV, Toh Z, Clutterbuck EA, Balloch A, Marimla RA, Tikkanen L, et al. No long-term evidence of hyporesponsiveness after use of pneumococcal conjugate vaccine in children previously immunized with pneumococcal polysaccharide vaccine. J Allergy Clin Immunol. 2016;137:1772–9.
43. van den Biggelaar AHJ, Richmond PC, Fuery A, Anderson D, Opa C, Saleu G, et al. Pneumococcal responses are similar in Papua new Guinean children aged 3-5 years vaccinated in infancy with pneumococcal polysaccharide vaccine with or without prior pneumococcal conjugate vaccine, or without pneumococcal vaccination. PLoS One. 2017;12: e0185877.
44. Roca A, Bojang A, Bottomley C, Gladstone RA, Adetifa JU, Egere U, et al. Effect on nasopharyngeal pneumococcal carriage of replacing PCV7 with PCV13 in the expanded Programme of immunization in the Gambia. Vaccine. 2015;33:7144–51.
45. Roca A, Hill PC, Townend J, Egere U, Antonio M, Bojang A, et al. Effects of community-wide vaccination with PCV-7 on pneumococcal nasopharyngeal carriage in the Gambia: a cluster-randomized trial. PLoS Med. 2011;8: e1001107.
46. Anttila M, Eskola J, Ahman H, Kayhty H. Avidity of IgG for Streptococcus Pneumoniae type 6B and 23F polysaccharides in infants primed with pneumococcal conjugates and boosted with polysaccharide or conjugate vaccines. J Infect Dis. 1998;177:1614–21.
47. Bogaert D, Sluijter M, De Groot R, Hermans PW. Multiplex opsonophagocytosis assay (MOPA): a useful tool for the monitoring of the 7-valent pneumococcal conjugate vaccine. Vaccine. 2004;22:4014–20.
48. Wiertsema SP, Corscadden KJ, Mowe EN, Zhang G, Vijayasekaran S, Coates HL, et al. IgG responses to pneumococcal and *Haemophilus influenzae* protein antigens are not impaired in children with a history of recurrent acute otitis media. PLoS One. 2012;7:e49061.
49. World Health Organization Pneumoccal Serology Reference Laboratories. Training manual for enzyme linked immunosorbent assay for the quantitation of *Streptococcus pneumoniae* serotype specific IgG (Pn PS ELISA). University of Alabama Website [Available from: https://www.vaccine.uab.edu/uploads/mdocs/ELISAProtocol(007sp).pdf.
50. van den Biggelaar AH, Pomat W, Bosco A, Phuanukoonnon S, Devitt CJ, Nadal-Sims MA, et al. Pneumococcal conjugate vaccination at birth in a high-risk setting: no evidence for neonatal T-cell tolerance. Vaccine. 2011;29: 5414–20.
51. Papua New Guinea Department of Health and Paediatric Society of Papua New Guinea. Standard treatment for common illnesses of children in Papua New Guinea. A manual for nurses, community health workers, health extension officers and doctors. 9th ed. Port Moresby: Department of Health; 2011. p. 148.
52. Smith-Vaughan HC, Byun R, Nadkarni M, Jacques NA, Hunter N, Halpin S, et al. Measuring nasal bacterial load and its association with otitis media. BMC Ear Nose Throat Disord. 2006;6:10.
53. Odutola A, Ota MO, Antonio M, Ogundare EO, Saidu Y, Foster-Nyarko E, et al. Efficacy of a novel, protein-based pneumococcal vaccine against nasopharyngeal carriage of *Streptococcus pneumoniae* in infants: a phase 2, randomized, controlled, observer-blind study. Vaccine. 2017;35: 2531–42.
54. Phuanukoonnon S, Reeder JC, Pomat WS, Van den Biggelaar AHJ, Holt PG, Saleu G, et al. A neonatal pneumococcal conjugate vaccine trial in Papua New Guinea: study population, methods and operational challenges. PNG Med J. 2010;53:191–206.
55. Blyth CC, Ford R, Sapura J, Kumani T, Masiria G, Kave J, et al. Childhood pneumonia and meningitis in the eastern Highlands Province, Papua New Guinea in the era of conjugate vaccines: study methods and challenges. Pneumonia. 2017;9:5.
56. Pomat W, Richmond P, Francis J, Wana S, Solomon V, Ford R, et al, editors. Immunogenicity of 10-valent and 13-valent pneumococcal conjugate vaccines given at 1–2-3 months of age in Papua new Guinean infants: a randomised controlled trial. In: Program and Abstracts. Tenth International Symposium on Pneumococci and Pneumococcal Diseases. Glasgow; 2016. Abstract no. 702.
57. Kakazo M, Lehmann D, Coakley K, Gratten H, Saleu G, Taime J, et al. Mortality rates and the utilization of health services during terminal illness in the Asaro Valley, eastern Highlands Province, Papua New Guinea. PNG Med J. 1999;42:13–26.
58. Aipit S, Aipit J, Laman M. Malnutrition: a neglected but leading cause of child deaths in Papua New Guinea. Lancet Glob Health. 2014;2:e568.
59. Peters HR, Kemiki AD, Vince JD. Child adoption in the western Highlands Province of Papua New Guinea. PNG Med J. 2000;43:98–104.
60. Pameh W, Ripa P, Vince J, Mueller I. Adoption and hospital admission in Port Moresby, Papua New Guinea. J Trop Pediatr. 2002;48:264–9.

61. Rero A, Aipit J, Yarong-Kote T, Watch V, Bolnga JW, Vei R, et al. The burden of child maltreatment leading to hospitalization in a provincial setting in Papua New Guinea. J Trop Pediatr. 2016;62:282–7.
62. Martinon-Torres F, Wysocki J, Center KJ, Czajka H, Majda-Stanislawska E, Omenaca F, et al. Circulating antibody 1 and 2 years after vaccination with the 13-valent pneumococcal conjugate vaccine in preterm compared with term infants. J Trop Pediatr. 2017;36:326–32.

Permissions

All chapters in this book were first published in PNEUMONIA, by BioMed Central; hereby published with permission under the Creative Commons Attribution License or equivalent. Every chapter published in this book has been scrutinized by our experts. Their significance has been extensively debated. The topics covered herein carry significant findings which will fuel the growth of the discipline. They may even be implemented as practical applications or may be referred to as a beginning point for another development.

The contributors of this book come from diverse backgrounds, making this book a truly international effort. This book will bring forth new frontiers with its revolutionizing research information and detailed analysis of the nascent developments around the world.

We would like to thank all the contributing authors for lending their expertise to make the book truly unique. They have played a crucial role in the development of this book. Without their invaluable contributions this book wouldn't have been possible. They have made vital efforts to compile up to date information on the varied aspects of this subject to make this book a valuable addition to the collection of many professionals and students.

This book was conceptualized with the vision of imparting up-to-date information and advanced data in this field. To ensure the same, a matchless editorial board was set up. Every individual on the board went through rigorous rounds of assessment to prove their worth. After which they invested a large part of their time researching and compiling the most relevant data for our readers.

The editorial board has been involved in producing this book since its inception. They have spent rigorous hours researching and exploring the diverse topics which have resulted in the successful publishing of this book. They have passed on their knowledge of decades through this book. To expedite this challenging task, the publisher supported the team at every step. A small team of assistant editors was also appointed to further simplify the editing procedure and attain best results for the readers.

Apart from the editorial board, the designing team has also invested a significant amount of their time in understanding the subject and creating the most relevant covers. They scrutinized every image to scout for the most suitable representation of the subject and create an appropriate cover for the book.

The publishing team has been an ardent support to the editorial, designing and production team. Their endless efforts to recruit the best for this project, has resulted in the accomplishment of this book. They are a veteran in the field of academics and their pool of knowledge is as vast as their experience in printing. Their expertise and guidance has proved useful at every step. Their uncompromising quality standards have made this book an exceptional effort. Their encouragement from time to time has been an inspiration for everyone.

The publisher and the editorial board hope that this book will prove to be a valuable piece of knowledge for researchers, students, practitioners and scholars across the globe.

List of Contributors

Eileen M. Dunne
Pneumococcal Research, Murdoch Childrens Research Institute, Parkville, VIC, Australia

Kylie Carville
Victorian Infectious Disease Reference Laboratory at the Peter Doherty Institute for Infection and Immunity, Melbourne, VIC, Australia

Thomas V. Riley
Microbiology & Immunology, School of Pathology & Laboratory Medicine, The University of Western Australia, Crawley, WA, Australia
Department of Microbiology, PathWest Laboratory Medicine, Queen Elizabeth II Medical Centre, Nedlands, WA, Australia

Jacinta Bowman
Department of Microbiology, PathWest Laboratory Medicine, Queen Elizabeth II Medical Centre, Nedlands, WA, Australia

Amanda J. Leach
Child Health Division, Menzies School of Health Research, Darwin, NT, Australia

Allan W. Cripps
School of Medicine and Menzies Health Institute Queensland, Griffith University, Southport, QLD, Australia

Denise Murphy
Public Health Bacteriology Laboratory, Centre for Public Health Sciences, Coopers Plains, QLD, Australia

Peter Jacoby and Deborah Lehmann
Telethon Kids Institute, The University of Western Australia, Subiaco, WA, Australia

I. Brent Masters and Alan F. Isles
Department of Respiratory and Sleep Medicine, Lady Cilento Children's Hospital, South Brisbane, QLD, Australia

Keith Grimwood
School of Medicine and Menzies Health Institute Queensland, Gold Coast campus, Griffith University, Building G40, Southport Gold Coast, QLD, Australia
Departments of Infectious Diseases and Paediatrics, Gold Coast Health, Southport Gold Coast, QLD, Australia

Ashleigh Trimble
Crosshouse Hospital, Kilmarnock Road, Crosshouse KA2 0BE, UK
Respiratory Infection Group, Liverpool School of Tropical Medicine, Pembroke Place, Liverpool L3 5QA, UK

A. M. Collins
Respiratory Infection Group, Liverpool School of Tropical Medicine, Pembroke Place, Liverpool L3 5QA, UK
Respiratory Research Group, Royal Liverpool and Broadgreen University Hospital Trust, Prescot Street, Liverpool L7 8XP, UK

V. Moffat
Aintree Hospital, Longmoor Lane, Liverpool L9 7AL, UK

Christopher C. Blyth
School of Paediatrics and Child Health, The University of Western Australia, Princess Margaret Hospital for Children, Roberts Road, Subiaco 6008, WA, Australia
Wesfarmers Centre for Vaccines and Infectious Diseases, Telethon Kids Institute, University of Western Australia, West Perth 6872, WA, Australia
Department of Infectious Diseases and PathWest Department of Microbiology, Princess Margaret Hospital for Children, Roberts Road, Subiaco 6008, WA, Australia

Deborah Lehmann and William Pomat
Wesfarmers Centre for Vaccines and Infectious Diseases, Telethon Kids Institute, University of Western Australia, West Perth 6872, WA, Australia
Papua New Guinea Institute of Medical Research, Goroka 441, Eastern Highlands Province, Papua New Guinea

Rebecca Ford, Joycelyn Sapura, Tonny Kumani, Geraldine Masiria, John Kave, Lapule Yuasi and Amanda Lang
Papua New Guinea Institute of Medical Research, Goroka 441, Eastern Highlands Province, Papua New Guinea

Andrew Greenhill
Papua New Guinea Institute of Medical Research, Goroka 441, Eastern Highlands Province, Papua New Guinea
School of Applied and Biomedical Sciences, Federation University Australia, Gippsland Campus, Northways Road, Churchill 3842, VIC, Australia

Ilomo Hwaihwanje
Eastern Highlands Provincial Hospital, Goroka 441, Eastern Highlands Province, Papua New Guinea

Nguyen T. K. Phuong
Respiratory Department, Da Nang Hospital for Women and Children, Da Nang, Vietnam
Infectious Disease Team, The Children's Hospital at Westmead and Discipline of Paediatrics and Adolescent Medicine, University of Sydney, Sydney, NSW, Australia

Tran T. Hoang
Neonatal Department, Da Nang Hospital for Women and Children, Da Nang, Vietnam

Pham H. Van
Microbiology Department, The University of Medicine and Pharmacy, Ho Chi Minh, Vietnam

Lolyta Tu
Antimicrobial Stewardship Team, The Children's Hospital at Westmead, Sydney, Australia

Stephen M. Graham
Centre for International Child Health, University of Melbourne and Murdoch Children's Research Institute, Melbourne, Australia

Ben J. Marais
Infectious Disease Team, The Children's Hospital at Westmead and Discipline of Paediatrics and Adolescent Medicine, University of Sydney, Sydney, NSW, Australia

Helen E. Jenkins
Department of Biostatistics, Boston University School of Public Health, Boston, MA 02118, USA

Breanne M. Head and Adriana Trajtman
Department of Medical Microbiology, University of Manitoba, Winnipeg, Canada

Zulma V. Rueda
Facultad de Medicina, Universidad Pontificia Bolivariana, Medellin, Colombia

Lázaro Vélez
Grupo Investigador de Problemas en Enfermedades Infecciosas, Universidad de Antioquia UdeA, Medellin, Colombia

Yoav Keynan
Department of Internal Medicine, University of Manitoba, Winnipeg, Canada
Department of Community Health Sciences, University of Manitoba, Winnipeg, Canada
Department of Medical Microbiology, University of Manitoba, Winnipeg, Canada

Serena Tricarico
Faculty of Medicine, University of Southampton, Southampton, United Kingdom
Institute for Life Sciences, University of Southampton, Southampton, United Kingdom
University of Southampton Malaysia Campus, Johor, Malaysia

Victor Lim
International Medical University, Kuala Lumpur, Malaysia

Mohd Nor Norazmi
Universiti Sains Malaysia Health Campus, Kelantan, Malaysia

C. Patrick Doncaster
Centre for Biological Sciences, Faculty of Natural and Environmental Sciences, University of Southampton, Southampton, United Kingdom

Deirdre A. Collins
School of Medical and Health Sciences, Edith Cowan University, Perth, WA, Australia
Wesfarmers Centre of Vaccines & Infectious Diseases, Telethon Kids Institute, University of Western Australia, Perth, WA, Australia

Anke Hoskins, Thomas Snelling, Kalpani Senasinghe and Deborah Lehmann
Wesfarmers Centre of Vaccines & Infectious Diseases, Telethon Kids Institute, University of Western Australia, Perth, WA, Australia

Jacinta Bowman and Natalie A. Stemberger
Division of Microbiology & Infectious Diseases, PathWest Laboratory Medicine WA, Perth, WA, Australia

Amanda J. Leach
Menzies School of Health Research, Charles Darwin University, Darwin, Northern Territory, Australia

Lidwien A. M. Smit and Dick Heederik
Institute for Risk Assessment Sciences (IRAS), Division Environmental Epidemiology, Utrecht University, 3508 TD Utrecht, The Netherlands

Gert Jan Boender and Thomas J. Hagenaars
Central Veterinary Institute, Wageningen University and Research Centre, Lelystad, The Netherlands

Gonnie Nodelijk
Central Veterinary Institute, Wageningen University and Research Centre, Lelystad, The Netherlands
Current address: GD Animal Health, Deventer, The Netherlands

Wouter A. A. de Steenhuijsen Piters and Debby Bogaert
Department of Paediatric Immunology and Infectious Diseases, The Wilhelmina Children's Hospital/ University Medical Center Utrecht, Utrecht, The Netherlands

Elisabeth A. M. Sanders
Department of Paediatric Immunology and Infectious Diseases, The Wilhelmina Children's Hospital/ University Medical Center Utrecht, Utrecht, The Netherlands
National Institute for Public Health and the Environment, Bilthoven, The Netherlands

Elisabeth G. W. Huijskens
Department of Medical Microbiology, Albert Schweitzer Hospital, Dordrecht, The Netherlands
Laboratory of Medical Microbiology and Immunology, St.Elisabeth Hospital, Tilburg, The Netherlands

John W. A. Rossen
Laboratory of Medical Microbiology and Immunology, St.Elisabeth Hospital, Tilburg, The Netherlands
Department of Medical Microbiology, University of Groningen, University Medical Center Groningen, Groningen, The Netherlands

Marion Koopmans
Department of Virology, Erasmus Medical Centre, Rotterdam, The Netherlands

Joris Yzermans
NIVEL, Netherlands Institute for Health Services Research, Utrecht, The Netherlands

Erica J. Shaddock
Division of Pulmonology and Critical Care, Department of Internal Medicine, Area 552 Charlotte Maxeke Johannesburg Academic Hospital, Jubilee Road, Parktown, Johannesburg 2193, South Africa
Faculty of Health Sciences, University of the Witwatersrand, Johannesburg, South Africa

Esther Muthumbi
KEMRI-Wellcome Trust Research Programme, Center for Geographical Medicine Research Coast, Kilifi, Kenya

Brett S. Lowe
KEMRI-Wellcome Trust Research Programme, Center for Geographical Medicine Research Coast, Kilifi, Kenya
Centre for Tropical Medicine & Global Health, University of Oxford, Oxford, UK

J. Anthony G. Scott
KEMRI-Wellcome Trust Research Programme, Center for Geographical Medicine Research Coast, Kilifi, Kenya
Department of Infectious Disease Epidemiology, London School of Hygiene & Tropical Medicine, London, UK

Cyprian Muyodi and Esther Getambu
Coast Provincial General Hospital, Mombasa, Kenya

Fergus Gleeson
Department of Radiology, Churchill Hospital, University of Oxford, Oxford, UK

Lena M. Mayer
School of Medicine, University of Basel, Klingelbergstasse 61, 4056 Basel, Switzerland
Division of Infectious Diseases & Hospital Epidemiology, Kantonsspital St. Gallen, Rorschacherstrasse 95, 9007 St. Gallen, Switzerland

Christian Kahlert
Children's Hospital of Eastern Switzerland, Claudiusstrasse 6, 9006 St. Gallen, Switzerland
Division of Infectious Diseases & Hospital Epidemiology, Kantonsspital St. Gallen, Rorschacherstrasse 95, 9007 St. Gallen, Switzerland

Frank Rassouli
Clinic for Pulmonology & Sleep Medicine, Kantonsspital St. Gallen, Rorschacherstrasse 95, 9007 St. Gallen, Switzerland

Pietro Vernazza and Werner C. Albrich
Division of Infectious Diseases & Hospital Epidemiology, Kantonsspital St. Gallen, Rorschacherstrasse 95, 9007 St. Gallen, Switzerland

Pierre Goussard
Department of Pediatrics and Child Health, University of Stellenbosch and Tygerberg Academic Hospital, Cape Town, South Africa

Helena Rabie
Department of Pediatrics and Child Health, University of Stellenbosch and Tygerberg Academic Hospital, Cape Town, South Africa
Childrens Infectious Diseases Clinical Research Unit (KidCRU), University of Stellenbosch, Cape Town, South Africa
Division of Infectious Diseases, Department of Paediatrics and Child Health, Faculty of Medicine and Health Sciences, Stellenbosch University, PO Cape Town 8000, South Africa

Geetha Nagaraj, Feroze Ganaie, Vandana Govindan and Kadahalli Lingegowda Ravikumar
Central Research Laboratory, KIMS Hospital and Research Centre, KR Road, VV Purum, Bangalore, Karnataka 560 004, India

Rebecca Nightingale, Tim Colbourn and Carina King
Institute for Global Health, University College London, London, UK

David Mukanga
Science and Health Impact Group (SHI), Kampala, Uganda

Limangeni Mankhambo
Parent and Child Health Initiative, Lilongwe, Malawi

Norman Lufesi
Acute Respiratory Infection Unit, Ministry of Health, Lilongwe, Malawi

Eric D. McCollum
Department of Pediatrics, Division of Pulmonology, Johns Hopkins School of Medicine, Baltimore, USA

Keiko Konomura and Manabu Akazawa
Public Health and Epidemiology, Meiji Pharmaceutical University, 2-522-1, Noshio, Kiyose, Tokyo 204-8588, Japan

Hideaki Nagai
Center for Pulmonary Diseases, National Hospital Organization Tokyo National Hospital, 3-1-1 Takeoka, Kiyose-shi, Tokyo 204-8585, Japan

Katharine Yang, Robert L. Kruse and Weijie V. Lin
Baylor College of Medicine, Houston, TX 77030, USA

Daniel M. Musher
Baylor College of Medicine, Houston, TX 77030, USA
Infectious Disease Section, Michael E. DeBakey Veterans Affairs Medical Center, 2002 Holcombe Boulevard, Houston, TX 77030, USA

Hirotaka Nakashima and Yusuke Suzuki
Centre for Community Liaison and Patient Consultations, Nagoya University Hospital, 65 Tsurumai-cho, Showa-ku, Nagoya, Aichi 466-8560, Japan
Department of Geriatrics, Nagoya University Hospital, Nagoya, Japan

Kazuhisa Watanabe and Hiroyuki Umegaki
Department of Community Healthcare and Geriatrics, Nagoya University Graduate School of Medicine, Nagoya, Japan

Masafumi Kuzuya
Department of Community Healthcare and Geriatrics, Nagoya University Graduate School of Medicine, Nagoya, Japan
Institute of Innovation for Future Society, Nagoya University, Nagoya, Japan

Biswajit Chakrabarti and Joseph Somers
Aintree University Hospital NHS Foundation Trust, Liverpool, UK

Dan Wootton
Institute of Infection and Global Health, University of Liverpool, Liverpool, UK
Department of Respiratory Research, Aintree University Hospital NHS Foundation Trust, Liverpool, UK

Steven Lane
Institute of Translational Medicine, University of Liverpool, Liverpool, UK

Elizabeth Kanwar and Nancy Prospero
Advancing Quality Alliance, Manchester, UK

Jacyln Proctor
Warrington and Halton Hospitals NHS Foundation Trust, Warrington, UK

Mark Woodhead
Department of Respiratory Medicine, Central Manchester University Hospitals NHS Foundation Trust, Manchester, UK
Manchester Academic Health Science Centre and Faculty of Medical and Human Sciences, University of Manchester, Manchester, UK

Carlos M. Luna, Laura Pulido, Alberto Casey, Diego Burgos and Sebastián D. Leiva Agüero
Department of Medicine, Pulmonary Diseases Division; Hospital de Clínicas, Universidad de Buenos Aires, Ayacucho, 1850, piso 5 dto B, 1112 Buenos Aires, Argentina

Alejandra Grosso, Evangelina Membriani and Andrea C. Entrocassi
Department of Medicine, Pulmonary Diseases Division; Hospital de Clínicas, Universidad de Buenos Aires, Ayacucho, 1850, piso 5 dto B, 1112 Buenos Aires, Argentina
Department of Chemical Biochemistry, Immuno-Serology Section, Faculty of Pharmacy and Biochemistry; Hospital de Clínicas, Universidad de Buenos Aires, Buenos Aires, Argentina
Department of Chemical Biochemistry, Section Microbiology, Faculty of Pharmacy and Biochemistry; Hospital de Clínicas, Universidad de Buenos Aires, Buenos Aires, Argentina

Marcelo Rodríquez Fermepin
Department of Chemical Biochemistry, Immuno-Serology Section, Faculty of Pharmacy and Biochemistry; Hospital de Clínicas, Universidad de Buenos Aires, Buenos Aires, Argentina

Carlos A. Vay, Susana Garcia and Angela Famiglietti
Department of Chemical Biochemistry, Section Microbiology, Faculty of Pharmacy and Biochemistry; Hospital de Clínicas, Universidad de Buenos Aires, Buenos Aires, Argentina

Michael S. Niederman
Pulmonary and Critical Care, New York Presbyterian/ Weill Cornell Medical Center, New York, USA

Deborah Lehmann, Anita H. J. van den Biggelaar and Peter Jacoby
Telethon Kids Institute, University of Western Australia, 100 Roberts Road, Subiaco, WA 6008, Australia

William S. Pomat
Telethon Kids Institute, University of Western Australia, 100 Roberts Road, Subiaco, WA 6008, Australia.
Papua New Guinea Institute of Medical Research, Homate Street, Goroka, Eastern Highlands Province 441, Papua New Guinea

Andrew Greenhill
Telethon Kids Institute, University of Western Australia, 100 Roberts Road, Subiaco, WA 6008, Australia.
Papua New Guinea Institute of Medical Research, Homate Street, Goroka, Eastern Highlands Province 441, Papua New Guinea
School of Applied and Biomedical Sciences, Federation University, Northways Road, Churchill, VIC 3842, Australia

Lea-Ann Kirkham and Peter C. Richmond
Telethon Kids Institute, University of Western Australia, 100 Roberts Road, Subiaco, WA 6008, Australia.

School of Paediatrics and Child Health, University of Western Australia, Roberts Road, Subiaco, WA 6008, Australia

Wendy Kirarock, Gerard Saleu, Geraldine Masiria, Birunu Nivio, Tilda Orami, Jacinta Francis, Rebecca Ford and Vela Solomon
Papua New Guinea Institute of Medical Research, Homate Street, Goroka, Eastern Highlands Province 441, Papua New Guinea

Megan Passey
The University of Sydney, University Centre for Rural Health, School of Public Health, 61 Uralba Street, Lismore, NSW 2480, Australia

Index

A

Acute Respiratory Syndrome, 29-31, 37

Aminoglycosides, 35, 177

Amoxicillin, 51, 53, 56-57, 160-161, 166, 178, 182, 198

Antibiotic Therapy, 10-11, 22-24, 111, 113, 124, 132-133, 136, 192-193, 197-200

Antimicrobial Susceptibility, 1-4, 6, 9, 40, 50, 55-56, 96, 222

Antimicrobial Therapy, 35, 46, 185, 203

B

Bacterium, 33-35, 67, 69, 123, 133, 177

Bronchopleural Fistulae, 10-11, 25

C

Cardiac Failure, 108, 192, 194-196, 198-199

Childhood Pneumonia, 26-27, 39-40, 46, 49, 54-55, 63, 85, 119, 166

Chlamydophila Pneumoniae, 30, 65-66, 70

Chloramphenicol, 4-5, 50, 56, 182

Cilostazol, 185-191

Coccidioidomycosis, 30-31, 35-36

Community-acquired Pneumonia, 8, 11, 14, 25-28, 34, 50-51, 55, 70, 98, 105-106, 113-114, 121, 137-138, 147, 167, 172, 175-177, 183, 192-193, 199-201, 207-208

Comorbidity, 63, 169, 192-194, 196, 199

Conjugate Vaccine, 1, 8-9, 14, 16, 25-28, 40, 47, 50, 54, 72-74, 84, 86-87, 96-97, 144, 147, 157-158, 168, 201-202, 207-208, 210, 213, 220-223

Coronary Artery Disease, 185

Corticosteroids, 107, 167, 179, 200

Corynebacteria, 177-178, 180-182, 184

Coryneform Bacteria, 180, 183-184

Cotrimoxazole, 4-5, 50-51, 87, 91, 93-94

D

Diabetic Ketoacidosis, 115

Diphtheria, 30-31, 34, 38, 81, 84, 177-178, 180, 184, 213

Diphtheroids, 177, 179-180, 182, 184

Drug Therapy, 49

E

Empyema, 10-19, 23-27, 111, 113, 144, 147, 178-181, 183-184, 202

Eosinophilia, 30-31, 36, 38

Erythromycin, 4-5, 69, 71, 87, 91, 93, 182
230-232

F

Fluoroquinolones, 32, 52, 69, 142, 197

G

Gastroenteritis, 216

Gentamicin, 32, 43, 56, 182

H

Haemophilus Influenzae, 14, 18, 25, 30, 39-40, 48, 50, 54-56, 65, 69, 84-85, 93, 96, 129, 147, 177, 184, 198, 213, 220-222

Helminths, 36

Hemorrhages, 189

Histoplasmosis, 30-31, 36, 38

Hydatidosis, 30-31, 36

I

Immunoglobulin, 70, 222

Intracranial Hemorrhages, 189

K

Kynurenine, 112-113

L

Legionella, 18, 30, 38, 65, 67-69, 71, 129, 138

Leptospirosis, 30-31, 34, 38

Lymphadenopathy, 36

M

Measles-rubella, 40

Melioidosis, 22, 29-31, 35, 37-38

Meningitis, 39-45, 47-48, 50, 60, 62, 64, 73, 115, 144, 149, 157, 169, 202, 204, 210-211, 215, 222

Morbidity, 2, 15, 23, 30, 40, 48, 58-60, 62, 65, 69, 71, 73, 75, 81-83, 98, 101, 114, 139, 143, 146-149, 177, 193-196, 198-199, 202, 211, 214-215, 221-222

Mortality, 8, 12, 17, 25, 27, 30-37, 40, 46, 48, 50, 56, 68, 71, 73, 75, 81, 83, 98, 105, 121, 136, 143, 145, 147, 149, 160, 166-167, 177, 179, 185, 204, 206, 208, 210-211

Mycoplasma Pneumoniae, 18, 26-27, 30, 56, 65-66, 70-71, 129

N

Nasopharyngeal Swab, 213-214

Necrotizing Pneumonia, 10, 12-16, 20, 22, 25-27, 178

O

Otitis Media, 1-2, 8-9, 25, 73, 95-96, 149, 157, 202, 211, 215, 221-222

P

Penicillin, 2, 4-5, 15, 23, 50-51, 85, 87, 89, 91, 93, 181-182, 204, 222

Peripheral Arterial Disease, 185

Pertussis, 24-25, 28, 30-31, 34, 38, 40, 54, 62, 81, 213

Pneumococcal Carriage, 2-3, 5-9, 55, 87-88, 93-95, 97, 158, 207, 210-211, 221-222

Pneumococcal Vaccine, 8, 121, 201, 206-207, 210, 221-222

Pneumococci, 1-7, 10-11, 17-18, 20, 22-23, 73, 94-96, 149-150, 157, 177, 221-222

Pneumococcus, 2, 9, 64, 74, 85, 89-91, 93-95, 157, 167, 175, 183-184, 210

Pneumonia, 2, 4, 8-30, 32-37, 39-41, 43-58, 61-63, 65-73, 81-82, 84-85, 88, 98-99, 104-109, 124-128, 141, 157, 159-164, 175-195, 206-208, 216, 219

Primary Care, 57, 108-109, 113, 134, 137, 166, 192-194, 197-198

Pulmonary Infections, 27, 29-31, 36, 66, 69-70, 147

Pyopneumothorax, 10, 23

R

Renal Disease, 180-181, 192, 194-196, 198

Respiratory Infections, 37, 52, 56-57, 70, 99, 104, 113-114, 121, 137, 147, 166

Respiratory Tract Infection, 40, 49-50, 54, 57, 112, 115, 121, 123, 125, 127-128, 136, 139, 148, 193, 199

S

Serotypes, 1-9, 11, 13, 15-17, 24-26, 50, 55, 73, 85, 87-97, 144, 149-150, 154, 156-158, 202, 206-213, 215, 219-220, 222

Staphylococcus Aureus, 9-11, 14, 25-28, 43, 50, 54, 56, 65, 69, 94, 104, 129, 147, 183

Streptococcus Pneumoniae, 1, 8-11, 15-16, 25-26, 48, 65, 69, 85-88, 92-93, 96-98, 106, 129, 144, 147, 149, 153, 175, 183, 191, 207-208, 210, 222

Streptomycin, 32

T

Tachycardia, 189

Tetracycline, 4-5, 34, 87, 91, 93, 124, 182

Tryptophan, 112-113

Tuberculosis, 22, 29-31, 38, 50, 56, 58-60, 62-65, 110-111, 115-116, 118-120, 129, 139, 141-143, 145-147, 179, 216, 220

Tularemia, 30-31, 34-35, 38

V

Vaccination, 3, 5-6, 8-9, 26-27, 31, 34-35, 39-42, 44-46, 51, 56, 59, 63-64, 75, 87-90, 105, 119-121, 148, 157, 161, 168, 174-176, 206-209, 216, 219

Vancomycin, 4, 15, 23, 51, 54, 56, 177-178, 181-182

www.ingramcontent.com/pod-product-compliance
Lightning Source LLC
LaVergne TN
LVHW080733210926
848485LV00003B/551